Antimicrobial Drugs

Antimicrobial Drugs

Chronicle of a Twentieth Century Medical Triumph

David Greenwood
Emeritus Professor of Antimicrobial Science
University of Nottingham Medical School, UK

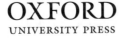
OXFORD
UNIVERSITY PRESS

OXFORD

UNIVERSITY PRESS

Great Clarendon Street, Oxford OX2 6DP

Oxford University Press is a department of the University of Oxford.
It furthers the University's objective of excellence in research, scholarship,
and education by publishing worldwide in

Oxford New York

Auckland Cape Town Dar es Salaam Hong Kong Karachi
Kuala Lumpur Madrid Melbourne Mexico City Nairobi
New Delhi Shanghai Taipei Toronto

With offices in

Argentina Austria Brazil Chile Czech Republic France Greece
Guatemala Hungary Italy Japan Poland Portugal Singapore
South Korea Switzerland Thailand Turkey Ukraine Vietnam

Oxford is a registered trade mark of Oxford University Press
in the UK and in certain other countries

Published in the United States
by Oxford University Press Inc., New York

A catalogue record for this title is available from the British Library
Data available

Library of Congress Cataloging in Publication Data
Greenwood, David, 1935-
  Antimicrobial drugs : chronicle of a twentieth century medical triumph /
David Greenwood.
     p. ; cm.
  Includes bibliographical references and index.
  ISBN-13: 978-0-19-953484-5 (alk. paper) 1. Anti-infective agents—
History—20th century.
  [DNLM: 1. Anti-Infective Agents—history. 2. History, 20th Century.
QV 250 G816a 2008] I. Title.
  RM263.G74 2008
  615'.1—dc22
     2007041196

Typeset by Cepha Imaging Private Ltd., Bangalore, India
Printed in Great Britain
on acid-free paper by
Biddles Ltd., King's Lynn, Norfolk, UK

ISBN 978-0-19-953484-5

10 9 8 7 6 5 4 3 2 1

Whilst every effort has been made to ensure that the contents of this book are as complete,
accurate and-up-to-date as possible at the date of writing. Oxford University Press is not able to
give any guarantee or assurance that such is the case. Readers are urged to take appropriately
qualified medical advice in all cases. The information in this book is intended to be useful to the
general reader, but should not be used as a means of self-diagnosis or for the prescription of
medication.

"Well," said Pooh, "we keep looking for Home and not finding it,
so I thought that if we looked for this Pit, we'd be sure *not* to find it,
which would be a Good Thing, because then we might find something
that we weren't looking for, which might be just what we're
looking for really.

A.A. Milne, *The House at Pooh Corner*, Chapter 7

For the incomparable Hanni,
with love and gratitude

Preface

In a remarkable decade between 1935 and 1944—a period more notorious for the spread of dictatorships, the Holocaust, and the prosecution of horrific wars in Europe and the Far East—a revolution took place that must rank as among the most important in history. Within those 10 years the face of medical practice was changed by the demonstration of the extraordinary antibacterial properties of Prontosil, the first of the sulphonamides (in Germany), penicillin (in Britain), and streptomycin (in the United States). The period has a particular poignancy for me since 1935 was the year in which I was born. It was in February of that year that details of Prontosil, the first really effective antimicrobial agent, were published in the *Deutsche Medizinische Wochenschrift* (1). Later in the year the discovery was described to a British audience at a meeting of the Royal Society of Medicine in London (2). Fleming's original description of penicillin had been published in 1929 (3), but was not followed up with any conviction at the time. The seminal paper by Howard Florey and his colleagues at Oxford outlining the amazing potential of Fleming's discovery appeared in *The Lancet* in August 1940 (4) and the Oxford team's dramatic report of penicillin's unparalleled ability to alter the course of infection in seriously ill patients appeared in the same journal almost exactly one year later (5). Selman Waksman's paper describing streptomycin followed in 1944 (6).

The discovery of sulphonamides, penicillin, and streptomycin triggered a frantic hunt for more antimicrobial drugs that was to yield an abundant harvest in an astonishingly short space of time. By the early 1960s more than 50 antibacterial agents were available to the prescribing physician and, largely by a process of chemical modification of existing compounds, this number has more than tripled today. So used have we become to the ready availability of these relatively safe and highly effective 'miracle drugs' (the popular epithet seems, for once, appropriate), that it is now hard to grasp how they transformed the treatment of infection. Before their introduction, serious systemic bacterial disease was virtually untreatable and millions died prematurely from pneumonia, tuberculosis, typhoid fever, meningitis, and many other bacterial infections. As Lawrence Paul Garrod observed in 1968, looking back on a lifetime in medicine:

> No one recently qualified, even with the liveliest imagination, can picture the ravages of bacterial infection which continued until little more than thirty years ago (7).

To take just one example: in the mid-1930s maternal mortality in England and Wales stood at around 40 per 10,000 births, a figure that had remained essentially unchanged for a century (8). About half these deaths were due to childbed fever caused by the highly virulent bacterium, *Streptococcus pyogenes* (9). The introduction of sulphonamides in 1935 had an immediate effect in saving the lives of young mothers (see Chapter 3). The subsequent development of penicillin, which has phenomenal activity against

Streptococcus pyogenes—the microbe is killed by a concentration of around one hundred-millionth of a gram of penicillin per millilitre of solution (0.01 μg/ml)—completed the triumph so that by 1970 maternal death due to perinatal streptococcal infection was a very uncommon event, at least in the developed world. Other bacterial diseases similarly responded to the new drugs: the availability of sulphonamides and penicillin gave doctors the means to treat most of the common life-threatening bacterial pathogens except tuberculosis. In 1944, with the report of the discovery of streptomycin this devastating condition was added to the list and victory over bacterial disease seemed complete.

Of course, the introduction of effective antibacterial chemotherapy is only one part of the story. For one thing, bacteria are not the only infectious enemies of mankind; many viruses, fungi, protozoa, and helminths can cause equally serious disease. The antimalarial drug quinine has been available in the form of cinchona bark since the seventeenth century and several anthelminthic agents have been known since antiquity. Moreover, the incidence of many bacterial diseases including scarlet fever, diphtheria, typhoid fever, and tuberculosis, was declining in the richer nations long before sulphonamides appeared. It is likely that improved nutrition, housing, and general hygiene standards were largely responsible for this decline; in the case of tuberculosis the removal of infected patients from the community into sanatoria also contributed greatly. Vaccination against smallpox, diphtheria, and a number of other diseases similarly played a crucial role in the fight against infection.

Today, much is heard of an impending 'post-antibiotic' era, owing to an inexorable rise of microbial drug resistance that some predict will undermine all that has been achieved. While there is little doubt that the unrestrained use of antibiotics has led to grave problems that we are only now seriously beginning to face, fear of such a gloomy prognosis should be tempered by the fact that there is little chance that we will return to that pre-antibiotic age in which doctors had daily to stand helpless by the bedside of children dying from the ravages of infectious diseases.

The story of antibiotics and other antimicrobial agents is a fascinating one. Discoveries have sometimes been made by pure serendipity; sometimes by logical experimentation that produced the right result for what turned out to be the wrong reason; sometimes by a process of random screening that might be described as 'planned serendipity'. Certainly, Lady Luck was never far from the scene, as she has been in many other therapeutic breakthroughs (10). But luck is sterile without the wit and invention needed to recognize and exploit it. As Louis Pasteur memorably put it,

> Dans les champs de l'observation le hasard ne favorise que les esprits préparés.*

This book offers a comprehensive account of the development of antimicrobial agents of all kinds: antibacterial, antiviral, antifungal, antiprotozoal, and antihelminthic compounds. But it is more than just a chronology of antimicrobial chemotherapy; it is also a celebration

---

* In the field of observation, chance favours only the prepared mind.

of a twentieth century miracle and of the men and women who made it happen. And celebration there should certainly be—with trumpets, drums, flags, and fireworks; for antimicrobial agents, with their ability to achieve not only palliative effects, but also permanent cure (still an uncommon outcome of most pharmacological intervention), have surely led to the relief of more human and animal suffering than any other class of drugs in the history of medical endeavour. They are truly the stuff that dreams are made on.

References

1. Domagk G (1935). Ein Beitrag zur Chemotherapie der bakteriellen Infektionen. *Dtsch Med Wochenschr* **61**, 250–3.
2. Hörlein H (1935). The chemotherapy of infectious diseases caused by protozoa and bacteria. *Proceedings of the Royal Society of Medicine* **29**, 313–24.
3. Fleming A (1929). On the antibacterial action of cultures of a penicillium, with special reference to their use in the isolation of B. influenzae. *British Journal of Experimental Pathology* **10**, 226–36.
4. Chain E, Florey HW, Gardner AD, *et al.* (1940). Penicillin as a chemotherapeutic agent. *Lancet* **2**, 226–8.
5. Abraham EP, Chain E, Fletcher CM, *et al.* (1941). Further observations on penicillin. *Lancet* **2**, 177–89.
6. Schatz A, Bugie E, Waksman SA (1944). Streptomycin, a substance exhibiting antibiotic activity against Gram-positive and Gram-negative bacteria. *Proceedings of the Society of Experimental Biology and Medicine* **55**, 66–9.
7. Garrod LP, O'Grady F (1968). *Antibiotic and chemotherapy*, 2nd ed. Churchill Livingstone, Edinburgh.
8. Loudon I (1992). *Death in childbirth*. Clarendon Press, Oxford.
9. Loudon I (2000). *The tragedy of childbed fever*. Oxford University Press, Oxford.
10. Le Fanu J (1999). *The rise and fall of modern medicine*. Little Brown & Co, London.

Contents

Acknowledgements

This is not really a historian's history, since I have not sieved through private papers, notebooks, or pharmaceutical company archives; nor have I tried to record the social impact of antimicrobial agents, though that would be a fascinating study. My aim has simply been to chronicle the development of antimicrobial agents through the twentieth century. The chief impetus was curiosity: although I have spent the best part of my professional life carrying out research and teaching in the field of antimicrobial chemotherapy, my knowledge of how the numerous agents arrived on the scene was fragmentary at best. Much of the information has been gleaned from researching the original literature; from the copious books and scientific publications dealing with antimicrobial agents and their development (what historians dismissively refer to as 'secondary sources'); from dredging the internet; from the numerous helpful conversations I have had over the years with those who have lived on the front line of the events described; and from long hours spent in lecture halls listening to the great and the good. I knew that the story would be interesting, but some aspects of it turned out to be even more fascinating than I had ever imagined.

I had arrogantly hoped to dispense with the customary long list of individual acknowledgements, since this book was intended to be all my own work, 'warts and all'. While that assertion remains valid in terms of responsibility for the content, the naïve assumption that I could produce a worthwhile narrative without outside help soon revealed itself as a patent absurdity. Many colleagues were necessarily consulted to check facts, to seek supplementary information or to find elusive papers. The road to eventual publication was itself considerably eased by help from the British Society for Antimicrobial Chemotherapy, notably the President, Peter Davey, the Executive Officer, Tracey Guest and the Editor-in-Chief of the *Journal of Antimicrobial Chemotherapy*, Alan Johnson. Their crucial backing helped to persuade Oxford University Press that the book might have a viable commercial future.

In addition I need to express my sincere thanks to the following, who have provided help in various ways, with profound apologies to anyone I may have inadvertently overlooked: Lisa Bayne, Archivist, Eli Lilly and Company; Dr Michael Carlile of Bridgwater, Somerset; Professor Patrice Courvalin (and his secretary, Sylvie Murguet) of the Institut Pasteur, Paris; Dr Simon Croft of the London School of Hygiene and Tropical Medicine; Dr Hugh Field of Queens' College, Cambridge; Mary Forrest, Managing Editor of the *Journal of Chemotherapy*, Florence; Dr Hajo Grundmann of the Centre for Infectious Diseases Epidemiology, Bilthoven, the Netherlands; Professor Jeremy Hamilton-Miller formerly of the Royal Free Hospital Medical School; Miss Rose Heatley, London; Dr Satoshi Hori of Juntendo University Graduate School of Medicine, Tokyo; Dr Fred Falkiner, Professor Hilary Humphreys, and the late Dr Stanley McElhinney, all of Dublin;

Dr William C. Hutchison of Draco, Perthshire; Professor John E. Lesch of the University of California, Berkeley; Professor Francis O'Grady, Emeritus Professor of Microbiology at the University of Nottingham; Dr Eric Sidebottom, Archivist, Sir William Dunn School of Pathology, Oxford; Dr Tilli Tansey of the Wellcome Trust Centre for the History of Medicine; Professor Richard Whitley of the University of Alabama at Birmingham; and Dr Morimasa Yagisawa of the Japanese Antibiotics Research Association. Moreover, it would be negligent if I were not to recognize the patient assistance of countless librarians, a group of people characterized in my experience by almost compulsive helpfulness. Georgia Pinteau and her colleagues at OUP also deserve praise for their exemplary skill and efficiency, to which I had already become accustomed during the gestation of the fifth edition of the student textbook, *Antimicrobial Chemotherapy* (Greenwood D, Finch RG, Davey PG, Wilcox MH, Oxford University Press, Oxford, 2007). Finally, I must record my heartfelt gratitude for the unfailing support of my wife Johanna (Hanni) to whom the book is rightfully dedicated, and to our daughter Dr Anna Crozier—a genuine medical historian—for constant help beyond the call of filial duty in locating and obtaining many obscure references.

Personalia

The public appetite needs heroes to celebrate in connection with great human achievements, and the twentieth century triumph over infectious disease is no exception. Alexander Fleming, of course, has come in for much adulation, though he was not the first to recognize antibiotic activity in micro-organisms and was certainly not responsible for the therapeutic exploitation of his discovery, penicillin. Ehrlich, Domagk, Waksman, and one or two others have also received a share of the limelight, though these days they are chiefly celebrated among the microbiological cognoscente. Folk memories naturally grow dim with the passage of years and in time even these names will fade into history so that future generations, if they encounter them at all, will acknowledge them only as one-dimensional figures rather than as real people. Such is the fate of the famous.

It is perhaps better so, if justice is to be done. Scientific advance is a complex process in which many hands and many minds participate and few receive any tangible recognition. Some are the early precursors of future advances whose time had not yet come: the giants on whose shoulders future workers stand, to paraphrase Isaac Newton. Some, to be sure, seem to have been mere puppets manipulated by an unseen and capricious hand, as the following chapters will amply demonstrate. Others were driven by a need to know and to do and the lucky few among these workhorses found their perseverance and efforts rewarded by success. Still others—the vast majority—were simply a cross-section of society, more, or sometimes less gifted than their contemporaries, but destined to be involved in multifarious ways in an enterprise of inestimable benefit to mankind. All have their part to play in the story of antimicrobial agents.

This book attempts to celebrate as many of the antimicrobial pioneers as possible and hundreds of individual names are herein recorded and listed below. Not all the names on the list were directly involved, but most contributed to, witnessed, or prefigured the events that unfolded in the twentieth century. But even this formidable list is grossly incomplete. Quite apart from the researchers and investigators whose role has been overlooked by unintentional omission, there are countless men and women—scientists, doctors, nurses, technicians, secretaries, bottle-washers, tea ladies, and long-suffering patients among them—who were essential to the process of bringing the medical advances to fruition, and whose names will never be known.

Chapter 1

Agents of infection

I saw with as great wonderment as ever before an unconceivably great number
of little animalcules. These animalcules, or most of them, moved so nimbly
among one another that the whole stuff seemed alive and moving…there are
more animals living in the scum on the teeth in a man's mouth than there are
men in a whole kingdom.

Antoni van Leeuwenhoek, *Letter to the Royal Society*
of London, 17 September, 1683

Evolving insights

Before the 'germ theory' took hold towards the end of the nineteenth century, the concept of infection and its spread had no doubt puzzled humankind since the dawn of
reflective thought. Problems became evermore acute as settlements were founded, towns
and cities grew, civilizations emerged, and trade routes began to offer the paths for unexpected visitations of epidemic disease (1). The unmistakable but apparently random
transmission of disease between family members, communities, and their domestic animals was attributed to retribution from the gods, activities of malign spirits, or noxious
emanations (miasmata) arising from stagnant pools and marshes, middens, decaying
corpses, or other environmental sources.

The devastating and essentially indiscriminate spread of the characteristic signs and
symptoms of plague, smallpox, and many other diseases fostered numerous speculations
as to what might cause epidemic and pandemic transmission of infection, while the
acquisition of disease by contact with, or proximity to, obviously infected persons, inani-
mate objects or places, gave rise to theories of contagion (2). Some early observers,
notably the sixteenth century Veronese scholar and physician, Girolamo Fracastoro came
remarkably close to realizing the true nature of infection, but without microscopy the
concept could be only dimly perceived and was incapable of proof. Fracastoro published
several works, including the poem *Syphilis sive morbus Gallicus* (1530), from which the
disease syphilis derives its name (and in which he describes possible treatments, including mercury and guaiacum, the heartwood—known as lignum vitae—or gum resin of an

aromatic Caribbean tree popularly believed to have curative properties) (3). But, it was in a later work *De contagione et contagiosis morbis et curatione* (1546) that he expanded earlier theories of 'seeds' of disease, and proposed three chief methods by which they are transmitted: by direct contact with an infected person; by contact with infected clothing or other contaminated materials; and through the air. The 'seeds', which clearly needed the power to multiply in some fashion, we would now call micro-organisms or, more popularly, 'germs'.

After his death, Fracastoro's ideas lay virtually dormant, but the notion that invisible, but animate creatures might be responsible for infectious disease were revived when a humble draper living in Delft, Antoni van Leeuwenhoek, took up the hobby of grinding magnifying lenses and used them to examine rain water, pepper infusions, gingival scrapings, faeces; indeed, whatever materials his insatiable curiosity could find (4). The world he discovered was an astonishing one, and included incredible numbers of obviously living creatures ('animalcules') invisible to the naked eye.

From 1673, until his death 50 years later, Leeuwenhoek submitted a stream of letters to the newly established *Royal Society of London* (founded in 1660) and his startling findings, illustrated with his own drawings, were published in their *Philosophical Transactions*. The richness and diversity of the world that was revealed by these publications soon aroused feelings of awe and raised speculations about the nature of microscopic creatures and their relationship to infectious disease. Conjecture about their origin was to add fuel to the intense debate about 'spontaneous generation'—for example of maggots arising from putrid flesh—that had simmered since ancient times. The Italian physician Francesco Redi exposed the basic fallacy of this belief in the seventeenth century by showing that maggots did not develop in meat protected from invasion by flies, but disproving the spontaneous emergence of microscopic organisms was more difficult. Controversy continued to rage throughout the eighteenth century, despite convincing evidence against spontaneous generation produced by the eminent Italian experimentalist, Lazzaro Spallanzani. The great French chemist and pioneering bacteriologist Louis Pasteur was eventually to settle the matter by a series of conclusive experiments conducted in the early 1860s that finally established his reputation as one of the outstanding scientists of his age (5).

Slowly, evidence began to emerge of the role of micro-organisms to explain the specific nature of many contagious diseases. The Italian naturalist Agostino Bassi is usually credited with the first crucial observation: that muscardine, a serious disease of silkworms was invariably associated with the presence of a fungus, now known as *Beauveria* (*Botrytis*) *bassiana*. Bassi's findings were first made known at a demonstration held at the University of Pavia in 1834 and published in two monographs during the next two years (6). Other discoveries followed and, once Robert Koch, while still a country doctor in Eastern Germany, had succeeded in establishing the role of *Bacillus anthracis* as the cause of anthrax in 1876 (7), the floodgates opened to a golden age of microbial discovery. Koch went on to discover the causes of tuberculosis (1882) and cholera (1883) and made technological advances that were instrumental in putting bacteriology on a sound scientific footing.

As a student in Göttingen, Koch had studied under the pioneer pathologist Jakob Henle, who had himself, with remarkable foresight, put forward a theory of the role of germs in disease. Henle had outlined a series of criteria that should be met in establishing microbial aetiology, which Koch later refined into what became known as 'Koch's postulates':

◆ The microbe must be found in all cases of the disease.

◆ It must be obtained in pure culture from a case of the disease and maintained in a series of pure cultures outside the body.

◆ Pure subcultures of the organism should be able to produce disease symptoms when inoculated into a healthy animal.

◆ The organism should be again recovered from the diseased animal.

In the event it turns out that Koch's postulates cannot always be fulfilled precisely, but in the early days of bacteriology the concept was very important in establishing the causative role of specific micro-organisms in individual infectious diseases.

By the end of the nineteenth century, the germ theory was firmly entrenched, although powerful dissenting voices remained. In Britain, these included the eminent gynaecologist, Lawson Tait (8) and the Cambridge anatomist-turned-historian, Charles Creighton, who notwithstanding his scepticism over the role of germs was able to write a comprehensive, if idiosyncratic, history of epidemic disease in Britain (9). Before we dismiss such historical 'losers' as wilfully blind to scientific advance, we should remember that early enthusiasm for the germ theory led to numerous false claims that were the subject of much legitimate dispute. Moreover, the theory failed to offer satisfactory answers to many epidemiological puzzles about the prevalence of infectious disease and vagaries of susceptibility among populations. Thus, when the German medicinal chemist and hygienist, Max von Pettenkofer drank a diluted culture of the cholera vibrio in defiance of the theories of Robert Koch, he was not entirely discounting the role of the organism in cholera, but seeking to reinforce his own view, based on epidemiological evidence, that the disease was produced by noxious emanations resulting from changes wrought by the organism in soil (10).

Such opposition, however, was swept aside by the weight of evidence in favour of the new doctrine and general acceptance of the germ theory gave an enormous fillip to the search for interventions that might be successfully used to treat diseases caused by specific micro-organisms. Some drugs, notably quinine and emetine (see Chapter 2) predated the recognition of the causative agents of the diseases—malaria and amoebic dysentery, respectively—the symptoms of which they so effectively controlled, but once the enemy had been identified efforts could be focused more precisely on targeting therapy at the microbe. At the forefront of these endeavours was the brilliant German pathologist, immunologist, and founding father of antimicrobial chemotherapy, Paul Ehrlich, who, as early as 1891 was experimenting with the dye methylene blue in human malaria (11) (see Chapter 3).

Malaria and amoebic dysentery are, of course, protozoal, not bacterial infections. Among other infective agents that we are aware of today, helminths (worms), which are visible to the naked eye, had been recognized since antiquity as unwelcome parasites of human beings. Acknowledgement of fungi as human pathogens owed much to the pioneering work of the eccentric Hungarian David Gruby through his mid-nineteenth century investigations of diseases such as ringworm and thrush (12). In the last decade of the nineteenth century a new kind of infectious particle—the virus—further complicated the picture, when the young Russian researcher Dimitri Ivanowsky and, independently, the Dutch bacteriologist, Martinus Willem Beijerinck, demonstrated that mosaic disease of tobacco was transmissible by an agent capable of passing through filters that withheld even the smallest bacteria. In 1901, the American Army bacteriologist Walter Reed and his colleagues made similar observations in the human infection, yellow fever, in the course of studies in Cuba that also proved (by allowing infected mosquitoes to feed upon volunteers, one of whom died) that the disease was spread by mosquitoes (13).

Recognition of the diverse structures and life cycles of the organisms responsible for infectious disease quickly made it plain that finding cures would require equal diversity in the weapons to be used. Further understanding of the complexities that exist within the different groups of infective agents revealed the task to be even more formidable than could have been imagined. Fortunately, as will emerge, Lady Luck was on hand to aid, and sometimes confound, the ingenuity of humankind.

Bacteria

Bacteria have a reputation as the true villains of the microbial world, owing to their involvement in the devastating visitations of the plague and cholera and their role in many other traditionally feared diseases—tuberculosis, leprosy, diphtheria, scarlet fever, childbed fever, typhoid, typhus, tetanus, gangrene, gonorrhoea, and syphilis to name but a few. Given this terrible criminal record, it may need an effort of will to appreciate the incontrovertible, but seldom acknowledged fact that the vast majority of species of this most ancient and successful form of life are not only innocuous to human beings, but are in many cases positively beneficial. Indeed, it could hardly be otherwise. In the lower gut, 1 g of colonic faeces contains around 10^{12} (1 million million) bacteria, and our skin and external orifices similarly teem with these organisms. It has been calculated that bacterial cells outnumber all other cells in the human body by a factor of at least 10, so that, in terms of the number of cells we harbour, each of us is less than 10 per cent human!

Nature and morphology of bacteria

Bacteria are nature's miracles of micro-engineering. Few bacterial cells are larger than 2–4 µm (thousandths of a millimetre) in diameter or length. Within that minute cell they fit a circular deoxyribonucleic acid (DNA) genome that may be well over 1-mm long by condensing it down and twisting it into a 'supercoiled' state. Specific enzymes are available to temporarily relax this strained structure by nicking the double helix in a controlled fashion, unwinding it, and then repairing the damage, thus enabling the genetic information to be transcribed and the DNA itself to be replicated. Faithful duplication of all the complex structures of the cell including the DNA, protein synthesizing work benches (ribosomes) and cell envelope, together with their segregation into two independent daughter cells can, under optimal conditions, be accomplished in as little as 20 min, or even less.

The cellular organization of bacteria is much simpler than that found in mammals and other higher organisms; indeed certain structures of more complex cells, such as mitochondria, may have originated as parasitic bacteria. In bacteria the nucleus (genome) lies free within the cytoplasm and there are none of the organelles characteristic of fungi, protozoa, and cells of higher organisms. This type of cellular organization is described as prokaryotic. The bacterial cytoplasm is enclosed within a lipid membrane similar to that found in mammalian cells, limiting the opportunity for antimicrobial agents to act selectively at this site without damaging the host. However, external to the cell membrane in all bacterial pathogens of man except mycoplasmas there is a rigid, shape-maintaining, carbohydrate-rich layer, known as peptidoglycan, which protects the cell from external stress. This layer is not present in mammalian cells and is thus a prime target for the selective toxicity that is a feature of the most successful antibacterial agents. Penicillins and cephalosporins (Chapter 4) act by interfering with the synthesis of peptidoglycan.

Morphologically, bacteria tend to be relatively conservative, but there is plenty of scope for ingenious diversity to suit the various lifestyles of individual organisms. In most cases the shape is that of a spherical coccus or a cylindrical bacillus. A few, like the spirochaetes of syphilis, have evolved a more complex corkscrew shape and others display a variant of the basic bacillary form: for example, the cholera vibrio adopts a 'comma' shape and the diphtheria bacillus is characteristically club-shaped. Some bacteria, like the anthrax bacillus and the clostridia that cause tetanus and gas gangrene solve the problem of survival in hostile environments by producing highly resistant spores allowing the microbes to remain dormant for long periods before recognition of favourable external stimuli triggers a process of germination, allowing them once more to grow and multiply. Certain bacteria such as the Rickettsiae that cause typhus and the Chlamydiae that are responsible for trachoma and other diseases are adapted to an obligatory intracellular existence, relying on the host cell for many of their metabolic functions.

Bacteria divide by transverse binary fission. Some cocci divide in random planes to form irregular clumps of individual cells looking under the microscope like bunches of grapes (staphylococci). Others always divide in the same plane, giving rise to chains of cells of varying length (streptococci). A few tend to remain in pairs, looking rather like beans, lying side-by-side or end-to-end depending on the species. Most bacilli simply elongate, constrict in the middle and separate into two daughter cells. Unusually, one group of bacilli, the actinomycetes, give rise to lateral branches as they extend and may produce a type of mycelium not unlike fungi. These organisms are abundant in soil and only a few species have been incriminated in human disease. They commonly produce antibiotic substances and many, notably those belonging to the *Streptomyces* genus, will be encountered throughout this book as the source of therapeutically valuable antibiotics. The mycobacteria that cause tuberculosis and leprosy are distantly related to the actinomycetes, but they do not normally branch.

Identification of bacteria

The infinite variety of bacteria makes their exact identification laborious and time-consuming, but medical bacteriologists have learnt many tricks to identify individual species or genera of bacteria quickly and with an acceptable degree of accuracy: after all, it is little use to the infected patient if their doctor is told with pinpoint precision what the sufferer has already recovered (or possibly died) from several weeks earlier. An experienced microscopist can often provide a vital clue to the identity of a pathogen within a few minutes and allow life-saving therapy to be instituted, for example in bacterial meningitis. Differential staining is frequently useful and nothing has been of more value than the now classic stain, developed more than a century ago, that bears the name of a young Danish doctor, Hans Christian Gram.

Within a few weeks of arriving on a study visit to Berlin in 1884, Gram fortuitously discovered that bacteria stained with the purple-blue aniline dye, gentian violet, could be differentially decolourized with an alcoholic solution of iodine and potassium iodide (14). Gram published the work (15), but soon returned to Denmark to pursue a career as a Professor of Pharmacology in Copenhagen, and carried out no further work on his discovery. However, a modification of his method has become one of the most frequently used techniques in bacteriology. The beauty of Gram's stain is that it distinguishes most bacteria as belonging to one of two types: those that resist decolourization after staining with gentian violet (or a similar aniline dye)—appearing purple under the microscope and designated as Gram-positive—and those that are easily decolorized and can for convenience be counterstained with a red dye and designated Gram-negative. Staphylococci and streptococci belong to the former kind and are thus called Gram-positive cocci, while many other organisms, including the typhoid bacillus and *Escherichia coli*, a very common cause of cystitis and, sometimes, more serious infection, are easily decolorized and are Gram-negative bacilli. Gram-negative cocci (e.g. the gonococcus and meningococcus) and Gram-positive bacilli (e.g. the organisms responsible for anthrax, diphtheria, tetanus, and gas gangrene) are also recognized. The technique is not only of taxonomic value. It turns out that the difference between Gram-positive and Gram-negative correlates with possession (by Gram-negative bacteria) of a external membrane-like structure covering the peptidoglycan layer, which effectively excludes many potential antibiotics from reaching their site of action within the cell. This is one of the principal factors to influence the spectrum of activity of various antibacterial agents.

Another extremely useful staining technique is used to recognize *Mycobacterium tuberculosis* and *Mycobacterium leprae*, the causative organisms of tuberculosis and leprosy, respectively. The cell wall of these bacteria contains waxy molecules—mycolic acids—that make them not only difficult to stain, but also impervious to many of the antibiotics used to deal with other bacteria. These organisms can be stained adequately only by hot, concentrated phenolic dyes. Once the dye has penetrated they are subsequently resistant to decolorization by mineral acids, such as hydrochloric and sulphuric acids; hence the term often used to describe the bacilli of tuberculosis and leprosy: 'acid-fast bacilli'. The acid-fast property is the basis for the Ziehl–Neelsen technique, an ingenious staining method that evolved in Germany from one described by Robert Koch, modified by Paul Ehrlich and then refined first by Franz Ziehl and later by Friedrich Neelsen. Clinical material, for example sputum in a suspected case of pulmonary tuberculosis, is stained with a hot solution of strong carbol fuchsin* which stains the entire preparation, along with any mycobacteria; all the background material, including any other bacteria present, can then be decolorized by application of acid (and methylated spirits, which also fails to remove the stain from most mycobacteria) and counterstained with a blue or green dye to provide a contrasting background. Since the bacteria of tuberculosis are very slow growing and those that cause leprosy cannot be cultivated artificially, the Ziehl–Neelsen technique is very valuable in rapidly establishing the diagnosis, allowing early treatment of these two very important infections.

Most other bacteria can be easily grown in nutrient broth—essentially a meat soup—usually solidified by a seaweed extract called agar–agar, generally abbreviated to just 'agar'. Horse or sheep blood is added to allow the growth of some of the more demanding pathogens. It was Robert Koch who popularized the use of agar as a solidifying agent and developed the method of obtaining pure cultures of bacteria that is still in use today (16). Earlier he used gelatin as the solidifying agent, but it had the disadvantage of liquefying at the optimum temperature (35–37°C; close to human body temperature) for the growth of bacterial pathogens. The suggestion of using agar came from Walther Hesse, a country physician interested in the new science of bacteriology, who spent a short time in Koch's laboratory in 1881 (17). Hesse's wife, Fanny (née Eilshemius) had the original idea. Fanny Eilshemuis had been born in New Jersey of German immigrants and had gone to her parents' homeland in 1874, where she met and married Walther Hesse. Her mother had learned of the use of the seaweed extract as a gelling agent from Dutch friends who had lived in Java, where the substance was widely used for culinary purposes.

Agar plate culture—originally literally on flat glass plates; later in the familiar Petri dishes—was a brilliant solution to the problem of isolating individual species of bacteria from sites with a mixed flora, since each individual colony that develops on the surface (provided the inoculum is sufficiently diluted and distributed) represents the progeny of a single bacterium. Koch and others had at first used slices of boiled potato to achieve the same effect, but agar plates were reusable, easier to handle and provided a much more elegant solution to the pure culture problem.

Petri dishes perpetuate the name of Richard Julius Petri, who had worked as an assistant in Koch's laboratory, and described his brainchild in a paper published in 1887: 'Eine kleine Modifikation des Kochschen Plattenverfahrens' (18) (a small modification of Koch's plate method). However, an English chemist, Percy Faraday Frankland, described a similar dish one year before Petri while working as a young Demonstrator at the Royal College of Chemistry in London and may have priority for the invention (19). Percy Frankland, son

---

* A fluorescent dye, auramine is now often preferred. This allows the specimen to be examined in a fluorescence microscope, making scanty bacilli easier to pick out.

of the eminent chemist, Sir Edward Frankland,* became an equally distinguished Professor of Chemistry and subsequently Dean of the Science Faculty at Birmingham University (20). Frankland senior was official analyst for the metropolitan water supply in London and a campaigner for safe water. It was probably under his father's encouragement that Percy, together with his wife Grace—an early supporter of women's rights—carried out some of the first studies on the bacteriology of water.

At the present time, molecular methods of bacterial diagnosis are slowly replacing the time-honoured techniques of microscopy, culture, and identification that established the discipline of medical bacteriology in the late nineteenth century. The change is inevitable, but few of the newer procedures, though ingenious and often adaptable to automation, require the skill and experience demanded by the elegant methods that evolved in the early days of bacteriology. Nor do they provide the intellectual satisfaction of recognizing the characteristic features of individual pathogens under the microscope or on the agar plate. Fortunately, a place still remains for the old-fashioned ways: nothing, for example, is more rapidly helpful to a doctor caring for a child with suspected bacterial meningitis, than a Gram-stained smear of cerebrospinal fluid interpreted by an experienced bacteriologist.

Bacteria as pathogens

Most members of the normal bacterial flora of the human body coexist with us quite happily and rarely cause disease. The infamous Mary Mallon, 'typhoid Mary' of early twentieth century New York, is an example of an unsuspecting carrier of a serious bacterial infection—and one who must have had questionable habits of personal hygiene—but relatively few of the classic bacterial pathogens regularly inhabit otherwise healthy persons. None the less, some of the resident flora can cause disease if they are given the right conditions. Thus hair follicles and minor abrasions in the skin may become infected with *Staphylococcus aureus*, which is often found in the nose or moist areas such as the armpits, to cause the familiar boils or more serious carbuncles and wound infections.

Infections caused by *Staphylococcus aureus* and another bacterium that can be harmlessly carried in the nose and throat, *Streptococcus pyogenes*, were rightly feared before the advent of penicillin and other antibiotics. These organisms can produce an amazing array of virulence factors (attributes that allow them to achieve a pathogenic effect) and strains possessing these factors can be formidable pathogens. *Streptococcus pyogenes* is often responsible for pharyngitis and impetigo, but much more seriously causes life-threatening diseases such as scarlet fever, childbed fever, and erysipelas. A rare manifestation is necrotizing fasciitis—the 'flesh-eating bug' disease of the popular press. Some strains of *Streptococcus pyogenes* may also give rise to serious effects on the heart (rheumatic fever) or kidneys (glomerulonephritis) probably caused by autoimmune reactions

---

* Among his other achievements, Edward Frankland first proposed the theory of valency bonds in chemical reactions. He was a friend of Michael Faraday, who became godfather to his son Percy; hence his son's middle name.

to shared antigens in the bacteria and host tissues. These diseases have declined in frequency in most countries since the introduction of penicillin, but have not completely disappeared. A related pathogen that is found among the normal throat flora in healthy individuals is *Streptococcus pneumoniae*, the commonest cause of pneumonia acquired outside hospital as well as other serious infections, including meningitis. It was seemingly miraculous cures of staphylococcal and streptococcal infections that led to sulphonamides and penicillin being hailed as 'miracle drugs'.

Several bacterial diseases, including tetanus, gas gangrene, scarlet fever, and diphtheria are the result of extremely potent toxins produced by the causative organisms. The spores of some Gram-positive bacilli can withstand boiling and, if present in food, may subsequently germinate and give rise to food poisoning. One such bacterium *Clostridium botulinum* produces a toxin that is the most poisonous substance known in nature: the lethal dose has been calculated to be about 1 ng (one thousand millionth of a gram) per kg.* The poison can persist even if the producer organism is subsequently killed and many deaths have been caused by improperly canned foods and other preserved products. Strains of *Staphylococcus aureus* that produce a particular enterotoxin may cause a form of food poisoning in which vomiting rather than diarrhoea predominates; others are responsible for 'toxic shock syndrome', which has been associated with the use of highly absorbent tampons in menstruating women. Babies occasionally experience 'scalded skin syndrome' another toxin-mediated disease associated with strains of staphylococci that produce an epidermolytic substance that causes extensive blistering. Antimicrobial therapy is, of course, unlikely to be of primary value in the treatment of infectious disease caused by poisons that the microbes excrete into the tissues, although antimicrobial drugs may be able to abort the production of such toxins.

Viruses

In its original sense 'virus' simply meant a poison. The meaning subsequently became extended to include any unspecified morbid principle capable of producing a poison and thereby initiating disease. In the early days of bacteriology it was sometimes used indiscriminately to describe infectious agents, so that when Louis Pasteur said that 'every virus is a microbe' he was merely going slightly over the top in his enthusiasm for the germ theory of disease. Nowadays, *virus* (aside from the usage in computing and the slipshod phraseology of journalists who refer to 'the e-coli virus') properly refers to infectious, non-cellular particles that can multiply only within living cells of a host organism. Even such a definition is becoming stretched as the nature of anomalous entities such as viroids (which are essentially protein-free viruses) and the prions responsible for transmissible spongiform encephalopathies such as Creutzfeldt–Jakob disease are revealed.

---

* When carefully controlled high dilutions of botulinum toxin—commonly known as 'Botox'—are injected into selected muscles it has the effect of immobilizing or weakening them. It has achieved popularity in some quarters as a cosmetic anti-wrinkle treatment. A more important use is in the control of facial tics, blepharospasm and other distressing conditions.

Although the birth of virology can be traced back to the early work of Ivanowsky, Beijerinck, Reed, and others in the late nineteenth century, the nature of the infective agent remained obscure and controversial for many years and it has been cogently argued that the true origins of virology as an independent discipline had to await developments that did not emerge until the mid-twentieth century (21). A major stumbling block in earlier studies was that, apart from the larger pox viruses, the agents could not be seen with even the most powerful microscopes that depended on light to visualize the image. The advent of the electron microscope, developed by the German physicist Ernst Ruska in the 1930s allowed the structure of these extraordinary particles to be revealed (22). The other major problem was that, unlike bacteria, viruses could not be grown in artificial culture media, since they depend on living cells for their propagation. Animal inoculation was seldom successful in the case of human viruses because most are species specific, though rabies virus is an important exception.

Much of the early work on viruses depended on growth of the infectious particles in whole organ culture or embryonated chicken eggs. By the beginning of the Second World War methods of establishing cultures of certain individual tissues for the propagation of viruses in the laboratory had been worked out. Foremost among workers developing these techniques were three remarkable Nobel laureates: a French émigré to the United States, Alexis Carrel; an American, Peyton Rous; and an Australian, Frank Macfarlane Burnet. Carrel, a brilliant, but controversial figure,* joined the Rockefeller Institute of Medical Research as an associate member in 1906; by 1912 he had been awarded the Nobel Prize for his pioneering work on vascular surgery and organ transplantation. He was also very active in developing tissue culture techniques and as early as 1911 established a culture of chicken heart cells that was perpetuated for over 30 years. Also in 1911, Peyton Rous used chick embryos to demonstrate the existence of a transmissible agent responsible for sarcoma in chickens—the first example of a virus-induced tumour—although Rous sarcoma virus as it is now known could not be visualized at that time. Macfarlane Burnet was instrumental in further exploring the use of chick embryos for the growth of viruses after being recruited in late 1931 by Henry Dale, Director of the National Institute of Medical Research Laboratories in Hampstead, London. In 1934 Burnet moved back to Melbourne as head of virology and Assistant Director of the Walter and Eliza Hall Institute. This incredibly productive scientist not only made many important advances in medical bacteriology and virology, but also radically changed the focus of his research in 1957 and became one of the pioneers of modern immunology. He received his Nobel Prize with Peter Medawar in 1960 for their researches into acquired immunological tolerance, but is perhaps better known for his revolutionary clonal-selection theory of antibody production.

---

* Alexis Carrel professed contentious right wing views, which included espousing Nazi policies on eugenics. He returned to France in 1941 and became a supporter of the Vichy government. After his death, his dubious past his seems to have been overlooked in favour of his scientific achievements. Streets in French cities were named after him, but were later changed when his beliefs were invoked by politicians of the extreme right. See: Weksler ME (2004). Naming streets for physicians. 'L'affaire Carrel'. *Perspect Biol Med* **47**, 67–73.

With the availability of antibiotics after Second World War problems of contamination that had bedevilled the growth of viruses in tissue culture were considerably alleviated. In 1949 John Franklin Enders and his colleagues, Thomas Huckle Weller and Frederick Chapman Robbins at the Children's Medical Center, Boston, Massachusetts succeeded in growing poliovirus in tissue culture opening the way for the development of effective vaccines against polio (see p. 366). The trio were jointly awarded a Nobel Prize in Physiology or Medicine in 1954. Tissue culture became the preferred method of propagating viruses, opening the way for an explosion in viral research and the amazing success of preventive vaccines against viral diseases.

Viruses have succeeded in reducing the problem of survival and replication to its most basic form; indeed, the question of whether they qualify for the epithet 'living' is a matter of scholarly debate. In most cases, the complete virus particle (virion) consist of no more than a strand of either ribonucleic acid (RNA) or DNA—never both—surrounded by a self-assembly coat of protein (the capsid) made up of numerous identical units (capsomeres) arranged with geometrical precision in icosahedral (having 20 equilateral triangular faces) or helical symmetry. Some viruses surround themselves with an envelope largely derived from the host cell in which they replicate. In certain viruses that are specialized to infect bacteria (bacteriophages) the nucleocapsid carries a cylindrical tail bearing filaments that allows it to dock onto the surface of the bacterial cell; the tail then contracts, injecting the nucleic acid into the bacterium rather in the manner of a hypodermic syringe.

Notwithstanding their minimalist character viruses are remarkably diverse (Table 1.1). The enterovirus group, which includes the polioviruses, are among the smallest and simplest. They are only around 25 nm in diameter (a nanometre is one millionth of a millimetre) and contain the bare minimum of nucleic acid needed to ensure their replication in the host cell. At the other extreme, the poxviruses, which include smallpox (but not chickenpox, which is a member of the herpesvirus group), are complex enveloped structures containing a relatively large genome in a virion that is around 300 nm in size and therefore just discernable in stained preparations in the light microscope.

Peter Medawar once described viruses as 'bad news wrapped in a protein coat'. Few would disagree, but the good news is that many of the viruses that afflict human beings give rise to diseases that have unpleasant symptoms, but are normally not life-threatening: upper respiratory infections such as sore throat and the common cold; childhood diseases like chickenpox, mumps, and rubella; diarrhoeal disease in children and adults. Others, like the yellow fever virus, the influenza viruses, the measles virus, and the hepatitis viruses, may cause more serious, even fatal disease, either directly or through the consequences of chronic infection. One potentially fatal viral disease, smallpox, was finally eradicated in 1977 through the Herculean efforts of the World Health Organization and another, poliomyelitis, is on the verge of following in its wake. Other viruses, of which the prime example is human immunodeficiency virus (HIV), the cause of acquired immune deficiency syndrome (AIDS), have emerged to cause worldwide problems that are devastating many communities. Some potentially lethal viruses, such as Lassa fever, Ebola, and similar haemorrhagic fever viruses, arise sporadically but have so far not managed to gain a foothold outside the areas in which they are endemic.

Table 1.1 Principal types of virus causing human infection

Virus family	Examples	Principal diseases
RNA viruses		
Orthomyxoviruses	Influenza A and B viruses	Influenza
Paramyxoviruses	Mumps virus	Mumps
	Measles virus	Measles
	Respiratory syncytial virus	Bronchiolitis
Rhabdoviruses	Rabies virus	Rabies
Arenaviruses	Lassa virus	Lassa fever
Filoviruses	Marburg and Ebola viruses	Haemorrhagic fever
Togaviruses	Rubella virus	German measles
Flaviviruses	Arboviruses	Yellow fever, dengue, etc.
	Hepatitis C virus	Hepatitis
Picornaviruses	Enteroviruses	Polio, meningitis
	Hepatitis A	Infectious hepatitis
	Rhinoviruses	Common cold
Retroviruses	Human immunodeficiency viruses	AIDS
Reoviruses	Rotaviruses	Infantile diarrhoea
Caliciviruses	Norwalk virus	Gastroenteritis
DNA viruses		
Poxviruses	Variola virus	Smallpox
	Vaccinia virus	Smallpox vaccine
Herpesviruses	Herpes simplex virus	Cold sores, genital herpes
	Varicella-zoster virus	Chickenpox, shingles
	Cytomegalovirus	Intrauterine infection
	Epstein–Barr virus	Glandular fever
Adenovirus	Many types	Conjunctivitis, etc.
Papovavirus	Papillomavirus	Warts, cervical cancer
Hepadnavirus	Hepatitis B virus	Serum hepatitis
Parvovirus	Parvovirus B19	Erythema infectiosum

Viruses are not only of importance in disease of human beings, animals, and plants; they have played a crucial part in the development of molecular genetics, notably through the meticulous work on bacteriophage of the German-born American, Max Delbrück, the American bacteriologist, Alfred Hershey, and the Italian-born American, Salvador Luria. These studies, which have had profound ramifications, were eventually rewarded by the award of a Nobel Prize which they shared in 1969.

The lifestyle of viruses, existing in an intimate relationship with the cells on which they depend for survival, has made them a much more difficult target than bacteria for selectively active therapeutic agents. Very few antiviral agents were available until the HIV pandemic concentrated the minds of scientists inside and outside the pharmaceutical industry, and even now few, if any, of the agents available to the prescriber are reliably curative (see Chapter 8).

Much more success in the control of viral disease has been achieved by the development of vaccines, the relatively simple antigenic structure of the organisms lending themselves peculiarly well to this preventative approach. Structural simplicity together with the high multiplication rate of viruses also has the consequence of increasing the likelihood of the appearance of variants that are able to survive and spread. Such mutants may display new and unexpected characteristics as the recent outbreak of severe acute respiratory syndrome (SARS) reminds us.

Fungi

Few organisms have had enjoyed such universal acclaim as the fungi. Long enjoyed as culinary delights in the shape of edible mushrooms (mushroom hunting is still a regular autumn ritual in many parts of continental Europe, though strangely neglected in Great Britain), it was then discovered in the nineteenth century that their cousins, yeasts, were responsible for the leavening of bread and for the fermentation so widely appreciated in wine making. When, in 1928, Fleming discovered that a fungus was able to produce a powerful antibiotic substance, later hailed as the wonder drug, penicillin, the fungal triumph was complete.

Like protozoa, fungi exhibit a eukaryotic cell structure (as opposed to the prokaryotic form of bacteria), with a distinct nucleus surrounded by a nuclear membrane, and various organelles common to mammalian and other living cells. They come in three basic types:

◆ Yeasts, which are thick-walled unicellular organisms that reproduce asexually by developing daughter cells that bud off and eventually detach from the parent.

◆ Filamentous fungi (moulds), which grow by elongation and branching, eventually forming masses of threads known as a mycelium. Some of the higher fungi produce the large fruiting bodies that are familiar to us as mushrooms and toadstools.

◆ Dimorphic fungi, which, amazingly, can adapt to a yeast or mycelial type of lifestyle depending on the conditions of growth in which they find themselves.

Despite the versatility of fungi and their ubiquity, these organisms have traditionally managed to maintain a relatively low profile as human pathogens, though many species can cause disease of varying degrees of severity. The most common problem caused by yeasts is the white discharge accompanying infection of the mucous membrane of the vagina—and, in infants, the elderly, immunocompromised individuals and denture wearers, the mouth—known as thrush. Sometimes antibiotic therapy that depletes the normal bacterial flora paves the way for opportunistic infection by yeasts that are unaffected by antibacterial drugs. A much more serious, but fortunately much less common infection than thrush is a form of meningitis caused by a yeast, *Cryptococcus neoformans*, which is carried by pigeons and grows luxuriantly in their faeces.

Filamentous fungi are responsible for the widespread infections of the nail, skin, and hair of man and animals known as ringworm. The infections are unsightly, irritating and contagious, but otherwise benign. A proportion of chronic ear infections are caused by common environmental fungi such as *Aspergillus niger*, and related species are responsible for some allergies. In parts of the world where ill-protected rural agricultural workers frequently suffer lacerations from thorns or other sharp-edged vegetation, serious disfiguring fungal infections may be acquired.

The group of fungi with dimorphic credentials are mostly restricted to endemic areas of North and South America and parts of Africa, where they cause conditions that range from self-limiting cutaneous lesions to serious pulmonary infections or fatal disseminated disease.

Most other fungal infections are mercifully rare, except in individuals whose normal host defences are seriously impaired by disease or medication. Such persons are prone to a wide variety of systemic infections and the yeasts or other fungi that may be encountered include many species that are otherwise unknown to cause human disease.

Protozoa

Protozoa are single-cell organisms with a eukaryotic cellular structure fundamentally organized on the same pattern as fungal, helminthic and, indeed, mammalian cells. There the resemblance stops. Protozoa are the flamboyant show-offs of the microbial world, flaunting a diversity that combines elegance with a wonderful plasticity of form.

Take the parasites that cause malaria: in the course of evolution they have developed a lifestyle that involves three distinct multiplicative phases in two different hosts and a level of antigenic diversity that has continually frustrated efforts to produce an effective vaccine. In the species of *Anopheles* mosquito that transmit the disease to man, male and female gametocytes are ingested with the blood of the infected mammalian host. In the gut of the mosquito the male gametocyte reveals himself to be composed of several separate gametes, which swim free and fertilize the females. Zygotes thus formed penetrate the mid-gut wall of the insect and settle on the body cavity side of the gut, where they undergo division within a cystic structure (the oocyst) to give rise to numerous sporozoites, which escape when the mature cyst ruptures and find their way to the insect's salivary glands. These sporozoites are the infective form, which are injected when the insect next takes a blood meal. In the mammalian host the sporozoites first invade cells of the liver, undergoing a cycle of asexual multiplication in which thousands of individual malaria parasites (merozoites) are formed. When the infected liver cell eventually ruptures the parasites are released and find a new home in circulating red blood cells, adopting a shape which, in stained preparations, resemble small signet rings. These ring-form trophozoites grow and multiply yet again, this time producing about 8–24 new merozoites, which infect fresh red blood cells and set up an ongoing cycle that continues to increase the number of circulating parasites. It is this phase of multiplication in the bloodstream that eventually leads to the symptoms of acute malaria. With one of the species that infects man, *Plasmodium falciparum*, the red blood cells harbouring developing parasites become sticky and block the capillaries of the brain. The patient rapidly becomes comatose and unless given urgent treatment with suitable antimalarial drugs, dies. To ensure the long-term survival of the parasite, some merozoites do not enter the multiplicative phase in the bloodstream, but instead differentiate into male and female gametocytes to await the opportunity provided by a hungry mosquito to complete the sexual stage of their life cycle.

Malaria parasites are formidable pathogens of humankind, responsible for uncountable episodes of debilitating fevers and a death toll that has been variously estimated— the true incidence is not known (23)—at between 1 and 2.5 million each year, chiefly, but not exclusively, among young children in the tropics. Certain other protozoa, while less widely distributed, are equally fearsome and scarcely less complex. Trypanosomes of the *Trypanosoma brucei* group are transmitted by various species of tsetse flies in tropical Africa. Some subspecies of this trypanosome cause an economically important disease, nagana, in cattle. Others attack human beings and, in areas in which the tsetse fly vectors are present in East and West Africa, give rise to a relentlessly fatal disease, sleeping sickness, in which the parasite eventually invades the central nervous system. The East African variety *Trypanosoma brucei rhodesiense*, which is transmitted by tsetse flies inhabiting the savannah lands that are the home to wild game, causes a relatively acute human infection in which death may ensue in weeks or months. In contrast, West African sleeping sickness, caused by *Trypanosoma brucei gambiense* usually follows a slow progressive course lasting months or years. The vectors live in the riverine areas of the tropical rain forest and, while important locally, the *gambiense* variety of the disease poses a hazard only to the most intrepid western tourists.

Another type of trypanosome, found exclusively in South America, causes Chagas' disease, a chronic condition involving the muscle of the heart and other organs. It is transmitted by reduviid bugs, which are about 3-cm long and are known as 'kissing bugs' or 'assassin bugs' because of their habit of landing on the face of an unsuspecting sleeper and taking a blood meal from around the mouth. The trypanosomes are not injected with the bite as they are in African trypanosomiasis, but are passed in the insect's faeces, which the unwitting sleeper rubs into the irritating bite wound after the bug has departed.

Related parasites are responsible for leishmaniasis, which is transmitted by sandflies, mainly in India, Africa, South America and coastal regions of the Mediterranean. There are three forms: cutaneous leishmaniasis, which is usually localized and self-limiting; mucocutaneous leishmaniasis, a disfiguring condition restricted to parts of Central and South America; and kala azar, a systemic disease which is usually fatal unless treated.

While malaria, trypanosomiasis, and leishmaniasis are essentially tropical diseases, other protozoal infections are found in all parts of the world. Two distant cousins of the malaria parasites, *Toxoplasma gondii* and *Cryptosporidium parvum*, are both very prevalent in man and animals in most countries. Serological evidence shows that human infection with *Toxoplasma gondii* is very common and increases with age. Acquisition of the parasite is normally unsuspected and may persist, probably for life, without causing any obvious symptoms. Undercooked meat is a common source of infection and the parasites are also frequently acquired from kittens, which often harbour the oocysts and excrete them in their faeces. Infection with toxoplasma is normally benign, though ocular problems sometimes occur and infection acquired by the developing foetus during pregnancy may give rise to congenital abnormalities or even stillbirth. Patients with compromised immune systems, including those with AIDS, may develop cerebral toxoplasmosis, apparently by recrudescence of dormant parasites normally held in check by immune defences.

Cryptosporidium parvum displays certain features that betray its ancestral relationship with toxoplasma, but infection with this protozoon leads to quite different problems. Much the most common symptom is profuse watery diarrhoea, often following contact with farm animals or ingestion of contaminated water. Symptoms usually abate after a few days in otherwise healthy subjects but may be intractable and life threatening in those that are immunocompromised.

Several other species of protozoa commonly cause diarrhoeal disease of varying degrees of severity. Among the most important, especially in areas of poor sanitation, is the amoeba that causes amoebic dysentery and amoebic liver abscess, *Entamoeba histolytica*. More common worldwide, but usually responsible for less serious disease, is the flagellate protozoon, *Giardia lamblia*, a cause of 'failure to thrive' in infants and chronic diarrhoea in all age groups.

One of the commonest causes of vaginal discharge in women (and sometimes urethritis in their male consorts) throughout the world is another type of flagellate protozoon called *Trichomonas vaginalis*. Unlike *Entamoeba histolytica* and *Giardia lamblia*, which can survive outside the body by surrounding themselves with a protective wall to form a resistant cyst that is responsible for transmitting infection, *Trichomonas vaginalis* has no cyst form and must rely on venereal transmission in its quest for new pastures.

Worms

Strictly speaking, helminths are not microbes, since the adult worms are visible to the naked eye. None the less they certainly cause infection (helminthologists rightly object to the term 'infestation'), which is often detected microscopically by the presence of their eggs or larvae. As befits well-adapted parasites, most live in harmony with their hosts and light infections seldom give rise to symptoms. Their pathogenic potential follows chiefly from their numbers, their size, and their location in the body. Some species are particularly unpleasant and on a global scale they are responsible for much morbidity and mortality.

Helminths come in three main kinds: nematodes (roundworms), trematodes (flukes), and cestodes (tapeworms). Any doubt about their importance can be easily dispelled by a consideration of the figures calculated (with many inevitable caveats) by the American helminthologist Norman Stoll for his Presidential address, entitled *This wormy world* to the American Society of Parasitologists in December 1946 (24). Stoll calculated that among the world population that then numbered around 2.2 billion people, 457 million harboured hookworms, 644 million *Ascaris lumbricoides* (the common roundworm), and 355 million *Trichuris trichiura* (the whipworm). Among some of the parasites causing serious deep-seated disease, the figures were: schistosomes (bilharzia), 114 million; and the filarial worms that cause 'river blindness' and elephantiasis, 778 million. Lest these figures be considered outdated, The British parasitologist David Crompton updated Stoll's calculation for the end of the twentieth century, when the world population had risen to over 6 billion (25). Crompton's estimates taken from literature published in the preceding few years were: hookworm infections, 1298 million; *Ascaris*, 1472 million; *Trichuris*, 1049 million; and schistosomiasis, 200 million. Only filariasis, calculated to affect around 138 million people, had markedly declined. Despite their reputation for relative harmlessness, hookworm, ascaris, and whipworm are probably still responsible for at least 135,000 deaths a year.

Nematodes

Many of the most common nematodes, such as hookworm, ascaris, whipworm, and threadworm, are confined to the intestinal tract, but can none the less cause considerable mischief. The hookworms, *Ancylostoma duodenale* and *Necator americanus* are important causes of anaemia; *Ascaris lumbricoides*, owing to its abundance and large size—the female worm can reach a length of at least 35 cm—can cause intestinal blockage; whipworm and ascaris have been associated with retarded educational development in areas where they are highly prevalent; and *Enterobius vermicularis* (the threadworm or pinworm) is responsible for the perianal itching that many readers will have suffered from as children.

More severe symptoms are caused by nematodes that invade tissues (Table 1.2). The filarial worm, *Onchocerca volvulus*, which is transmitted by biting blackflies in tropical Africa and parts of South America is responsible for 'river blindness', so-called because the flies breed in the vegetation on the banks of fast-flowing rivers. Heavy infections with another filarial worm, *Wuchereria bancrofti*, which is spread by mosquitoes throughout the tropics, give rise to the horrific deformities, usually of the legs or scrotum, known as elephantiasis. The leishmaniasis expert Philip Marsden tells of how Patrick Manson, lauded as the 'father of tropical medicine' and discoverer of the mosquito transmission of filariasis, was once unsuccessfully sued by a Chinaman whom he had operated on in Amoy:

> The plaintiff used to spread a cloth over his elephantoid scrotum and sell sweetmeats from it to passers-by. Manson took it off, leaving the Chinaman with a sadly depleted sales pitch (26).

Brugia malayi, a related species found, as the name suggests in South-East Asia, is also implicated in elephantiasis. Other filarial worms cause fewer problems, although the adult worms of one species, *Loa loa*, found exclusively in West Africa, cause local reactions as they migrate round the body under the skin and may disconcertingly travel across the front of the eye.

Table 1.2 Principal tissue nematodes causing human infection

Species	Disease	Transmission	Geographical distribution
Wuchereria bancrofti	Elephantiasis	Mosquitoes	Tropical belt
Loa loa	'Calabar' swellings	Deerflies	West and Central Africa
Brugia malayi	Elephantiasis	Mosquitoes	South-East Asia
Mansonella perstans	Non-pathogenic	Biting midges	Tropical Africa, S. America
Mansonella ozzardi	Non-pathogenic	Biting midges	West Indies, S. America
Onchocerca volvulus	River blindness	Blackflies	Tropical Africa, Central America
Dracunculus medinensis	Guinea worm disease	Water fleas	Africa, Indian subcontinent
Trichinella spiralis	Trichinosis	Infected pork	Worldwide

Uniquely, *Trichinella spiralis*, which is usually acquired by eating infected pork products (or, less commonly, poorly cooked meat from other sources, including bears and walruses), is a short-lived intestinal worm that produces numerous larvae. The larvae penetrate the gut wall and migrate to skeletal muscle producing during the migratory phase an alarming, sometimes fatal, reaction, but in muscle the larvae settle into a quiescent phase awaiting ingestion by the next host (clearly unlikely in the case of human infection!). *Trichinella spiralis* has the distinction of being the first pathogenic worm to be definitively identified in human beings—and by that much-maligned species, the first year medical student: on 2 February 1835, James Paget, who later became a renowned surgeon eponymously remembered for his description of the bone disease, osteitis deformans, found the larvae of the worm encysted in muscle of a body of an Italian man, Paolo Bianchi, that he was dissecting at St. Bartholomew's Hospital in London (27). He himself recalled the discovery in his memoirs:

> My share was the detection of the 'worm' in its capsule; and I may justly ascribe it to the habit of looking-out and observing, and wishing to find new things, which I had acquired in my previous studies of botany. All the men in the dissecting-rooms, teachers included, 'saw' the little specks in the muscles: but I believe that I alone 'looked-at' them and 'observed' them: no one trained in natural history could have failed to do so (28).

To see what others have missed is an important instrument of progress in all forms of learning and one that is often insufficiently valued.

Trematodes (flukes)

The flukes that infect human beings (Table 1.3) have a complex life cycle with a primary intermediate host, which is always a particular species of snail; most also spend time in a secondary intermediate host found in the aqueous environments where the snails live: freshwater fish in the case of *Clonorchis sinensis,* the Chinese liver fluke; crabs and crayfish with *Paragonimus westermani,* the lung fluke. *Fasciola hepatica,* the sheep liver fluke, which also infects human beings in the UK and other countries where sheep are reared,

Table 1.3 Principal trematodes (flukes) causing human infection

Species	Transmission	Geographical distribution
Clonorchis sinensis (Chinese liver fluke)	Infected fish	Far East
Fasciola hepatica (Sheep liver fluke)	Infected vegetation	Worldwide
Fasciolopsis buski (Intestinal fluke)	Water chestnuts	Far East
Paragonimus westermani (Lung fluke)	Crabs and crayfish	Mainly Far East
Schistosoma mansoni (Bilharzia)	Infected water	Africa, West Indies
Schistosoma haematobium (Bilharzia)	Infected water	Africa
Schistosoma japonicum (Bilharzia)	Infected water	Far East

is sometimes found in wild watercress in contaminated pastures inhabited by the snail vector, *Lymnaea* species. The geographical distribution of the parasites is restricted to those areas in which the intermediate hosts are found.

The most important of the trematode parasites of man are the schistosomes also known as blood flukes, often called bilharzia in commemoration of the German physician Theodor Maximilian Bilharz who first described *Schistosoma haematobium* in Cairo in 1851. The schistosomes are chiefly restricted to Africa (*Schistosoma haematobium* and *Schistosoma mansoni*) and the Far East (*Schistosoma japonicum* and *Schistosoma mekongi*). *Schistosoma mansoni* is also found in parts of the West Indies and South America, where it was carried by the slave trade.

Most flukes are hermaphrodite, but in the schistosomes the sexes are separate. Although the life cycle includes a snail intermediate host, schistosomes have dispensed with the secondary intermediate host, the infective larvae (cercaria) being simply shed by the snails into water, where they attach themselves to the skin of those swimming or paddling in the water. The schistosomula penetrate the skin and find their way to the liver where they grow to maturity, before migrating to the small veins of the bladder (*Schistosoma haematobium*) or rectum (*Schistosoma mansoni*, *Schistosoma japonicum*, and *Schistosoma mekongi*). How they manage to survive in the bloodstream as foreign invaders was long a puzzle, but it has been found that they coat themselves with antigens from the host so that they are not recognized by the immune system. They can live for many years passing their eggs through the mucosa of the bladder or rectum into the urine or colonic faeces. The adult worms themselves cause little problem, but in heavy infections eggs become deposited in the liver and elsewhere causing fibrosis, gross enlargement of the liver and spleen, and sometimes initiating cancerous changes.

Cestodes (tapeworms)

Cestodes also belong to the flatworm group. Infection with the two most familiar tapeworms, *Taenia saginata* and the much less common *Taenia solium*, is acquired from eating undercooked beef and pork, respectively. The larvae are freed from the muscle by digestion in the gut and attach themselves to the intestinal wall, the individual segments (proglottids) developing to maturity as they grow backwards from the head until the worm achieves a length of 10 m or more. The worms are hermaphrodite and cross-fertilization occurs between different segments. The terminal segments are virtually just bags of thousands of eggs, which detach from the end of the worm as it continues to grow and are passed in faeces, to await ingestion by cattle or pigs. It is suspected that birds foraging on sewage farms may be responsible for carrying the eggs to pasture land. Very occasionally, *Taenia solium* eggs develop in the human host and may lodge in the brain, giving rise to a condition resembling epilepsy, known as cerebral cysticercosis.

Contrary to their reputation, and despite their enormous size, intestinal infection with the beef and pork tapeworms is benign. The principal problems are caused by the alarming discovery of segments of the worm in underwear and bedclothes. The segments that become detached from the end of the worm are slippery and weakly motile, and they sometimes escape through the anus to the consternation of the infected host who has usually not suspected infection. Infection with most of the other tapeworms that are occasionally encountered is similarly generally asymptomatic, though the fish tapeworm *Diphyllobothrium latum,* which is found in lakeland areas where raw fish is consumed, has been associated with vitamin B_{12} deficiency.

In a reversal of the customary parasitic role, human beings can become an accidental intermediate host of *Echinococcus granulosus,* a tapeworm harboured by dogs and other canine species. Sheep normally act as the intermediate host and human infection is usually acquired from sheepdogs in sheep-farming areas. After ingestion of the egg, the larvae hatch and penetrate the gut wall to enter the bloodstream. The liver usually filters out the circulating larval forms and they settle there, surrounding themselves with a cyst wall, the so-called hydatid cyst, within which new larvae are produced. Sometimes infection is asymptomatic and the cyst may spontaneously regress, but often it grows inexorably. Unless it is removed surgically—a procedure not without risk—the size can seriously compromise liver function and will eventually cause death.

****

It will be evident from this brief overview of the diversity of micro-organisms and the infections that they cause, that no single type of remedy is likely to be effective, even against all members of any one group. This expectation has been more than met by experience, so that it has been necessary to assemble a large armoury of drugs to meet the microbial threat. As will be seen in the subsequent chapters, success has not been uniform. Many thousands of agents that are active against bacteria have been discovered or invented, and about 250 of them have reached the world market place. In contrast, the total number of drugs available to the prescriber for use against viral, fungal, protozoal, and helminthic infection falls far short of this figure. In some cases, no effective remedy has yet been found. Much has been achieved in the development of safe and effective therapies for infectious diseases, but much more remains to be done.

References

1. McNeill WH (1979). *Plagues and peoples*. Penguin Books, Harmondsworth.

2. Bulloch W (1938). *The history of bacteriology*. Oxford University Press, London.

3. Hudson MM, Morton RS (1996). Fracastoro and syphilis: 500 years on. *Lancet* **348**, 1495–6.

4. Porter JR (1976). Antony van Leeuwenhoek: tercentenary of his discovery of bacteria. *Bacteriol Rev* **40**, 260–9.

5. Dubos R (1960). *Louis Pasteur. Freelance of science*. Da Capo Press, New York.

6. Porter JR (1973). Agostino Bassi bicentennial (1773–1973). *Bacteriol Rev* **37**, 284–8.

7. Koch R (1876). Die Aetiologie der Milzbrand-Krankheit begründet auf die Entwicklungsgeschichte des Bacillus anthracis. *Beiträge zur Biologie der Pflanzen* **2**, 277–310.

8. Greenwood A (1998). Lawson Tait and opposition to germ theory: defining science in surgical practice. *J Hist Med Allied Sci* **53**, 99–131.

9. Creighton C (1881 and 1884). *A history of epidemics in Britain*, Vols. 1 and 2. Cambridge University Press; reprinted (1965): Frank Cass, London.

10. Locher WG (2001). Max von Pettenkofer—life stations of a genius on the 100th anniversary of his death (February 9, 1901). *Int J Hyg Environ Health* **203**, 379–91.

11. Guttmann P, Ehrlich P (1891). Ueber die Wirkung des Methylenblau bei Malaria. *Berliner Klinische Wochenschrift* **28**, 953–6.

12. Rosenthal T (1932). David Gruby (1810–1898). *Ann Med Hist* **4**, 339–46.

13. Goodwin LG, Gordon Smith CE (1996). Yellow fever. In: Cox FEG, ed. *Illustrated history of tropical diseases*, pp. 142–7. Wellcome Trust, London.

14. Jacobson W (1983). Gram's discovery of his staining technique. *J Infect* **7**, 97–101.

15. Gram C (1884). Ueber die isolierte Färbung der Schizomyceten in Schnitt- und Trockenpräparaten. *Fortschritte der Medicin* **2**, 185–9.

16. Brock TD (1988). *Robert Koch. A life in medicine and bacteriology*, pp. 94–104. Science Tech Publishers, Madison, WI.

17. Gröschel DHM (1981). 100 years of agar use in microbiology. *Am Soc Microbiol News* **47**, 391–2.

18. Petri RJ (1887). Eine kleine Modification des Kochschen Plattenverfahrens. *Centralblatt für Bakteriologie und Parasitenkunde* **1**, 279–80; cited by Mochmann H, Köhler W (1997). *Meilensteine der Bakteriologie*, 2nd edn., p. 333. Wötzel, Frankfurt.

19. Wainwright M (1998). Who invented the Petri dish? *Soc Gen Microbiol Quart* **25**, 98–9.

20. Mackie R, Roberts G, Percy Faraday Frankland (2006). *Biographical database of the British chemical community 1880–1970*. Open University, Milton Keynes. Available at: http://www5.open.ac.uk/Arts/chemists/person.cfm?SearchID=3677

21. van Helvoort T (1996). When did virology start? *Am Soc Microbiol News* **62**, 142–5.

22. Ruska H, von Borries B, Ruska E (1940). Die Bedeutung der Übermikroskopie für die Virusforschung. *Archiv der Gesamte Virusforschung* **1**, 155–9.

23. Snow RW (2004). The invisible victims. *Nature* **430**, 934–5.

24. Stoll NR (1947). This wormy world. *J Parasitol* **33**, 1–18; reprinted in *J Parasitol* 1999; **85**, 392–6.

25. Crompton DWT (1999). How much helminthiasis is there in the world? *J Parasitol* **85**, 397–403.

26. Marsden PD (1993). Obstructive lymphatic filariasis. *BMJ* **306**, 136.

27. Campbell WC (1979). History of trichinosis: Paget, Owen and the discovery of *Trichinella spiralis*. *Bull Hist Med* **53**, 520–52.

28. Paget S (ed.) (1902). *Memoirs and letters of Sir James Paget*, p. 55. Longmans, Green and Co., London.

Chapter 2

Out of darkness

I wish I could repeat the very sound of those groans and of those exclamations that I heard from some poor dying creatures when in the height of their agonies and distress, and that I could make him that reads this hear, as I imagine I now hear them, for the sound seems still to ring in my ears.

Daniel Defoe. *A Journal of the plague year*, 1722 (1).

For those of us fortunate enough to live in the industrially developed countries of the twenty-first century western world it is hard to envisage the all-pervading fear of infection that has existed through most of mankind's urban history—and still dominates many poor communities excluded from or unable to afford the benefits of modern medicine. Before the therapeutic revolution of the twentieth century, grieving parents regularly buried young infants who had succumbed to infectious diseases such as measles, diphtheria, scarlet fever, whooping cough, and dysentery in the very dawn of their life. Unhappily they still do in some parts of the world: even now around 10 million children a year scandalously die from preventable diseases (2). Similarly, until the last century, the death of bread-winners and young mothers in the prime of life from pneumonia, tuberculosis, childbed fever, and other infections was a common experience, mirrored today by the death toll from HIV-related illness in many countries. A visitation of the plague could decimate whole communities within a few weeks; cholera could kill in a day.

All this changed in the twentieth century, when mortality from infectious diseases in the United States fell from 797 deaths per 100,000 population in 1900 to 36 per 100,000 in 1980 (3). Improved social conditions accounted for some of the decrease, but the introduction of specific treatments and prophylactic measures undoubtedly had a major impact. The most marked decline occurred after the introduction of sulphonamides in the late 1930s. A similar picture has been described in the Netherlands (4).

Combating infection before the twentieth century

Little could be done before the true nature of infection was recognized. It was only in the sixteenth and seventeenth century that understanding of the specificity of infectious disease gradually began to emerge (see Chapter 1). Before then, fevers were mostly undifferentiated, beyond being characterized as intermittent or continuous; epidemics (pestilence) tended to be lumped together as visitations of divine wrath, although the symptoms described were sufficiently characteristic for them sometimes to be recognizable from contemporary records as specific diseases such as bubonic plague. That there was some appreciation of contagion is evident from the restraints forced on those actually or supposedly suffering from leprosy, and the *Quaranta giorni* (40 days) restrictions imposed on presumptively infected persons entering Venice in the fourteenth century, which gave rise to the modern term, *quarantine*. The Venetians could have had little idea of whether the period of restriction was appropriate; it was probably chosen to represent the biblical 40 days that Jesus spent in the wilderness. It nevertheless allowed ample time for death or recovery of those already infected and covered the incubation period of most communicable diseases.

In the earliest times infections had perforce to be treated empirically. Without a proper understanding of the underlying causes of disease there was little opportunity for a rational approach to afflictions that were generally believed to follow from divine retribution, demonic possession or other factors beyond mere human powers of intervention. General ignorance of the causes of disease did not, of course, prevent the search for effective cures. From the earliest times mankind has struggled to mitigate the effects of disease, and bizarre though some ancient remedies seem to us today—often including ingredients that would not be out of place in Shakespeare's witches' cauldron—the efforts to influence disease merely reflect the perplexing world that confronted humanity deprived of modern insights. In fact some remedies used by early civilizations are not so strange even in the light of more modern knowledge. The disinfectant properties of wine and vinegar seem to have been appreciated by the early Egyptians, and possibly before. Honey was used for many purposes in the ancient world, including application to suppurating sores and ulcers, a use that has some scientific basis and is still in vogue in some places (5).

Prayers, sacrifice, and priestly intercession naturally feature prominently in early attempts to seek relief from infectious disease, especially when the help of physicians was clearly ineffectual. Often pious practices were combined with natural remedies. In her fascinating account of the life of Francesco di Marco Datini, the fourteenth century 'Merchant of Prato', Iris Origo describes the usual array of strange nostrums that were prescribed for the sick by Tuscan physicians at the time. But, when the chips were down, as when Francesco's wife Margherita was confined to bed with a double tertian fever (probably severe malaria), the advice of doctors was set aside and their friend Domenico di Cambio offered his own infallible cure:

> If she would be healed speedily, let three sage-leaves be picked at morn before sunrise, and let the man who picks them do so on his bended knees, saying three Our Fathers and three Hail Marys in honour of God and the Holy Trinity, then send the leaves here in a letter, and I will write some words on each. And as the fever approaches, let her say an Our Father and a Hail Mary, and then eat a leaf, and so for each one of the three. And when she is done with eating them, she will be rid of the fever. But she must have faith, for if she has not, they will be of no avail (6).

Use of herbs, with or without divine assistance, is a feature of medicine in all cultures and has yielded a considerable number of effective medicines that are of undisputed value. Indeed, the reputable scientific discipline of pharmacognosy still seeks to discover yet more untapped resources from the natural world. The systematization of plant products in western medicine is largely attributable to Pedanius Dioscorides, a Greek physician from Anazarbus in Roman-occupied Asia Minor, who flourished in the first century of the present era. His *Materia Medica*, written around AD 60, was used and developed in the following century by another highly influential Greek physician, Galen of Pergamum, as well as later Islamic philosophers, like the great polymath, Avicenna (ibn Sina).

On St John's day (24 June) 1527, the volatile Swiss physician (though whether he was actually qualified is disputed), surgeon, and alchemist, Theophrastus Philippus Aureolus Bombastus von Hohenheim, better known by his adopted name, Paracelsus, famously burned the books of Avicenna on the students' annual bonfire in the market place of Basle. Paracelsus favoured the use of chemical compounds over the largely botanical remedies preferred by the prevailing medical doctrines. The theories he propounded owed more to alchemy and 'vital forces' than to rational experimentation (7). Among substances he promoted were mercury, lead, arsenic, and antimony compounds. Some of these had, in fact, been recommended for certain medicinal purposes by earlier authorities, including Dioscorides and Galen (8), but had largely fallen into disuse, being correctly regarded as poisons by the medical establishment. Not surprisingly, Paracelsus's ideas were opposed in many academic circles, but in the intellectual ferment of the sixteenth century he found many converts, and chemical medicine based on paracelsian principles was widely, if controversially, practised throughout Europe by the early seventeenth century. How many of these early remedies had any efficacy is subject to conjecture, but it is safe to say that, like many 'alternative' medicines peddled today, very few would have had any effect beyond that of a placebo and many are likely to have done more harm than good.

With the emergence of 'enlightenment' thought in the eighteenth century came a belief in a more rational approach to disease and its cure. Hospitals and dispensaries were opened in the major cities and the medical profession consolidated its elite position as the purveyors of medical care based on qualified and, eventually, registered practitioners.*

Unfortunately, reason is powerless without knowledge and the medical profession had few reliable resources on which to base an effective approach to the many infectious diseases that were rife within society. Quacks flourished and were often vilified by qualified practitioners. But as the medical historian Roy Porter has pointed out it is a mistake to see a clear-cut distinction between knowledgeable regular doctors practising rational medicine on one hand and unscrupulous, trash-dispensing, mountebanks on the other (9). For one thing, many of the nostrums peddled by quacks were based on the same ingredients used by qualified doctors. In an age when few reliable remedies were available, the prescriptions

---

* In Britain, the General Council of Medical Education and Registration, the forerunner of the General Medical Council, was established in 1858.

dispensed by or on behalf of medical practitioners were likely to be as futile as those of the most dubious of charlatans. Moreover, conventional doctors were not shy of the sort of self-advertisement of which they disparagingly accused their so-called 'bastard brethren'.

Those derided, as quacks were not a homogeneous group. They ranged from the outright crooks and get-rich-quick merchants that every society throws up, to unqualified, but basically ethical practitioners fulfilling a genuine social need to those unable to afford doctors fees. Some are impossible to pigeon-hole. The self-styled 'Chevalier' John Taylor, son of an apothecary, operated on the fringes of regular practice in the eighteenth century. He travelled widely as an itinerant oculist achieving by his undoubted skill entrée into the courts of much of the nobility of Europe. He operated on the failing eyesight of Johann Sebastian Bach during his last illness and may have contributed to his death (10).

Glimmers of light

Gradually, experimentation and careful observation started to sort the wheat from the chaff. Slow, but perceptible progress began to be made in understanding ways in which infection could be treated or avoided. When a pandemic of Asiatic cholera struck Britain in 1831—the first recognized case died in Sunderland on 26 October that year—a 22-year-old Irish graduate of Edinburgh University, William Brooke O'Shaughnessy travelled to Newcastle-on-Tyne, a few miles north of Sunderland, to see for himself the features of the disease. What awaited him shocked him to the core:

> On the bed lay an expiring woman...presenting an attitude of death which...I never saw paralleled in terror...On the floor extended on a palliasse...lay a girl of slender make and juvenile height, but with the face of a superannuated hag (11).

O'Shaughnessy was an ingenious and resourceful young man.* He had already expounded views on the treatment of cholera at a meeting of the Westminster Medical Society on 3 December 1891 (12) shortly before travelling north. After analysing blood drawn from cholera patients he attended there, he noted that they suffered a catastrophic loss of water and neutral saline ingredients from the bloodstream and concluded that they would benefit if given copious amounts of tepid water infused with salts.† It was a remarkably prescient observation, which was taken up with success by Thomas Latta a physician practising in Leith near Edinburgh (13). Others attempted to use fluid injections,

---

* O'Shaughnessy left England and joined the Bengal army in 1833 as an assistant surgeon and was soon appointed professor of chemistry and medicine at Calcutta Medical College. He showed his astonishing versatility by establishing an extensive telegraph service in India, something that had been considered almost impossible because of the geography and climate. He is also credited with introducing cannabis into England for use in medicine. He was knighted in 1856. See: Prior K. Brooke, Sir William O'Shaughnessy (1808–1889). *Oxford Dictionary of National Biography*, Oxford University Press, 2004 [http://www.oxforddnb.com/view/article/20895] and Cosnett (11).

† A Dr Jaenichen in Moscow, where cholera was also raging, reached the same conclusion at about the same time. See: Sheehy TW (1989). Origins of intravenous therapy. *Lancet* 1, 1081.

too, and there were reports of miraculous results, with moribund patients sitting up and chatting within minutes, only to relapse as the relentless catastrophic diarrhoea reasserted itself. However, the time was not ripe for the introduction of this life-saving therapy. Intravenous injections of chemically unstandardized, impure, and unsterile solutions were at that time extremely hazardous. Moreover, the method went against the prevailing medical wisdom and was roundly condemned by many practitioners. The use of intravenous fluids in cholera patients did not begin to be taken seriously until Leonard Rogers, a distinguished member of the Indian Medical Service, who helped to establish a School of Tropical Medicine in Calcutta (14), demonstrated the value of the procedure in Calcutta in the first decades of the twentieth century. In the meantime the wretched sufferers from cholera in a series of pandemics that swept along trade routes from their endemic focus in the Ganges delta into Europe, North America, and elsewhere in the nineteenth century continued to be subjected to blood-letting, emetics, calomel (mercurous chloride; a favourite Victorian panacea with purgative properties—as if that were necessary in cholera!) or, if they were lucky, simple neglect.

Cholera also played a part in establishing the importance of careful epidemiological investigation in the mid-nineteenth century. During the third cholera pandemic of 1853–54, John Snow, a Yorkshire-born doctor whose main interest was in expanding understanding of the new-fangled techniques of anaesthesia, acted on his theory, already expounded in 1849, that cholera might be a water-borne disease (15). When the dreaded infection struck Soho in London, close to where Snow was living, he famously deduced the source of the local outbreak by examining the distribution of cases and aborted the epidemic by removing the handle of the Broad Street pump (16). Whether the dramatic action was really a vindication of his ideas is unclear, since the epidemic was already on the wane.

Snow's theories prompted fierce debate, but failed to convince the medical establishment. Nor were his local critics convinced. Among them was the curate of St Luke's church in Soho, the Reverend Henry Whitehead. He decided to carry out his own investigations of the Broad Street outbreak. Much to his chagrin, but to his great credit, he was led to admit that Snow's conclusions had been correct. Whitehead became one of Snow's most enthusiastic supporters after he died in 1858. At a dinner given for the Reverend Whitehead in a Fleet Street tavern in 1874, on the occasion of his leaving London for a country living, he gave a 3 h after-dinner speech—described in *The Times* as 'probably the longest after-dinner speech on record'—in which he described the events in Soho and heaped praise on Snow and his work (17).

A further development of the nineteenth century was the gradual acceptance of the value of various specific germicides. By the end of the century, numerous types of compound were in regular use. Metals, notably silver and mercury, were acknowledged to have properties that rendered them useful in reducing contagion. The antiseptic properties of chlorine, discovered by the Swedish scientist Carl Wilhelm von Scheele in 1774, also came to be recognized.

The related halogen, iodine, discovered fortuitously by the Frenchman Bernard Courtois in 1811, and developed further by his compatriot Jean Guillaume Auguste Lugol, was widely used as a disinfectant during the American Civil War (18). In 1834 Friedlieb Ferdinand Runge, professor of chemistry in Breslau, isolated phenol (carbolic acid) from coal tar.* These and other germicides were all far too toxic to be used except as topical antiseptics and disinfectants, though this did not stop doctors from occasionally attempting cures by injecting them.

In Vienna in 1847 the lugubrious Hungarian, Ignaz Philipp Semmelweis, commenced work which showed that doctors could reduce the incidence of childbed fever by the simple expedient of washing their hands in chloride of lime between the post-mortem and lying-in rooms. Few believed him, but a seed of truth had been sown (19). Semmelweis's views on the role of contagion in puerperal fever had been anticipated by the Scottish general practitioner, Alexander Gordon during his investigation of an epidemic of puerperal fever in Aberdeen that reached its peak in 1790 (20). Others, including the physician and author Oliver Wendall Holmes in Boston, Massachusetts, had much the same idea about the transmissibility of the disease.

But it was Louis Pasteur's ground-breaking studies on alcoholic fermentation and his convincing rebuttal of the doctrine of spontaneous generation in the mid-nineteenth century that provided the key to understanding the relationship between microbes and infectious disease and created a paradigm shift in attitudes to infection and its avoidance. It was Pasteur's work that inspired the Scottish surgeon Joseph Lister to seek ways of preventing germs from causing their mischief. Lister realized that a single airborne microbe, landing on an unprotected wound, could initiate infection. Working first in Glasgow, and moving to Edinburgh in 1869, he initiated the work on the use of antiseptics that was to revolutionize surgical practice. In 1871 he introduced the famous carbolic spray that transformed the likelihood of surviving a devastating bacterial infection during a surgical operation. Lister's house surgeon and later successor, the fellow Scot William Watson Cheyne enthusiastically promoted and extended Lister's ideas (21).

Another preventative intervention that is still in use today was introduced in the last quarter of the nineteenth century by Carl Siegmund Franz Credé, a German obstetrician working in Leipzig. Credé—who had strenuously opposed Semmelweis's views on puerperal fever—popularized the instillation of silver nitrate into the eyes of newborn babies and succeeded, between 1874 and 1880, in reducing the incidence of ophthalmia neonatorum (a potentially blinding eye infection of babies born to mothers with gonorrhoea) from 13.6 per cent to almost zero in the Leipzig maternity hospital (22).

It may have been the work of Credé that inspired the American doctor and chemist, Albert Coombs Barnes to exploit the germicidal properties of silver commercially. After completing his medical studies in Philadelphia, where he had been born in poverty, Barnes travelled to Berlin and Heidelberg to gain further experience. Back in the United States he devised a colloidal preparation of silver together with the German chemist, Herman Hille, whom he had met in Heidelberg. The pair set up a company to market a topical antiseptic product, which they called Argyrol. The enterprise succeeded beyond

---

* Runge also isolated aniline, which was exploited in the dyestuffs industry and was to have a profound influence on the development of antimicrobial agents (see Chapter 3, p. 50).

all expectation. In 1907, Barnes bought out his partner after a court case and proceeded to make a fortune out of Argyrol, which he spent on amassing a formidable collection of artworks, including many impressionist and post-impressionist paintings, for which he had an unerring eye. In 1922 he established the Barnes Foundation to promote the advancement of education and the appreciation of the fine arts (23).

Further useful innovations were introduced at the end of the nineteenth century. In 1895 Arthur Nicolaier a doctor in the University clinic of Göttingen, described the use of Hexamine (also known as methenamine) for the treatment of urinary infection (24). Hexamine breaks down in the acidic conditions usually prevailing in infected urine to liberate formaldehyde and is still occasionally prescribed for the prevention of recurrent cystitis. Nicolaier had already made his reputation in 1884 as a 22-year-old medical student by his discovery of the tetanus bacillus. He died in Berlin, aged 80, in 1942, probably by his own hand under threat of imminent transportation to Theresienstadt prison camp north of Prague. In 1899, a few years after Nicolaier's introduction of Hexamine, Rudolf Emmerich and Oscar Loew described, in unwitting anticipation of the later discovery of antibiotics, an extract of the bacterium then known as *Bacillus pyocyaneus* (now *Pseudomonas aeruginosa*), which inhibited many pathogenic micro-organisms, but unfortunately proved too toxic for systemic use. This substance, pyocyanase, was still in use in Germany in the 1930s as a throat spray for the treatment of diphtheria.

Aside from these isolated examples, there was really very little that could be done to save the hapless sufferer from infection as the nineteenth century closed. Most of the pills and potions—of qualified practitioners of medicine or of unscrupulous quacks alike—were useless. The pre-twentieth century therapeutic cupboard was not, however, completely bare. Herbal remedies that expelled worms visible to the naked eye were recognized to be effective from the earliest times. Paracelsus's use of mercury for syphilis was sufficiently effective for its use to continue until more reliable drugs became available in the twentieth century. Chaulmoogra oil, from *Taraktogenos kurzii* and various species of *Hydnocarpus*, a traditional treatment for leprosy in India, was introduced into European medicine in the nineteenth century (see Chapter 5). Most significantly of all, two fruits of the European colonization of South America, cinchona bark and ipecacuanha root, contained active ingredients that stood the test of time: quinine and emetine. From the seventeenth century, these substances provided (when properly used) effective remedies against two very important diseases: malaria and amoebic dysentery.

Remedies against intestinal worms

Santonin

The ability of certain plant products to rid the body of worms present in the intestinal tract was known to Dioscorides and Galen. Among the most effective preparations were those obtained from the tiny unexpanded flower buds (capitula) of *Artemisia maritime* var. *stechmanniana*, known as wormseed (though they did not in fact contain seeds), *semen cinae* or *semen contra* (short for *semen contra vermes*; seeds against worms). Wormseed is an effective vermifuge for the common roundworm, *Ascaris lumbricoides*; less so for the common threadworm of children, *Enterobius vermicularis*. Originally, the flower heads themselves were used. The plants were known as santonica and the best examples were considered to be those growing in the steppes of the southern Russian empire or the Levant. Until the Bolshevik revolution of 1917 most supplies were imported from Russia. The active ingredient, santonin, was first obtained independently in 1830 by two German druggists (Apotheker), one from Düsseldorf and identified only as 'Apotheker Kahler'; the other Joachim August Alms, a student pharmacist from Penzlin, a small town in north-east Germany, who later qualified as a doctor. The results were published together, an apparent coincidence that came about because of a delay in publication of Kahler's findings. In April 1830 he submitted a paper 'Ueber einen neuen Stoff im Semen Cinae' (on a new substance in semen cinae) outlining his results— together with a sample of the crystals he had obtained by ether extraction—to Rudolph Brandes, a prominent apothecary in Salzuflen, a spa town south-west of Hanover. Brandes had founded the *Archiv des Apotheker-vereins im Nördlichen Teutschland* (sic) (Archives of the Society of Apothecaries in northern Germany) in 1822 to promote the work of pharmacists,* but he held back publication of Kahler's paper until he himself had confirmed the finding. In August 1830, a report entitled 'Ueber einen neuen Stoff im levantinischen Wurmsamen' ('On a new substance in Levantine wormseed') arrived from August Alms, making similar claims to those of Kahler. Brandes promptly published both reports together in the same issue of his journal (25). By 1844, word of the isolation of santonin had filtered through to *The Lancet* in England, and an annotation appeared in the edition of 11 May (26).

Oil of *Chenopodium*

In America an infusion of the fruit of a common plant, *Chenopodium ambrosioides* var. *anthelminticum* (American wormseed or Mexican tea), has been used for centuries by Mexican farmers and became a popular folk remedy against ascaris and hookworm throughout the United States. Like many other treatments for intestinal complaints it was often given with castor oil, that sovereign aid to regular bowel movements, which remained the bane of children's lives well into the twentieth century. Crude American wormseed preparations were replaced in the early twentieth century by oil of *Chenopodium*, a distillate of the crushed seeds, which yields a mixture of various essential oils including the active principle, ascaridole. Although the traditional treatment and the oil seem to be effective, the precise role of the active principle is unclear. It has been pointed out that oil of *Chenopodium* is itself a mild purgative that could cause the expulsion of worms. Moreover, the spontaneous passage of worms is a common occurrence in areas of high prevalence, and folk remedies with supposed vermifuge properties easily acquire a spurious reputation (27).

---

* The publication Rudolph Brandes founded, continues today as *Archiv der Pharmazie*. The Apotheke (pharmacy), which he inherited from his father, Johann Gottlieb Brandes remains in family hands and still trades from the same building in Bad Salzuflen. See: http://www.brandessche-apotheke.de/index1.htm.

Male fern

Dryopteris filix-mas (male fern) a plant widespread in northern temperate countries was used in antiquity to rid the body of tapeworms, but the remedy seems to have fallen into disuse among medical men until the eighteenth century, when it was revived by Madame Nouffer, the widow of a surgeon from Murten (known in French as Morat), Switzerland. Madame Nouffer acquired considerable celebrity in Europe through her secret remedy for the expulsion of tapeworms. The treatment, which turned out to be an enema followed by administration of powdered root of male fern, scammony (a gum resin with a strong purgative action) and gamboge (another gum resin imported from south-east Asia) was so successful that she was able to sell the recipe to the French king Louis XVI for a handsome sum in 1775. Male fern subsequently became widely used for the expulsion of tapeworms. The dried root or rhizome contains the active ingredient filicin and was used until oily extracts were introduced during the late nineteenth century. Correctly used, extract of male fern is undoubtedly effective and it continued in use as the standard treatment for tapeworms in medical practice until the 1960s.

Other worm remedies

Many other plant extracts, oils, and resins—pomegranate bark, jalap, *Quassia* wood, turpentine, and croton oil among them—have been used through the centuries to expel worms and were much favoured by nineteenth century practitioners. Mercury in the form of calomel (mercurous chloride), a pet nostrum of Victorian doctors, was also popular. Insofar as they worked at all, most of these interventions functioned chiefly by virtue of their purgative action often helped along by the co-administration of castor oil or other laxatives. Few could be relied on to achieve the desired effect.

In the case of threadworms, traditionally diagnosed by eagle-eyed mothers keeping watch for the tell tale short 'threads'—adult female worms—on the surface of their offsprings' stools, drugs were sometimes considered unnecessary. As the Victorian physician Thomas Watson noted in his lectures to medical students of King's College, London:

> Thread-worms may be scooped out of the rectum, with the finger. Old women fish for them with a piece of fat meat, or a candle, wherewith the entangled worms are drawn out of the bowel (28).

Such manipulations, even if successful, may have effected temporary relief, but would not prevent reinfection, since the numerous eggs produced by the female worm and laid in the perianal region remain directly infectious to the child and his companions.

Quinine

The famous voyage of Christopher Columbus in which he fortuitously discovered the New World of the Americas while looking for a westward route to the East Indies changed the world for ever. Europeans may prefer to forget much of what ensued, not least the exploits of the Spanish conquistadors, the horrors of the slave trade and the introduction of deadly viruses, such as those of smallpox, measles, and yellow fever, which devastated the indigenous populations and facilitated colonization (29). But over 100 years after Columbus's epic voyage of 1492 an event occurred that was to be of unquestionable benefit for mankind: sometime between the death of Shakespeare in 1616 and the birth of Antoni van Leeuwenhoek in 1632, the curative properties of the bark of the *Cinchona* tree, later found to contain the antimalarial agent quinine were discovered in Spanish-administered Peru (30). To lay down some other historical markers, it was the time of the Thirty Years War in Europe and of the intrepid journey of the Pilgrim Fathers to seek a new life in what was to become New England.

How the discovery was made is unclear. Legend has it that an infusion of the bark, long known to the Peruvian Indians, was used to treat Francisca Henriquez de Ribera, wife of the Spanish Viceroy in Peru, the fourth Count of Chinchón,* who was suffering from a malignant tertian fever. The Countess is said to have staged a remarkable recovery and returned to Spain to broadcast the virtues of the miraculous remedy. This romantic story is almost certainly false in every particular.

For a start, malaria was most probably absent from pre-Columbian America, though it was rife throughout much of Europe. Biological and molecular evidence suggests that strains of malaria parasite found in South America are recent introductions from Africa (31). Early records fail to mention intermittent fevers similar to those that are characteristic of malaria among the first Spanish settlers or the populations they encountered (32); nor does the bark feature among the surveys of local medicinal plants that were prepared by order of the Spanish crown, although a substance called quina-quina does.[†] Thus, even if *Cinchona* bark was used by the indigenous peoples before the Spanish invasion, it is unlikely to have been for malarial fevers—in fact, when malaria and the therapeutic value of the bark did emerge, the local populace were extremely reluctant to use it for that purpose.

The legend of the 'Countess's powder' has also been refuted by contemporary documents (33). A very detailed diary of the Viceroy and his family was kept by his secretary, Don Antonio Suardo, and it is clear that the Countess was in robust health during the time of the supposed cure. Moreover, she died in 1641—possibly of yellow fever—at Cartagena in Bolivia on the way back to Spain at the end of her husband's tour of office in 1639, so she certainly did not return to Spain to popularize the cure.

The true origins of the discovery of the medicinal properties of *Cinchona* bark will probably never be known. One possibility, for which there is some documentary support in the works of seventeenth century Spanish doctors, is that Peruvian mineworkers in the province of Quito (now in Ecuador) were observed to use hot infusions of the powdered

---

* Linnaeus (Carl von Linné), the great Swedish botanist and inventor of the Latin binomial classification system universally used today, gave the genus name *Cinchona* to the fever-bark tree in honour of the Countess, but unfortunately misspelt her name.

† This substance is thought to be Peru balsam, *Myroxylon peruiferum*, an aromatic substance that was the subject of much early confusion. It is still found in some haemorrhoid preparations and other products.

bark to counteract shivering when they emerged cold and damp from the river that they were obliged to swim across on the way to their work in the local silver mines. The infusion may indeed have had some effect, since quinine has muscle-relaxing properties and is still used, with modest benefit, to treat nocturnal leg cramps (34). The Jesuit missionaries who first witnessed the use of *Cinchona* in this way are then said to have taken the bark to an apothecary in the Peruvian capital, Lima; there it was dispensed to physicians (including the Viceroy's personal physician, Juan de Vega) who used the bark according to the prevailing doctrine of analogy to counteract the shivering attacks characteristic of malarial rigors. To their surprise, they discovered that the 'hot' stage that normally followed in intermittent fevers was also suppressed. Perhaps for the first, but certainly not for the last time, a major discovery was found to succeed for the wrong reasons!

It soon became clear that the remedy often produced remarkable results in tertian and quartan fevers. Not surprisingly, since both the diagnosis and the dosage were very imprecise, relapses were also recorded. Juan de Vega did not trust the new remedy sufficiently to risk it on such an important personage as the Viceroy, who, during several episodes of intermittent fever between 1630 and 1638, was always subjected to the usual treatment of blood-letting.

Introduction of the bark in Europe

After the successful trials in Lima, samples of the bark were shipped to Seville, possibly by Juan de Vega, who is credited by some contemporary authorities in introducing the bark after returning to Spain. However, there is conflicting evidence that de Vega remained in Lima and was apparently still signing documents there in 1650 shortly before he died. Whatever the truth of the matter, the bark eventually reached Rome, courtesy of the Jesuits, sometime—probably on several occasions—between 1630 and 1645. Rome was the centre of the Christian world. It was there that the Spanish Jesuit priest, Juan de Lugo, who was born in Madrid, but had spent his early life in Seville, was installed as a professor at the Gregorian University where he was elected Cardinal in1643. Although he had no medical training, Cardinal de Lugo heard about the bark and became convinced of its benefits. He purchased large quantities for free distribution to the poor through the college's apothecary and the Ospedale di Santo Spirito, where a fresco was commissioned to commemorate the discovery and the Cardinal's act of charity.

News of the discovery soon spread throughout Europe, though its nickname 'Jesuit's bark' did not encourage its use in protestant lands. Nevertheless, the bark had reached England by 1650 and although the influential Thomas Sydenham, often called the father of English medicine, at first opposed its use, he was eventually persuaded to change his mind perhaps because of—or despite—the success obtained by an enterprising apothecary, Robert Talbor. The medical fraternity regarded Talbor as a quack, but he was an enterprising man and an effective self-publicist. He published his *Pyretologia, a rational account of the cause and cure of agues* in 1672, and had the good fortune to successfully use his 'secret remedy' to cure King Charles II, who rewarded him with a knighthood.

Talbor went on to repeat his success by curing the son of Louis XIV of France and the Queen of Spain. Louis XIV bought the recipe for 2000 livres and after Talbor's death the secret ingredient was disclosed to be *Cinchona* bark.

Popularization of *Cinchona* in books written by such influential physicians as Sydenham in England, Francesco Torti in Italy, and other contemporaries, ensured that the reputation of the bark was secure (35). That the reputation should survive unscathed despite uncertainties of diagnosis, inappropriate use, inevitable variability of quality of the bark, and unscrupulous adulteration of supplies, is perhaps surprising—or may be a tribute to the erudition of seventeenth and eighteenth century physicians, whose professional acumen is often underrated.

Isolation of quinine

Some of the uncertainties about *Cinchona* bark were relieved in 1820, when two young professors at the newly established École de Pharmacie in Paris, Pierre Joseph Pelletier and Joseph Bienaimé Caventou, succeeded in isolating two alkaloids, quinine and cinchonine, from samples of the bark. The stereoisomers, quinidine and cinchonidine, which are also naturally present, were identified later but synthesis of the natural products on a commercially viable scale proved difficult and has still not been achieved. All the alkaloids have some antimalarial activity and quinidine, which is more usually used in conditions of abnormal heart rhythm, is an effective alternative if quinine is not at hand. Cardiac effects of *Cinchona* bark were recognized in the late seventeenth century, but quinidine itself was not used for arrhythmias until 1918, when Walter Frey introduced the treatment in Austria (36).

Pelletier and Caventou's work enabled defined salts of quinine to be manufactured and ushered in a period during which proper dosages were established. The development came none too soon for a medical profession intent on establishing a rational scientific basis for therapy. As the eminent Victorian physician Thomas Watson observed in lectures to medical students:

> ...I am old enough to be aware of the infinite superiority of the salt over the actual bark. To obtain the desired effect, it was often necessary to give it in such quantities as almost justified Mr. Abernethy's sarcastic way of speaking of it and of physicians. He said the doctors talked of throwing in the bark, as if it were to be pitched into the stomach with a shovel (37).

By the end of the nineteenth century, when the identity of the parasites responsible for malaria had been identified, and microscopical diagnosis became possible, the pre-eminent place of quinine in the therapy of malaria was undisputed, save for a few dissenters who favoured arsenic or other nostrums. Anton Chekhov, who probably carried quinine in his doctor's bag, celebrated its efficacy by naming one of his two dachshunds Quina (the other was called Brom, German for bromine) (38). Patrick Manson, the 'father of tropical medicine', in the first edition of his classic textbook *Tropical Diseases* (1898), would write:

> In serious cases, to use any drug to the exclusion of quinine is culpable trifling (39).

Securing supply

Quinine was the first genuinely effective antimicrobial agent. It was not only important in domestic medicine, but became essential for the protection of armed forces, officials, and colonialists throughout the world. The European powers were particularly anxious to secure supplies of the drug for the protection of their citizens in highly malarious areas of their burgeoning empires in Africa, India, and elsewhere.

The natural habitat of *Cinchona* trees lay in the high slopes of the Andes in the Spanish colonies that were to become Peru, Ecuador, Bolivia, and Columbia. Naturally enough, such a valuable commodity as the bark was jealously guarded and costs for importing countries were high. As the nineteenth century progressed, uncertainties of supply caused to some extent by overexploitation of the plantations, but more importantly by the political instability that swept through the area, caused the problem to become ever more acute. Obtaining control of the trade by establishing plantations of their own became a priority for European colonial powers. Several expeditions were dispatched in the mid-nineteenth century to identify the best varieties of *Cinchona* and to bring back seeds for germination and propagation in areas that would ensure reliable supplies. Unfortunately great confusion existed over the classification of *Cinchona* species, owing to its propensity to form hybrids by cross-pollination (40). The best bark was thought to come from *Cinchona calisaya, Cinchona officinalis*, and *Cinchona succirubra*.

The hardships and adventures endured by the early plant hunters, including the Frenchman, Hugues Weddell, the German, Karl Hasskarl (working on behalf of the Dutch), and the Englishmen, Richard Spruce, Sir Clements Markham, and Charles Ledger have been graphically described in the books of Mark Honigsbaum (41), Fiammetta Rocco (42), and Gabriele Gramiccia (43). Weddell's specimens, germinated at the Jardin des Plantes in Paris, yielded little quinine; similarly, Hasskarl's seeds, though they grew well in Dutch plantations in Java, yielded only small quantities of the drug. Markham's collection of young plants, obtained at great personal cost and painstakingly transported, all died before they could be propagated, but some of his seeds of *Cinchona officinalis, Cinchona succirubra*, and *Cinchona calisaya* were germinated in India. Spruce, who was sponsored by the Royal Botanic Gardens at Kew, obtained samples of *Cinchona succirubra* from which successful plantations were eventually established in the Nilgiri hills in Madras.

But the greatest success was achieved by the English merchant adventurer, Charles Ledger, who had the benefit of the phenomenal knowledge of *Cinchona* trees of his faithful servant Manuel Incra Mamani, a Bolivian Indian. The journeys undertaken by this intrepid pair are the stuff of Hollywood at its most imaginative and improbable. Ledger was interested only in making money, and was as concerned to exploit the commercial value of alpacas and their wool as *Cinchona* bark.

Thanks to Mamani, Ledger was able to obtain a mixture of seeds, some of the highest quality, from carefully selected varieties of *Cinchona calisaya* harvested at the most favourable time. In 1865 he dispatched 20 lb of the seeds to his brother George in London, hoping to sell them at a good profit to the British government. However, the time was not opportune. The British plantations in Madras were proving a success and the offer was refused. On the advice of a London quinine manufacturer, John Eliot Howard, George Ledger turned to the Dutch Consul, who agreed to buy 1 lb of the seeds for 100 guilders (about £20). The remainder were sold for £50 to an Anglo-Indian plantation owner, but they failed to thrive in the Indian climate.

The seeds sold to the Dutch proved an unparalleled success. By 1872, when seedlings planted in Java had grown sufficiently for tests to be carried out on the bark, the yield of quinine from some of the trees was found to exceed all expectations. The trees were identified as an unusual variety of *Cinchona calisaya*, later granted species status and renamed as *Cinchona ledgeriana*. Nearly all the quinine used today comes from this species, grafted on to hardier *Cinchona succirubra* roots.

Apart from the honour of having a species named after him, Charles Ledger gained little from his immense contribution to medicine. For many years he divided his time between South America and Australia, where he tried to promote his alpaca trade. In 1891 fate struck a double blow, when his wife died of influenza and he lost his savings in a banking collapse. Attempts to obtain a small pension from the Dutch authorities were rebuffed, but support from Markham and others eventually persuaded them to change their mind and in 1897 he was granted an annuity of 1200 guilders. He died in relative poverty aged 87 in 1905.

As for Manuel Incra Mamani, he had already lost his life in tragic circumstances around 1871.* At Ledger's request he had made another journey into the high Andes to collect a further supply of seed. On his way back he was apprehended by the police, who demanded to know the reason why he was carrying such a quantity of seed. Faithful to the last, Mamani refused to betray his master. All his possessions were confiscated and he was put into prison, where he was beaten and half-starved. After 20 days he was released, but he died at home a few days later.

The impact of quinine

Historically, malaria is not a tropical disease. It existed in temperate climates well into the last century and was common throughout the whole of Europe, including Finland and northern Russia (44). Strenuous efforts in the mid-twentieth century eventually managed (in 1975) to rid Europe of this scourge, but attempts to eradicate malaria from the hyperendemic areas of the tropics and subtropics met with only modest success. Even today, it is estimated that there are 300–500 million cases of malaria each year and up to 2 million deaths from the disease, mainly, but certainly not exclusively, in tropical Africa (45).

Malaria is so widespread, and in its most virulent form so dangerous, that quinine and the related antimalarial alkaloids in the natural bark can surely claim to have saved more lives and alleviated more serious suffering than any other drug in the pharmacopoeia. Throughout its 350-year history it has been widely used both for the treatment

---

* 1871 is the date given by Gramiccia (43); Rocco (42) dates Mamani's death to 1865; and Honigsbaum (41) to 1877.

of intermittent fevers—and many other conditions in which it is unlikely to have had any value, such was its reputation as a wonder drug—and for prevention.

Without quinine, the history of the world would have been quite different. Malaria itself has shaped the destiny of nations from the earliest times of recorded history (46), but the availability of *Cinchona* bark from the seventeenth century significantly blunted its impact. For those fortunate enough to have access to the drug it vastly improved the chances of surviving a debilitating and often fatal disease.

The Holy See was among the first to benefit. Situated in the notoriously unhealthy Roman Campagna (a likely candidate for the origin of the term *mal'aria*), living in or visiting Rome was always a risky business. During the Papal conclave of July 1623, just before *Cinchona* bark became known, 8 of the 55 Cardinals and 30 secretaries died of the fever that was raging in the city at the time (47). Malaria in the Campagna was not brought under control until the Pontine marshes were drained in the 1930s, as part of one of the most grandiose and successful land reclamation and resettlement schemes initiated by *il duce*, Benito Mussolini. Visiting Rome was never to be quite as dangerous again, save for a short period after 1943, when the Italian army changed sides and retreating German troops deliberately sabotaged the pumps and tide gates to reflood the area with the brackish water that favoured the main local vector, *Anopheles labranchiae*. Erich Martini, an eminent medical entomologist from the Tropical Institute in Hamburg* who was a Nazi party member and adviser to the regime, probably masterminded the plan, which led to a massive epidemic of malaria in the region. Though the primary intention of the flooding is likely to have been to hinder the Allied advance, as an entomologist, Martini must have been aware of its other consequences.

Rome was not the only important administrative centre to benefit from the ability to treat local outbreaks of malaria: at least one other was the malarious marshland on the Virginia/Maryland border by the Potomac river (now Washington, DC) to which the national seat of government of the United States was transferred from Philadelphia in 1800. Similarly, St Petersburg, the beloved city of Peter the Great of Russia, which was founded in 1703 on the marshes of the Neva river delta, was notorious for a high incidence of malaria. Thousands of peasants died during construction of the city, with malaria as a contributing factor, and the tsar was careful to ensure a ready supply of *Cinchona* bark for his own family.

Exploration and colonial development in Africa, India, and other highly malarious regions would have been much more difficult, if not impossible, if *Cinchona* bark and, later quinine, had not been available. Malaria contributed largely to the reputation of West Africa as 'the white man's grave', and many other parts of the European colonies were infamous for their dangerous intermittent fevers. Supplies of the drug and—once the vector had been identified—mosquito netting became part of the essential kit of all Europeans working in these areas.

---

* Known since 1942 as the Bernhard-Nocht-Institut für Tropenmedizin in tribute to its founder, Bernhard Nocht.

Some of our drinking habits were also modified: quinine is very bitter and has, from the earliest times, been administered with wine or spirits. The Scottish physician William Buchan in his popular treatise *The Domestic Medicine*, first published in 1769, recommended a typical recipe for the prevention of agues:

> Take an ounce of the best Peruvian bark, Virginia snake root, and orange peel, of each half an ounce; bruise them all together, and infuse for five or six days in a bottle of brandy, Holland gin, or any good spirit; afterwards pour off the clear liquor, and take a wine glass of it twice or thrice a day (48).

Buchan was born in Ancrum, near Jedburgh in Roxburghshire and studied medicine in Edinburgh. He later practised in Yorkshire before returning to Edinburgh, where his book was written, probably together with his friend, the botanist and printer, William Smellie.* *The Domestic Medicine* was one of the most prominent of many self-help books that were aimed at a health-conscious Georgian and Victorian readership. It went into many editions in Britain and America (where it remained in print until 1913) and was translated into several languages (49). Like many of his contemporaries, Buchan was a firm advocate of bitter remedies apparently on the grounds that if it tasted nasty, then it must be doing you good. Several cocktail ingredients, such as Angostura bitters were originally developed because of their supposed medicinal properties.

The practice of mixing gin with quinine solution became popular during colonial times and 'Indian tonic water' containing quinine was a favourite mixer for the traditional 'sundowner' gin and tonic. It is doubtful whether this had any real effect in keeping malaria at bay. Certainly, for present-day Indian tonic water to be effective several litres would need to be imbibed, even if it contains the statutorily required level of not less than 57 mg quinine sulphate per litre.[†]

Introduction of quinine into India had not been straightforward. Although *Cinchona* bark was brought to Calcutta within 20 years of it becoming available in Europe and was successfully used for over a century, it fell into disrepute at the beginning of the nineteenth century. In 1804, a ship's surgeon, James Johnson stopped off in Calcutta during a voyage to the East Indies aboard *HMS Caroline* (50). It was only a brief visit, but it had profound implications. He arrived at the height of the malaria season and the first case he treated with *Cinchona* bark failed. His second case was treated with leeches and, as luck would have it, recovered. On the strength of this dubious evidence, Johnson advised that use of *Cinchona* should be abandoned in favour of bleeding, purging, and large doses of mercury. When another doctor, Edward Hare, arrived in India in 1839 to work

---

* Smellie was interested in medicine and attended lectures on the subject in Edinburgh, but did not qualify. His name appears as the printer of the first edition, but some think he also helped to write the book. Most likely, he edited down William Buchan's verbose style before publication. See: Lawrence CJ. William Buchan: medicine laid open; ref. 49.

† Anthony Freeman, a consultant physician in Swindon treating elderly patients for nocturnal cramps, discovered from a manufacturer that the concentration was, in fact, 30 mg per litre. See: Freeman, AG. On nocturnal cramps. *Lancet*; 1995; 345: 1188.

in the foothills of Nepal where the most virulent form of malaria was rife, he was appalled to discover how ineffective the recommended treatment was:

> The patients all died, no remission took place, there were head symptoms, and I durst not give quinine; in fact it was so utterly forbidden by all authorities that it never occurred to me to give it.

By chance, Hare discovered some old medical writings by James Lind—the ship's surgeon who introduced the use of orange and lime juice in the prevention of scurvy, a feared disease of long sea voyages, in a famous treatise published in 1753—in which he described the curative effect of *Cinchona* bark in malarial fevers. Quinine, by then replacing use of the bark, was reintroduced with great success and during the next 9 years, in which Hare treated nearly 7000 cases of malaria during his service with European regiments, mortality was less than 0.5 per cent (51).

For colonial powers and army strategists, quinine was an essential weapon of conquest. In many military conflicts deaths from disease vastly outnumbered casualties inflicted by the enemy and malaria was usually one of the major incapacitating causes. It has been estimated that the annual incidence of malaria suffered by British units stationed in tropical countries during the nineteenth century ranged from 59–870 per 1000 (52). Famously, during the First World War, the French, British, and German armies in Macedonia were immobilized by malaria for 3 years.

Although the use of quinine for treatment was undisputed by the mid-eighteenth century, opinion was divided on its value as a prophylactic (53). The petulant, but very influential Ronald Ross, who demonstrated the role of mosquitoes in the transmission of malaria in 1898, favoured the use of mosquito netting and anti-mosquito measures such as drainage of marshy areas and clearance of mosquito habitats. Others strongly promoted the use of quinine, but sometimes its use was distinctly half-hearted: during the American Civil War (1861–65), army surgeons recommended 'the administration of half a gill of whisky, containing quinine in a concentration of 2–4 grains [130–260 mg], served twice daily to every man in the command'. When the Government proved unwilling to provide a sufficient quantity of the whisky, the Sanitary Commission undertook to supply it. Perhaps unsurprisingly, 'the quinine and whisky were sometimes employed together; sometimes the whisky was given alone' (54).

By the time of the First World War, the proponents of prophylaxis were in the ascendancy, but supplies of quinine were inadequate and the Dutch had a virtual monopoly of the bark. Vast quantities of the drug were being consumed throughout the world, a situation exacerbated in the last year of the war by the mistaken belief that it might be of use in the developing influenza epidemic. It was only on 3 September 1918, 10 weeks before the armistice was signed, that the British authorities—led by H. S. Abrahamson, managing director of the Association of Quinine Manufacturers in Allied Countries—succeeded in concluding a 'War Agreement' with the Kina Bureau, a consortium of plantation owners in Java. This belatedly guaranteed the Allies sole rights to the Dutch supplies for the duration of the war (55). Once the war was over, the agreement lapsed and world quinine prices leapt (56).

Demand for quinine was not confined to use in malaria. When a drug is shown to be reliably successful in some particular disease, claims for its value in unrelated illnesses often multiply, and this was especially true in those early days when so little prescribed medication actually worked. As noted above, quinine was widely used during the great 'Spanish flu' pandemic. A collection of multilingual papers on quinine published by the Bureau tot Bevordering van het Kinine-gebruik (Bureau for the promotion of quinine use) in the Netherlands in 1925 contains articles extolling the virtues of the drug in many other conditions, including pneumonia, haemorrhoids, lumbago, cancer, and syphilis (57). It was availability and price that largely influenced the search for alternatives to quinine in Germany in the years following the end of the Great War (see Chapter 7).

Despite the development of synthetic antimalarial agents quinine is still, after more than 350 years, widely used as the drug of choice in acute malaria, especially the most dangerous form caused by *Plasmodium falciparum*, which can rapidly kill. But the impact of quinine extends far beyond its use as an antimalarial agent, as will emerge in the next chapter.

Emetine

Dysentery—literally, affliction of the bowels—can have many causes, but usually refers to inflammation and invasion of the colonic mucosa, with profuse diarrhoea, classically caused by bacteria of the *Shigella* genus (bacillary dysentery) or the amoeba, *Entamoeba histolytica* (amoebic dysentery). Both types can be severe to the point of being life-threatening; *Entamoeba histolytica* can also cause invasive disease of other organs, usually the liver. It was the association of the colonic lesions of amoebic dysentery with liver abscesses that helped to fuel suspicion that two forms of 'bloody flux' existed, well before the true aetiological agents were discovered in the late nineteenth century (58).

Amoebic dysentery is a serious disease with a high mortality. It has undoubtedly existed since ancient times and must have been responsible for much of the epidemic dysentery described in military campaigns—including the Napoleonic, Crimean, and Boer Wars—throughout history. That the dysentery was amoebic rather than bacillary can be deduced from the fact that it was not generally regarded to be particularly contagious, except in the insanitary circumstances of slave ships and in crowded prisons. The bacteria that cause dysentery rely on direct transmission from infected persons (commonly via microscopic faecal contamination of the immediate environment) and often cause explosive outbreaks. In contrast, the protozoa responsible for amoebic dysentery are able to form cysts that persist in the environment to give rise to sporadic infection acquired from drinking contaminated water or from unhygienic practices.

Reliable therapy of severe bacillary dysentery had to await the coming of antibiotics, but amoebic dysentery has been treatable with a natural remedy, extract of ipecacuanha root, since the seventeenth century. Perhaps because sufferers from other forms of acute diarrhoea and true bacillary dysentery often recover spontaneously, except in the most severe cases, the reputation of the remedy extended to all forms of dysenteric disease. Successful treatment of hepatic amoebiasis was not possible until more accurate diagnosis became available, though this did not preclude at least one unusual cure. Sir George Ballingall, a nineteenth century military surgeon of some repute, in an account of dysentery and liver disease suffered by European troops in India tells of 'A story very generally current in India, of an officer on the Madras establishment having had an abscess of the liver opened by his adversary's ball, in fighting a duel, and by this means obtaining a complete cure' (59).

Ballingall (a delightfully appropriate name for the purveyor of this tale!) recognized two forms of dysentery: 'colonitis' an acute form restricted to the intestinal canal; and 'hepatic flux', a more chronic variety in which the liver was involved. His treatise, written in 1818, provides an insight into how dysentery was treated in the early nineteenth century, before the efficacy of ipecacuanha was generally accepted. Among the procedures he recommends for the acute form are:

- *General blood-letting*: 'Of this remedy I have to express a very favourable opinion. I must, however, candidly own, that the opinion is grounded more on the ravages of inflammation so universally apparent in the dead, than on any repeated or extensive experience of its beneficial effects on the living'.

- *Topical bleeding*: application of leeches to the abdomen or rectum. '...the practice was attended with decided benefit; the pain and tension, as well as the bloody discharges by stool being immediately diminished'.

- *Purgatives*: 'to ascertain that his intestinal canal is not overloaded with faeculent matter'.

- *Emetics*: 'to remove from the stomach any deleterious substance recently swallowed and to give the other medicines one wishes to administer a better chance of success'.

- *Blisters*: 'I have never known them fail to be attended by a diminution of the internal pain, the frequency of stools, and tenesmus'.

- *Injections* (enemas): 'If thrown up in sufficient quantity, and with a tolerable degree of force, they will reach every part of the large intestines, and from thus coming in immediate contact with the seat of the disease, their beneficial effects are greatly augmented'.

- *Sudorifics* (opium and ipecacuanha): 'To which I am disposed to assign the most powerful and salutary effects.

Mercury was also in very general use, but in Ballingall's view was seldom useful in the acute form of the disease. He was, however, unstinting in its praise in 'hepatic flux':

> If, in treating of the acute form of flux, I have refrained from an indiscriminate, and, as I conceive, unmerited commendation of this powerful medicine, it is only in hopes of being able to urge its employment with double force [in hepatic flux]; to ascribe an almost unlimited power to it in this disease; and to express an opinion that it will seldom disappoint our most sanguine hopes.

One can only feel for the poor patients having to undergo the recommended regimens, especially as cure was by no means guaranteed.

The ipecacuanha plant, *Cephaëlis (Psychotria) ipecacuanha*, is a native of Brazil, where it grows abundantly in moist, shady situations in the Amazon and Atlantic forest areas. Portuguese and Dutch settlers colonized Brazil in the sixteenth century and the cumbersome name is a Portuguese transliteration of the Tupi-Guarani word for the plant, ipe-kaa-guéne, literally meaning low or creeping plant causing vomit (60). This indicates that the emetic properties of the shrub were well known to the indigenous population, but whether they were aware of its effect in dysentery is less clear. The plant is listed as a priority species for conservation (61).

The value of ipecacuanha root in dysenteric disease was certainly recognized by Europeans in the seventeenth century and was mentioned as early as 1625 by Samuel Purchas, the rector of St Martin's Ludgate, London, in a famous book about early voyages of discovery based on manuscripts written by his predecessor at St Martin's, Thomas Hakluyt (62). A description of the root also appeared in an early account of medicinal plants in Brazil by the Dutch physician Willem Piso, who introduced it to Europe around 1658. By 1686 it was being touted round Paris by a young physician, Jean-Adrien Helvétius, who had the good fortune to attract the attention of Louis XIV, when his son the Dauphin and other members of the court were suffering from dysentery. The treatment was a success, and after further successful trials at the Hôtel-Dieu, the king paid Helvétius 1000 Louis-d'or for the secret of the remedy (63). The story has striking similarities with Talbor's experience with *Cinchona* bark.

An alkaloid, which was given the name emetine, was isolated from ipecacuanha root in 1817 by the French physiologist, François Magendie in collaboration with Pierre-Joseph Pelletier, who later went on to isolate quinine (see p. 34). However, Magendie's solution was later shown to be a crude mixture of several alkaloids, and despite the efforts of Pelletier himself and of several other nineteenth century chemists to separate the various components of the mixture, emetine proper was not obtained in pure form until the British chemists, Benjamin Horatio Paul, and Alfred John Cownley formally characterized the different constituents in 1894 and 1895 (64). Francis Lee Pyman, professor of chemistry at Manchester College of Science and Technology, finally put forward a structure for emetine in 1927 shortly before he moved to Nottingham to become director of research for the Boots Pure Drug Company.* One of the major alkaloids, cephaeline, also has antiprotozoal activity, but is an even more powerful emetic than emetine itself. Emetine, unlike quinine, was not used in Victorian medicine, perhaps because of uncertainties about the purity of available formulations. Indeed, an authoritative account of dysentery written in the last decade of the century fails to mention emetine as an alternative to the root (65).

By the nineteenth century ipecacuanha root was firmly established in medical practice, though it was more widely used as a relatively mild and safe emetic than as a specific for dysentery. In most European countries bacillary dysentery was much more common than the amoebic variety and inability to distinguish between the two gave ipecacuanha an unreliable reputation. The substance was also widely prescribed to promote perspiration and expectoration; indeed, the effect of ipecacuanha in promoting coughing and the expulsion of mucus secretions from the respiratory tract made it a popular remedy for whooping cough. The drug appeared (and still does) in many patent medicines purporting to alleviate this condition. A popular formulation—for children as well as adults—was

* Pyman started his research career with Burroughs Wellcome in 1906; he was director of research at the Wellcome Chemical Research Laboratories during the First World War and moved to Manchester in 1919. In 1943 he was appointed chairman of the Therapeutic Research Corporation (see p. 103). His proposed structure for emetine was basically correct although minor modifications were later made.

ipecacuanha wine, obtained by macerating the powdered root in sherry for 7 days. In dysentery ipecacuanha was used together with opium, partly in order to suppress the emetic effect and allow higher doses to be given, but also because opium has a constipating effect on its own. Some physicians preferred to prescribe *ipecacuanha sine emetina* (ipecacuanha without emetine) thus depriving the drug of its most important constituent. Opium—often administered as an alcoholic tincture, laudanum, or the aromatic mixture paregoric—was the omnicompetent nostrum of Victorian physicians; Waring's *Manual of Practical Therapeutics* (1871) devotes nearly 30 pages to the drug, recommending it for everything from hay fever to whooping cough (66). It may not have exerted much therapeutic benefit, but at least it alleviated pain, which is more than can be said for most medical interventions before the twentieth century.

Ipecacuanha and opium were the chief ingredients of Dover's powder, a proprietary remedy that remained popular until at least the mid-twentieth century. It was originally formulated for the treatment of gout, but became popular as an analgesic and diaphoretic. The inventor, Thomas Dover, was a physician from Bristol, who had been a student of Thomas Sydenham. He joined a privateering expedition to the South Seas in 1708 and was a member of the shore party that discovered Alexander Selkirk (the real-life model for Robinson Crusoe) in 1710 (67). The recipe for his *pulvis ipecacuanhae compositus* appeared in his book *The Ancient Physician's Legacy* in 1732.

The pure substance, emetine, became the drug of choice for amoebic dysentery only after the publication in 1912 of a study by Leonard Rogers in Calcutta. The paper, which starts engagingly with the sentence 'Ipecacuanha is a drug with an interesting past and a brilliant future', described three cases in which cure of amoebic dysentery or acute amoebic hepatitis was achieved after administration of emetine hydrochloride by hypodermic injection (68). Two of the three cases also received ipecacuanha at some stage, but standards of proof in those days were less important than the endorsement of an eminent tropical expert. Emetine was thereafter widely used in preference to the native compound, but because of its toxic effect on the heart it was normally administered only in hospital, where the patient could be kept rested and under supervision. Although emetine is very effective against active amoebae, it does not suppress the cyst form of the protozoon. Moreover, its emetic properties required it to be given by injection. A compound form of emetine in which it is complexed with bismuth iodide was introduced by Andrew Grover Du Mez, director of the Philippine School of Pharmacy, Manila, in 1915. Emetine bismuth iodide is more successful against the cysts; unlike the parent compound, emetine, it is administered by mouth in gelatine capsules, but it remains a powerful emetic and is extremely unpleasant to take.

Emetine, latterly in the form of a somewhat less toxic derivative, dehydroemetine (first synthesized in 1959), is still available for the treatment of amoebic dysentery in some parts of the world, but has been generally superseded by safer and more reliable remedies (see p. 310). Ipecacuanha remains in the pharmacopoeia as a relatively mild and useful emetic for the emergency treatment of some types of poisoning. It also survives in many simple remedies sold to the public for coughs and colds; such products probably do little harm and equally little good.

References

1. Defoe D (1966). *A journal of the plague year*, p. 120. Penguin English Library edition, Harmondsworth.
2. UNICEF. *The state of the world's children 2006*. UNICEF 2005. Available at: http://www.unicef.org/ (Published annually).
3. Armstrong GL, Conn LA, Pinner RW (1999). Trends in infectious disease mortality in the United States during the 20th century. *J Am Med Assoc* **281**, 61–6.
4. Mackenbach JP, Looman CWN (1988). Secular trends of infectious disease mortality in the Netherlands, 1911–1978: quantitative estimates of changes coinciding with the introduction of antibiotics. *Int J Epidemiol* **17**, 618–24.
5. Zumla A, Lulat A (1989). Honey: a remedy rediscovered. *J R Soc Med* **82**, 374–5.
6. Origo I (1963). *The merchant of Prato*, p. 302. Penguin Books, Harmondsworth.
7. Ball P (2006). *The devil's doctor. Paracelsus and the World of Renaissance Magic and Science.* Heinemann, London.
8. McCallum RI (1999). *Antimony in medical history*. Pentland Press, Edinburgh.
9. Porter R (1989). *Health for sale. Quackery in England 1660–1850*. Manchester University Press, Manchester.
10. Wolff C (2001). *Johann Sebastian Bach. The learned musician*. Oxford University Press, Oxford.
11. O'Shaughnessy WB, letter to the *Lancet*, 1831; cited in Cosnett JE (1989). The origins of intravenous fluid therapy. *Lancet* **1**, 768–71.
12. O'Shaughnessy WB (1831–32). Proposal of a new method of treating the blue epidemic cholera by the injection of highly oxygenised salts into the venous system. *Lancet* **1**, 366–71.
13. Cosnett JE (1989). The origins of intravenous fluid therapy. *Lancet* **1**, 768–71.
14. Power, H (1996). The Calcutta School of Tropical Medicine: institutionalizing medical research in the periphery. *Med Hist* **40**, 197–214; Manson-Bahr P. Major-General Sir Leonard Rogers, KCSI, CIE, FRCP, FRCS, FRS (IMS ret) (1956). In: *History of the school of tropical medicine in London 1899–1949*, pp. 149–50. HK Lewis, London.
15. Snow SJ (2004). Snow, John (1813–1858). *Oxford dictionary of national biography*, Oxford University Press; Available at: http://www.oxforddnb.com/view/article/25979.
16. Snow J (1855). *On the mode of communication of cholera*. Churchill, London,. Available at: University of California, Los Angeles, Department of Epidemiology, School of Public Health http://www.ph.ucla.edu/epi/snow/snowbook.html.
17. Chave SPW (1958). Henry Whitehead and cholera in Broad Street. *Med Hist* **2**, 92–109.
18. Forrest RD (1982). Development of wound therapy from the Dark Ages to the present. *J R Soc Med* **75**, 268–73.
19. Loudon I (2000). *The tragedy of childbed fever*. Oxford University Press, Oxford.
20. Loudon I (1996). Alexander Gordon, puerperal fever and antisepsis. *Aberdeen University Review* **56**, 285–300.
21. Cheyne WW (1885). *Manual of the antiseptic treatment of wounds for students and practitioners.* Smith, Elder & Co, London. See also: http://www.watson-cheyne.com/.
22. Oriel JD (1991). Eminent venereologists 5: Carl Credé. *Genitourin Med* **67**, 67–9.
23. The Barnes foundation. Available at: http://www.barnesfoundation.org/.
24. Nicolaier A (1895). Ueber die therapeutische Verwendung des Urotropin (Hexamthelenetetramin). *Dtsch Med Wochenschr* **21**, 341–3.
25. Kahler (1830). Ueber einen neuen Stoff im Semen Cinae. *Archiv des Apotheker-vereins im Nördlichen Teutschland* **3**, 318–9; Alms A (1830). Ueber einen neuen Stoff im levantischen Wurmsamen. *Archiv des Apotheker-vereins im Nördlichen Teutschland* **3**, 319–20; Brandes R (1830). Nachricht zu vorstehenden beiden Abhandlungen. *Archiv des Apotheker-vereins im Nördlichen Teutschland* **3**, 320.

See also: Schröder W (1960). Die pharmazeutisch-chemischen Produkte deutscher Apotheken zu Beginn des naturwissenschaftlich-industriellen Zeitalters. *Veröffentlichung aus dem Pharmaziegeschichtlichen Seminar der Technischen Hochschule Braunschweig, Band 3*, pp. 134–41. Braunschweig.

26. Annotation (1844). A tasteless worm medicine. *Lancet* **1**, 226.

27. Kliks MM (1985). Studies on the traditional herbal anthelmintic *Chenopodium ambrosiodes* L.: ethnopharmacological evaluation and clinical field trials. *Soc Sci Med* **21**, 879–86.

28. Watson T (1857). *Lectures on the principles and practice of physic*, 4th edn., Vol. II, p. 579. John W. Parker & Son, London.

29. Naranjo P (1992). Epidemic hecatomb in the New World. *Allergy Proc* **13**, 237–24.

30. Duran-Reynals ML (1947). *The fever bark tree. The pageant of quinine*. WH Allen, London.

31. Dunn FL (1965). On the antiquity of malaria in the western hemisphere. *Hum Biol* **37**, 385–93; Conway DJ, Fanello C, Lloyd JM, *et al.* (2000). Origin of *Plasmodium falciparum* malaria is traced by mitochondrial DNA. *Mol Biochem Parasitol* **111**, 163–71.

32. Guerra F (1977). The introduction of cinchona in the treatment of malaria. *J Trop Med Hyg* **80**, 112–8 and 135–40.

33. Haggis AW (1941). Fundamental errors in the early history of cinchona. *Bull Hist Med* **10**, 417–59 and 568–92.

34. Diener HC, Dethlefsen U, Dethlefsen-Gruber S, Verbeek P (2002). Effectiveness of quinine in treating muscle cramps: a double-blind, placebo-controlled, parallel-group, multicentre trial. *Int J Clin Pract* **56**, 243–6.

35. Jarcho S (1993). *Quinine's predecessor. Francesco Torti and the early history of cinchona*. The Johns Hopkins University Press, Baltimore.

36. Prinz A (1990). Discovery of the cardiac effectiveness of cinchona bark and its alkaloids. *Wien Klin Wochenschr* **102**, 721–3.

37. Watson T (1857). *Lectures on the principles and practice of physic*, 4th edn., Vol. I, p. 781. John W Parker and Son, London.

38. Nabokov N (1969). *Speak memory*, p. 40. Penguin Books, Harmondsworth.

39. Manson P (1898). *Tropical diseases*, p. 110. Cassell, London.

40. Gramiccia G (1987). Notes on the early history of cinchona plantations. *Acta Leiden* **55**, 5–13.

41. Honigsbaum M (2001). *The fever trail. The hunt for the cure for malaria*. Macmillan, London.

42. Rocco F. Quinine (2003). *Malaria and the quest for a cure that changed the world*. Harper Collins, London; published in the United States as *The miraculous fever tree*.

43. Gramiccia G (1988). *The life of Charles Ledger (1818–1905). Alpacas and quinine*. Macmillan Press, Basingstoke.

44. Bruce-Chwatt LJ, de Zulueta J (1980). *The rise and fall of malaria in Europe*. Oxford University Press, Oxford.

45. Guerin P, Nosten F, White NJ. Malaria: an essential R & D agenda. Available at: http://www.neglecteddiseases.org/1-1.pdf.

46. Poser CM, Bruyn GW (1999). *An illustrated history of malaria*, pp. 5–9. Parthenon Publishing, New York.

47. Ott M. Urban XIII. Available at: http://www.newadvent.org/cathen/15218b.htm.

48. Buchan W (1785). *The domestic medicine, Chapter XIV: of intermitting fevers and agues*, 2nd edn. Available at: http://www.americanrevolution.org/medicine.html.

49. Lawrence C (1975). William Buchan: medicine laid open. *Med Hist* **19**, 20–3.

50. Greenhill WA (2004). 'Johnson, James (1777–1845)' (Harrison M, revised) *Oxford dictionary of national biography*, Oxford University Press,. Available at: http://www.oxforddnb.com/view/article/14891.

51. Rogers L (1919). *Fever in the tropics*, 3rd edn. Oxford University Press, Oxford.

52. Bruce-Chwatt LJ (1971). Malaria and its prevention in military campaigns. *Zeitschrift für Tropenmedizin und Parasitologie* **22**, 370–90.

53. Curtin PD (1989). *Death by migration. Europe's encounter with the tropical world in the nineteenth century*, pp. 132–40. Cambridge University Press, Cambridge.

54. Woodward JJ (1863). *Outlines of the chief camp diseases of the United States armies as observed during the present war: a practical contribution to military medicine*. Lippincott, Philadelphia; reprinted Hafner Publishing Company, New York, 1964.

55. Anonymous ('X.F.O.') (1919). Quinine as an economic weapon. *Chemist and Druggist*, 20 September 1919, pp. 61–3; Abrahamson HS (1919). Quinine as an economic weapon (correspondence). *Chemist and Druggist* 27 September, p. 94.

56. Anonymous (1919). The quinine situation. *Chemist and Druggist*, 4 October, p. 81.

57. Bureau tot Bevordering van het Kinine-gebruik (1925). *Chininum. Scriptiones collectae anno MCMXXIV editae*. Amsterdam.

58. Bray RS (1996). Amoebiasis. In: Cox FEG, ed. *Illustrated history of tropical* diseases, pp. 170–7. Wellcome Trust, London.

59. Ballingall G (1818). *Practical observations on fever, dysentery and liver complaints, as they occur amongst European troops in India*, pp. 64–89 and 103. John Brown, Edinburgh.

60. *Oxford English dictionary* (1989), 2nd edn. Oxford University Press, Oxford.

61. Vieira RF (1999). Conservation of medicinal and aromatic plants in Brazil. Symposium: perspectives on new crops and new uses. Available at: http://www.hort.purdue.edu/newcrop/proceedings1999/pdf/v4-152.pdf.

62. Purchas S (1625). *Hakluytus posthumus, or purchas his pilgrims*, Vol. IV, p. 1311. Fetherstone, London.

63. Pereira J (1857). (Taylor AS, Rees GO, eds). *The elements of materia medica and therapeutics*, 4th edn., Vol. II, Part II, pp. 55–6 Longman, Brown, Green and Roberts, London.

64. Janot MM (1893). The ipecac alkaloids. Cited in Manske RHF, Holmes HL, eds. *The alkaloids: chemistry and physiology*, Vol. III, pp. 363–94. Academic Press, New York.

65. Davidson DM, Davidson A (1893). Dysentery. In: Davidson A, ed. *Hygiene and diseases of warm climates*, pp. 546–611. Pentland, Edinburgh.

66. Waring EJ (1871). *A manual of practical therapeutics*, pp. 448–76. Churchill, London.

67. Osler W (1908). Thomas Dover, physician and buccaneer. In: *An Alabama student and other biographical essays*, pp. 19–36. Oxford University Press/Humphrey Milford, London.

68. Rogers L (1912). The rapid cure of amoebic dysentery and hepatitis by hypodermic injections of soluble salts of emetine. *BMJ* **1**, 1424–5.

Chapter 3

From quinine to sulphonamides (by way of Serendip)

I once read a silly fairy tale called *The Three Princes of Serendip*: as their highnesses travelled, they were always making discoveries, by accident and sagacity, of things which they were not in quest of.

Horace Walpole (1717–1797). *Letter to Horace Mann, British Envoy in Florence*, 28 January 1754.

In addition to its formidable reputation as a specific for the treatment of intermittent fevers, *Cinchona* bark was fated to play a vital part in several unconnected events that were to have far-reaching consequences. As is well known (I assume) to practitioners of homeopathy, its founder Samuel Hahnemann formulated his controversial therapeutic theories after dosing himself with *Cinchona* bark and suffering symptoms reminiscent of the ague (the popular name for malarial fevers), possibly engendered by an idiosyncratic allergy to the drug. Whether this chance observation represented the major insight that Hahnemann proposed is a moot point, but Lady Luck was not to stake her reputation on this event; she was busy forming liaisons with quinine that were to revolutionize fashion, medicine, the pharmaceutical industry, and ultimately—as though she were just weaving a convoluted thread to lead humankind from one effective antimicrobial drug to another— the treatment of infectious disease.

Cinchona bark and willow bark

In 1763, the Reverend Edward Stone,* a former Dean of Wadham College, Oxford, wrote to the President of the Royal Society from his home in Chipping Norton, Oxfordshire, describing the successful use of willow bark to alleviate agues and other distempers (1). Stone had reasoned from the bitterness of *Cinchona* bark that the bitter bark of other trees might offer a cheaper substitute and that the common white

---

* The name is often given as Edmund Stone, but this is an error arising from confusion with a contemporary of that name (1).

willow, *Salix alba*, which he had accidentally tasted and found to fit the bill, was the one to go for:

> As this tree delights in a moist and wet soil where agues abound, the general maxim that natural remedies carry their cures with them was so very appropriate that I could not help applying it; and that this was the intention of Providence I must own had some weight with me (2).

Despite this optimism, Stone's remedy failed to live up to his aspirations that it might offer a cure for the ague, but its bitterness and astringency appealed to medical opinion of the time and it seemed to be of help in some other conditions. The idea was not new. Willow bark had been recommended for fevers as far back as the time of Hippocrates, and Dioscorides had written of its medicinal properties, but use of the bark had fallen into disuse no doubt because of its lack of clear efficacy. Stone's contribution was to bring the remedy back to the attention of the scientific community by having his letter accepted for publication in the *Transactions of the Royal Society*. Species other than white willow—the more bitter the better—were also brought into use during the nineteenth century and the barks found a regular place in Victorian materia medica as serviceable if undistinguished drugs.

The active principle of willow bark, salicin, was first crystallized in 1829 by Pierre-Joseph Leroux, a pharmacist practising in Vitry-le-François on the Marne in north-east France, but it was not until 1838 that Raffaele Piria, an Italian chemist working in Paris, succeeded in synthesizing salicylic acid. Salicylic acid was extensively used in pain relief and as an antiseptic (though it lacks antibacterial properties). In 1874 the German chemist Friedrich von Heyden set up a factory, 'Salicylsäurefabrik F v Heyden', in Radebeul on the outskirts of Dresden specifically to manufacture the substance. The factory flourished and soon expanded into other products.* Situated in the heart of Saxony in eastern Germany, von Heyden's firm has had a chequered history, eventually becoming a 'Volkseigener Betrieb' (People's factory) in the German Democratic Republic. After German reunification in 1990, it re-emerged as a private company, Arzneimittelwerk Dresden (Pharmaceutical works, Dresden), and was acquired by the West German chemical concern, Degussa AG. In 2001 the pharmaceutical division was sold to the Croatian pharmaceutical company Pliva (see footnote p. 239). The factory still stands in Radebeul.

The principal disadvantage of salicylic acid is that it is nauseating to take and harmful to the stomach. An acetylated derivative, which is much safer, was subsequently synthesized in 1853 by the French organic chemist Charles Frédéric Gerhardt. Millions of tablets of acetylsalicylic acid—aspirin—are now swallowed daily, but Gerhardt was unaware of the analgesic, antipyretic, and anti-inflammatory properties of the compound

---

* The Heyden company's most famous achievement was a process, discovered in 1941 by Richard Müller, which paved the way for the production of silicones. The discovery was the accidental outcome of research Müller had started in 1932 with the quixotic aim of manufacturing an 'artificial fog' to protect whole towns from air attack. The process was independently discovered around the same time in America by Eugene Rochow and is known as the Müller–Rochow synthesis.

and he joins the ranks of those (we will meet several others on the course of this book) who were blissfully ignorant of the value of a substance that they held in their hands.

Acetylsalicylic acid was resynthesized in 1897 by Felix Hoffmann in the laboratories of Friedrich Bayer and Company at Elberfeld in the Rhineland area of Germany.* He was reputedly seeking a better-tolerated substitute for the irritant salicylic acid as a palliative for his father's crippling rheumatism. A patent application for acetylsalicylic acid was disallowed in Germany, but Bayer registered the trade name 'Aspirin'† ('spir' from *Spiraea ulmaria*—meadowsweet—a plant from which Raffaele Piria had synthesized salicylic acid). The launch of aspirin was delayed until 1899 because the influential director of pharmacological research, Heinrich Dreser mistakenly believed it to have a harmful effect on the heart; moreover, he favoured another recent Bayer discovery, the 'heroic' drug, heroin. When aspirin was eventually marketed it was an immediate hit and became one of the most widely used remedies of all times. Nearly 50 years later, another derivative of salicylic acid, *para*-aminosalicylic acid, was to play a major part in the battle against tuberculosis (see p. 164). Towards the end of the twentieth century, hitherto unsuspected properties of aspirin in the prevention of heart disease and strokes were uncovered, and there are even suggestions that it might protect against certain forms of cancer.

The Bayer Company had been formed in 1863 as a partnership between a dye salesman, Friedrich Bayer and a master dyer, Johann Friedrich Wescott. Their expertise lay in natural dyes, but the company they founded was set up to exploit the vast potential of the exciting synthetic aniline dyes that were beginning to appear. After the early death of the two founders (both died when they were only 55), the company started to diversify into pharmaceuticals as potentially useful by-products of dye manufacture. The policy quickly paid off in 1888 when one of its young chemists, Carl Duisberg, who was to become Managing Director in 1912, and his collaborator Oskar Hinsberg discovered an analgesic, phenacetin (3).

Aniline dyes transformed the dyestuffs industry and were a major influence in the genesis of industrial research laboratories (4). Several dyestuff producers besides the Bayer Company were to metamorphose into pharmaceutical firms that would eventually become multinational giants of the worldwide ethical drug market. The synthetic dye that contrived this revolution emerged not in Germany, but in London. It was another fruit of the love affair between quinine and Lady Luck.

From quinine to aniline dyes

Easter 1856: an 18-year-old assistant at the Royal College of Chemistry in London had the hare-brained idea (as teenagers do) that he could upstage the Director of the College, the distinguished German chemist August Wilhelm von Hofmann, by producing quinine

---

* The full name of the company after 1881was: 'Aktiengesellschaft Farbenfabriken vormals [formerly] Friedrich Bayer & Co'. In 1929 Elberfeld, together with the neighbouring town of Barmen and some smaller communities, amalgamated to form Wuppertal.

† After the First World War Bayer's assets in Britain, France, Russia, and the United States were seized and aspirin became a generic name. Elsewhere it is still used as a Bayer brand name.

from coal tar products. He probably kept the idea to himself, for he carried out the experiments in a makeshift laboratory that he had constructed at home. Instead of obtaining quinine he accidentally discovered the first synthetic aniline dye and went on to make his fortune.

The young assistant was William Henry Perkin, youngest son of a building contractor in Shadwell, East London. His father had wanted him to become an architect, but the lad found himself attracted to chemistry through the influence of his form master Thomas Hall at the City of London School. Hall had himself studied chemistry under Hofmann at the Royal College and encouraged his pupil to follow his example (5). Perkin enrolled in the College in 1853 at the age of 15 and was such a diligent student that by 1855 Hofmann appointed him as an assistant.

Chemistry was still in its infancy at this time, but its importance was being boosted by the demands of industry. Gaslight was becoming a standard fixture in streets, houses, and factories, and among pressing concerns was the need to find uses for the noxious by-products of gas production, tons of which, in London, were dumped annually in the Thames (6). The early chemists throughout Europe had seized upon coal gas and the most distasteful and intractable of all the by-products, coal tar, as rich sources of organic substances such as benzene and toluene, which became known as aromatic hydrocarbons. In 1824 the Scottish chemist, Charles Macintosh, used naphtha—a crude coal-tar derivative—to produce waterproof materials from rubber, including his celebrated mackintosh raincoat.

Aniline was first obtained in Oranienburg a few miles north of Berlin by Friedlieb Runge, formerly the professor of chemistry in Breslau. Runge had established a factory in a former royal palace, Schloss Oranienburg, to manufacture stearine and paraffin wax candles. In his chemical laboratory he continued to investigate products of the distillation of coal tar and in 1834 hit upon both phenol (see p. 27) and aniline, which he originally called kyanol. In fact, Otto Unverdorben a chemist-apothecary from Dahme, south of Berlin had unwittingly obtained aniline earlier (1826) through distillation of the vegetable dye indigo, but it was only later that Hofmann showed the substance to be identical to aniline. Runge, one of the foremost organic chemists of his day, had noted that kyanol reacted with chloride of lime to produce a blue colour, but he does not seem to have realized the practical implications of the finding. Nevertheless, the discovery of aniline had a profound impact on the development of the German chemical industry. By 1865 Friedrich Engelhorn had established the Badische Anilin und Soda Fabrik (BASF), which grew to be a leading chemical supplier. In 1867, the chemists Paul Mendelssohn-Bartholdy* and Carl Alexander von Martius established a factory in Rummelsburg near Berlin, later called Aktien-Gesellschaft für Anilin-Fabrikation, or AGFA.

One of Hofmann's pet theories was that coal-tar derivatives might provide the key to a prize to which many chemists of the time aspired: the synthesis of quinine. Coal tar seemed at least to contain the right elements, though nothing was known at the time

* Son of the composer, Felix Mendelssohn-Bartholdy.

about their molecular arrangement in any of its components or in quinine. No doubt the dream of producing synthetic quinine was widely debated among students and staff of the Royal College of Chemistry.

At Easter 1856, just after his eighteenth birthday, William Henry Perkin settled into his ill-equipped amateur laboratory to try his luck at proving Hofmann's theory correct. He did not succeed, but the experiments he performed were to change his life and eventually the course of medicine. His Big Idea was to obtain quinine by oxidizing allyl-*o*-toluidine with potassium dichromate, but when he did this all he got was a nondescript reddish precipitate. Undeterred, he decided to try aniline instead of toluidine and this time the precipitate was black. However, when the dried and washed precipitate was dissolved in alcohol a rich purple solution was obtained. Perkin was an enthusiastic amateur painter and the colour captured the young man's imagination sufficiently for him to try to use it to stain a silk cloth. To his surprise—for artificial dyes that lacked such properties had been tried before by others—the colour remained rich and attractive even after washing and exposure to sunlight.

Perkin clearly had a nose for business. He knew he was on to something, but had no experience of how to exploit it. Hofmann was not consulted, but a friend of William Perkin's elder brother, Thomas, suggested sending a sample of dyed cloth to Pullar's dye works in Perth Scotland, which in 1852 had been awarded a royal warrant as silk dye makers. The choice was providential. Robert Pullar, son of John Pullar, who had founded the firm in 1824, was an ambitious and open-minded young man of only 28 and was intent on expanding the business. On receipt of the dyed cloth, he sent an encouraging reply to Perkin, who immediately filed a patent application, offered his resignation to Hofmann, and started to make plans to set up a manufacturing unit with no capital and no commercial experience whatsoever (7).

Surprisingly, the only person to oppose this seemingly foolhardy scheme was Hofmann, who naturally considered that a talented young chemist was throwing away a safe career in scientific research. Most supportive were his friends and family. His brother Thomas dropped the idea of taking over the existing family business as had been planned and joined William in setting up the dye works; their father sank most of his savings into his sons' venture to provide the capital. A small factory was built at Greenford Green near Harrow, suitable equipment was installed, problems of scaling up the laboratory process were overcome, and within 6 months of the opening of the factory in 1858 the new dye was on the market. Several names were suggested for the new colour—Tyrian purple, aniline purple, and mauveine among them—but it was mauve, from the French for mallow, a plant with purple flowers that was to capture the public's imagination.

Mauve was a fashion sensation; even Queen Victoria wore the new colour. Soon colour chemists in continental Europe were vying with each other to produce new and vivid dyes from aniline and other organic residues (8). The modern dyestuff era had begun and the seeds of many pharmaceutical products had been sown. The progression from dyes to drugs owes much to a diminutive cigar-smoking German Jewish Doctor who has become known as the 'father of chemotherapy': Paul Ehrlich.

Ehrlich and the foundation of chemotherapy

Dyes in the service of medicine

Dyes had always fascinated Paul Ehrlich. As a young man he had experimented with the staining of tissues with his cousin on his mother's side, Carl Weigert, who was himself a pioneer of the use of aniline dyes in bacteriology and histology. After a peripatetic student career in Breslau, Strasbourg, Freiburg-im-Breisgau, and Leipzig, Ehrlich graduated MD in 1878 on submission of a thesis entitled 'Beiträge zur Theorie und Praxis der histologischen Färbung' (Contributions to the theory and practice of histological staining). In his first post at the famous Charité Hospital in Berlin one of his main preoccupations was the observation of the action of various dyes on tissues, outside the body and in living animals. He also developed staining methods that were to provide the foundations for future haematological and histological advances.

Around 1887, Ehrlich began to show symptoms of tuberculosis and he spent much of 1888 and 1889 in Italy and Egypt, where the climate seems to have effected a cure. On his return Ehrlich first set up a small private laboratory, but was soon offered an assistantship in the Institute for Infectious Diseases that had been established in Berlin with Robert Koch as Director. Here he started to establish his reputation in the newly fashionable field of immunology and began a fruitful collaboration (which later turned sour) with Emil von Behring, the discoverer of diphtheria antitoxin and a pioneer of serotherapy. Von Behring, who was Ehrlich's junior by just one day, was, with Ehrlich and Koch, the third member of the great German scientific triumvirate, which, supported by many talented colleagues, outshone even the Pasteurian French school at this time (9).

By 1896, Ehrlich's reputation was sufficient for him to be appointed Director of a new Institut für Serumforschung und Serumprüfung (Institute for serum research and testing) in Steglitz, Berlin. According to his biographer Martha Marquardt, his devoted secretary between 1902 and 1915,* this was a happy and productive period, but facilities in what had reputedly been a bakery were inadequate (10). In 1899 arrangements were made for him to transfer to more opulent surroundings in the newly opened Royal Prussian Institute for Experimental Therapy in Frankfurt. This was extended in 1906, through the munificence of Franziska Speyer, the widow of a Frankfurt banker, by the adjacent construction of a Research Institute for Chemotherapy: the Georg-Speyer Haus.

In 1908 Ehrlich shared the Nobel Prize for Physiology or Medicine with the great immunologist, Ilya Metchnikov, for his work on bacterial toxins, the standardization of

---

* The biography, written in English and based on an earlier German version (most copies of which were destroyed during the Nazi years) is unashamedly laudatory, but offers an affectionate, human, and largely accurate portrayal of Ehrlich's life. Martha Marquardt spent the Second World War in occupied Paris and, at the invitation of Almroth Wright, came to England in 1946. Here she wrote the biography and spent her remaining years deciphering and collating Ehrlich's papers for publication together with another German émigré, Fred Himmelweit.

antitoxin concentrations in serum and the formulation of his 'side-chain' theory of immunity. The theory was an attempt to account for the action of toxins and the specific nature of antitoxins. He postulated (to oversimplify what was an elaborate hypothesis) that all cells have receptors ('side-chains') that are able to bind certain toxins in a 'lock and key' arrangement. The specificity of the interaction depends on the stereochemical structure of the receptor so that only certain cells bind particular toxins—for example, tetanus toxin bound only to nerve cells. According to the theory, antitoxins represented a gross excess of the receptors that are liberated into the bloodstream where they mop up circulating toxins (11). The side-chain theory as Ehrlich expounded it to explain immune phenomena has turned out to be fairly wide of the mark. Nevertheless, it was a brave attempt to reconcile many puzzling features of the immune response and contained a sufficient grain of truth to represent a remarkable insight for the time.

Despite the acclaim that attended his serological work, Ehrlich never abandoned his interest in dyes. Indeed, the origins of the side-chain hypothesis lay in his earlier work with vital stains, in which he had observed that bacterial, protozoal, or tissue cells exhibited specific affinities for different dyes. He had also made the crucial connection between the ability of dyes to stain microbes while sparing surrounding tissues and the possibility of achieving selective toxicity—the necessary basis for effective antimicrobial chemotherapy.

Theory had been turned into action shortly after he joined Robert Koch's laboratory in 1890. Noting the ability of methylene blue to stain malaria parasites within red blood cells, he decided to try the dye as a treatment for malaria. Together with a colleague, Paul Guttmann, he administered a chemically pure preparation of methylene blue (gelatine capsules of 0.1 g given at intervals of 1–3 h) to two patients diagnosed with malaria at the Moabit Hospital in Berlin, where he had a part-time clinical post (12). Both patients recovered and suffered no ill effects apart from irritation of the bladder, which, mixing scientific advance with folk medicine, they treated with a little grated nutmeg—a measure that they felt obliged to explain:

> Massgebend für diese Präventivanwendung der Muskatnuss ist die in Süddeutschland, zumal in München, vielfach gebräuchliche Praxis, dysurischen Beschwerden, wie sie durch den Genuss frischen Bieres hervorgerufen werden können, durch das Gebrauch dieses Gewürzes vorzubeugen. [Justification for the prophylactic use of nutmeg is the common practice in south Germany, especially Munich, of using this spice to prevent dysuria caused by the enjoyment of fresh beer.]

This was Ehrlich's first published paper on the use of dyes and other chemicals to treat infection, a practice to which he later gave the name 'specific chemotherapy' ('specific' to distinguish it from the more general use of chemical substances). It was a small beginning, but was to have great consequences.

Ehrlich's success in treating malaria with methylene blue alerted dye manufacturers to the possibility of a new market and dyes specifically designed against microbial pathogens began to be investigated. Ehrlich himself was naturally in the forefront of this work and set up an animal model for the investigation of the treatment of trypanosomiasis, the life-threatening cause of sleeping sickness, which was as important in the

German-administered territories in Africa as it was to the British colonies there. In Frankfurt, Ehrlich was able to establish links with local dyestuff manufacturers, Meister, Lucius und Brüning, at Hoechst-am-Main (later known as Farbwerke Hoechst) and Leopold Cassella and Company in Frankfurt. In 1906 Hoechst, Cassella, and a third company, Kalle and Company, joined forces in a 'dreiverband', a precursor of what was to become, with Bayer and several other firms, IG Farbenindustrie from 1925 until its disbandment at the end of Second World War.

Germany and France were at this time magnets attracting young medical scientists from all over the world who wished to visit, and if possible work in, the laboratories where so many brilliant discoveries were being made. Among them were a number of Japanese bacteriologists intent on carrying back the new techniques to their country, which was anxious to modernize its economy. One of the visitors to Paul Ehrlich's laboratory was Kiyoshi Shiga, a graduate of the Imperial University Medical School in Tokyo, who arrived in 1901 with a young wife and newborn child (13). He was an enthusiastic microbiological pioneer already becoming known for his discovery in 1898 of the bacilli causing dysentery, which were named *Shigella* in his honour. Shiga was a protégé of Shibasaburo Kitasato, who had worked with Robert Koch and Emil von Behring in Berlin; in 1892 he had set up a similar Institute of Infectious Diseases in Tokyo, financed by one of the prominent modernizers of Japan, Yukichi Fukuzawa. The institute later came under government control and in 1914, Kitasato resigned in protest against its policies. He set up a private research organization, the Kitasato Institute, which was to become a leading player in the early days of antibiotic research in Japan.

In Ehrlich's laboratory Shiga was given the task of investigating the activity of azo dyes in a mouse model of trypanosomiasis and had found one called trypan red to be the most effective. The dye was one of those provided by Arthur von Weinberg, who was Head of Research of the Cassella company (14); he later suffered persecution under the Nazis and died in Theresienstadt, the Czech Jewish ghetto run along concentration camp lines by the German SS (15). Around the same time as Shiga's investigations, Félix Mesnil and Maurice Nicolle in the Pasteur Institute in Paris sought support from Bayer in Elberfeld to carry out similar experiments with dyes (16). Two of them, supplied by Bayer, trypan blue, and afridol violet proved to be the most promising. Like Shiga's trypan red, the compounds were tried in the treatment of trypanosomiasis in Africa, but were soon abandoned. Trypan blue was most successful, at least in cattle, but meat from treated animals could not be sold since the dye turned it bright blue.

Arsenic

Meanwhile Paul Ehrlich's attention was turning from dyes to arsenical derivatives. Arsenic, notwithstanding its reputation as a poison, was in medical use before the time of Hippocrates and, as a substance favoured by Paracelsus, had become a favourite nostrum among physicians by the eighteenth century. Its purported properties were not confined to medicinal benefits: it was alleged to improve strength and sexual prowess in men, while women sometimes used it to improve their complexions (17). Arsenic eating, like opium eating, became fashionable in some quarters. In turning to arsenic as a solution to her problems, Madame Bovary was using a readily available and popular vehicle for suicide or murder.

The popularity of arsenic in nineteenth century medicine was given added impetus by the availability of a water-soluble form, liquor arsenicalis (potassium arsenite) introduced in 1786 by Thomas Fowler, Physician to Stafford Infirmary, and generally known as Fowler's solution. Like opium, it was in universal use in Victorian medicine, and was sometimes prescribed in heroic doses (the hapless patient being the hero!). The esteem in which these two substances was held may be gauged from a quotation from the 1880s:

> If a law were passed, compelling physicians to confine themselves to two remedies only in their entire practice, arsenic would be my choice for one, opium for the other. With these two I believe one could do more than with any two of the pharmacopoeia (18).

Even Patrick Manson, though dismissing those who relied on arsenic for the treatment of malaria, recommended it as a blood restorative after fever (19).

How arsenic came to be considered as a treatment for trypanosomiasis is unclear. It is likely that the first person to use it in a trypanosomal disease was none other than the missionary–explorer David Livingstone. In a letter to the *British Medical Journal* in March 1858 (20) Livingstone describes using arsenic around 1847–1848 to treat a mare that became ill after having been bitten by tsetse flies. The horse was probably suffering from a trypanosomal infection known as nagana, though the cause of the disease was unknown at that time—the role of trypanosomes in human sleeping sickness and various animal diseases was established only towards the end of the nineteenth century.

In his letter to the *British Medical Journal* Livingstone draws attention to the effect of arsenic in making the sick animal's coat smooth and glossy and it is tempting to speculate that others had noted the curative effect of arsenic when old nags were given the drug to improve their general appearance before sale by adding lustre to the coat; arsenic was certainly widely used in this fashion in Europe and elsewhere. Much more likely, however, arsenic was used empirically for its general 'restorative' properties and was discovered, no doubt with surprise, to work. Later it was formally demonstrated that the drug cleared protozoa from the bloodstream.

For want of anything better, arsenicals were sometimes used to treat human sleeping sickness in Victorian times, though the patient was almost as likely to die from the treatment as from the disease. The first arsenical derivative with a claim to be sufficiently safe for regular use was a compound optimistically named 'atoxyl' even though the lack of toxicity was merely relative. This chemical derivative had originally been described in 1863 by Antoine Béchamp, a controversial French biologist whose ideas are claimed by some to have been plagiarized by Pasteur (the claim has been convincingly dismissed as tendentious propaganda). Although it became universally known as atoxyl, the designation was actually the trade name for the commercial product manufactured by a firm called Lanolinfabrik, founded by the chemist Benno Jaffé in the Charlottenburg district of Berlin (21). Around the turn of the twentieth century it was introduced into medicine for conditions in which other arsenicals were commonly prescribed. Ehrlich himself tested the compound *in vitro* against trypanosomes and rejected it as having no effect on the viability of the protozoa, but in 1905 the Canadian physician, Harold Wolferstan Thomas described the efficacy of atoxyl in a mouse model of trypanosomiasis (22).

Thomas had turned to atoxyl after finding that other arsenicals were highly toxic in the animal experiments he was conducting at the Liverpool School of Tropical Medicine with his fellow Canadian John Todd, who succeeded him in 1905 as Director of the School's Research Laboratories in Runcorn, Cheshire,* and his Austrian colleague Anton Breinl, who in 1910 moved on to become Director of the Australian Institute of Tropical Medicine in Townsville, Queensland. In the happy-go-lucky atmosphere of research at that time Thomas had '...tried the drug in high doses intravenously on myself without ill effects'. The experiments were a success, but Thomas was aware that he had not found the ideal non-toxic solution to sleeping sickness:

> ...nor do I think atoxyl is a perfect preparation from its toxic effects on certain canines and felines, but it is an advance on arsenious acid, and if further efforts be made to produce a substance like trypan red, but less irritating in action, the combination ought to be of service in the treatment of trypanosomiasis (22).

By 1906 apparent success in the treatment of African sleeping sickness with atoxyl was being reported by Robert Koch, by the Portuguese Physician, Ayres Kopke, and by the Belgian tropical expert Emile van Campenhout (who recommended using the drug together with strychnine and cold baths (23)) among others. The military doctor, Paul Uhlenhuth, later professor of hygiene and bacteriology at the University of Strasbourg, similarly recommended atoxyl for the treatment of trypanosomiasis (dourine) in horses.

Paul Ehrlich visited the Liverpool School of Tropical Medicine in 1907, an event documented for posterity by a request for reimbursement of his train fare (24). He probably took the opportunity to visit the Liverpool School while in England to deliver the Harben Lectures at the Royal Institute of Public Health in London. He returned to Germany sufficiently convinced of the potential of arsenical drugs to direct much of his subsequent research effort to these compounds. Ehrlich reasoned that the success of atoxyl in treatment must result from changes to the drug in the bloodstream since the drug had no effect in the test tube. A similar phenomenon had been observed previously with some dyes, which are converted to colourless reduction products in tissues. The formal structure of atoxyl was unknown when it was first described, but the French chemist, Ernest Fourneau, had described the molecule as an arsenical derivative of aniline in which the arsenic atom was pentavalent (i.e. the arsenic combined with other groups through five atomic bonds; Fig. 3.1). Ehrlich confirmed that the compound was a pentavalent arsenical, but showed that Fourneau's structure was crucially incorrect in that the arsenic molecule was attached to a carbon of the benzene ring of aniline, leaving a reactive amino group free to undergo modification in the formation of new derivatives. He went on to postulate that in the body the compound was reduced to a trivalent derivative and, indeed, trivalent arsenical compounds turned out to be active *in vitro* as well as *in vivo*.

....

* Thomas left Liverpool in 1905 to lead a School expedition to Manáos in Brazil. Todd was, in turn, succeeded as Director of the Runcorn laboratory by Anton Breinl (ref. 24, p. 26 and 49).

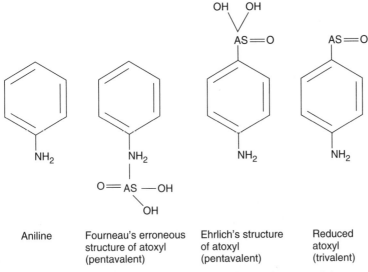

Aniline | Fourneau's erroneous structure of atoxyl (pentavalent) | Ehrlich's structure of atoxyl (pentavalent) | Reduced atoxyl (trivalent)

Fig. 3.1 The aniline molecule and two proposals for the structure of the arsenical derivative, atoxyl. Ehrlich's structure proved correct and he rightly deduced that the antimicrobially active compound was a trivalent derivative produced within the body.

Salvarsan, the imperfect magic bullet

Ehrlich's chemotherapeutic dream was to create a 'magic bullet' that would home in on its microbial target and destroy the infective agent without causing any damage to the host. The phrase has become synonymous with antimicrobial chemotherapy, though no substance has yet been found that completely fits the bill (penicillin is the closest). Ehrlich was fond of dramatic similes and metaphors and he probably first used the term 'magic bullet' (in German 'Zauberkugel') during an address on the occasion of the opening of the Georg-Speyer Haus in 1906 (25). It first appeared in English in one of Ehrlich's Harben Lectures to the Royal Institute of Public Health in London in 1907. The lectures were translated by Carl Prausnitz, a German doctor who was working as a demonstrator at the Institute and was bilingual, having spent part of his childhood in England.* According to Dr David Hide, Prausnitz, who, like Ehrlich, had studied medicine at Breslau, actually gave one of the lectures: Ehrlich had been unable to deliver it himself because he had injured his eye on a shirt stud (26).

---

* Prausnitz's maternal grandmother was English. He worked at the Royal Institute of Public Health from 1906 until 1910, when he returned to Germany to work with Richard Pfeiffer in Breslau. When Hitler came to power in 1933, he emigrated to England and became a British citizen, adding 'Giles' (his mother's maiden name) to his surname (*see* Hide 1992; ref. 26).

The term 'Zauberkugel' no doubt also featured in Ehrlich's address on chemotherapeutics to the seventeenth International Congress of Medicine, held in London in August 1913, the appropriate part of which appeared in *The Lancet* as follows:

> A remedy provided with such a haptophoric group would be entirely innocuous of itself, as it is not fixed by the organs; it would, however, strike the parasites with full intensity, and in this sense would correspond to the immune productions, to the anti-substances discovered by Behring, and which, after the manner of the bewitched balls, fly in search of the enemy (27).

This reads like a translation, and probably is, since Ehrlich, although he could read English, was never fluent; but it was 'magic bullets' not 'bewitched balls' that subsequently caught the popular imagination. The nearest to a magic bullet that Ehrlich had been able to find by the time he gave this address was far from the ideal, but it was to be hailed as a triumph and was to confirm his reputation in the scientific pantheon.

Since Ehrlich's visit to England in 1907, his chemist at the Georg-Speyer Haus, Alfred Bertheim, had been charged with the task of producing numerous derivatives of arsenicals, which were then tested against trypanosomes in mice. The aim was to find a compound with an acceptable therapeutic index: the ratio of the curative to the toxic dose. Hundreds of derivatives were tested and in late 1908 Ehrlich was able to report that one—arsenophenylglycine; compound number 418—was proving promising. By this time a new type of organism was coming under scrutiny as a possible target: the spirochaetes, which were responsible for diseases such as syphilis and relapsing fever (an infection transmitted by ticks or lice) in man and spirillosis in chickens.

Spirochaetes had been described in 1905 by Friedrich (Fritz) Schaudinn and Erich Hoffmann in lymph node exudate from a case of syphilis (28). Spirochaetes were not at first recognized to be bacteria because of their unusual corkscrew-like appearance under the microscope. One theory was that they were related to the trypanosomes, which also have a rather serpentine motion because of the way their flagellum—the organ of motility—is attached to the body of the parasite. It was probably this erroneous association of spirochaetes with trypanosomes that led Ehrlich to decide to test his arsenical derivatives against these organisms.

The decision was a providential one, but Ehrlich was also setting his team formidable problems. The spirochaete of syphilis, *Treponema pallidum* (originally called *Spirochaeta pallida*; the pale spirochaete) is extremely difficult to handle in the laboratory: it is an unusually delicate bacterium which dies very quickly outside the body (hence the requirement for venereal transmission); moreover, laboratory animals are, in the ordinary sense, refractory to infection and the microbe cannot, even today, be grown reliably in cell-free culture in the test tube or Petri dish. These problems did not deter a new Japanese visitor to the Georg-Speyer Haus, Sahachiro Hata, who arrived at an opportune moment in Spring 1909. Hata was another prize pupil of Kitasato's and had discovered a way of propagating the spirochaete of syphilis in the testes of rabbits. He soon had the model set up in Frankfurt and was testing the arsenicals that Bertheim continued to provide. By the end of 1909 he was able to tell Ehrlich that compound 606—dihydroxydiamino arsenobenzene dihydrochloride (Fig. 3.2); later known as arsphenamine—was by far the most effective one that he had tested.

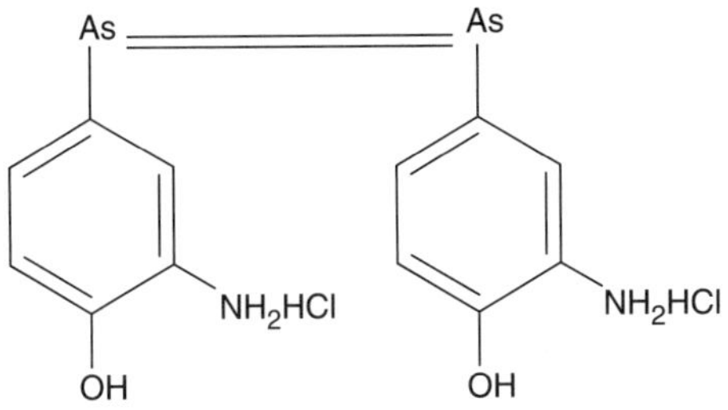

Fig. 3.2 Structure of arsphenamine (Salvarsan).

Compound 606 had already been in existence for about 2 years and had been rejected in favour of an earlier one, compound 418, arsenophenylglycine, which was already in tentative clinical trial. However, Hata was adamant that 606 was better and Ehrlich, who had a hunch that this compound would come good (29), cautiously arranged for a few trusted colleagues to test it in patients. Credit for the first therapeutic use of compound 606 in human beings goes to Professor Julius Iversen, a Finnish doctor working in the Obuchow Hospital in St. Petersburg, who used it to treat patients with relapsing fever. Most probably the first syphilitic patients to receive the drug were those suffering from tertiary syphilis—otherwise known as general paralysis of the insane—under the care of Professor Konrad Alt in the psychiatric hospital in Uchtspringe (30), a village lying north of Magdeburg in Sachsen-Anhalt. Other colleagues with whom Ehrlich was in contact in Magdeburg, Sarajevo, and Pavia were given the drug to treat cases of early syphilis.

Arsphenamine was not easy to handle: it spontaneously oxidized unless kept under vacuum and was very insoluble, so that it had first to be dissolved in alkali and then neutralized. Also it was not absorbed when given by mouth and intramuscular injections caused pain and tissue necrosis, so it had to be given by slow injection directly into the bloodstream—an uncommon procedure at the time. Ehrlich was able to mitigate some of the problems of arsphenamine by further derivatization to form a soluble salt, neoarsphenamine (compound 914) in 1912. Despite all the problems, arsphenamine was immediately, and perhaps prematurely, hailed as a success and Ehrlich was able to announce his discovery at the Congress for Internal Medicine held in Wiesbaden in April 1910. His fame among fellow scientists now extended to the general public and though he was inundated with requests for his 'miracle cure' he insisted that the drug must first be much more widely tested.

Facilities at the Georg-Speyer Haus were inadequate to synthesize arsphenamine (and later neoarsphenamine) in sufficient quantity and an arrangement was made with Farbwerke Hoechst to manufacture the drugs, which they named 'Salvarsan' and 'Neosalvarsan'.* Supplies were sent all over the world and were initially provided free of

---

* It was later marketed by Burroughs Wellcome as 'Kharsivan'; the firm also manufactured neoarsphenamine (Neosalvarsan) under the name Neo-Kharsivan. Another version of Neosalvarsan, Novarsenobillon, was produced by May & Baker in collaboration with Poulenc Frères in France.

charge. Among the recipients was Almroth Wright, the irascible Director of the Institute of Pathology and Research at St. Mary's Hospital, Paddington, and creator in 1907 of the famous 'Inoculation Department', which was financially independent and operated autonomously.* Wright was a champion of serum therapy (on which the finances of the Inoculation Department depended) and a friend of Ehrlich's; his book *Studies on Immunisation* (31) is dedicated to Metchnikov and Ehrlich.

Wright, like most of his contemporaries, but more vehemently than some, had little faith in specific chemotherapy as a possible route to the control of infectious disease. He naturally passed the drug on to his young assistants, Alexander Fleming and Leonard Colebrook (later Wright's biographer), who were to play such an important part in the realization of the dream of antimicrobial chemotherapy as it eventually unfolded. Ever inventive, Fleming and Colebrook devised a method to facilitate the intravenous delivery of the drug and proceeded to treat 46 patients suffering from primary, secondary, and tertiary syphilis. In a cartoon Ronald Gray, an artist friend of Fleming's who had introduced him to the Chelsea Arts Club, portrayed him in a kilt, cigarette in mouth and holding an enormous syringe, as 'Private 606'. Fleming and Colebrook's assessment of Salvarsan might be taken as typical of medical opinion at the time:

> Whether the new drug will displace mercury in the treatment of syphilis remains to be seen, and we do not venture to express any opinion on this subject. It, however, certainly has a remarkable effect in causing the lesions [of syphilis] to disappear, and especially is this seen in some cases which have resisted mercurial treatment. Much has been made of the dangers inherent in the administration of the drug, but so far as we have gone we have not seen the slightest trace of the evil effects which have been written about in any case which has been injected intravenously (32).

The dangers of Salvarsan use were, however, all too apparent. In 1918 the Medical Research Committee (later Medical Research Council) set up a 'Salvarsan Committee' partly in response to concerns about toxicity. A comprehensive survey published by the Committee in 1922 found a number of adverse events, some of which the investigators attributed simply to the known harmful effects of arsenic. Damage to the liver was a prominent finding, sometimes leading to death. With hindsight many of these cases were probably attributable to viral hepatitis, though the Salvarsan Committee—having no knowledge of the virus—reasonably argued that the relationship to Salvarsan treatment was too frequent to be merely accidental. The overall incidence of fatalities was found to be only around 1 in 5000 to 1 in 10,000 (33). Of course, at this time, as now with cancer or AIDS, side effects of treatment were more acceptable, when little else was on offer. As the Salvarsan Committee lucidly observed:

> The patient who is suffering from syphilis, and the doctor who proposes to treat him, have to choose between two risks. On the one hand is the more or less measurable risk attendant on the arsenobenzol treatment which offers the most hopeful prospect of cure; on the other the risks, that cannot so accurately be measured, which may attend uncured syphilis.

---

* The Wright–Fleming Institute business was sold in 1959 to the firm of CL Bencard, a subsidiary of Beecham Research Laboratories (see p. 124).

Not everyone was enthusiastic about Salvarsan and Neosalvarsan. Reports of the harmful effects of treatment, and general suspicion of the use of artificial chemicals, particularly those based on known poisons such as arsenic, led to condemnation of the new treatment in some quarters. One trenchant critic was Victor Mentberger from the dermatological clinic* of the University of Strasbourg, who in a monograph surveying the place of arsenic therapy in syphilis, published in 1913, described as many as 274 fatalities after the use of Salvarsan (34). In another famous incident in 1914, the Director of the Frankfurt dermatological clinic, Karl Herxheimer was accused by a Frankfurt newspaper, *Der Freigeist*, of having used the drug forcibly on his patients, including prostitutes, some of whom had died. Ehrlich himself was vilified and was called to testify in the subsequent libel trial. The editor of *Der Freigeist*, Karl Wassmann was found guilty and jailed for 1 year, though he served only 2 months, being released on a general amnesty at the start of the First World War (35). In 1933, with the rise of the Nazis, Herxheimer was forbidden to enter the Frankfurt clinic and was, like von Weinberg, later deported to the Theresienstadt ghetto, where he died (36).

Paul Ehrlich died from a stroke in August 1915. He had been showered with honours and his fame was assured, but his final years were clouded with worries: his country was at war and the work of his institute consequently disrupted; the Wassmann affair had left a sour taste; and his health was failing. Above all the chemotherapy work was unfinished. He was well aware that Salvarsan was far from being the solution to the treatment of infection. Quite apart from its very limited spectrum of activity—confined to spirochaetal diseases such as syphilis, yaws, and relapsing fever—it was far from fulfilling his dreams of *therapia sterilisans magna*;† that is, a therapy that would eliminate the microbes in one, or at the most two, doses and thus prevent them from developing resistance, a phenomenon that he had already observed in his work with the effects of trypan red on trypanosomes.

Ehrlich's legacy

Although Paul Ehrlich fully deserves the epithet 'father of chemotherapy', in truth his direct influence on antimicrobial chemotherapy as it was to develop in the decades after his death was relatively small. In the light of subsequent experience, the arsenical compounds for which Ehrlich and his colleagues were responsible were not an unqualified success, though they remained in clinical use in some quarters beyond the introduction of penicillin. It became clear early on that the drugs were only reliably curative in the early stages of syphilis and had little benefit in the late stages of the disease.

....

* In Germany and some other countries of continental Europe, sexually-transmitted diseases are often dealt with by specialists in dermatology.

† Ehrlich ended his Nobel lecture in 1908 with the words: 'For with the help of this substance [arsenophenylglycine] it is really possible in every animal species and with every kind of trypanosome infection to achieve a *complete cure* with *one* injection, a result which corresponds to what I call *therapia sterilisans magna*'.

Many attempts were made to improve on the efficacy of Ehrlich's Salvarsan and Neosalvarsan. In England, Burroughs Wellcome marketed a substance called Kharsulphan; similar compounds that were put on sale included Metarsenobillon (May & Baker in collaboration with Poulenc Frères in France), and Sulpharsenol (Laboratoire de Biochimie Médicale). In America a derivative called Mapharsen (oxaphenarsine) was introduced in the 1930s by Parke, Davis and company, and was subsequently widely used for the treatment of syphilis by American physicians until penicillin superseded it during the Second World War. The molecule had originally been investigated by Paul Ehrlich, but was rejected on the grounds of toxicity. It was revived by the chemist Arthur Tatum* when he took over the chair of pharmacology and toxicology at the University of Wisconsin from Arthur S Loevenhart, who died suddenly in 1929. Tatum had inherited a collaborative programme on arsenicals for use in syphilis and trypanosomiasis that his predecessor had negotiated with Parke, Davis and Frank Whitmore of Northwestern University. Whitmore provided the Mapharsen—a name coined by Tatum—and it turned out to be much less toxic than had been believed (37).

Among other arsenical compounds that found some advocates in the interwar years were sulfarsphenamine and sulfoxylsalvarsan (Myosalvarsan), but neither survived into regular therapeutic use. Since results with all the arsenical compounds were often disappointing, combination therapy, in which arsenicals were used together with the former standard treatment, mercury, or with bismuth or silver, was commonly recommended.

Some efforts to find antibacterial compounds that would fulfil Ehrlich's chemotherapeutic ambitions continued after his death. Julius Morgenroth, an assistant, who had accompanied Ehrlich to Frankfurt from Steglitz, remained a leading proponent of chemotherapy and continued to pursue research in this field after he moved back to Berlin in 1905 to become head of the bacteriology section of the Pathological Institute at the Charité. In 1911 he synthesized a series of quinine derivatives (another quinine connection!), with a view to uncovering useful antibacterial activity or improving the potency against malaria parasites. One of these compounds, ethylhydrocupreine (Optochin), had a marked inhibitory action against pneumococci in the test tube and in mice. Unfortunately, when human trials were started, it proved toxic, causing irreversible damage to the optic nerve. The risk of severe side effects was no barrier to use in a condition such as pneumonia, which carried a mortality of at least 25 per cent, and Optochin or its soluble ethyl carbamate salt, Solvochin, continued to be used sporadically until safer drugs became available. Almroth Wright, one of the first investigators to use Optochin, was more cautious. He was in South Africa investigating antipneumococcal vaccines in gold mine workers among whom pneumonia was common. When he learnt from Morgenroth of the possibility of blindness, and some of his earliest patients showed signs of optic damage, he quickly abandoned the trial. The failure did nothing to improve his

---

* Father of the biochemist and microbial geneticist, Edward Lawrie Tatum (1909–1975; Nobel laureate 1978).

scepticism about the potential of antibacterial chemotherapy. Optochin has survived into present day use, not as a therapeutic drug, but as a reagent for the laboratory identification of pneumococci, which are much more sensitive to its action than other streptococci. Similar quinoline derivatives, including Eucupin and Vuzin reached the market in Germany, but interest faded once sulphonamides and penicillin appeared.

The British bacteriologist, Carl Browning pursued an interest in dyes that he had acquired while working with Ehrlich in Frankfurt. Among the substances he had worked with there was a yellow dye, trypaflavine, a derivative of acridine orange that was active against trypanosomes. On his return to the United Kingdom, Browning showed that trypaflavine, which he called acriflavine, and a precursor compound, proflavine, were effective germicides when applied to wounds; moreover, they had the benefit over other local antiseptics that they were not inactivated by serum. Browning and his colleagues published their findings in 1917; it was an opportune time to test the effectiveness of acriflavine in field hospitals and it soon proved its value (38).

Morgenroth also experimented with acridine derivatives and produced a compound called Rivanol, which claimed to be less irritant than acriflavine. It enjoyed a short vogue in the treatment of amoebic dysentery, but was soon abandoned. It can still be found as a component of some proprietary medicines in continental Europe. Later acridines were intensively investigated for antimalarial activity by the chemists of the Bayer organization, eventually leading to the discovery of the antimalarial drug, atebrin (see p. 291).

In America, Hugh Young, a genito-urinary surgeon at the Johns Hopkins Hospital in Baltimore who had been stimulated by Ehrlich's ideas when he attended his address to the International Medical Congress in London in 1913, introduced a compound called mercurochrome just after the end of First World War (39). It was originally intended as a urinary antiseptic for instillation into the bladder, but speculative intravenous use in septicaemia appeared to produce some impressive cures and it enjoyed a short vogue, especially in the United States, before it was discarded for systemic infections. Leonard Colebrook and Ronald Hare tested mercurochrome in Almroth Wright's Inoculation Department at St. Mary's Hospital shortly before Alexander Fleming's discovery of penicillin (40), but the substance evoked little impact in Britain.

Meanwhile, at the Institut Pasteur in Paris, Albert Frouin was fruitlessly trying to harness metals into service as antimicrobial compounds. One such compound, stannoxyl, a mixture of tin and stannous oxide, was briefly championed in Britain by a Royal Army Medical Corps captain, Arthur Compton, who had earlier worked with Frouin at the Institut Pasteur. He treated several patients, who had been referred to him for the preparation of autogenous vaccines* for the management of boils or acne, with tablets of stannoxyl obtained from France (41). Although he claimed remarkable success and went on to repeat the exercise in some poorly characterized cases of so-called 'mixed infection'

* Autogenous vaccines—killed suspensions of organisms isolated from the patient that were suspected of being the cause of a problem—were widely used between the wars in the belief that they would boost the body's immunity. They were still occasionally being used in Harley Street in the 1960s.

accompanying pulmonary tuberculosis (42), few were impressed and the drug fell into well-deserved obscurity.

Despite these desultory reports and the acknowledged success of arsenical compounds in syphilis, the prevailing view of systemic antibacterial chemotherapy, or 'inner disinfection' as it was often called, remained profoundly sceptical. Most informed opinion in the interwar years took the view that attacking bacteria within the complex environment of the human body without causing unacceptable toxicity was likely to be extremely difficult, if not impossible.

Some seemingly authoritative statements from this period are heavy with dramatic irony. In a lecture to the Harvey Society of New York delivered on 8 December 1923, the distinguished American pharmacologist Walter A Jacobs of the Rockefeller Institute* opined:

> At present the data available seem quite barren of suggestion...In the case of bacterial infections, experience has presented us with too few points of contact between our knowledge of chemical structure and whatever biological properties may be required in the exhibition of a therapeutic effect to present a rational basis for the search for curative substances (43).

Little did Jacobs know that a potent antibacterial compound was already available in his laboratory. The Director of the Rockefeller, Simon Flexner, had in 1912 chosen Jacobs to head the Institute's chemotherapy research effort. Together with his colleague Michael Heidelberger he investigated hydrocuprein derivatives and *Cinchona* alkaloids as well as analogues of Ehrlich's arsenicals (and discovered one, tryparsamide, which was to prove useful in African sleeping sickness; see p. 278). One of the intermediates they were using to modify these compounds was a chemical called *p*-aminobenzenesulphonamide, which had been synthesized in 1908 in Vienna by the chemist, Paul Gelmo. This substance—later known as sulphanilamide—turned out to be the major breakthrough in antimicrobial chemotherapy that would point the way to further chemotherapeutic triumphs. Jacobs and Heidelberger, writing of their researches in 1919 had noted that 'Many of the substances described in this paper were highly bactericidal *in vitro*, a property which will be discussed in the appropriate place by our colleague Dr Martha Wolstein' (44). Martha Wollstein (her name was misspelt in Jacobs and Heidelberger's paper) was a medically qualified bacteriologist at the Rockefeller, with a particular interest in children's diseases. The promised publication never materialized, perhaps because she became preoccupied with the bacteriology of Spanish flu, which was raging at the time. It is, in any case, unlikely that *p*-aminobenzenesulphonamide, a substance used only as a reagent in the Rockefeller investigations, would be among those tested for antibacterial activity, but a

---

* The Rockefeller Institute (now Rockefeller University), founded in 1901, was established through the generosity of the remarkable American entrepreneur and philanthropist, John D Rockefeller. Medical research in the United States and elsewhere benefited enormously from the generosity of Rockefeller (whose father had been a travelling quack) and his son, John D Rockefeller Jr, as will be clear from many references throughout this book.

major discovery was tantalizingly close at hand to scientists working in a laboratory dedicated to chemotherapy in one of the most prestigious research institutes in the world. Fickle Lady Luck sometimes likes to tease.

Carl Browning perhaps showed more culpable ignorance in delivering the presidential address to the Royal Medico-Chirurgical Society of Glasgow on 4 October 1935 (45). Reviewing progress in chemotherapy over the previous 30 years, he could point only to a handful of antiprotozoal compounds, 'an almost miraculous spirochaeticide'—Salvarsan—and a few antiseptics. For the systemic treatment of bacterial infections the cupboard was bare (spirochaetes were an atypical exception). Though he spoke and read German, Browning was plainly not keeping up with developments in Germany. Even as he addressed the worthies of Glasgow, the first (even more miraculous) results with a new red dye were filtering through to an incredulous medical profession. Only the previous day—3 October 1935—the properties of the dye had been revealed at a notable meeting of the Royal Society of Medicine in London (46).

From dyes to sulphonamides

Although general enthusiasm for Ehrlich's ideas soon waned in the years after his death, interest continued in German dyestuff companies, which held around 80 per cent of the world market for dyes at the time of the First World War. Before the war the growing strength of these firms had already encouraged them to diversify into pharmaceuticals and other products. Following Ehrlich's lead, arsenicals and other metallic compounds came under scrutiny, but, quite naturally, his ideas on the potential of dyes and dye derivatives occupied much of their attention. Particularly appealing to them was the idea that dyes with specific binding affinities that were 'parasitotropic', rather than 'organotropic'—two of Ehrlich's favourite adjectives—might lead to compounds suitable for treatment of human disease.

Dyes themselves were known to possess antibacterial activity, even in high dilution, and attempts were sometimes made in the spirit of Guttmann and Ehrlich's work with methylene blue in malaria to use them for systemic therapy. These forays met with little success, but some acidic dyes proved useful when applied topically and were once widely used for purposes as diverse as treatment of infected burns and pre-operative skin sterilization. Methylene blue itself enjoyed a short and unrewarding vogue as a urinary antiseptic. Those with memories that stretch back to before the 1950s will remember the common sight of children with impetigo lesions brightly stained with crystal violet (gentian violet). Crystal violet paint is still available for topical application, but it is now seldom used for skin infections; similarly, use in yeast infections of the mouth or vagina (thrush), which was also once common, is now discouraged because of the risk of causing mucosal ulceration. The bright red paint devised by the mercurial Italian physician Aldo Castellani for use in superficial fungal infections was also widely used. The preparation owed its colour to a red dye, basic fuchsin, but the antifungal activity was as likely to be due to other ingredients, which included phenol, resorcinol, and alcohol, and modern preparations are usually colourless.

The first fruits of the search for dye derivatives that might be useful in human disease were in the field of tropical medicine, chiefly in the form of antiprotozoal agents for the treatment of African sleeping sickness and malaria (see Chapter 7). Remarkably, methylene blue itself was still occasionally being recommended for the treatment of malaria as late as 1925 (47). Hope of finding a dye that would be useful for the systemic treatment of bacterial infection was pursued most energetically within the Bayer organization—from 1925 to 1945 part of IG Farbenindustrie.*

Success eventually came in 1932, but in the most extraordinary fashion. In perhaps the clearest example in medical history of scientific theory being turned on its head, investigation of a dye led to the discovery of a powerful antibacterial agent that was already sitting unsuspected on the chemists' shelves. In the process the fate of dyes as potential therapeutic compounds was virtually sealed.

The discovery of Prontosil

In 1927 Heinrich Hörlein, director of research at IG Farben's Elberfeld plant, recruited a 32-year-old doctor called Gerhard Domagk, to head a new Institute of Experimental Pathology (expanded in 1929 to Experimental Pathology and Bacteriology). Domagk was born the son of a teacher in Lagow in Mark Brandenburg, Eastern Germany (now Łagów, Poland). He enrolled in medicine at the University of Kiel in 1914, but his studies were interrupted by the outbreak of war and he soon found himself learning the trade at first hand serving as a medical orderly on both the western and eastern fronts. The experiences of wound trauma and infections on the battlefield made a profound impression on him. On resuming his studies and qualifying after the war, he established his reputation in the field of pathological anatomy in Kiel City Hospital and the University of Greifswald, where he investigated the interaction of bacteria with the reticulo-endothelial system. By 1927 he was a lecturer at the Institute of Pathology of the University of Münster, where his interests also included tumour pathology. The contract he signed with IG Farben was initially for 2 years, since he was firmly set on an academic career and had obtained leave of absence from Münster as part of the arrangement. In the event he stayed at Elberfeld until his retirement in 1960. Domagk's studies had convinced him of the primacy of host immunity in defence against bacterial infection. Consequently—and, as it turned out, fortunately—when systematic investigation of potential antibacterial compounds began in 1929, substances received from the chemists were not only tested *in vitro*, but were also tested in animals, where they could support highly efficient host defence mechanisms. Domagk's favoured model was infection of mice with a very virulent strain of *Streptococcus pyogenes* originally isolated from a patient suffering from septicaemia.

....

* A loose amalgamation between AGFA, BASF, and Bayer had been established in 1904; this was expanded in 1916 to include the Hoechst group and two chemical firms, Weiler-ter Meer and Griesheim-Elektron. The arrangement was formalized as 'Interessengemeinschaft der Deutschen Teerfarbenindustrie AG', in 1925.

The chemists charged with synthesizing compounds for Domagk to test were Fritz Mietzsch and Josef Klarer. The first substances Domagk received were arsenicals, antimonials, the currently fashionable gold salts (at least one of which was subjected to a limited clinical trial) or acridine derivatives. Some exhibited antibacterial activity, but were too feeble or too toxic to excite further interest (48). Soon the chemists turned their attention to basic azo dyes. The approach was thoughtful and systematic.

A red dye called chrysoidine had been synthesized in 1875 by Heinrich Caro,* Head of Research at the Badische Anilin und Soda Fabrik (BASF)—he was also responsible for the synthesis of methylene blue—and independently by Otto Witt, an émigré German who worked for the dyestuff firm of Williams, Thomas & Dower in Brentford, North London.† This compound was known to possess germicidal properties; it had been used as an antiseptic and had briefly attracted the attention of Paul Ehrlich. The structure was that of a diazo compound (i.e. it contained an N=N linkage) with a diamino substituted benzene ring attached to one nitrogen (forming the coloured part of the molecule) and a simple benzene ring attached to the other (Fig. 3.3). Related compounds had been prepared by various workers and even used clinically as urinary antiseptics or in the treatment of gonorrhoea.

Hörlein had experimented with sulphonamide derivatives of azo dyes as early as 1909. It had transpired that the sulphonamide component improved the binding of the dyes to natural fibres, enhancing their colour fastness. Realizing that the same type of substitution might increase the affinity of dyes to bacterial cells, it was decided to synthesize chrysoidine analogues in which the simple benzene ring was substituted with a sulphonamide grouping (SO_2NH_2). One of these compounds, synthesized by Josef Klarer (substance Kl 695), in which a rather complex diethyl substitution had been made to the chromophore, proved effective and safe in Domagk's mouse model, though puzzlingly it had no useful activity in the test tube. A much simpler derivative, compound Kl 730, a sulphonamide-substituted version of chrysoidine, solutions of which resembled red ink, was passed to Domagk's laboratory for testing in December 1932. According to the pathologist Ekkehard Grundmann, who knew Domagk and had access to his diaries,‡

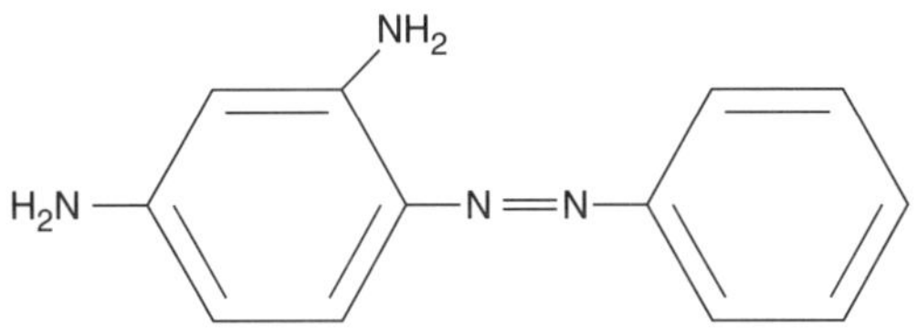

Fig. 3.3 Structure of chrysoidine.

---

* Caro had learnt his trade in England and was a friend of William Henry Perkin.

† Both Caro and Witt probably relied on information from Johann Peter Griess another expatriate German who worked as a chemist for Allsopp's Brewery at Burton-on-Trent. He had discovered a simple way of making diazo compounds as a student in Magdeburg and continued to make azo dyes in his spare time while working for Allsopp's (see Ref. 4).

‡ Grundmann succeeded Domagk at Bayer a few years after his retirement in 1960; he later became Director of the Gerhard Domagk Institute for Pathology at the University of Münster.

he was away at a scientific meeting at the time and a laboratory technician, Margarete Gerresheim, was the first to observe the astonishing results in tests of Kl 730 in mice (49). Intrigued, but sceptical on hearing of the results on his return, Domagk set about repeating the experiment himself, starting on 20 December 1932 and continuing over the Christmas period. The outcome was crystal clear. Klarer's compound was amazingly effective: 26 mice had been infected with the highly virulent *Streptococcus*; 12 that had received various dilutions of Kl 730 by mouth were all alive and healthy 8 days later, while the 14 untreated control mice had all died within 72 h (Fig. 3.4).

Streptokokkenversuch vom 20. XII. 1932

infiziert mit 1:1000 verdünnter Eibouillonkultur, 0,3 ccm i. p; behandelt $1\frac{1}{2}$ Stunde nach der Infektion

Nr.	Gewicht	Präparat Nr.	%	Dosis	Art der Behdlg.	21. XII.	22. XII.	23. XII.	24. XII.	25. XII.	26. XII.	27. XII.	28. XII.
201	14 g					m	kr.	kr.	†				
202	14 g					m	†						
203	14 g	Anfangskontrollen				m	†						
204	17 g					m	†						
205	19 g					m	†						
206	14 g					m	m	†					
303	18 g	Prontosil	0,01%	0,2	per os	m	m	m	m	m	m	m	m
304	19 g			0,2		m	m	m	m	m	m	m	m
305	18 g			1,0		m	m	m	m	m	m	m	m
306	14 g			1,0		m	m	m	m	m	m	m	m
307	16 g		0,1 %	0,2		m	m	m	m	m	m	m	m
308	15 g			0,2		m	m	m	m	m	m	m	m
309	17 g			1,0		m	m	m	m	m	m	m	m
310	17 g			1,0		m	m	m	m	m	m	m	m
311	14 g		1,0 %	0,2		m	m	m	m	m	m	m	m
312	17 g			0,2		m	m	m	m	m	m	m	m
313	18 g			1,0		m	m	m	m	m	m	m	m
314	14 g			1,0		m	m	m	m	m	m	m	m
315	18 g					m	kr.	†					
316	16 g					m	†						
317	15 g					m	†						
318	14 g	Endkontrollen				m	†						
319	15 g					m	†						
320	14 g					m	†						
321	15 g					m	†						
322	17 g					m	†						

m = munter, kr. = krank, † = tot

Fig. 3.4 Domagk's mouse experiment of 20 December 1932 in which the efficacy of Prontosil against *Streptococcus pyogenes* was first demonstrated. From: Domagk G (1935) Ein Beitrag zur Chemotherapie der bakteriellen Infektionen. *Deutsche Medizinische Wochenschrift* 61, 250–3. Reproduced courtsey of Georg Thieme Verlag, Stuttgart. m, healthy; kr, sick; †, dead.

As a dedicated pathologist, Domagk carried out histological examination of the mice and came to the conclusion that Kl 730 (later called streptozon and given the trade name Prontosil rubrum) had caused a degenerative effect on the streptococci allowing them to be effectively ingested and cleared by phagocytic cells, apparently explaining the lack of effect in the test tube.

Mietzsch and Klarer lost no time in filing a patent application for Prontosil and related substances on Christmas day 1932; the full patent was eventually granted on 2 January 1935 (50). In the meantime, further safety tests were carried out in mice, rabbits, and cats and tentative clinical trials were started. The first report of the effectiveness of Prontosil (while it was still known as streptozon) was made to a meeting of the Vereinigung Düsseldorfer Dermatologen (Union of Düsseldorf dermatologists) on 17 May 1933—a time better remembered in German history as being shortly after Hitler had come to power as Reichskanzler. The patient was a 10-month-old boy* dying of a staphylococcal septicaemia. He had been treated with various medications available at that time, including a dubious vaccine preparation known as Streptosan, but his condition continued to deteriorate. At the end of March 1933 he was close to death and was speculatively given half a tablet of streptozon by mouth twice a day (with short interruptions) for 3 weeks. After 4 days his temperature had gradually reverted to normal and his general condition was good. Several weeks later the child was discharged from hospital. The case was, subsequently published as a short report in *Zentralblatt für Haut- und Geschlechtskrankheiten*; the name of the doctor making the historic presentation to the assembled dermatologists is revealed only by his surname, Foerster (51).† The meeting Chairman, Professor Hans Theodor Schreus, director of the skin clinic of the Düsseldorf medical academy (and, by inference, Dr Foerster's superior), added the comment that by chance he had just received the drug from IG Farben for clinical testing. Although streptozon was intended for use in streptococcal infection, it was decided to try it on the staphylococci infecting this moribund infant. (*Are you still alive, fortunate child? Or did you perhaps succumb to some later childhood illness, or to the terrible bombing that reduced the population of Düsseldorf by half between 1939 and 1945?*)

Several other preliminary reports followed in 1934, but it was in the 15 February 1935 issue of *Deutsche Medizinische Wochenschrift*, soon after the Prontosil patent was awarded, that Domagk described his experimental results (52). The same issue carried the first detailed clinical reports from Philipp Klee's department in Wuppertal (53) and from Schreus in Düsseldorf (54), the professor this time reserving the glory for himself. In December 1935 Domagk's 6-year-old daughter, Hildegard, became another early beneficiary of Prontosil treatment. She had fallen down the stairs at home and a needle she was holding penetrated her hand and broke. The needle was removed surgically, but, as was

---

* In Theodor Schreus's 1935 description of the first use of Prontosil (54)—apparently the same case— the child is described as 1.5 years old.

† Daniel Bovet, in his account of the discovery of sulphonamides, *Une chimie qui guérit: histoire de la découverte des sulfamides* (Editions Payot, 1988) gives Foerster's first name as Richard. I am indebted to John Lesch of the University of California, Berkeley for this information.

common at the time, the wound became badly infected and Domagk persuaded the surgeon to allow him to administer Prontosil by mouth and rectally (55). The drug probably saved her from amputation of the arm, if not from death.

With the discovery of the remarkable safety and efficacy of Prontosil rubrum and the development a little later of the soluble disodium salt, 'Prontosil solubile', which was suitable for injection, the IG Farben executives must have thought they had found a goldmine. They could certainly congratulate themselves: the discovery had been made through unrivalled expertise and brilliant teamwork; patents conferring sole rights had been secured in the major trading nations. But Lady Luck, who often seems intent on exposing the efforts of mere mortals to ridicule, had other ideas.

The French connection

After the publication of Domagk's paper in February 1935, scientists in France were quick off the mark in following up the findings. A request to IG Farben for a sample of the drug was turned down, probably because the firm of Rhône-Poulenc was party to the discussions between Heinrich Hörlein and Ernest Fourneau—head of the therapeutic chemistry laboratory of the Institut Pasteur and close associate of the Poulenc brothers—and the issue was still commercially sensitive. However, although Prontosil was subject to a patent, French law did not recognize the patenting of medicinal products and it was synthesized under the name 'Rubiazol' by André Girard, a chemist at Rhône-Poulenc. On 6 May the Romanian-born immunologist, Constantin Levaditi and his collaborator Aron Vaisman at the Institut Alfred Fournier in Paris were able to report the activity in laboratory animals at a meeting of the Académie des Sciences (56). Later that year, Jacques Tréfouël and his wife Thérèse, together with Daniel Bovet and his brother-in-law, Federico Nitti, examined a series of analogues of Prontosil and found that only those containing a sulphonamide group were active. They proposed that the diazo bond of Prontosil was split in the body and when each component was separately synthesized, p-aminobenzenesulphonamide itself (sulphanilamide) was found to be the active moiety (57)—the chromophore on which the work of Klarer and Mietzsch had been based was revealed to play no part whatsoever in the antibacterial activity. The two structures are compared in Fig. 3.5.

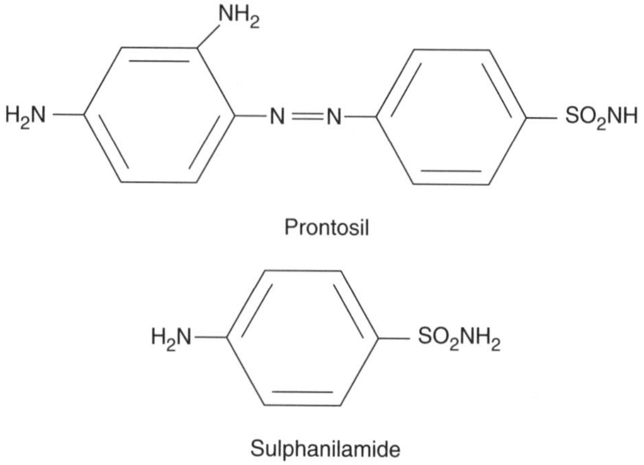

Prontosil

Sulphanilamide

Fig. 3.5 Structures of Prontosil and sulphanilamide.

Sulphanilamide was subject to no patent restrictions. By the start of the Second World War, it was widely available under at least 33 different trade names and chemists everywhere were trying to improve upon it.

None the less, the big breakthrough had been made in Domagk's laboratory and it was his report that alerted the discovery to the world. In 1938 he was nominated for the Nobel Prize and in October 1939 he received a telegram from Stockholm telling him that the nomination was successful. Adolf Hitler had other ideas. When Carl von Ossietzky, the editor of the pacifist newspaper *Weltbühne* had been awarded the Peace Prize in 1935,* Hitler had decreed that no German citizen should accept the honour. After an altercation with the Gestapo during which he was briefly imprisoned, Domagk reluctantly wrote to the Nobel Committee that 'In accordance with the law of which I have now been fully advised, I am obliged to decline the prize offered to me'.

After the war, Domagk was able to travel to Sweden to receive his Nobel Prize, though he did not get the prize money, which had been returned to the general fund according to the rules. For the ceremony he wore his wedding suit since he had lost his dress suit in the aftermath of war; his brother-in-law lent him a suitable waistcoat and tie.

Few would begrudge Domagk the award of this high accolade, especially as he received no monetary benefit from it. But in reality, Domagk did not discover, or invent Prontosil. It was an Elberfeld team effort aided and abetted by a sizeable contribution from Lady Luck. In actual fact, the attention focused on Gerhard Domagk rankled with his colleagues, not least with Josef Klarer, who had synthesized Prontosil and whose health had suffered during the frequent bombing raids of the war. He remained unrecognized beyond receiving, together with his chemist colleague Fritz Mietzsch, an honorary doctorate from the University of Münster. Heinrich Hörlein, who had initiated the project that led to Prontosil, was even less fortunate. As a member of the board of management of IG Farben he was arraigned before the war trial court at Nuremberg. Thirteen of his 23 fellow directors were sentenced to terms of imprisonment, but Hörlein's record of scientific achievement provided him with a successful defence and he was acquitted. Although he had joined the National Socialist Party in 1934, cogent reasons were adduced that this was a ploy to put himself in a better position to protect the company, which had been the subject of suspicion and direct attack by sections of the party because of the use of animals in research (the Nazis preferred human beings for their bizarre experiments) and production of treatments for tropical diseases, which benefited the enemies of the Fatherland (see p. 276). In fact, Hörlein had an unblemished record of opposition to many aspects of party activities and there is no evidence that he collaborated in providing material for unethical human experiments (58).

The sulphonamide phenomenon

The discovery of sulphonamides as potent antibacterial agents altered the perception of science and medicine to the possibilities of the effective treatment of infection and paved

* Ossietzky was at that time in a Concentration camp in Germany. He was officially said to be free to go to Norway to receive the prize, but was refused a passport. He was released into a civilian hospital and died of tuberculosis in 1938.

the way for the antibiotic revolution. After Heinrich Hörlein described the properties of Prontosil to a British audience at a meeting of the Section of Tropical Diseases and Parasitology of the Royal Society of Medicine on 3 October 1935 (46), the *Lancet* reported that the president of the meeting Philip Manson-Bahr had remarked, no doubt with the customary politeness of such occasions, but with unwittingly prescient understatement '...that a contribution to chemotherapeutics had been made by Prof. Hörlein which might indeed prove to be monumental' (59).

Hörlein had stressed that the activity of Prontosil was virtually restricted to *Streptococcus pyogenes* (and, perhaps, staphylococci), a much-feared pathogen responsible for scarlet fever, puerperal fever, erysipelas, septicaemia, and rheumatic fever among other things. From the start, then, it was natural that it was the antistreptococcal activity that received the greatest attention. The first clinical results in England came from Queen Charlotte's Maternity Hospital, which had opened on a new site in Chiswick in West London in 1930.* The new hospital incorporated a special unit for the treatment of cases of puerperal fever, a complication of childbirth as greatly feared then as it had been in Victorian times, and included a laboratory, known as the Bernhard Baron Research Laboratory after the memorial fund that had provided most of the money for the venture. The natural choice for Director of the new laboratory was Leonard Colebrook— universally known as 'Coli'—who had a special interest in puerperal fever and was one of the few medical scientists in the country interested in chemotherapy. He had collaborated with Fleming in testing Salvarsan (see p. 60) and, having noted that associated streptococcal infections often cleared up when treating syphilitics, had investigated the possibility of treating streptococcal infections with arsenical compounds (60). Inexplicably, he does not seem to have taken any interest in trying out penicillin, which his former colleague at St. Mary's Hospital described in 1929 (see p. 92).

Coli was a cautious and meticulous worker. By 1935 he was convinced that the way forward lay in strict preventive measures rather than systemic chemotherapy and he was instrumental in introducing the use of a new disinfectant, chlorxylenol (Dettol), which he had learned of from a distant cousin who worked for the firm of Messrs Reckitts, and which proved to be very non-toxic when applied to skin. He was, however, alert to the new continental developments in chemotherapy. As early as mid-March 1935, scarcely a month after Domagk's landmark paper he had been in correspondence with Henry Dale, Director of the National Institute for Medical Research and Francis Green, Secretary of the Medical Research Council's Therapeutic Trials Committee offering to investigate the new drug (61).†

---

* Queen Charlotte's moved again in 2000 to a new unit on the Hammersmith Hospital site.

† According to his biographer, Bill Noble, Coli did not learn about Prontosil until some time after Hörlein's address to the Royal Society of Medicine in October 1935. News was supposedly conveyed by a postcard from a friend from his student days, Claude Lillingston, who then lived in Paris (62, p. 66). Whatever the role of this missive, research by the historian John Lesch (61) clearly shows that Colebrook knew about Prontosil in March 1935.

With some difficulty Coli obtained samples of Prontosil from Germany and the French equivalent from Paris. Some preliminary work in mice failed to confirm the activity, but Gladwin Buttle of the Wellcome laboratories had also been studying the new compound and had obtained encouraging results that persuaded Coli to attempt the first tentative clinical trial with the help of Méave Kenny, resident medical officer at Queen Charlotte's. The first patient, recorded in Coli's own notes, was:

> Mrs R. Admission 14/1/36 6th day after labour with scarlatinal erythema, especially on trunk and legs. Abdomen very suggestive of early generalized peritonitis, but tenderness mostly on right. Pulse 140, rising after admission to 150. Temperature 104–5°F. Prognosis very bad.

Mrs R recovered and the entry ends with the laconic statement: 'Seems likely that the drug may have helped' (62).

This case and 37 others, in which a mortality rate of 8 per cent was obtained, compared with around 25 per cent in similar cases during the previous year, was published in *The Lancet* (63), but there was still considerable doubt about the significance of the findings. Coli himself remained characteristically cautious, but pressed on with treating 26 more women with equally good results (64). However, there had been no untreated control group in either study, since Coli had considered this unethical, and he freely conceded that other factors—for example, a coincidental fall in virulence of streptococci involved in puerperal fever—might have been involved in their spectacular success. Reviewing the evidence, Colebrook's colleague, the obstetric surgeon Frederick Gibberd, who was an advisor in obstetrics to the Ministry of Health, and held appointments at Guy's Hospital and Queen Charlotte's, had similar doubts about the interpretation of the results, but was clearly impressed with the obvious decline in mortality since Prontosil had been introduced (65). Lawrence Paul Garrod, Professor of Microbiology at St Bartholomew's Hospital, in an unsigned editorial in the *British Medical Journal* written in early 1937* soon after the publication of Colebrook and Kenny's second study, was prepared to be more unequivocal:

> ...it may be said that the promised value of this treatment in streptococcal infections alone bids fair to place it among the major therapeutic discoveries of modern times (66).

The prediction was amply justified. In childbed fever alone the new treatment was to save the lives of countless young mothers. Between 1935, when Prontosil was first described and 1945, when penicillin became generally available, the maternal mortality rate—a rate that had scarcely altered in 100 years—showed a dramatic decline (Fig. 3.6). The fall in mortality from erysipelas was equally spectacular, though another important streptococcal disease, scarlet fever, was less strikingly affected, since the disease was already yielding to better nutrition and housing, combined, perhaps, to a decline in virulence of the causative organism (67).

Two of the earliest male beneficiaries of Prontosil treatment in England, were Coli's colleagues in the Bernhard Baron Laboratory, Ronald Hare, later to become professor of

---

* The year in which Garrod was promoted to the Chair of Bacteriology at Bart's.

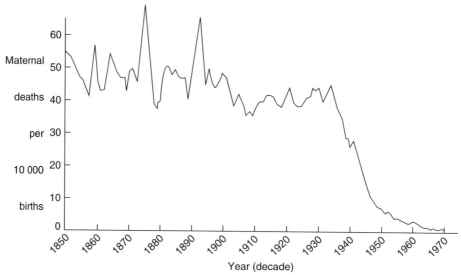

Fig. 3.6 Annual rates of maternal mortality in England and Wales, 1850–1970 (data from *Decennial Supplements*, Registrar General for England and Wales). Reproduced from: Loudon I. *Death in childbirth*. Clarendon Press, Oxford, 1992, p. 15.

microbiology at St. Thomas' Hospital, London and Winston Maxted, a laboratory technician, who later became an international expert on streptococci. Two days after the historical admission to hospital of Mrs R, Coli's first treatment success, Hare had cut himself with a sliver of glass contaminated with streptococci and was subsequently admitted to St. Mary's Hospital in a serious condition; 2 months later, Maxted developed a severe tonsillitis in the course of his work with virulent streptococci. Both men received intravenous Prontosil and turned a bright red colour, but both recovered (68).

Providentially, the Second International Congress of Microbiology took place in London in July 1936 just after publication of Colebrook and Kenny's first results. The Tréfouël's came from Paris to the Congress and took the opportunity to visit the laboratory at Queen Charlotte's. It may have been this visit that stimulated the laboratory chemist, Albert Fuller, to seek the metabolic products of Prontosil in urine and thus help to prove the theory that sulphanilamide alone was the active component of Prontosil as the Tréfouël's had proposed (69).

Another delegate at the 1936 Congress was Perrin Long, Professor of Medicine at the Johns Hopkins Medical School in the USA. Although Coli had enthusiastically described his results with Prontosil to the Congress, Long missed the paper because he was visiting a colleague who had been admitted to University College Hospital after a road traffic accident. Fortunately, he learnt about the puerperal fever findings when Ronald Hare mentioned Prontosil during a casual conversation at the meeting. According to Hare Long, realizing the potential importance of what he heard, immediately cancelled all his plans and returned to the States on the next available boat (70). Limited supplies of sulphanilamide were obtained from the DuPont Company and he and his colleague Eleanor Bliss were soon able to confirm the European results. By early 1937 they had published their own successful case reports (71), and Long was able to describe with clinical colleagues the successful use of a sulphonamide in meningitis—a report later reprinted as a 'landmark paper' in *The Journal of the American Medical Association* (72).

No doubt encouraged by Long, his professorial colleague in the Department of Pharmacology and Therapeutics at Johns Hopkins, Eli Kennerly Marshall, began to take an interest in sulphonamides. With his research group he developed techniques that measured the behaviour of sulphanilamide in the body. Linked to studies on toxicity, these investigations enabled the establishment of rational dosage schedules. Marshall was also instrumental in the clinical development of sulphaguanidine, a poorly absorbed sulphonamide that remained within the gut and was therefore particularly suitable for the therapy of bacillary dysentery (73). The drug, originally synthesized by Philip Winnek at the Stamford Research Laboratories of the American Cyanamid Corporation in 1940, was to play an important role in the war, especially in the Pacific theatre, where dysentery was a common cause of incapacitation. During the desperate defence of Port Moresby, New Guinea, in 1942, Australian troops were hit by an outbreak of severe dysentery and sulphaguanidine supplies were flown in to keep them in fighting condition.

Perrin Long and Eleanor Bliss wrote an important book on the sulphonamides, published in 1939 (74); together with Kennerly Marshall they were among the most powerful advocates of the new drugs in the United States. The medical press in America had been slow off the mark in noting the developments in Continental Europe, but the reports in *The Lancet* began to stimulate interest throughout the English-speaking world. Perhaps even more influential were reports in the New York Times in December 1936 that President Roosevelt's son, Franklin D Roosevelt Jr, having 'faced death' from a throat infection, was saved by a new drug, Prontylin (75), a version of sulphanilamide synthesized by the Winthrop Chemical Corporation. The fashionable Boston throat specialist, George L Tobey, administered the treatment.

Disappointingly, sulphanilamide turned out to have little value in pneumococcal pneumonia, a common and life-threatening disease for which there was no treatment other than serum therapy of doubtful efficacy. However, the distinguished physician and experimental pathologist, Lionel Whitby, showed in 1938 that a newly synthesized sulphonamide derivative, sulphapyridine, exhibited clear activity (76). Mary Evans and Wilfrid Gaisford (later a distinguished Professor of Paediatrics in Manchester) carried out the first clinical trial of this compound from March to June 1938 in patients with pneumonia at Dudley Road Hospital (now City Hospital) in Birmingham (77). Sulphapyridine was synthesized by a team of chemists led by Arthur Ewins, head of chemical research of the British firm May & Baker in Dagenham, Essex.* The product

---

* An old established firm, in which the Poulenc Frères (later Rhône-Poulenc, then Aventis) in France had acquired a controlling interest in 1927.

was later marketed as Dagenan in recognition of its provenance, but was always known in Britain by its laboratory code 'M & B 693', or simply as 'M & B'. Ewins' group included Montague Phillips, who devised an important step in the synthesis of sulphapyridine and later complained that his contribution was never properly acknowledged, though his name appears with that of Ewins on the patent. Ewins, the son of a railway signalman, was originally recruited by Burroughs Wellcome as a laboratory technician straight from school in 1899. He had been a Scholarship boy at Dulwich College, where he was privileged to be taught chemistry by Herbert Baker, who was to become professor of inorganic chemistry at Oxford and a Fellow of the Royal Society. Ewins later worked with Henry Dale at the Medical Research Council, helping to synthesize Salvarsan during First World War before joining May and Baker after the war (78).

Sulphapyridine was almost certainly the drug used to treat Winston Churchill when he developed pneumonia in North Africa in December 1943. Robin Pulvertaft, later professor of clinical pathology at the Westminster Hospital Medical School, was in charge of the Central Medical Laboratory in Cairo at the time. He was summoned to Tunisia to attend a sick dignitary who turned out to be Churchill. Pulvertaft had been using crude home-made penicillin for the topical treatment of battle wounds and the question of treating Churchill with the new drug was discussed. However, it was felt improper to experiment on the Prime Minister and Churchill's Physician, Lord Moran treated the great man successfully with a sulphonamide (79).

Within a few years of the discovery of sulphanilamide and sulphapyridine the effectiveness of the drugs was firmly established. Sulphathiazole and sulphadiazine emerged as less toxic rivals to sulphapyridine and numerous other variants on these themes soon followed. Sulphathiazole was first reported by Russel Fosbinder and Lewis Walter from the Maltbie Chemical Company* in 1939 (80), but was simultaneously synthesized in several other laboratories, including May and Baker, where it was listed as M & B 760. Sulphadiazine was, like sulphaguanidine, synthesized by Philip Winnek and his colleagues in 1940 at American Cyanamid (81).† Sulphacetamide emerged in 1938 from Max Dohrn's laboratory at the Schering company in Berlin—a firm founded by the pharmacist Ernst Schering in 1871—and was marketed as Albucid. James Sprague's group at Merck synthesized sulphamerazine and sulphamethazine in the early 1940s. Many of these compounds were independently synthesized elsewhere and became the subject of acrimonious patent disputes.

---

* Founded around the turn of the twentieth century in West Orange, New Jersey by Birdsey L Maltbie, a graduate of Albany School of Pharmacy.

† American Cyanamid was originally a manufacturer of fertilizers. During the great depression of the 1930s, it acquired the Lederle Antitoxin Company (see footnote p. 126) and a dyestuffs firm, the Calco Chemical Company, in order to diversify its business. It eventually became part of Wyeth in 1994. See: Travis AS (2005). From color science to polymers and sulfa drugs. Calco Chemical Company and American Cyanamid between two world wars. *Chemical Heritage* **23**, 8–13 (available at: http://www.colorantshistory.org/CalcoArticle.html). Wyeth was originally founded in Philadelphia in 1860 by the brothers, John and Frank Wyeth.

It had already become clear by the start of Second World War that sulphonamides were valuable in many bacterial infections other than those caused by streptococci and staphylococci. Soon sulpha drugs were '...available at pharmacies in all manner of ointments, sprays, nose drops and medicated bandages, or in tablets to be consumed like aspirin' (82). One sulphonamide preparation, Elixir Sulfanilamide, marketed to pharmacies in 1-gallon bottles by a small company in Tennessee founded by Samuel E Massengill,* proved a disaster. In 1937, Massengill's chief chemist, Harold Watkins had been asked to formulate a palatable liquid preparation and had come up with one that included as a solvent, diethylene glycol. The preparation had been approved for distribution after tests of appearance, flavour, and smell, but was not tested for safety, although diethylene glycol was known to be poisonous. A total of 105 of 353 people who had received the drug died. Watkins was subsequently fired and later shot himself. The incident had one positive outcome: legislation was enacted to strengthen the notoriously lax 1906 Food and Drug Act; the Food and Drug Administration (FDA; formed in 1930 from the Bureau of Chemistry in the Department of Agriculture) was given increased powers, including the requirement for pharmaceutical companies to disclose all active ingredients and submit safety testing information before marketing any new drug (83).

The Elixir Sulfamilamide affair was not the only sulphonamide-associated drug scandal. In 1940 the Winthrop Chemical Company in New York, who had a cartel agreement with the Bayer arm of IG Farben in Germany (see p. 291), marketed a batch of sulphathiazole tablets that were contaminated with phenobarbitone (phenobarbital), leading to over 300 deaths or injuries. Once more the FDA intervened, this time to formulate the first regulations for 'Good Manufacturing Practice' (84).

On a happier note, perhaps the strangest use to which sulphonamides were put during Second World War was revealed by the Austrian-born protein chemist from Cambridge, Max Perutz in an obituary of the biochemist Reinhold Benesch:

> His first piece of research was a contribution to the British war effort. When asked to develop a way of packing eggs for the troops more tightly, he fed hens with sulphanilamide, which inhibited the enzyme carbonic anhydrase that is essential for calcification of their eggshells; the shell-less 'floppy' eggs could be packed like matchboxes. Benesch never told me whether the army adopted his invention (85).

If the story did not come from such an eminent source it might be passed off as fabrication, especially as Benesch was well known for his sense of humour, but sulphonamides do inhibit carbonic anhydrase and the tale may well be true.

Another use of a sulphonamide certainly had an unexpected benefit. Nanna Svartz, Professor of Medicine at the Karolinska Institute in Stockholm, used a modification of sulphapyridine, sulphasalazine, manufactured in Sweden by AB Pharmacia, in patients with rheumatic polyarthritis. Svartz was a rheumatologist who was convinced of the

---

* The Massengill business was acquired by Beecham Inc. in 1970 and formally merged with the Company the following year. See Lazell HG (1975). *From pills to penicillin. The Beecham story*, pp. 180–8. Heinemann, London.

infective basis of rheumatoid arthritis then, as now, a disease of uncertain aetiology (86). One of the patients that she treated with sulphasalazine also suffered from ulcerative colitis, which seemed to respond to the therapy. Treatment of other ulcerative colitis cases confirmed the effect (87). In a replay of the discovery of sulphonamides, it turned out that the effect is not due to the supposedly active component: in sulphasalazine, 5-aminosalicylic acid is linked to sulphapyridine in a diazo linkage and this is split by gut bacteria to liberate 5-aminosalicylic acid, which, used alone, was later shown to be just as active (88).

The analogy with Prontosil is uncanny: Prontosil owed its activity to a sulphonamide substituent, which was attached to a supposedly essential feature in a diazo linkage. In sulphasalazine a sulphonamide was, in its turn, modified by addition of a new substituent, again through a diazo linkage, retaining a supposedly essential antibacterial feature; the substituent proved to be the active ingredient and the antibacterial part of the molecule was shown to be unnecessary. That the drug should have been found serendipitously to be useful in ulcerative colitis by treating a patient with rheumatoid arthritis makes it even more astonishing. Sulphasalazine is still used in inflammatory bowel disease although 5-aminosalicylic acid (also known as mesalazine; mesalamine) is just as effective. Sulphapyridine is no longer used as an antibacterial agent because of problems of side effects.

By the end of the Second World War more than 5000 sulphonamide derivatives had been synthesized; at least a dozen were on the market and the scope for successful therapy of various bacterial diseases was well established (89). Elmore Northey, a distinguished organic chemist at American Cyanamid who was very closely involved with sulphonamide research, wrote a comprehensive monograph on this important group of compounds in 1948 detailing the extensive progress that had been made since their discovery more than a decade earlier (90).

Gerhard Domagk was meanwhile picking up the pieces of his work in a shattered research laboratory* and was turning his attention to antituberculosis agents (see Chapter 5). Leonard Colebrook had moved on to the Birmingham Accident Hospital, where he became expert in the control of hospital infection and a pioneer in the employment of Infection Control Nurses. He spoke little of his achievements. His second wife, Vera, whom he had married in 1945 (his first wife, Dorothy, died during the war), recalls his embarrassment when she read of his work at Queen Charlotte's in a medical book:

> I went looking for my husband who was chopping up a fallen tree in our woodland in Farnham Common. "Is there another Leonard Colebrook?" I asked, puzzled. "Not to my knowledge" he replied. "Why?" "Then—did you do this work?" My tone was full of awe and admiration. He ducked his head in embarrassment. "Er—yes—well yes, I had something to do with it" he muttered and hurriedly went on chopping (91).

Sulphonamides are little used today, except as adjuncts to diaminopyrimidines (see p. 255) with which they interact synergically. This property is chiefly made use of in the

---

* The occupying forces had dissolved the IG Farben consortium, but the Elberfeld and Leverkusen sites were allowed to continue, trading once again under the name of Bayer.

prevention and treatment of infection with *Pneumocystis carinii*, a fungus that causes a form of serious pneumonia in immunocompromised patients, including those with acquired immune deficiency syndrome (AIDS), and in the prevention of malaria. Otherwise, sulphonamides still find only occasional use in urinary tract infection and in some topical preparations.

Almost as soon as the sulphonamides had established their effectiveness, the new 'miracle drug' penicillin started to overshadow them. But it was Prontosil and its active component sulphanilamide that created the first real breakthrough in the treatment of bacterial infection, effectively signposting the way ahead for the remarkable events that were to follow. Even before penicillin became available it was possible for the historian Frank Sherwood Taylor—Curator of the Museum of the History of Science in Oxford and from 1950 the Director of the Science Museum, South Kensington—to publish a book with the supremely confident title: *The Conquest of Bacteria* (92).

References

1. Pierpoint WS (1997). Edward Stone (1702–1768) and Edmund Stone (1700–1768): confused identities resolved. *News and records of the Royal Society, London*, Vol. **51**, pp. 211–17. Available at: http://www.journals.royalsoc.ac.uk/media/5g04842utg6yukcg9j4k/contributions/1/g/e/g/1geg1uj0kb39rbdu.pdf
2. Stone E (1763). An account of the success of the bark of the willow in the cure of the agues. *Philos Trans R Soc* **53**, 195–200; cited in: Gibbs DD (1985). Quinine, willow bark and Thomas Bewick. *J R Coll Phys Lond* **19**, 173 and 178.
3. Dünschede H-B (1971). *Tropenmedizinische Forchung bei Bayer*, pp. 1–9. Michael Triltsch Verlag, Düsseldorf.
4. Beer JJ (1958). Coal tar dye manufacture and the origins of the modern industrial research laboratory. *Isis* **49**, 123–31.
5. Greenaway J (1932). In: *The life and work of William Henry Perkin*. The Chemical Society, London, 1932, pp. 7–38. [This book is about Perkin's son (1860–1929), also a distinguished chemist, but contains useful information about his father's early life.]
6. Burke J (1978). *Connections*, pp. 200–2. Macmillan, London.
7. Garfield S (2000). *Mauve. How one man invented a colour that changed the world*. Faber and Faber, London.
8. Rose FL (1963). The origin and rise of the synthetic drugs. In: Poynter FNL *Chemistry in the service of medicine*. Pitman, London, pp. 179–197.
9. Mochmann H, Köhler W (1997). *Meilensteine der Bakteriologie*. Edition Wötzel, Frankfurt am Main.
10. Marquardt M (1949). *Paul Ehrlich*, pp. 41–8. Heinemann, London.
11. Ehrlich P (1908). *Nobel lecture*. http://www.nobel.se/medicine/laureates/1908/ehrlich-lecture.pdf
12. Guttmann P, Ehrlich P (1891). Ueber die Wirkung des Methylenblau bei Malaria. *Berliner Klinische Wochenschrift* **28**, 953–6.
13. Trofa AF, Ueno-Olsen H, Oiwa R, Yoshikawa M (1999). Dr. Kiyoshi Shiga: discoverer of the dysentery bacillus. *Clin Infect Dis* **29**, 1303–6.
14. Ehrlich P, Hata S (1911). *The experimental chemotherapy of spirilloses*, p. 118. Rebman, London.
15. Johann Wolfgang Goethe-Universität Frankfurt am Main (2007). Arthur von Weinberg. http://www.anorg.chemie.uni-frankfurt.de/AK_Fink/priv/frankfurt/weinberg/weinberg.htm

16. Dünschede H-B (1971). *Tropenmedizinische Forschung bei Bayer*, p. 20. Michael Triltsch Verlag, Düsseldorf.

17. Haller SJ (1975). Therapeutic mule: the use of arsenic in the nineteenth century materia medica. *Pharm Hist* **17**, 87–100.

18. Crawcour IL. Journal, Louisiana State Medical Society. Cited in: Haller SJ (1975). Therapeutic mule: the use of arsenic in the nineteenth century materia medica. *Pharm Hist* **17**, 87–100.

19. Manson P (1898). *Tropical diseases*. Cassell, London.

20. Livingstone S (1858). Arsenic as a remedy for the tsetse bite. *BMJ* **1**, 360–1. Available at *Livingstone Online* http://www.livingstoneonline.ucl.ac.uk/view/transcript.php?id=LP104

21. Moore B, Nierenstein M, Todd JL (1907). On the treatment of trypanosomiasis by atoxyl (an organic arsenical compound), followed by a mercuric salt (mercuric chloride) being a bio-chemical study of the reaction of a parasitic protozoon to different chemical reagents at different stages of its life-history. *Biochem J* **2**, 300–24.

22. Thomas HW (1905). Some experiments in the treatment of trypanosomiasis. *BMJ* **1**, 1140–3.

23. Breinl A, Todd JL (1907). Atoxyl in the treatment of trypanosomiasis. *BMJ* **1**, 132–4.

24. Power HJ (1999). *Tropical medicine in the twentieth century. A history of the Liverpool School of Tropical Medicine, 1898–1990*, p. 27. Kegan Paul, London.

25. Sykes R (2000). Towards the magic bullet. *Int J Antimicrob Agents* **14**, 1–12.

26. Hide DW (1992). Carl Prausnitz—father of clinical allergy. *Southampton Med J* **8** (2). Available at: http://www.39springhill.freeserve.co.uk/cpg.htm.

27. Ehrlich P (1913). Chemotherapeutics: scientific principles, methods and results. *Lancet* **2**, 445–51.

28. Schaudinn FR, Hoffmann E (1905). Ueber Spirochaetenbefunde im Lymphdrüsensaft Syphilitischer. *Deutsche medizinische Wochenschrift* **31**, 711–14.

29. Marquardt M (1949). *Paul Ehrlich*, pp. 168–9. Heinemann, London.

30. Wendt H. Gedanken zu "100 Jahre Uchtspringe". http://www.uchtspringe.de/100wendt.htm

31. Wright AE (1909). *Studies on immunisation*. Constable, London.

32. Fleming A, Colebrook L (1911). On the use of Salvarsan in the treatment of syphilis. *Lancet* **1**, 1631–4.

33. Medical Research Committee (1922). *Special report series no. 66. Reports of the Salvarsan Committee II. Toxic effects following the employment of arsenobenzol preparations*. His Majesty's Stationery Office, London.

34. Mentberger V (1913). *Entwicklung und gegenwärtiger Stand der Arsentherapie der Syphilis mit besonderer Berücksichtigung des Salvarsans (Ehrlich–Hata 606) und des Neosalvarsans*. G Fischer, Jena.

35. Marquardt M (1949). *Paul Ehrlich*, pp. 234–8. Heinemann, London.

36. University Hospital Giessen and Marburg (2006). Station Herxheimer. http://www.med.uni-marburg.de/d-einrichtungen/derst1/

37. Swann JP (1985). Arthur Tatum, Parke Davis and the discovery of Mapharsen as an antisyphilitic agent. *J Hist Med Allied Sci* **40**, 167–87.

38. Browning CH, Gulbransen R, Thornton LHD (1917). The antiseptic properties of acriflavine, proflavine and brilliant green; with special reference to suitability for wound therapy. *BMJ* **2**, 70–5.

39. Lesch JE (2007). *The first miracle drugs. How the sulfa drugs transformed medicine*, pp. 20–34. Oxford University Press, New York.

40. Colebrook L, Hare R (1927). On the bactericidal power of mercurochrome. *Br J Exp Pathol* **8**, 109–14.

41. Compton A (1918). The treatment of staphylococcal infections by stannoxyl: furunculosis and acne. *Lancet* **1**, 99–100.

42. Compton A (1918). The treatment of staphylococcal infections by stannoxyl: "mixed infection" of pulmonary tuberculosis. *Lancet* **2**, 234–6.

43. Jacobs WA (1923). The chemotherapy of protozoan and bacterial infections. *Harvey Lect* **19**, 67–95.

44. Heidelberger M, Jacobs WA (1919). Studies in the cinchona series III. Azo dyes derived from hydrocupreine and hydrocupreidine. *J Am Chem Soc* **41**, 2131–47.

45. Browning CH (1935–1936). Chemotherapy—the progress of thirty years and the prospect. *Trans R Medico-Chirurgical Soc Glasgow* **30**, 1–16.

46. Hörlein H (1935). The chemotherapy of infectious diseases caused by protozoa and bacteria. *Proc R Soc Med* **29**, 313–24.

47. Pitschugin PI (1925). Das Methylenblau bei Behandlung von Malaria bei Kindern. *Jahresbericht für Kinderheilkunde* **108**, 347–53.

48. Domagk G (1947). *Pathologische Anatomie und Chemotherapie der Infektionskrankheiten*, pp. 11–12. Georg Thieme Verlag, Stuttgart.

49. Grundmann E (2004). *Gerhard Domagk—the first man to triumph over infectious diseases*, pp. 45–6. LIT Verlag, Münster.

50. Schreiber W (1985). Vor 50 Jahren: Entdeckung der Chemotherapie mit Sulphonamiden. *Deutsche Medizinische Wochenschrift* **110**, 1138–42.

51. Foerster (1933). Sepsis im Anschluß an ausgedehnte Periporitis, Heilung durch Streptozon. *Zentralblatt für Haut- und Geschlechtskrankheiten* **45**, 549–50.

52. Domagk G (1935). Ein Beitrag zur Chemotherapie der bakteriellen Infektionen. *Deutsche Medizinische Wochenschrift* **61**, 250–3.

53. Klee P, Römer H (1935). Prontosil bei Streptokokkenerkrankungen. *Deutsche Medizinische Wochenschrift* **61**, 253–5.

54. Schreus H (1935). Chemotherapie des Erysipels und andere Infektionen mit Prontosil. *Deutsche Medizinische Wochenschrift* **61**, 255–6.

55. Domagk G (1936). Chemotherapie der Streptokokkeninfektionen. *Klinische Wochenschrift* **15**, 1585–90.

56. Levaditi C, Vaisman A (1935). Action curative et préventive du chlorhydrate de 4′-sulfamidi-2, 4-diaminoazobenzène dans l'infection streptococcique expérimentale. *Comptes Rendu de l'Academie de Sciences, Paris* **200** 1694–6

57. Tréfouël J, Tréfouël Mme J, Nitti F, Bovet D (1935). Activité du p-aminophénylsulfamide sur les infections streptococciques expérimentales de la souris et du lapin. *Comptes Rendu des Séances de la Société de Biologie et des ses Filiales* **120**, 756–8.

58. Lesch JE (2007). *The first miracle drugs. How the sulfa drugs transformed medicine*, pp. 108–21. Oxford University Press, New York.

59. Anonymous (1935). Chemotherapy in streptococcal infections. *Lancet*, **2**, 840.

60. Colebrook L (1928). *A study of some organic arsenical compounds with a view to their use in certain streptococcal infections*. Medical Research Council Special Report Series 119. His Majesty's Stationery Office, London.

61. Lesch, JE (2007). *The first miracle drugs. How the sulfa drugs transformed medicine*, p. 132. Oxford University Press, New York.

62. Noble WC (1974). *Coli: great healer of men*, p. 67. Heinemann, London.

63. Colebrook L, Kenny M (1936). Treatment of human puerperal infections, and of experimental infections in mice, with Prontosil. *Lancet* **1**, 1279–86.

64. Colebrook L, Kenny M (1936). Treatment with Prontosil of puerperal infections due to haemolytic streptococci. *Lancet* **2**, 1319–22.

65. Gibberd GF (1937). Prontosil and similar compounds in the treatment of puerperal haemolytic streptococcus infections. *BMJ* **2**, 695–8; Loudon I. The use of historical controls and concurrent

controls to assess the effects of sulphonamides, 1936–1945. The James Lind Library (www.james-lindlibrary.org). Available at: http://www.jameslindlibrary.org/trial_records/20th_Century/1930s/colebrook_lancet_june_1936/colebrook_lancet_june_commentary.php

66. Editorial (1937). Therapia sterilisans magna. *BMJ*; 1, 79. Reprinted in: Waterworth PM (1985). LP Garrod on Antibiotics. *J Antimicrob Chemother* 15 (Suppl. B), 6–7.

67. Loudon I (2000). *The tragedy of childbed fever.* Oxford University Press, Oxford.

68. Hare R (1970). *The birth of penicillin and the disarming of microbes*, pp. 138–9. George, Allen & Unwin, London.

69. Fuller A (1937). Is *p*-aminobenzene sulphonamide the active agent in Prontosil therapy? *Lancet* 1, 194–8.

70. Hare R (1970). *The birth of penicillin and the disarming of microbes*, pp. 141–2. George, Allen & Unwin, London.

71. Long PH, Bliss EA (1937). Para-amino-benzene-sulfonamide and its derivatives. Experimental and clinical observations on their use in the treatment of beta-hemolytic streptococcic infection. *J Am Med Assoc* 108, 32–7.

72. Schwentker FF, Gelman S, Long PH (1937). The treatment of meningococcic meningitis with sulphanilamide. *J Am Med Assoc* 108, 1407–8. Reprinted in: *J Am Med Assoc* 1984; 251, 788–90.

73. Harvey AM (1976). The story of chemotherapy at Johns Hopkins: Perrin H. Long, Eleanor A. Bliss, and E. Kennerly Marshall, Jr. *Johns Hopkins Med J* 138, 54–60.

74. Long PH, Bliss EA (1939). *The clinical and experimental use of sulphanilamide, sulfapyridine and allied compounds.* Macmillan, New York.

75. Anonymous (17 December 1936). Young Roosevelt saved by new drug. *New York Times*; Anonymous (18 December 1936). Conquering streptococci. *New York Times*; Kaempfert W (20 December 1936). New control for infections. *New York Times*.

76. Whitby LEH (1938). Chemotherapy of pneumococcal and other infections with 2-(*p*-aminobenzenesulphonamido) pyridine. *Lancet* 1, 1210–12.

77. Evans GM, Gaisford WF (1938). Treatment of pneumonia with 2-(*p*-aminobenzenesulphonamido) pyridine. *Lancet* 2, 14–19.

78. Dale HH (1958). Arthur James Ewins 1882–1958. *Biograph Memoirs Fellows R Soc* 4, 81–91.

79. Scadding JG (1993). A summons to Carthage, December 1943. *BMJ* 307, 1595–6; Bickel L (1972). *Rise up to life*, p. 211. Angus and Robertson, London.

80. Fosbinder R, Walter LA (1939). Sulfanilamido derivatives of heterocyclic amines. *J Am Chem Soc* 61, 2032–3.

81. Roblin RA, Williams JH, Winnek PS, English JP (1940). Chemotherapy II. Some sulfanilamido heterocycles. *J Am Chem Soc* 62, 2002–5.

82. Craft W (1944). The miracles of penicillin. *Am Mercury*; 59, 157–62; cited by Whorton JC (1980). Antibiotic abandon: the resurgence of therapeutic rationalism. In: Parascandola J, ed. *The history of antibiotics—a symposium*, pp. 125–36. American Institute for the History of Pharmacy, Madison.

83. Wax PM (1995). Elixirs, diluents, and the passage of the 1938 Federal Food, Drug and Cosmetic Act. *Ann Intern Med* 122, 456–61.

84. Unot SW (2004). "God, motherhood and the flag". *Implementing the first pharmaceutical current good manufacturing practices (CGMPs) regulations.* Available at: http://www.fda.gov/oc/history/makinghistory/ firstgmps.html

85. Perutz M (1987). Reinhold Benesch (1919–1986). *Nature* 325, 576.

86. Svarz N (1941). Erfarenheter med salazopyrin. *Nordisk Medicin* 11, 2261–4; Svartz N (1942). Salazopyrin, a new sulfanilamide preparation. *Acta Med Scand* 110, 577–98.

87. Svartz N (1948). The treatment of 124 cases of ulcerative colitis with salazopyrine and attempts at desensitization in cases of hypersensitiveness to sulfa. *Acta Med Scand* 139 (Suppl. 206), 465–72;

Korelitz BI (1992). Where do we stand on drug treatment in ulcerative colitis? *Ann Intern Med* **116**, 692–4.

88. Azad Khan AK, Piris J, Truelove SC (1977). An experiment to determine the active moiety of sulphasalazine. *Lancet* **2**, 892–5.

89. Hawking F, Green FHK (1945). *The medical uses of sulphonamides*, 2nd edn. Medical Research Council War Memorandum No. 10. His Majesty's Stationery Office, London.

90. Northey EH (1948). *The sulfonamides and allied compounds*. Reinhold Publishing, New York.

91. Colebrook V (1974). Foreword. In: Noble WC. *Coli: great healer of men*, pp. 8–9. Heinemann, London.

92. Taylor FS (1940). *The conquest of bacteria; from 606 to 693*. Secker and Warburg, London.

Chapter 4

Wonder drugs

> If Florey had not turned in 1939 from experimental pathology to chemotherapy where should we be now?
>
> Medicine's debt to Florey. *British Medical Journal*, 2 March 1968, p. 529*

Successful though the sulphonamides were in curing previously untreatable bacterial infections, nothing could have prepared the world for penicillin. Several hundred times as active as sulphonamides against streptococci (including pneumococci), staphylococci, gonococci, and meningococci among other bacteria, and—aside from idiosyncratic hypersensitivity—virtually free from side effects, it was the nearest thing before or since to the magic bullet of which Ehrlich had dreamed. Indeed the reliability and safety, when used in the treatment of syphilis, was so much greater than that of Ehrlich's Salvarsan that penicillin effectively superseded it overnight once its activity had been formally established.

The story of penicillin is a strange one: discovered 4 years before Prontosil (there may even have been earlier intimations), it remained a laboratory curiosity until taken up by a team at Oxford in the late 1930s. It was originally revealed as a life-saving drug in England, but its commercial development largely took place in America.

Unlike sulphonamides penicillin is a naturally occurring substance—an antibiotic in the true sense of the word—and was just the first of a family of compounds known as β-lactam antibiotics because of an essential molecular feature on which their activity depends. Chemical modifications of these structures have led to the description of hundreds of derivatives, about 80 of which are still on the world market.

Penicillin

Paving the way: Fleming and St Mary's

Nineteen twenty-eight was a relatively quiet year in Britain: the economic times were hard, with high unemployment and massive social deprivation,† though the Wall Street crash and the Great Depression were yet to come. During the year women in Britain celebrated

---

* Leading article written after Florey's death on 21 February 1968, published anonymously, but written by LP Garrod. See: Waterworth PM (1985). LP Garrod on antibiotics. *Journal of Antimicrobial Chemotherapy* 15, Supplement B.

† Vividly described by George Orwell (Eric Arthur Blair; 1903–50). It was in the winter of 1927–28 that the Eton educated, disillusioned, ex-colonial administrator exchanged his suit for tramp's clothes and set out to live for 2 years *Down and out in Paris and London* before setting out on *The Road to Wigan Pier*.

extension of the franchise to those over 21; aficionados of the new jazz craze enjoyed Louis Armstrong's latest hit, *West End Blues*; and the Hungarian chemist Albert von Szent-Györgyi discovered vitamin C while working with Sir Frederick Gowland Hopkins at the Sir William Dunn Institute of Biochemistry at Cambridge. But it was a seemingly insignificant event that took place in a West London hospital that was eventually to make the year truly memorable.

It was on Monday, 3 September 1928 (or possibly the following day) that Alexander Fleming, newly awarded the title of Professor of Bacteriology, interrupted a holiday to return to St Mary's Hospital, Paddington to advise a surgical colleague on a difficult infection (1). While there, he went into his small second floor laboratory overlooking Praed Street. In the course of a conversation with a young colleague, Merlin Pryce, who, until moving to another department in February that year, had been helping him with studies of staphylococcal variants (2), he picked up a discarded Petri dish that he had inoculated with staphylococci several weeks earlier. The plate was contaminated with a mould around which colonies of staphylococci appeared to be undergoing lysis.

Few events in the history of medicine have been raked over so minutely as this incident and its ramifications. Despite the fact that the main protagonists, and several well-placed observers, have recorded their recollections of what happened, the events have become interwoven with fanciful myths, and uncertainties remain in the official accounts that have never been entirely dispelled. What is clear is that the unusual observation of lysis of staphylococci in the vicinity of a contaminating mould intrigued Fleming sufficiently for him to immediately reach for a platinum loop, such as bacteriologists routinely use to inoculate their cultures, take a sample of the mould that was contaminating the plate and subculture it in broth. He considered the observation sufficiently important to photograph it and to preserve the culture by exposure to formalin vapour, a technique that he often used for other demonstration plates. After a lapse of nearly 2 months—on 30 October 1928 according to his own notebooks—he began some experiments to investigate the phenomenon. By following up this finding and recording the results of his experiments in a paper published in a scientific journal (3), Fleming deserves the lasting gratitude of mankind even though the true value of the discovery was only fully realized by others.

Alexander Fleming was an archetypical taciturn Scot; it has been said that having a conversation with him was like playing tennis with a man who, every time you served the ball, put it in his pocket. This is not, perhaps, surprising. He had been born and brought up on the remote Lochfield Farm (the farmhouse still stands, as isolated as ever, with just an inscribed slab of granite to commemorate its claim to fame) high on the moors 4 miles north of Darvel, itself a tiny town in the Ayrshire countryside (4). His father, Hugh Fleming, was a farmer whose wife had died in 1874, leaving him with four young children. In March 1876 he married Grace Stirling Morton, the 28-year-old daughter of another local farmer. She bore him four more children, of whom Alec was the third. His mother, to whom he was very close, died in May 1927, 16 months before the event that was to make him famous.

In 1895, aged 14, Alec Fleming moved to London, where he joined his half-brother, Tom, who had studied medicine at Glasgow University and had finished up as an eye specialist with a London practice. His half-sister Mary acted as housekeeper, and they were also joined by two brothers (like Alec, sons of their father's second marriage), John and Robert, who eventually set up a successful optical business. After a spell studying at Regent Street Polytechnic, which had been opened a few years before by the philanthropist Quintin Hogg,* Alec worked for 4 years as a junior clerk in the office of a shipping company, the America Line in the City of London. In 1900 a £250 share in the legacy of his father's eldest brother, John, enabled him to escape from the boredom of the office and, after a successful and seemingly effortless year making up deficiencies in entry qualifications, he entered St Mary's Hospital Medical School—apparently chosen on the slender grounds that he had once played in a water polo match against the Mary's team and knew that they had an active swimming club—in October 1901 (5).

Alec was a diligent and successful student who carried off many student prizes. He had vague plans to become a surgeon when he qualified, but a member of staff of Almroth Wright's Inoculation Department, John Freeman, wanted to retain his skills as a member of the St Mary's rifle club, which was bidding for the Armitage Cup at Bisley in 1906. Consequently Fleming, as he himself later admitted (6), drifted into the field of bacteriology by being persuaded to join Wright's department; he was to stay there for the rest of his working life.

Flem (as he was universally known among his medical colleagues) worked with Wright (known in the department as 'the Chief') throughout the First World War, helping him, together with John Freeman, Leonard Colebrook, and others, in setting up a unit located in the casino in Boulogne as part of the British Army General Hospital in the town. Meanwhile, to everyone's astonishment, he had married an Irish Catholic nurse, Sarah (Sally, later Sareen) McElroy, who ran a nursing home with her twin sister Elizabeth in Baker Street close to the Fleming family flat in Clarence Gate Gardens.†

Fleming's work in Boulogne on the bacteriology of battle wounds had a profound effect on him and he was able to make a number of important observations on the influence of antiseptics on wound healing. He established a reputation for careful, precise work and technical ingenuity. By the time he returned to St Mary's after the war he was a valued member of Wright's team, recognized as the Chief's right-hand man.

In 1921 he accidentally discovered in his own nasal secretions and, subsequently, other body fluids, a substance that caused dissolution of a particular non-pathogenic variety of *Staphylococcus* (7). The properties of the substance, which Almroth Wright (who was renowned for his classical neologisms) called lysozyme, occupied him and his young

---

* The Royal Polytechnic Institution in Regent Street was originally founded in 1838, but was a financial failure. Hogg purchased the lease in 1882 and developed it as a Christian institution offering educational and other opportunities to young men and women to whom they would be otherwise denied. See: Woods G Hogg, Quintin (1845–1903), rev. Roger T. Stearn, *Oxford Dictionary of National Biography*, Oxford University Press, 2004 [http://www.oxforddnb.com/view/article/33926].

† How Alexander Fleming met his future wife is not known. Elizabeth later married Alec's elder brother, John.

assistant V. D. Allison* for several years and were still ongoing in 1928. Although they made little headway into understanding the nature of the substance, which they assumed was some sort of enzyme involved in resistance to infection, the discovery was to pave the way for Fleming's (and, curiously, Howard Florey's; see p. 95) later interest in penicillin.

Luck in a cold climate

By the mid-1920s Fleming had established sufficient reputation for him to be invited to contribute a chapter on staphylococci to a multi-volume book called *A System of Bacteriology in Relation to Medicine*, which was published by the Medical Research Council in 1929 (8). As part of the background work for this chapter he asked Merlin Pryce to repeat some work reported by Joseph Bigger, Professor of Microbiology at Trinity College, Dublin, on staphylococcal variants developing under different conditions of incubation. One of the things Fleming wanted to know was whether the properties of the variants that developed were stable. When asked by Fleming to confirm this point, Pryce felt that he had done insufficient work and said that he was unsure. Pryce had moved on to another department by this time, and Fleming had therefore to repeat the work himself. The famous 'penicillin' plate was probably one of the cultures he prepared for this purpose. If this is so, Pryce's later claim that, if his reply to Fleming's question had been 'yes', penicillin would not have been discovered, may well be true (2).

Fleming was far from being the first to observe the inhibition of bacteria by fungi (9), but he had the good fortune to encounter the right type of fungus and the nous to attempt to find out whether the phenomenon might be of use in the laboratory if not in the clinic. His first experiments revealed that the 'mould broth filtrate', for which he proposed the simpler term 'penicillin'—the name later adopted by Howard Florey's group for the specific active component—was highly active, had differential activity against common bacterial pathogens, was rather unstable, and appeared non-toxic to animals and human leucocytes. An account of the discovery was made at a meeting of the Medical Research Club on 13 February 1929, but Fleming was a notoriously soporific lecturer and, as had happened with his earlier revelation of lysozyme in the same forum, his description of the phenomenon generated no discussion or questions. More information was made known in a paper that he submitted to *The British Journal of Experimental Pathology* in early May 1929, and which was published with a speed that probably reflects the editor's lack of suitable material rather than any sense of its importance, in the June 1929 issue.

---

* Allison later worked at the Ministry of Health's bacteriology laboratory in Endell Street, Central London. In 1939, at the start of the Second World War, he was seconded to Cardiff to head one of the laboratories of the Emergency Public Health Laboratory Service. After the war this became the Public Health Laboratory Service, with its headquarters and most of its reference laboratories in Colindale, North London. Allison became director of the Streptococcal Reference Laboratory at Colindale with Winston Maxted as his head technician. See: Williams REO. *Microbiology for the Public Health. The Evolution of the Public Health Laboratory Service 1939–1980.* Public Health Laboratory Service, London, 1985.

The fungus that had contaminated Fleming's plate was *Penicillium notatum*, at first misidentified by Charles La Touche, a young Irish mycologist from University College Dublin,* who had been employed at St Mary's to investigate the role of fungi in allergy, as *Penicillium rubrum* (he later apologized for the mistake). Fleming tested numerous other fungi, but the only one that produced inhibition of bacterial growth was a strain of *Penicillium* obtained from La Touche, which is likely to have been identical to the original contaminant. It later transpired that Fleming's mould was one of the few *Penicillium* strains to produce penicillin in sufficient quantity to cause the effect he had observed.

Legend, perpetuated by an offhand and no doubt thoughtless remark made by Fleming himself, has it that the offending fungal spore had blown in through the window from Praed Street, on which St Mary's Hospital stands. Ronald Hare, who was an eye witness to the events, though not directly involved, has pointed out that this is extremely unlikely, since no bacteriologist works by an open window, especially when traffic is roaring by on the road below and, in any case, the windows of the laboratory could be opened only with great difficulty. Moreover, the particular species of fungus involved was to be found in La Touche's ill-equipped laboratory on the floor below and this is much more likely to have been the source (10).

Although the mould broth filtrate reliably exhibited potent antibacterial activity, the phenomenon observed on the original plate paradoxically proved difficult to replicate. Inoculating a suitable growth medium with staphylococci, artificially contaminating it with the fungus and incubating it in the normal way at 37°C does not produce inhibition of growth, let alone lysis of the bacteria. The reasons for this are complex: the fungus grows very slowly and needs time to produce an adequate quantity of penicillin, especially at 37°C; staphylococci, in contrast, grow slowly at normal room temperature, but flourish at body temperature to form visible colonies about 2–3 mm in diameter in less than 18 h. Moreover, luxuriant growth of the staphylococci depletes the medium of growth factors and in these conditions the fungus struggles to grow. Crucially, penicillin causes lysis of bacteria only when they are multiplying; when colonies are fully grown active multiplication more or less ceases.

In fact, the phenomenon Fleming observed occurred through an astonishing concatenation of fortuitous circumstances. Ronald Hare convincingly reconstructed the likely sequence of events in 1966. Hare realized that Fleming had probably deliberately left the staphylococcal cultures at room temperature for a prolonged period (following the technique Joseph Bigger had described) as part of his investigation of staphylococcal variants. Following up this hunch, Hare inoculated a nutrient agar plate with staphylococci and a few fungal spores and then left the Petri dish at room temperature for 5 days. The result, as he had hoped, was a faithful reproduction of Fleming's original observation.

* La Touche was a science graduate of University College Dublin (BSc 1924; MSc 1925), but became a licentiate of Apothecaries Hall, Dublin in 1946, a relatively undemanding way to obtain a medical qualification (data from *The Medical Directory*). He subsequently worked at the University of Leeds Medical School and became President of the British Society for Medical Mycology from 1976–78.

However, when Hare repeated the experiment, as every good scientist should, he failed to confirm his earlier finding. Fortunately, he had the foresight to keep a record of ambient temperatures during the tests and noted that the conditions during the second experiment had been much warmer than in the first. Further experiments established that the effect that Fleming had seen could be demonstrated only if the temperature did not exceed about 20°C. Hare went on to investigate temperatures in London at the time of Fleming's discovery. Meteorological records revealed that there had been a cold spell, with maximum temperatures below 20°C, between 27 July and 6 August 1928, then a spell of hot weather (temperatures reached around 25°C; hot by English standards!) ending abruptly on 28 August with temperatures reaching 20°C on only two occasions in the next 9 days (11).

In the absence of any other explanation, it seems likely that Fleming inoculated the plate with staphylococci before he went on holiday at the end of July; he purposely left it at room temperature and was unaware that it had been accidentally contaminated with a fungal spore. Because of the prevailing weather conditions the fungus was able to grow and start to produce penicillin, but the staphylococci remained dormant until the weather improved and they then started to multiply. Developing colonies that became exposed to penicillin as it diffused through the growth medium began to undergo lysis and those in the immediate vicinity of the contaminant fungus, where the penicillin concentration was high, failed to grow at all.

Fleming's discovery of penicillin is often presented as a classic example of serendipity. And so it was; but this time, Lady Luck had moved into overdrive, for the phenomenon that presented itself on the plate had come about by an extraordinary chain of chance events: the need for Fleming to repeat Pryce's work; the accidental contamination of the culture plate; Fleming's interrupted holiday; the casual circumstances in which the famous Petri dish was observed; the unusual nature of the contaminant; the fact that the culture was not incubated at body temperature as would usually happen; and last but not least, the vagaries of the English climate, without which the necessary conditions for the discovery would not have occurred.

The odds on these circumstances arising by chance are astronomical, but that is the nature of chance events. It was fortunate too that the observation was made by someone with the time and inclination to follow it up and report his findings in the scientific literature, albeit in a specialized pathology journal that did not have a particularly wide circulation.

Hare's account of the circumstances of Fleming's discovery have been questioned by Robert Scott Root-Bernstein of Michigan State University in his book *Discovering* (12). He puts forward instead a highly speculative theory that Fleming originally investigated the *Penicillium* mould as a possible lysozyme producer as part of his ongoing interest in the earlier compound. As Ronald Bentley has pointed out (13), this alternative scenario seems extremely fanciful given what is known of the circumstances of the discovery, and would scarcely be worth consideration if it had not been swallowed whole by Eric Lax in his popular account of the penicillin story (14). Fleming himself seemed unsure how the phenomenon he had stumbled upon came about (15), but the version put forward by Hare, who knew all the protagonists well, has the virtue of fitting the known facts and has been shown by experimentation to be entirely plausible.

The dormant miracle

The title of the paper Fleming wrote 'On the antibacterial action of cultures of a penicillium, with special reference to their use in the isolation of *B. influenzae*' reflected his view that penicillin might find its greatest use in selective culture media for the isolation of *Haemophilus influenzae*—known at the time as *Bacillus influenzae* and thought to be a secondary invader, if not the primary cause of epidemic influenza. However, he kept his options open by suggesting that '...it may be an efficient antiseptic for application to, or injection into, areas infected with penicillin-sensitive microbes'. According to Gwyn Macfarlane in his detailed and perceptive biography of Fleming, Almroth Wright wanted the reference to therapeutic use expunged as mere speculation, but Fleming stood his ground (16).

There were few grounds for believing that penicillin would be a breakthrough in treatment of bacterial infections. Conventional wisdom at the time was sceptical of the likelihood of developing effective antibacterial agents other than for topical use (see p. 64). Fleming himself seems to have been of this opinion; his boss, Wright, certainly was. In a paper in *The Lancet* in 1927, which is (at least to modern ears) a masterpiece of pedantry and pomposity masquerading as clear-sighted analysis of his friend Ehrlich's principles of chemotherapy, he failed spectacularly to predict the coming revolution in naturally occurring antibacterial compounds:

> Having realised how difficult it is for the chemist to produce (and, of course, we cannot reasonably expect nature to provide ready-made) effective pharmaco-chemical bactericidal agents, we may now turn to consider the further problem which confronts the physician who has to bring such agents into application, not only (for that is a comparatively simple matter) upon microbes circulating in the blood, but also (and this is what is really difficult) upon microbes dispersed throughout the organism (17).

Fleming himself, in a paper read at a meeting of the Royal Society of Medicine on 4 February 1928, just a few months before his momentous discovery, was slightly more open-minded, but clearly remained faithful to Wright's 'stimulate the phagocytes' philosophy. Antiseptics were fine, so long as they did not interfere with the normal bactericidal mechanisms of the blood, but:

> At present there seems little chance of any general antiseptic killing bacteria in the blood-stream but there is some hope that chemicals may be produced with special affinities for particular bacteria and may be able to destroy these in the blood although they may be quite without action on other and, it may be, closely allied bacteria (18).

He clearly had in mind his other brainchild, lysozyme (for which he managed to get in a plug in his talk), which was only active against certain non-pathogenic bacteria and had not proved to be of any therapeutic value.

Fleming's therapeutic ambitions for penicillin were limited to possible topical use. Tests of its effect on phagocyte function were similar to those he had performed with flavines and other antiseptics with the aim of investigating whether normal phagocytic processes in superficial infections would be compromised. He did not test penicillin in any animal protection tests of the kind that Domagk was later to perform with Prontosil. The possibility of oral use—which, in any case, we now know would be unlikely to work—does not seem to have been considered, perhaps because ingesting a filtered culture fluid seemed outlandish, though the meat broth used to grow the fungus is not much different from a culinary meat stock.

Attempts to apply the mould broth filtrate topically were restricted to a few tentative cases: The first documented therapeutic use (recorded in Fleming's notes as occurring on 9 January 1929) was by installation into the nasal antrum of Fleming's colleague, Stuart Craddock, who had a sinus infection. The results were equivocal at best, but success was obtained in the topical treatment of an eye infection in Keith Rogers, a medical student who was captain of the London University rifle team (19). Crude broth filtrate was also used on a few patients in the hospital, but nothing that could be graced with the epithet of 'clinical trial' was ever carried out.

Surprisingly, Fleming's former collaborator, Leonard Colebrook, who had taken a prolonged interest in Salvarsan and later showed such awareness of the potential of Prontosil (see p. 72–4) seems to have paid no attention whatsoever to penicillin. He had ample opportunity to hear about the discovery: quite apart from his former association with the St Mary's department, his right hand man at Queen Charlotte's was Ronald Hare, who had joined him when the laboratory was opened in 1930. Furthermore, they were visited at Queen Charlotte's by a former St Mary's student, Cecil George Paine, who had been sufficiently impressed by Fleming's work to take a sample of the mould with him when he moved to Sheffield as an assistant pathologist. As early as 1930 Paine was providing colleagues at Sheffield Royal Infirmary with crude filtrates of cultures to use in skin and eye infections. Documentary evidence of the successful treatment of two cases of gonococcal eye infection in babies, the first a 3-week-old boy admitted on 28 August 1930 and started on penicillin on 25 November, was discovered in old case notes unearthed by Milton Wainwright and Harold Swan in 1984 (20). After carrying out his successful experiments with penicillin and before starting a new job as consultant pathologist at the Jessop Hospital for Women in Sheffield, Paine spent a month in Colebrook's department at Queen Charlotte's learning about puerperal fever, but if he mentioned his success with Fleming's mould it cannot have aroused much interest. Paine seems to have done no further work with penicillin and joined the ranks of those who regretted missed opportunities.

Penicillin would have been a godsend in puerperal fever in 1930 and would certainly have overshadowed the later use of Prontosil and the sulphonamides, the history of which might have been very different. Of course, such experience as there was at this time was with topical penicillin and this would have been of little avail in puerperal sepsis. Injection was out of the question. No one, least of all the ever-cautious

Colebrook, would try to inject a crude culture filtrate into a sick woman without irresistible evidence of likely benefit. The possibility of purifying penicillin does not seem to have arisen, although Colebrook had an experienced biochemist, Albert Fuller, on his staff.

Fleming did make some effort to purify the active ingredient of his mould juice, just as he had done with lysozyme. He loosely supervised the abortive attempts of his colleagues, Stuart Craddock and Frederick Ridley*—and, later, a chemist, Lewis Holt—to purify penicillin, but they made little material progress. Harold Raistrick, professor of biochemistry from 1929–33 at the London School of Hygiene and Tropical Medicine, newly constructed in Keppel Street, Bloomsbury, also took a keen interest in the compound as part of his researches into chemical substances produced by fungi. Raistrick had the assistance of a mycologist, Victor Charles—who would soon be tragically killed in a street accident—and it may have been Charles who cast doubt on the identity of Fleming's mould. A colleague, the biochemist Percival Clutterbuck, sent a culture of the fungus to Charles Thom, a mycologist at the United States Department of Agriculture. Thom had made his reputation studying the fungi involved in the ripening of cheeses such as Camembert and Roquefort, and had just published an authoritative book on the penicillia. It was he who formally identified the fungus as *Penicillium notatum*.

A further effort to purify penicillin was undertaken in the United States in the early 1930s. Roger Reid, a student at the State College of Pennsylvania (now Pennsylvania State University) was encouraged to study penicillin as a master's degree project by his supervisor, Joel A Sperry, professor of bacteriology at the associated agricultural college. The dissertation, entitled *A study of the bactericidal, bacteriolytic or inhibitory substance produced by molds and some factors which influence its production*, revealed a typical student project: diligently performed, but adding little to what was already known (21). The master's dissertation was submitted and accepted in 1931, but when Reid came to write his PhD thesis in 1935 the topic was *A study of factors influencing bacterial pigmentation* (22). Reid himself claimed that he was discouraged from making penicillin the study of his doctoral research by a sceptical supervisor who considered the curious substance to be an unsuitable subject for a PhD (23). Nevertheless, Reid continued his interest in penicillin while still working for his doctorate, presenting his findings at meetings of the Society of American Bacteriologists (now the American Society for Microbiology) and publishing a more extensive paper on the topic in the Society's *Journal of Bacteriology* in 1935 (24); but like others, he made little headway.

Much has been made of Fleming's failure to purify penicillin and more actively pursue its therapeutic potential. He himself put this down to lack of chemical expertise and others have pointed to aspects of the behaviour of penicillin in his early experiments that

---

* Ridley later became a consultant surgeon at Moorfields Eye Hospital in London.

discouraged belief that it might be of value in deep-seated infections (25). While this may be true, the environment in which Fleming worked must also have played a part. Until quite recently, and certainly in Fleming's time, such research as took place in hospital laboratories was pretty much an unregulated pursuit largely left to the resources of individuals imbued with the amateur spirit of discovery. Fleming's principal duties at St Mary's concerned the functions of Almroth Wright's semi-commercial Inoculation Department—itself an anomalous appendage of the Hospital and its Medical School—for which he had increasing administrative responsibility as the aging Wright took less interest in the day to day management. Penicillin and chemotherapy (a topic that was anathema to Wright) were very much side issues that could be pursued only in desultory fashion as inclination and other duties permitted.

In one way the circumstances of the discovery of penicillin were propitious. It is much more difficult now for dabblers, mavericks, and eccentric 'misfits', who have the capacity to radically alter thinking, to find a fertile environment in which to express their idiosyncratic talents. But the circumstances for validating and developing the discovery were certainly not favourable. Professor of bacteriology, Fleming might be, but the title did not carry the overtones of research excellence that it now does, at least in medical schools. The whole ethos of academic performance was then very different from what it is today. In Fleming's time advancement did not depend on the scramble for funds and the 'publish or perish' philosophy that now prevails. Moreover, the modern preference for highly focused strategic research by dedicated teams with a 'critical mass' of expertise in relevant fields hardly existed in Fleming's time; indeed, had it done so, it is highly likely that penicillin would have been ignored. In order to follow up his finding, a Fleming of today would be expected to apply for a research grant and, if successful, to assemble a team with the required skills to follow the discovery through. This line of action would hardly have occurred to Fleming, who preferred to encourage young colleagues to dabble with his weird and wonderful mould juice in splendid and largely undisturbed isolation. In any case, it is extremely unlikely that Fleming's historic observation would have been deemed worthy of funding by grant-awarding bodies at that time. Penicillin was a product of its time and that, perhaps, was the greatest good fortune of all.

It is, however, also fortunate that not all academic institutions in 1930s Britain had a laissez faire attitude to research. There were a few centres of research excellence where scientific advance was driven by individuals in whom intellectual ability was combined with vision, ambition, and the force of character to take ideas forward—always, of course, with the aid of what Paul Ehrlich insisted were the four essential 'Gs': Geld, Geduld, Geschick und Glück (money, patience, ability, and luck). Happily for the future of penicillin, all these qualities (though 'geld' was to be a constant problem) came together in the person of Howard Florey, who became Professor of Pathology in the University of Oxford in 1935.

Realizing penicillin's potential: Florey and Oxford

If St Mary's Hospital, Paddington is where penicillin was conceived by Lady Luck and Alexander Fleming, the Sir William Dunn School of Pathology in Oxford is where it was born. The midwife was a German refugee, the obstetrician an Australian, ably supported by a team of talented assistants. The extraordinary gifts of the infant became evident within a year of the birth, but it was in the United States that the talents of the prodigy were to be nurtured and presented to the world.

The Sir William Dunn School of Pathology was endowed by a grant awarded by the trustees of the estate of a wealthy Scot, Sir William Dunn, former Consul General of the Orange Free State in South Africa (26). It was opened in1927 with the Danish immunologist Georges Dreyer, who had overseen every aspect of its palatial design, as its head. The early years of the school were unremarkable, but in 1934 Dreyer died suddenly while on a visit to Denmark and the professorship was offered to Howard Florey. The distinguished physiologist, Sir Charles Sherrington, with whom Florey had earlier worked in Oxford, lent his authority to the appointment, but Florey had already established a considerable reputation in experimental pathology and he was eminently well qualified for the post (27).

To describe Howard Florey as being unlike Alexander Fleming is a gross understatement; they were cast in quite different moulds. Florey was a native of Adelaide, South Australia, the youngest son of a successful manufacturer of boots and shoes. He excelled both academically and on the sports field at school and subsequently as a medical student at Adelaide University. Even as a student he was attracted to scientific research. In 1920 he was awarded a Rhodes scholarship to study at Magdalen College, Oxford under Sherrington and despite financial problems—his father had died in 1918 and his business was by then in a state of financial collapse—he accepted and set sail for England immediately after taking his final examinations in December 1921.

After 3 years at Oxford, culminating with a stint as medical officer on an Oxford University arctic expedition, Florey moved to Caius College, Cambridge with a studentship in physiology. A year later he was on the move again, this time to the United States on a Rockefeller Foundation Fellowship that was to provide crucial contacts when the penicillin story began to unfold. On his return to England he completed his PhD at Caius College and worked briefly at the London Hospital, Whitechapel and again in Cambridge, before accepting an appointment as the Joseph Hunter Professor of Pathology in the University of Sheffield in 1931. It was at Sheffield that he met Cecil George Paine, who was a member of the pathology staff, and learned, with little obvious enthusiasm, of his trial of Fleming's mould juice.

Florey took up his appointment at the Sir William Dunn School of Pathology in Oxford on 1 May 1935 soon after Domagk had published his landmark paper on Prontosil (see p. 69). He set about the task of organizing the diverse and uncoordinated work of the school. New faces were brought in, including the future Nobel laureate Peter Medawar. The appointment of Arthur Duncan Gardner, head of the independent Standards laboratory that was accommodated within the school, was secured as Reader in Bacteriology.

Florey's own research plan was to investigate mysteries of the function of the lymphatic system and the properties of lysozyme and other natural antibacterial substances. He had started to take an interest in lysozyme and its role in the body's natural defences against infection while at Cambridge and continued to work on the problem in Sheffield. He was familiar with the work of Fleming, who had discovered the substance, and had submitted tissue specimens to him, probably for assay of their lysozyme activity. With the help of the eminent organic chemist Sir Robert Robinson he obtained a grant from the Medical Research Council in July 1935 and started work on lysozyme with Eric Roberts a young chemist from Robinson's department, and Brian Maegraith, another Australian Rhodes scholar, who was later to become a distinguished professor of tropical medicine in Liverpool.

What Florey's group lacked if they were to make any progress was an experienced biochemist, and a tentative enquiry was made to Sir Frederick Gowland Hopkins in the School of Biochemistry in Cambridge (also endowed with money from the estate of Sir William Dunn) to ask whether his protégé, Norman Pirie might be interested. Hopkins declined to release Pirie, but by chance he had just read a very impressive PhD thesis by one of his other students and strongly recommended him. Thus it was that, a young Jewish refugee from Hitler's Germany, Ernst Boris Chain, came to work in Florey's team.

Chain, son of a Russian father and a German mother, had arrived in Britain in April 1933 armed with a degree in chemistry and physiology and a DPhil gained for research carried out in the Institute of Pathology of the Charité Hospital in Berlin. He was a complex character, excitable, argumentative, and prone to periods of depression. He was also an accomplished pianist who had toyed with an alternative career in music and a fluent speaker of English, German, Russian, French, and Italian (28).

The 29-year-old Chain was an enzymologist by training and started work on enzymic properties of snake venoms, but Florey suggested that he should broaden his interests by undertaking a study of the mode of action of lysozyme. This sent Chain on a search of the literature for articles on other naturally occurring antibacterial products, one of which was Fleming's 1929 article in the *British Journal of Experimental Pathology*, a journal of which Howard Florey was one of the editors. Fleming's description of penicillin as a bacteriolytic substance led Chain to believe that it was, like lysozyme, an enzyme and he thought it would be instructive to compare their properties. Florey and Chain agreed to include penicillin in their studies—not a foregone conclusion; episodes of friction between the notoriously blunt Florey and the impetuous Chain often occurred—and in the late stages of 1938 or early 1939, work on the substance began. Fortuitously, but not crucially since it could have been obtained elsewhere, a culture of the *Penicillium* mould was found to be available in the School where one of the late Georges Dreyer's colleagues, Margaret Campbell-Renton, had maintained the strain after investigating it as a possible source of bacteriophage.

Neither Florey nor Chain had any inkling when they undertook their investigation that penicillin was likely to be of any therapeutic value. The aim was to understand the interaction between natural products and bacteria and to elucidate the mode of activity of naturally occurring enzymes, a class of compounds to which penicillin was thought to belong. It was in 1939 as the threat and then the reality of war began to descend that thoughts began to turn towards possible therapeutic use of the compounds they were studying.

The reasons for this change of emphasis are unclear, but the intention was first expressed in research grant applications. Florey's ambitions for the Dunn School were always threatened by the perennial problem of lack of funds and applications to the Medical Research Council had met with only small sums for Chain's salary and immediate expenses. It is of course commonplace for scientists to magnify the possible practical implications of their research when trying to obtain research funds (if only a fraction of the research grant applications that offered the expectation of a cure for cancers came to fruition, the diseases would have been conquered long ago), but other factors were at work to focus minds on potentially practical implications of their work. The success of sulphonamides had altered the mindset of scientists about the possibilities of antibacterial drugs. Moreover, in early September 1939, Florey (and, independently, Fleming) attended the Third International Congress for Microbiology in New York, where a young Frenchman, René Dubos, working at the Rockefeller Institute in New York, made a dramatic announcement of his discovery of an antibiotic, tyrothricin, produced by a soil bacterium, which was active against streptococci in mice (see p. 150–151).

It is unlikely that Florey actually attended Dubos's presentation, since war in Europe broke out while the New York meeting was underway and the British delegates rushed back across the Atlantic, but he always acknowledged his awareness of the work, which had also been described in a series of published papers. Certainly, tyrothricin aroused widespread interest and Florey was careful to cite Dubos's work in his applications for financial support.

Whatever the reason, by the outbreak of the Second World War Florey's interest had been stimulated to the point of investigating the possibility of getting clinical cooperation for testing any substances with therapeutic potential and he was actively canvassing the idea of penicillin as a possible chemotherapeutic agent. In a letter written 3 days after the outbreak of war to Sir Edward Mellanby, secretary of the Medical Research Council and a colleague during his time in Sheffield, Florey wrote, with blithe unconcern for embellishment of the known facts:

> Filtrates of certain strains of penicillium contain a bactericidal substance, called penicillin by its discoverer Fleming, which is especially effective against staphylococci, and acts also on pneumococci and streptococci. There exists no really effective substance acting against staphylococci *in vivo*, and the properties of penicillin which are similar to those of lysozyme hold out promise of its finding a practical application in the treatment of staphylococcal infections. Penicillin can be easily prepared in large amounts and is non-toxic to animals, even in large doses (29).

The immediate outcome of this plea was a promise of £25 for expenses, with the possibility of £100 to follow. As Gwyn Macfarlane sardonically notes in his biography of Florey: 'There cannot be many Government-sponsored schemes that have had a smaller initial investment and a larger return' (30).

Fortunately Florey was on good terms with the Rockefeller Foundation and was able to take advantage of a visit in early November 1939 from Harry M. Miller of the Natural Sciences Division to plead his case. Miller was sympathetic to Florey and offered his personal support to a request for funds. The consequent application to the Foundation in

New York yielded $5000 per year for 5 years—more than had been requested. This sum, around £1000 per year at the existing exchange rate, was manna from heaven to Florey, who was constantly frustrated by the need to spend so much valuable research time passing round a begging bowl with meagre results. Most importantly, the future of the penicillin project was now reasonably secure.

Chain set to work with an American Rhodes scholar, Leslie Epstein, who was originally employed to pursue research on lysozyme, the subject of his Oxford DPhil. Epstein was greatly influenced during his stay in England from 1937–40 by left wing intellectuals that he met and he was drawn into campaigns for social justice and the political debate over the impending war. On his return to the United States he changed his name to Falk and became a prominent supporter of the civil rights movement.

Although progress in the extraction and purification of penicillin from cultures of the mould was at first slow, it soon accelerated, aided and abetted by the technical ingenuity of Norman Heatley, who had been recruited by Florey in September 1936 from the Sir William Dunn Institute of Biochemistry in Cambridge, where he had been working under Joseph Needham.* Heatley had been awarded a Rockefeller Fellowship to work in Copenhagen, but was persuaded to remain in Britain in those uncertain times to join the penicillin project. Heatley found Chain a difficult customer to deal with and agreed to work with him only when it was made crystal clear that he would be answerable to Florey, not Chain. The retention of Heatley proved crucial. Not only did he suggest a critical step in the purification of penicillin, but he also developed a reliable quantitative method of assaying the activity of the substance, devised methods for the extraction of penicillin, and organized large scale cultivation of the fungus in flasks, bottles, trays, pie dishes, tins, and hospital bedpans (31). As Florey's successor as Professor of Pathology in Oxford, fellow Australian Henry Harris put it in his Florey Centenary Lecture in 1998:

> without Fleming, no Florey or Chain, without Chain no Florey, without Florey no Heatley, without Heatley, no penicillin (32).

By March 1940, sufficient crude penicillin had been obtained to start animal studies; at first toxicity tests—initiated by Chain, apparently dissatisfied with Florey's tardiness—and then pharmacological studies. Meanwhile, Duncan Gardner and Jean Orr-Ewing, a medical bacteriologist who had worked for Florey's predecessor, Dreyer† were discovering

---

* Needham was a biochemist and fellow of Caius College, who had established a reputation in chemical embryology. During the 1930s, three young Chinese researchers awoke in him an interest in the culture of their country, which led him to learn Chinese in order to undertake a study of the achievements of Chinese civilization. He wrote prolifically on the topic and became the foremost western sinologist of the twentieth century. See: Needham Research Institute. Joseph Needham (1900–95). http://www.nri.org.uk/joseph.html

* Jean Orr-Ewing, a fellow of Lady Margaret Hall, Oxford, and former student at the college, studied medicine at St Mary's Hospital from 1920–23, but as a clinical student may have escaped Alexander Fleming's notoriously inaudible lectures.

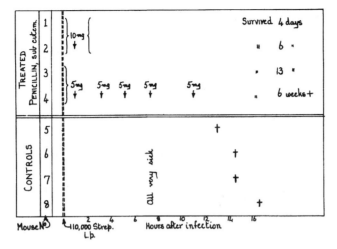

Fig. 4.1 First mouse protection test carried out in Oxford on 25 May, 1940. Chart drawn by Norman Heatley from his notes made at the time. Reproduced courtesy of Miss Rose Heatley.

penicillin's astonishing potency (far greater than that of the sulphonamides) against a range of pathogenic bacteria, despite the fact that the crude extracts at their disposal normally contained less than 1 mg of penicillin per litre. The time had come for the mouse protection tests that Fleming had omitted to carry out.

At 11 a.m. on Saturday, 25 May 1940, the day before the start of the evacuation of Dunkirk, Florey with the help of James Kent (Fleming's personal technician since his early days at Cambridge*) personally injected eight white mice intraperitoneally with a culture of a virulent *Streptococcus* prepared by Duncan Gardner. Heatley kept notes of the procedure and observed developments into the small hours of the following morning. Four mice remained untreated and all died within 16 h. Two received, after 1 h, a subcutaneous injection of 10 mg of crude penicillin; they survived for 4 and 6 days, respectively. The other two mice received 5 mg penicillin every 2 h for 10 h; one survived for 13 days, the other was still alive at 6 weeks (Fig. 4.1).

The design of the experiment was admirably economical, but scientifically inadequate compared with Domagk's similar test of Prontosil (see Fig. 3.4, p. 68). Nevertheless, the result was unequivocal and confirmatory tests rapidly followed. It has often been said that Florey was fortunate to have chosen mice rather than guinea pigs,

---

* J. H. D. Kent became Florey's personal technician in 1927 at the age of 14. He remained loyal to his boss for 40 years at Cambridge, Sheffield, and Oxford. He was one of the two witnesses to Florey's second marriage, to Margaret Jennings, on 6 June 1967 (the other was Margaret's housekeeper, Cecilia Little). Jim Kent was rewarded with an honorary Oxford M.A. in 1978. See: Williams TI. *Howard Florey. Penicillin and After*. Oxford University Press, 1984, p. 33, 373.

which are idiosyncratically susceptible to penicillin and sometimes die through an effect on the bacterial flora in the caecum. However, death in guinea pigs usually occurs only after oral administration of penicillin, and since Florey always used injection, this effect of penicillin may not, in any case, have been detected at this stage.

By August 1940 Florey sensed he had something special and enough information to publish preliminary results. The paper duly appeared in *The Lancet* on 24 August 1940 with the uncompromisingly optimistic title *Penicillin as a chemotherapeutic agent* (33). Seven members of the Oxford team were listed as authors in alphabetical order (which must have pleased Chain). In addition to Chain, Florey, Gardner, and Heatley, Margaret Jennings (a pathologist who became Florey's second wife in 1967 shortly before he died), Jean Orr-Ewing, and Gordon Sanders (a pathologist trained at St Thomas' Hospital, London) received due credit. The article also carried an acknowledgement of the otherwise unsung technical contributions of Donald Callow (Chain's technician), George Glister (the technician in charge of penicillin production), S. A. Cresswell, Jim Kent, and E. Vincent. A fairly phlegmatic editorial assessment accompanied the article (34).

Two weeks after the *Lancet* paper appeared the London blitz commenced,* but Oxford remained unscathed. After the successful animal experiments, Florey was looking to start human trials and approached Professor Leslie Witts, Nuffield Professor of Clinical Medicine at Oxford's Radcliffe Infirmary. During their discussions a young student, Charles Fletcher, later to become a professor of clinical epidemiology and a presenter of popular television programmes on medical topics for the BBC, turned up to visit his professor. He had just finished a stint as house physician and was looking for a research topic to suit his new position as a Nuffield research fellow. Witt suggested that Fletcher might like to look at the clinical use of penicillin, Florey agreed and Fletcher leapt at the chance.

The initial experiments on human volunteers were intended simply to confirm the safety and pharmacological properties of penicillin and a 50-year-old woman dying of disseminated breast cancer agreed to become the first to receive an injection of the drug. On Friday, 17 January 1941, Florey and Witts were on hand to witness Fletcher give the woman, Elva Akers, an intravenous injection of 100 mg of partially purified penicillin. She suffered a rigour, prompting the realization that pyrogenic impurities still needed to be removed from the preparations, but was otherwise unharmed (35).

Fletcher's patient was not, in fact, the first to receive an injection of penicillin. Two patients of an American physician, Henry Dawson of the College of Physicians and Surgeons, Columbia University, New York had already had this honour. In 1940 Dawson had read the report from the Oxford team in *The Lancet* and obtained a culture of the *Penicillium* mould from Roger Reid in Pennsylvania (see p. 93). With the

* The date of the commencement of the London blitz is usually given as 7 September 1940, although at least one bomb was dropped on Central London 2 weeks earlier during the weekend in which the *Lancet* paper appeared.

help of a biochemist, Karl Meyer* and a bacteriologist, Gladys Hobby, he obtained sufficient crude penicillin to attempt some injections. On 15 October 1940 he cautiously injected 0.1 ml of a crude extract in butyl alcohol into the skin of two patients, Aaron Alston and Charles Aronson in the Presbyterian Hospital, New York. Encouraged by the lack of any serious reaction each then received 1 ml, and on the following day 5 ml, subcutaneously. Alston subsequently received intramuscular, and beginning on 11 January 1941, a series of six daily intravenous injections. There appear to have been no harmful effects, but also—unsurprisingly given the small amounts of penicillin likely to have been present—no obvious clinical benefit. The findings, together with some satisfactory results in eye infections, were reported at a meeting of the American Society for Clinical Investigation on 5 May 1941 and attracted the attention of the press and a local chemical firm, Chas Pfizer and Co. (36).

Meanwhile, back in Oxford, further clinical studies quickly established the concentrations achieved in the bloodstream after injection of penicillin and the basic excretion characteristics of the drug. Remarkably, given the level of purity of the crude penicillin preparations, no further side effects were noted once the problem with pyrogens was overcome. By early February the Oxford team were ready to start their first therapeutic trial.

The patient was a 43-year-old Oxford policeman, later identified as Albert Alexander. In September the previous year he had developed a seemingly trivial sore on the corner of his mouth—reputedly from a rose thorn in his garden—which had evolved into a life-threatening suppurative infection with staphylococci and streptococci unresponsive to sulphonamide therapy. On 12 February 1941 he was started on a course of injections of penicillin: 200 mg at first, then 100 mg every 3 h. After 4 days, the patient's condition was strikingly improved, but on 17 February the supply of penicillin ran out, despite the fact that Fletcher was cycling to the Dunn Laboratories daily with the man's urine so that penicillin could be re-extracted. On 15 March, Albert Alexander died of an overwhelming staphylococcal pyaemia.

Four other patients, three of them children, had been treated with injections of penicillin by the end of May 1941. Most poignant was the fourth patient to receive intravenous penicillin, John Cox, a four and a half year-old boy (I was just 1 year older at the time, and here I am writing of it over 65 years later!) whose remarkable improvement was used as an illustration in the subsequent paper in *The Lancet*. John had developed a severe staphylococcal infection complicated by meningitis following an attack of measles. When started on penicillin he was semi-comatose, and virtually moribund. After 11 days treatment an extraordinary transformation in his condition was obvious: he was alert, playing with toys, and able to sit up in bed displaying an engagingly wistful smile (Fig. 4.2). He died from a ruptured artery in the brain on 31 May 1941, but the autopsy revealed no evidence of continuing infection.

---

* Meyer, a German born near Cologne, had earlier met Ernst Chain while studying medicinal chemistry in Berlin. Coincidentally he also developed a research interest in lysozyme. See: Simoni RD, Hill RL, Vaughan M, Hascall V. The discovery of hyaluronan by Karl Meyer. *Journal of Biological Chemistry* 2002; 277: e1–e2.

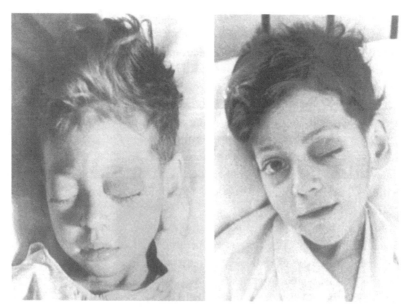

Fig. 4.2 John Cox, the fourth patient to be treated with penicillin by injection. Before (left) and 11 days after (right) treatment. From: Abraham EP, Chain E, Fletcher CM et al (1941). Further observations on penicillin. *Lancet* 2: 177–189. Reproduced by permission of Elsevier.

In this first trial five other patients received topical therapy for eye infections and one was given oral treatment for a urinary tract infection. All 10 cases were described in a paper that appeared in *The Lancet* almost exactly 1 year after the first (37). The effect of penicillin had been little short of miraculous and Florey was now sure of the importance of the discovery. Unlike the short earlier report, this was a long, detailed account of the properties of the mould, production methods, bacteriological results, and pharmacological data as well as the clinical findings. *The Lancet* seemed equally convinced and the editorial comment was now much more positive (38). Authorship of the paper was again alphabetical, but this time Chain was not top of the list: a chemist, Edward Abraham, had returned from Sweden, where he had been working on a Rockefeller Fellowship, and had joined the penicillin team. His immediate contribution had been to improve the purification process.

On 13 May 1940, 12 days before Florey's first animal protection experiment, Winston Churchill had told Parliament and the British people that he had '...nothing to offer but blood, toil, tears and sweat'. Less than 18 months later in August 1941 the war was still not going well, but something much more positive was on offer if production hurdles could be overcome: a life-saving drug the like of which had never before been seen.

Bringing penicillin to the world

Large-scale production was now the problem. This was clearly beyond the resources of the Dunn School, despite the ingenuity of Norman Heatley and the sterling efforts of the six 'penicillin girls'—Ruth Callow, Claire Inayat, Betty Cooke, Peggy Gardner, Megan

Lankaster, and Patricia McKegney*—who had been recruited to assist George Glister in providing enough material for the clinical trials. By this time, the *Penicillium* mould was being grown in 600 purpose made ceramic vessels, provided by the firm of James Macintyre and Company Limited, of Burslem, which had been approached on Florey's behalf by Dr Peter Stock, a local general practitioner[†] that he happened to know. The animal operating theatre of the Dunn School had been commandeered to accommodate the cultures and the unit was acting as a small penicillin factory. With this material a second trial, supervised by Florey's wife Ethel, was carried out at the Radcliffe Infirmary in 1942 (39) and Alexander Fleming scrounged enough penicillin from Florey to successfully treat a case of meningitis in St Mary's Hospital with intrathecal penicillin (40).

Approaches were made to British firms capable of commercial production, and one, Kemball, Bishop and Co., a small chemical firm (later taken over by Pfizer, with whom they had a long association) showed some interest. Despite their precarious position in the war-ravaged East End of London, they eventually started to produce crude filtrate for the Dunn School. Other initiatives came largely from the Therapeutic Research Corporation, a consortium of British pharmaceutical firms formed in 1941,[‡] with penicillin as one of their principal concerns (41). In February 1943, Glaxo took over and adapted a disused cheese factory belonging to the Nestlé Company in Aylesbury, Buckinghamshire for penicillin production with help from Burroughs Wellcome and the Ministry of Supply (42). By 1943 sufficient drug had been produced, predominantly by Kemball Bishop, ICI, and Glaxo, to meet some military needs, mostly for use in North Africa and during the advance through Italy. Florey himself took a close interest in this work, which was supervised by his former Oxford colleague (and fellow Rhodes scholar from Adelaide) Hugh Cairns, who was now a brigadier in the British Army (43). Until the end of the war only small quantities of penicillin were made available for civilian use in the United Kingdom (44).

With Britain at war and in danger of invasion, things were too uncertain to leave the question of supplies up to indigenous firms. Florey was ahead of the game and was already making plans in the spring of 1941, while the first clinical trials were under way, to visit the United States to drum up support. With the blessing of the Medical Research Council, and funding once more from the Rockefeller Foundation, Florey and Heatley set off on 27 June 1941—just 4 weeks after the setback of the death of John Cox—in a blacked out plane to fly to Lisbon en route for New York. Chain had not been told and was reportedly furious.

First stop in the United States, after a courtesy call to the Rockefeller Foundation, was the home of the physiologist, John Fulton, an old friend who had been a fellow Rhodes

---

* All, except Peggy Gardner receive an acknowledgement in Florey's 1941 paper (Reference 30).

† Stock later gave up general practice and became a cardiologist in Stoke.

‡ The original consortium was made up of Boots Pure Drug Company, British Drug Houses, Glaxo Laboratories, May & Baker, and the Wellcome Foundation. Imperial Chemical Industries (pharmaceuticals) joined after its formation from the parent company in 1942.

scholar at Oxford and who was looking after the Floreys' children for the duration of the war. Through various intermediaries, including Ross Harrison, chairman of the National Research Council and Charles Thom, the mycologist who had earlier correctly identified Fleming's mould (see p. 93), Florey and Heatley were finally directed to the Agriculture Department Research Laboratories in Peoria, Illinois, which had opened only in late 1940 and was known to have experience of fermentation techniques. It was an inspired and fateful choice: the situation of the laboratories, in the American corn belt, south-west of Chicago, and the expertise to be found there were to prove pivotal in the development of high yield penicillin cultures.

After making contact with Robert Coghill, chief of the Fermentation Division in Peoria, Florey left Heatley to collaborate with Coghill and his team and set off on a tour of the major drug companies to try to persuade them to produce enough penicillin to enable him to extend his clinical trials. It turned out at first to be a fruitless exercise. The distinguished Australian professor from Britain was cordially received, but he found that firms were unwilling at that time to turn over manufacturing facilities to an uncertain product involving a mould that might contaminate other production processes. In the end the only penicillin Florey subsequently received on his return to Oxford was a 5 g sample from Merck. Nevertheless American drug companies were not uninterested in what he had to say. In fact penicillin had already attracted more interest in the States than Florey had realized and some firms, notably Merck, Squibb (where an interest in penicillin had started as early as 1936), and Lilly, were already conducting tentative investigations of their own (23).

In Peoria, Heatley was assigned to work with the mycologist Andrew Moyer who was an expert in the cultivation of moulds. Moyer used the readily available corn steep liquor, a locally available by-product of the process of corn starch extraction, as the growth medium and adapted it for the optimum growth of the *Penicillium* mould. By use of this medium yields of penicillin were much greater than those obtained in Oxford. Later, at the suggestion of Orville May, director of the Peoria laboratory, a deep fermentation method rather than surface culture was developed, increasing yields further. Heatley, who had been fully open about the Oxford work, was surprised to find that Moyer was highly secretive about his methods. The reasons for this became clear when it was revealed that Coghill and Moyer had applied for patents* of the production process a moved that was to lead to an acrimonious dispute after the end of the Second World War. At that time, patenting of discoveries and inventions, especially those of benefit to health, was regarded in academic circles in Britain as being ignoble, if not downright unethical. When Chain (son of an industrial chemist) had suggested patenting penicillin he had been soundly rebuffed.

---

* These patents were assigned to the Department of Agriculture since, as government employees they were barred from taking out personal patents. However, the restriction did not extend to foreign patents and Moyer also took out a British patent on the production process.

On 7 August 1941 before returning to England (via the Connaught Laboratories in Toronto, where one of the workers he encountered was Ronald Hare, who had moved there from Queen Charlotte's) Florey visited an old friend, Alfred Newton Richards, a pharmacologist in whose Philadelphia laboratories Florey had worked in 1926. The meeting with Richards was to prove more productive than any other that he had during his frustrating time in the United States. In June 1941 a National Defense Research Committee had been set up under the direction of Vannevar Bush, an eminent electrical engineer later involved in the Manhattan Project. Medical matters were delegated to a Committee on Medical Research under the chairmanship of Richards. Florey managed to convince his old friend of the importance of penicillin and in October 1941 the Committee on Medical Research agreed that further research on penicillin would be desirable. Richards then approached the major pharmaceutical companies in the United States to seek their cooperation, promising government funds for the project.

On 7 December 1941 Japanese planes attacked the American Pacific Fleet in Pearl Harbor precipitating the American decision to enter the Second World War. Penicillin production became a national priority. Despite the reluctance to of the drug firms to share commercially sensitive information, and a fear of breaching US antitrust laws—a specific exemption was obtained for penicillin production in 1943—considerable cooperation between many American pharmaceutical firms, academic institutions, and government agencies was achieved once the United States had joined the war (45).

The first documented 'miracle' cure with penicillin in the United States took place in mid-March 1942 in the isolation unit of Yale's New Haven Hospital in Connecticut. The patient was a 31-year-old woman, Anne Sheafe Miller, wife of the university's director of athletics, Ogden Miller. Anne Miller had developed a septicaemia following a miscarriage and her physician, John Bumstead, had despaired of being able to save her life. By chance, another of Bumstead's patients in a nearby room was Howard Florey's old friend, John Fulton who was well aware of Florey's work with penicillin. Fulton used his influence to obtain 5.5 g of crude penicillin from Merck and intravenous injections were started on 14 March 1942. As with Albert Alexander, the patient's urine was collected and sent back to Merck for re-extraction but, more fortunate than the Oxford policeman, Anne Miller survived. She died 57 years later on 27 May 1999 at the age of 90 (46).

The project to produce penicillin in the United States during the war was outstandingly successful. All the major industrial players committed resources to the problem with the help of public funds and tax incentives. The brilliant Austrian-born organic chemist Oskar Wintersteiner* and his colleagues at Squibb succeeded in crystallizing the drug as early as 1943, allowing chemically pure penicillin to be produced. Many academic institutions received government contracts to pursue research on penicillin. Intensive work also continued at Peoria where a search was instituted for strains of mould that produced better yields of penicillin. The mycologist Kenneth Raper, who had earlier worked with

---

* Wintersteiner had earlier worked on insulin at Columbia University. After his success with penicillin at Squibb, he went on to crystallize streptomycin. Like Chain he was an accomplished pianist.

Charles Thom, looked after the laboratory's culture collection and was entrusted with this task. Samples of fungi were isolated from specimens sent from all over the world, but it was a spontaneous mutant of a strain of *Penicillium chrysogenum* isolated from a mouldy cantaloupe melon obtained from the local market in 1943—bought, according to legend, by a laboratory assistant, Mary Hunt, earning her the nickname 'mouldy Mary'—that was to prove a winner. The Croatian geneticist, Milislav Demerec working at the Carnegie Institution's Cold Spring Harbor Laboratory, New York, used X-ray mutagenesis to persuade the Peoria strain of *Penicillium chrysogenum* to produce even higher levels of penicillin. Workers at the University of Wisconsin further enhanced the yield by ultraviolet irradiation of spores of Demerec's improved strain.

In the meantime back in Oxford, Edward Abraham was busy trying to unravel the structure and chemistry of penicillin ably abetted by Robert Robinson, the Australian chemist John Cornforth, and Wilson Baker* at the nearby Dyson Perrins Laboratory, Oxford's centre of excellence in organic chemistry.

Elucidation of the structure of the penicillin molecule (or rather molecules, since it turned out that several closely related variants of penicillin were elaborated by the producer mould[†]) proved to be contentious and difficult. In the event it was not chemistry, but X-ray crystallography—a procedure by which the structure of crystallized molecules can be mathematically deduced according to interference patterns produced as the constituent atoms are deflected by X-rays—that cracked the problem. The technique was the speciality of Dorothy Crowfoot Hodgkin in Oxford.[‡] In 1945 she used it to prove that penicillin exhibited an unusual fused β-lactam–thiazolidine ring structure (Fig. 4.3). The β-lactam arrangement had originally been proposed by Abraham, but opposed by Robinson and Cornforth.

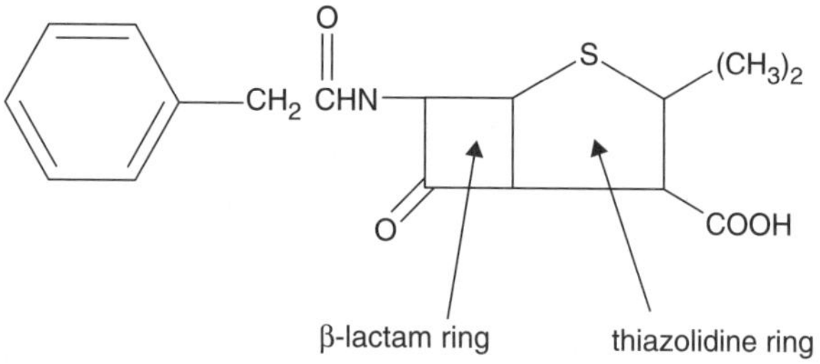

Fig. 4.3 Structure of benzylpenicillin (penicillin G).

---

* Baker was an accomplished organic chemist, but was also a pacifist and was much concerned at the time with helping to set up the Oxford Committee for Famine Relief, which later developed into Oxfam. He died in 2002, aged 102.

[†] These were: 2-pentenylpenicillin (penicillin F); benzylpenicillin (penicillin G); *p*-hydroxybenzylpenicillin (penicillin X); and n-heptylpenicillin (penicillin K). The four types were originally given the numbers I–IV in the United Kingdom. Penicillin F (I) is the substance produced by Fleming's original mould. The Peoria process favoured the production of penicillin G (II) and, since this variant appeared to exhibit the best properties, benzylpenicillin was the form that was developed and is the one now used therapeutically.

[‡] Where later one of her students was Margaret Thatcher.

The one goal that eluded everyone was the chemical synthesis of penicillin, which was universally assumed to be the route to mass production. By the time the structure had been worked out, the pharmaceutical companies were so efficient at mass producing the drug by fermentation processes that they were no longer interested in chemical synthesis, but John Sheehan of the Massachusetts Institute of Technology continued to work on the problem and in 1957 achieved the total synthesis of natural penicillin (47).

The first clinical trials of penicillin in the United States took place with the limited amount of drug then available in 1942. The studies were coordinated by a committee chaired originally by Perrin Long of Johns Hopkins, who had been instrumental in awakening American interest in sulphonamides (see p. 74–5). However, Long soon joined the US Army Medical Corps and was posted overseas. Chairmanship of the committee was taken over by the Boston Physician, Chester Scott Keefer. In spring 1943, as more supplies slowly came on stream, the studies were extended to military personnel at Bushnell General Hospital in Utah. By the D-day landings in Normandy in June 1944, production in the United States had increased to over 100 billion units* per month, sufficient for military and much civilian use. It was a remarkable achievement. All restrictions on sale were removed by the end of the war, by which time production had reached around 650 billion units per month.

In Australia, Howard Florey's birthplace, penicillin production for military use in New Guinea started in 1943 at the Commonwealth Serum Laboratories in Melbourne. Percival Bazeley (48), a veterinary scientist serving with the Australian Army, and a chemist, H. H. Kretchmar supervised the project. They flew to the United States to learn production methods in November 1943 and remarkably were able to have the first usable supplies ready by Christmas that year.

During the war attempts to produce penicillin were also pursued in many other countries, including, perhaps surprisingly, the USSR, the Netherlands, Germany, and Japan. The Russians were let into the secrets as war allies. Howard Florey and Gordon Sanders were entrusted with the mission of carrying cultures and technical know-how on the production and application of the new drug in a top secret operation in late 1943. Over Christmas and New Year they endured a nightmarish journey that took them to Moscow via Marrakesh, Cairo (where they met Robin Pulvertaft, just back from ministering to Churchill; see p. 76), Teheran (where Florey developed bronchopneumonia and was kept in the American Hospital for several weeks), Baku, and Stalingrad (49). They found that Russian scientists were already experimenting on a *Penicillium* mould of their own, but had made little progress. By 1944, with the additional information provided by

---

* One unit of penicillin was originally defined arbitrarily in Oxford by comparison to an early stock solution. Florey and Jennings later defined it more precisely for assay purposes as 'that amount of penicillin which when dissolved in fifty millilitres of meat extract just inhibits completely the growth of the test strain of *Staphylococcus aureus*.' The strain used was one kept in Oxford and known universally as 'the Oxford staphylococcus'. See: *Penicillin: its properties, uses and preparations*. The Pharmaceutical Press, London, 1946. A unit is now recognized to be equivalent to 0.6 µg (millionths of a gram).

Sanders, Florey, and American scientists, the Scientific Research Institute of Microbiology in Kirov was producing sufficient penicillin for use in front-line military hospitals.

In Holland, scientists at the Nederlandsche Gist- en Spiritusfabriek (Netherlands Yeast and Spirit factory),* led by a young microbial biochemist Adrianus Petrus Struyk, learnt about Florey's work during the summer of 1943, possibly through Dutch broadcasts from London. Working in Delft under difficult wartime conditions and in secret, Struyk's group succeeded in partially purifying small amounts of penicillin from a strain of *Penicillium baculatum* obtained from the Dutch culture collection at Baarn. The team were aided by advice from a Jewish physician, the medical biochemist Andries Querido of the University of Leiden. Despite being interned in a transit camp before being sent to Teresienstadt, Querido was allowed privileges as an 'essential worker' to attend scientific meetings at Delft. The active product obtained in Delft was given the name 'bacinol', partly because it was uncertain at that stage that it was actually identical to penicillin, but also to avoid raising awareness of the development to the occupying German forces (50). After the war the factory became an important producer of penicillin in the Netherlands (51).

Florey's *Lancet* papers reached Germany as early as 1942 through neutral Sweden. Several firms, including Schering in Berlin and the constituent companies of IG Farben attempted, with little success, to replicate the findings. Some work with antibiotic-producing moulds was carried out in Gerhard Domagk's laboratory in Elberfeld by the bacteriologist, Maria Brommelhues, but nothing of note was obtained. As in the United States, synthesis of penicillin was thought to be the best route to large-scale production. The Viennese-born chemist Richard Kuhn—like Domagk, a Nobel Prize winner who was prevented by Hitler from accepting the honour before the war—was charged with the task at the Kaiser-Wilhelm-Institut for Medical Research (now the Max Planck Institut) in Heidelberg, but lack of information on the correct structure prevented any real progress (52). A biochemist, Heinz Öppinger of Hoechst was able to obtain miniscule quantities of penicillin by late 1942, but it was insufficient even for basic animal tests. It took him a further 2 years to work out an improved method of production involving a rotating drum that provided conditions similar to those of submerged fermentation that were so successful in the United States. By this time facilities to pursue the research had collapsed. The technique came to light when Harold Raistrick interviewed Öppinger on behalf of the Allied Commission after the war (53).

Others in Germany worked on the penicillin project and some research on the new drug was undertaken in occupied Czechoslovakia at a firm in Olomutz (Olomouc) in Moravia that had been commandeered by the German authorities. 'Unofficial' research on penicillin was also carried out in Prague during the war at Jiří Fragner's pharmaceutical plant (now part of the Czech pharmaceutical group Zentiva) by a team that included the microbiologist Ivan Málek and the chemist Karel Wiesner,† who later emigrated to Canada where he

---

* Originally formed in 1870, the Nederlandsche Gist- en Spiritusfabriek later merged with Brocades and now trades as DSM-Gist.

† Jirí Fragner was an uncle of Wiesner's wife. See: Schneider WG, Valenta Z. Karel Frantisek Wiesner 25 November 1919–28 November 1986. *Biographical Memoirs of Fellow of the Royal Society* 1991; 37:463–490.

pursued a distinguished career at the University of New Brunswick (54). Hitler's personal physician, the disreputable Theodor Morell, considered by many of his colleagues to be a charlatan, may have used penicillin to treat the Führer after the 1944 assassination attempt, earning him an Iron Cross. The origins of Morell's penicillin (if indeed it was the genuine article) are obscure, but it probably came from the Czech laboratories in Olomutz. Certainly his claims to have access to significant amounts of the drug are almost certainly bogus.

In fact, enthusiasm for penicillin in wartime Germany is likely to have been muted. Although German physicians who were able to experience personally some remarkable cures welcomed Prontosil and the ensuing sulphonamides, Nazi ideology leant towards snake-oil preparations such as Omnadin, a non-specific 'immune stimulant' made from ill-defined lipids and proteins of animal origin. Surprisingly, Omnadin's dubious reputation survived the war and was touted for a time in combination with penicillin as 'Omnacillin'.

From Germany and Switzerland information about penicillin filtered through to Japan, where research started in early 1944 just as the US Marines were landing on the Gilbert and Marshall Islands as they kept up their island-hopping progress in the Pacific war. Japanese scientists were more successful than their German counterparts. By the time of the Japanese surrender on 15 August 1945, penicillin-producing strains of *Penicillium* had been isolated, an active product produced, a handful of cases successfully treated and production of penicillin (renamed hekiso: 'blue principle', presumably from the colour of the mould) started at the Banyu Pharmaceutical Company (55). In 1946 penicillin production continued and, indeed, flourished with the help American advice, notably from Jackson Foster of the University of Texas at Austin. Foster, one of Selman Waksman's former students at Rutgers (see p. 148) had worked on penicillin with another Waksman protégé, Boyd Woodruff, at Merck in Rahway, New Jersey before moving to Texas in 1946. By 1948 Japan was self-sufficient in penicillin production and started to export the drug the following year (56).

The American success in mass-producing penicillin during the Second World War owed much to the commercial exploitation of the deep-tank fermentation method, which much improved yields. First to adopt this technique on a large scale was the firm Chas Pfizer and Co. in New York, where the method was already used in the manufacture of citric acid. In autumn 1942, a chemical engineer working for the company, Jasper Kane, suggested exploiting the citric acid method for penicillin production and his colleague John McKeen, who later became chairman of the company, put this into effect (57). British firms did not adopt the American deep fermentation methods until after the war, but were none the less able to produce 25–30 million units per week by 1945. Towards the end of the war government money was provided through the Ministry of Supply to build penicillin plants at Barnard Castle, County Durham for Glaxo and at Speke in Liverpool for the Distillers Company.* Deep fermentation technology, licensed

---

* Distillers, as the name suggests, specialized in whisky and gin. Later they produced streptomycin and other drugs, one of which was thalidomide, which became notorious for causing serious birth defects and was removed from the market in 1961. In 1963 Eli Lilly bought the Speke site, retaining the Dista name that the previous owners had used on many of their products.

from the United States under favourable terms, was installed in both plants; Distillers enlisted technical expertise from the Commercial Solvents Corporation, which had helped to pioneer the deep fermentation method in the United States, and by 1946 was a major player in penicillin production in the United Kingdom.

While the level of production reached in Britain during the war fell short of the American feat it was a creditable accomplishment given the resources available in a country ravaged by war. All the same, the American success cannot be written off as simply due to more favourable circumstances. It came about because of the energy and determination of leaders of American industry and science and an unprecedented cooperation between government, academia, and commerce. It is lesson from which we could still learn.

Miracle drug: acclaim and hyperbole

Penicillin undoubtedly changed the face of infectious diseases. It had proved itself in war, especially in the treatment of shrapnel wounds that frequently led to gas gangrene or deep wound infections with other organisms; in burns that often became colonized with virulent streptococci; and in the rapid cure of venereal diseases (the response in gonorrhoea was 'like turning off a tap' (58)) that sometimes incapacitated fighting troops as effectively as bullets and bombs. Equally impressive activity against syphilis was demonstrated in 1943 by the work of John Mahoney, Director of the Venereal Disease Research Laboratory at Staten Island Marine Hospital in New York (59). Now that penicillin was more or less freely available in civilian hospitals its astounding ability to stop such dreaded diseases as pneumonia and meningitis in their tracks captured the imagination of a world exhausted by war.

The drug was a public sensation. In parts of Europe a black market in penicillin—or, often, worthless substitutes—briefly appeared (the trade was immortalized in the film made from Graham Greene's novella *The Third Man*), but quickly evaporated as cheap penicillin flooded the market. All the major drug houses in the United Kingdom were marketing penicillin by 1946, not only in injectable form, but also as ointments, creams, lozenges, and, in the case of May & Baker Ltd., as dental cones for insertion in sockets after tooth extraction. One enterprising doctor, Hans Enoch, a German émigré* who had established a business called *The International Serum Company* in England before the war, marketed crude preparations of penicillin—Vivicillin for injection and Pennotin for oral or topical use—harvested from liquid cultures of *Penicillium notatum*. The preparations, which alarmingly contained living fungal hyphae (so does blue cheese, but that is not injected!), were claimed to have several advantages: to be free from pyrogens and other

---

* Hans Enoch had a colourful life: as a front-line soldier in the German army in the First World War he was awarded the Iron Cross. He then studied medicine and chemistry in Heidelberg and subsequently worked in the Paul Ehrlich Institute. Along with other Jews he was barred from practice when the Nazis came to power and was imprisoned in 1934 for 7 months, fleeing to England after his release.

impurities; to contain useful antibacterial metabolites removed by other manufacturing processes; and (most fanciful of all) to prolong the activity for 36–48 h by continuation of the formation of penicillin *in vivo* (60). These products briefly aroused considerable interest, but were rightly shunned by the medical profession.

The amazing cures achieved by penicillin had already became widely known during the war, and once it was over Fleming was besieged by the media and universally lionized, whereas Florey and his team and the American corporate effort received little global publicity. To some extent this was due to the natural inclination for popular adulation to focus upon a single individual rather than the teamwork that characterized the work in Oxford and the United States, but it also reflected the differing temperaments of the main protagonists. Fleming, laconic and uncommunicative though he was by nature, paradoxically enjoyed being in the limelight. He seldom refused an invitation to be interviewed or to travel abroad to receive the huge number of honorary degrees and medals that were showered upon him after the war. He had been singled out by the media for praise as early as 1942, after Almroth Wright wrote to *The Times* claiming the glory of discovering penicillin for Fleming—and by extension St Mary's Hospital—with the characteristically classical flourish, *palmam qui meruit ferat* (61).* Although Robert Robinson at Oxford immediately countered, pointing out that if Fleming deserved a laurel wreath, Florey should receive a handsome bouquet, the tide of public acclaim drowned out his voice. Charles Wilson—more famous as Lord Moran, Churchill's physician—the dean of St Mary's, and popularly known as 'corkscrew Charlie' because of his political skills, encouraged the hospital, which was always in financial difficulties, to milk the exposure to public attention.

While Fleming did nothing to discourage media interest in the penicillin story, Florey found public adulation distasteful. Partly from a personal aversion to publicity and partly from a fear that the Oxford team would be inundated with requests for penicillin that could not be satisfied, Florey always shunned the media and paid the price of not being accorded the same public esteem. He was happy to address medical, scientific, and academic audiences, and did so tirelessly in Britain and on several foreign trips, but he strongly believed it to be inappropriate for scientists to court publicity.

The contribution of the Oxford team was always acknowledged in the many books on penicillin that appeared in the immediate post-war period, but the American contribution, without which the large-scale production of penicillin would have been much delayed, often received scant attention. The tone of these books reflects the general feeling at the time—a feeling that now, in the early twenty-first century, seems to have almost completely evaporated—that science and medicine were to be at the forefront of the better future that post-war euphoria confidently expected. Sometimes, medical

* Let him who has won it bear the palm. Taken from a poem by John Jortin (1698–1770) and used as a motto by Horatio Nelson (1758–1805).

authors who should have known better were almost as hysterical as the general public. The colourful Harley Street surgeon, George Bankoff, a Russian émigré who wrote popular science books under his own name and as George Sava or George Borodin, was moved to write:

> Soon young ladies will be able to buy their lipsticks impregnated with Penicillin. They still will have their lips made beautiful and inviting, but the danger of infection that every kiss potentially can transmit will be removed. Penicillin will be like a guardian angel ready to halt any intruder that is unwelcome. Be it an ordinary streptococcus, or the microbe of influenza, or even the dreaded microbe of syphilis; be it the unknown microbe of cancer, or the germ that infects our lung tissue, it will be quite immaterial. It will be arrested before it is able to do harm or cause damage, by the invisible amount of Penicillin spread on the lips together with the lipstick. Facial creams, mascaras and, of course, all tooth-paste will be impregnated with Penicillin too, thus preserving teeth healthy and unblemished...Penicillin given in sufficient doses to any would-be dictator, or any evil genius trying to discover more potent rockets or liquid air-bombs, will perhaps mellow their brain and subdue their evil desires (62)

He goes on to speculate that *Penicillium* moulds contaminating the waters of Lourdes might be responsible for the miraculous cures!

Bizarre though all this sounds, it gives some flavour of the response to the 'miracle' of penicillin in some quarters and helps to explain the adulation that Fleming received. Wherever he went round the world—and he was never slow to accept invitations—Fleming was greeted with scenes of near mass hysteria usually reserved for royalty and film stars. Florey was irritated by the acclaim Fleming received, especially when he was credited with work that had actually been done at Oxford, but he reserved his frustration to private remarks to colleagues and refrained from taking his misgivings into the public arena. The volatile Chain, meanwhile, predictably fumed. He was openly scornful of the popular veneration of Fleming, but no one took much notice. By the time Fleming hysteria was at its height after the war, Chain and Florey had the Nobel Prize under their belts and both were being wooed—Florey in Australia and Chain in Israel and Italy—for prestigious positions that would satisfy their professional ambitions.

Fleming, Florey, and Chain were jointly awarded the Nobel Prize for Physiology or Medicine in 1945. There had been pressure for Fleming alone to receive the prize for his role in making the original discovery. Others wanted Fleming and Florey to share the honour. Göran Liljestrand, secretary of the Nobel Committee of the Karolinska Institute, championed the inclusion of Chain. Nanna Svarz, another member of the Nobel committee charged with reviewing nominations for the medicine prize, argued that Fleming should receive half the prize with Florey and Chain sharing the other half. In the end common sense and good counsel prevailed and the prize was equally shared.

The Nobel Prize is popularly regarded as a reward for genius. It is a tricky word to define, but it is hard to conclude that Alexander Fleming was a true genius in any meaningful sense of the term. Certainly he was not the quiet visionary of popular myth, nor did he claim to be; he is better characterized as a highly competent and resourceful, but not particularly hard working bacteriologist (he was as much at home playing snooker in the Chelsea Arts Club as in his laboratory) who had the gumption to follow up an interesting

observation and the great fortune to see it finally mature into a discovery of lasting importance. It was Howard Florey, Ernst Chain, and their colleagues who we must thank for
uncovering the therapeutic benefit of penicillin. This is not to minimize the American
contribution, which was certainly crucial in bringing the benefits of penicillin to the world
so quickly, nor the efforts of the rest of the team at the Dunn School—above all the vital
input of Norman Heatley—whose role Florey was always punctilious in acknowledging.

The Dunn School achievement is an example, perhaps, of collective genius—or the
happy association of the right people in the right place at the right time led by two scientists of outstanding ability. As if to show that penicillin was not a fluke, within a few years
the school was to be instrumental in bringing another major antibiotic to the attention
of the world—but this time without Chain and with only minimal input from Florey.

Cephalosporins

The story of the first cephalosporins is as extraordinary in its own way as that of penicillin and again luck was to play a major role. By the end of the Second World War, the
work of René Dubos on tyrothricin, the remarkable success of penicillin and the discoveries of Selman Waksman (see Chapter 5) had awakened considerable interest in
microbes as a natural source of potent antibacterial compounds. Florey himself had
sought other natural products after the successful trials of penicillin and had investigated
two potential compounds: helvolic acid, produced by a variant of the common fungus
Aspergillus fumigatus; and patulin (also known as claviformin and clavulin among other
names) isolated from *Penicillium claviforme*. Neither of these antibiotics lived up to early
expectations because of problems of toxicity, although patulin enjoyed a brief vogue as a
possible cure for the common cold until a Medical Research Council trial in 1943–44
showed the claim to be bogus (63). The patulin trial was placebo controlled and double-
blind (neither patient nor doctor knew which was the 'active' treatment) with various
dosages or placebo allocated alternately according to a predetermined code. Although the
findings of the trial were disappointing, it served as an exemplary model for the future
conduct of drug efficacy trials (64).

Sea and Sardinia

One person to be enthused by the hunt for antimicrobial agents was an obscure Italian doctor, Giuseppe Brotzu. Brotzu was far from obscure in his own city, Cagliari, Sardinia, where
he held the positions of rector of its ancient University and director of the Institute of
Hygiene that now bears his name. Moreover, he was well known to the locals who suspected
him to be a harbinger of bad luck because of his predilection for black suits, in which he
stalked the streets even on the hottest day (65). He did not deserve this reputation, for he
was a devout, modest, and humane man who did much to promote the well-being of the
island community, notably in helping to rid it of the scourge of indigenous malaria (66).

As a hygienist Brotzu was well aware of the dangers of the discharge of untreated
sewage into the sea where the people of Cagliari collected mussels and the young

folk swam. Typhoid was, after all, endemic in Sardinia and he had tried to implement a ban on the harvesting and sale of mussels in the vicinity of local sewage outfalls. It was therefore a puzzle to him that the youngsters who swam in the polluted sea seldom contracted typhoid fever or other illnesses. The mystery deepened when he failed to isolate the salmonellae that cause typhoid from seawater samples, though faecal carriage of the organism must have been common in the community.

Brotzu speculated that the sewage might be self-sterilizing, possibly because of the presence of antibiotic-producing moulds, eschewing the more likely explanations that the combined effects of salinity, sunlight and massive dilution might be responsible. In summer 1945, as the world began the process of reconstruction after a devastating war, Brotzu and his assistant Antonio Spanedda, a professor of microbiology who later entered the priesthood, started to collect samples from the sewage outfall to see whether they could find organisms that might be responsible for killing pathogenic bacteria in the water. Numerous fungi were tested for antibiotic activity by allowing them to grow on agar in a Petri dish for 3 or 4 days and then streaking cultures of pathogenic bacteria radially from the mould to the edge of the dish; after further incubation inhibition of bacterial growth indicated antibiotic activity.

On 20 July 1945, a mould was isolated, after incubation of a sample at room temperature on ordinary nutrient agar, that was able to prevent growth of *Eberthella typhi* (an old name for the causative organism of typhoid fever, now known as *Salmonella enterica* serotype Typhi) and other important bacterial pathogens. Among the organisms against which Brotzu tested the mould—with alarming disregard for personal safety—were: *Pasteurella pestis* (the causative organism of bubonic plague, now known as *Yersinia pestis*); *Brucella melitensis* (the cause of Malta fever, notorious among bacteriologists for its propensity to cause laboratory acquired infections); *Shigella shiga-kruse* (cause of a particularly virulent form of bacillary dysentery and now known as *Shigella dysenteriae*); and *Vibrio cholerae* (the cause of Asiatic cholera).

These noteworthy results were published not in an international, nor even a national Italian journal, but in the house journal of the institute, *Lavori dell'Istituto d'Igiene di Cagliari* (67). It is often said that Brotzu actually founded the periodical for the purpose of publishing his paper, and that it was the only issue that ever appeared. Indeed, Edward Abraham claims to have heard this story from Brotzu himself (68). However, a series with this title* appeared as early as 1940; it seems to have been mainly a collection of reprints of works published by members of the Institute. Brotzu's paper was never published—or, so far as is known, even submitted—elsewhere and it seems likely that he had it privately printed locally (the paper bears the imprint 'Cagliari—Tip. [Tipografia] C.E.L. 1948') and inserted in the *Lavori* along with the others.

....

* Brotzu's paper is included in a collection described as 'Lavori dell'istituto d'igiene dell'università di Cagliari' in the Wellcome Library for the History and Understanding of Medicine in London. The holding, with slight variants of the title, covers the period 1940-54. Each consists of reprints.

Three years elapsed between the discovery and committing the results to print in 1948. Little is known of what happened in the intervening years other than what is revealed in the paper. Like Fleming before him, Brotzu found that he lacked the expertise to extract and purify the substance responsible for the antibacterial activity, but succeeded in obtaining a brownish-yellow concentrate after partially evaporating a filtrate of the culture fluid, precipitating out protein material with alcohol and then distilling the alcoholic solution under vacuum.

With cavalier disregard for ethical considerations remarkable even by the standards of the day, Brotzu apparently moved on to clinical trials without any prior animal tests. He used crude culture fluid to inject carbuncles, abscesses and superficial skin infections, and the crude concentrate to treat typhoid and paratyphoid fever and undulant fever (brucellosis) by the intravenous, intramuscular, and rectal routes. Unsurprisingly, intravenous administration produced a severe febrile reaction and intramuscular injections were painful. None the less, he claimed that uniformly satisfactory results were achieved, even in cases of ringworm (a fungal infection) treated with packs of the native fungal mycelium!

Brotzu's paper ends with the exhortation: 'Si è voluto riferire quanto sopra nella speranza che altri istituti meglio dotati di mezzi possano giungere ad un progresso maggiore nella selezione del micete, preparazione culturale dell'antibiotico, ed estrazione di esso'. [The above findings are reported in the hope that other, better-equipped institutes can achieve greater progress in the selection of the mould, cultural preparation of the antibiotic and its extraction.] It is hard to imagine anything better designed to consign a work to eternal obscurity than the course of action of publishing it in a house journal, but Brotzu did not let the matter lie. Some attempts were made to obtain funds to pursue research into his antibiotic, but these failed to evoke any interest (69), and he was left with the option of trying to interest others in the discovery through personal contacts. One such contact was a British public health doctor, Blyth Brooke, who had been stationed in Sardinia during the war.

Blyth Brooke might never have gone to Italy. As medical officer of health for the London Borough of Finsbury he had plenty of war work to do looking after casualty services, air raid shelter facilities, and wartime nurseries during the blitz. Having decided that he wanted to be involved in the overseas war effort, he offered his services to the war office hoping to go to the Far East, where he had family connections with the Rajah Brooke dynasty* in Sarawak (70). When he was rejected because of lack of tropical experience, he volunteered in 1942 to join the Royal Army Medical Corps and was commissioned and sent to Italy, serving in Rome, Sardinia, and Trieste, where he remained, with the rank of Major, until 1946 (71).

---

* The British adventurer, Sir James Brooke (1803–68) became Rajah of Sarawak in 1841 after putting down a rebellion. He and his successors—his nephew, Charles (Johnson) Brooke (1829–1917) and Charles' son, Vyner Brooke (1874–1963)—were known as the White Rajahs. Sarawak was invaded by Japan in 1941 and after the war the family ceded their rights to the British government.

By 1948 Brooke had resumed his work in Finsbury (and started to read law, eventually being admitted to the bar) but he was still in touch with Brotzu, who sent him a copy of his paper and asked for advice. Brooke contacted the Medical Research Council and the Secretary, Sir Edward Mellanby, naturally suggested that Howard Florey in Oxford was the person most likely to help.

Oxford: cephalosporin C

Things were changing at the Sir William Dunn School. The success of penicillin had made the school famous in scientific circles, if not in the public imagination. Florey was still nominally in charge, but was being wooed by the Australian authorities. He was actively involved in the setting up of the Australian National University in Canberra and (with Gordon Sanders) in planning the John Curtin School of Medical Research (72). Chain was becoming progressively disgruntled, among other things with the lack of the lavish facilities he would have liked. He, too, was being courted, including a tempting offer from the Weizmann Institute, named after its founder Chaim Weizmann, in Rehovot, Israel. He preferred, however, to accept an offer from the Italian Government to organize and direct a research centre for chemical microbiology at the Istituto Superiore di Sanità in Rome, which eventually opened with a staff of over 90 scientists in June 1951.

Chain left Oxford for Rome in October 1948, just after Brotzu had sent a culture of his mould to the Sir William Dunn School (would he have preferred to send it to Rome if he had known?). The mould was initially given to Norman Heatley to investigate. He carried out a few desultory experiments, but was more interested at the time in micrococcin, a thiopeptide antibiotic produced by bacteria (*Bacillus* and *Micrococcus* species), which it was hoped might have some activity in tuberculosis.* Edward Abraham, together with his colleague Harold Burton and a DPhil student, Guy Newton, took over the investigation as part of their general interest in peptide antibiotics and arranged for culture fluid material to be prepared at the Medical Research Council's Antibiotics Research Station, which had been set up in a large house at Clevedon, a seaside town on the Bristol Channel near Weston-Super-Mare.

The Clevedon unit played an important, but largely forgotten part in the penicillin story. The Royal Navy had originally bought the house in 1943 in order to produce penicillin for its own use. Cultures were grown in vessels stacked on shelves ranged from floor to ceiling in a long, narrow, high room. Access to the top shelves without disturbing the cultures was consequently difficult, but the problem was solved by raising the lady technicians in a specially installed bosun's chair said to be large enough to accommodate an elephant (73). The Clevedon house was acquired in 1946 by the Distillers Company, which was at the time using its expertise in fermentation for penicillin production encouraged by the Ministry of Supply (see p. 109). It was taken over by the Medical

---

* Many years later it was found to have antimalarial activity. See: Rogers MJ, Cundliffe E, McCutchan TF. The antibiotic micrococcin is a potent inhibitor of growth and protein synthesis in the malaria parasite. *Antimicrobial Agents and Chemotherapy* 1998; 42: 715–716.

Research Council in 1949 under the direction of the statistician Brendan K. Kelly who had formerly worked for the Distillers Company in Epsom. According to Ernst Chain it was Howard Florey who had insisted on a statistician being in charge so that results would be properly interpreted. The Medical Research Council pulled the plug on the operation in 1961. As Edward Abraham ruefully observed, the decision to close the unit was made just as the cephalosporins were beginning to show promise (68).

Brotzu had identified his mould as *Cephalosporium acremonium* (though this is revealed only in the 'conclusions' at the end of his paper and no details are given); it is now more commonly called *Acremonium chrysogenum*. In England, solvent extraction of culture fluids of the mould yielded an antibiotic that was active against only a few organisms, such as staphylococci and streptococci. These are Gram-positive bacteria and the substance was given the name cephalosporin P (for 'positive'). It turned out to be an antibiotic with a steroid-like structure, related to helvolic acid, which had previously been investigated at the Sir William Dunn School, but had been dropped because of toxicity problems.

Cephalosporin P could not account for the results that Brotzu had reported, but the Clevedon team, noting that a proportion of the activity in broth was lost in acid conditions and that extracts in amyl acetate differed in activity from broth cultures, reasoned that two, not one antibiotic must be present: one soluble in amyl acetate; the other water soluble and acid labile. Turning their attention to the aqueous phase, an antibiotic with the required spectrum of activity was detected; since it was also active against Gram-negative organisms the compound was called cephalosporin N (74). The new antibiotic was unstable and difficult to work with and it was some time before Abraham and Newton were able in 1954 to isolate it in a pure form and identify it as a new penicillin. It was renamed penicillin N and later called adicillin because the side chain contained a form of adipic acid (α-aminoadipic acid). An identical compound, named synnematin B, had been discovered in the United States. Both cephalosporin P and penicillin N (synnematin B) aroused some minor interest—the latter because of its activity against Gram-negative bacteria, which the original benzylpenicillin lacked—but neither survived early trials. In fact, it turned out that neither of these agents was the forerunner of the cephalosporins that are so widely used today.

After 6 years of investigation Brotzu's mould had yielded two antibiotics and its antibacterial activity had been accounted for. There the matter might have rested, but in their analysis of penicillin N, Newton and Abraham had, in September 1953, found evidence of another compound, which also showed antibacterial activity. This substance was christened cephalosporin C. The new substance was clearly related to penicillin N, since it had the same α-aminoadipic acid side chain, but in terms of antibacterial potency it possessed only about one-tenth the activity. Furthermore, it was produced by the mould in quantities that were too small to account for any of the activity that Brotzu had observed (75). Studies of penicillin N were by then ongoing, and, since it would be difficult to accumulate enough cephalosporin C to carry out proper studies, the Oxford workers might have been forgiven for ignoring this minor metabolite. That it was not relegated to obscurity as a curiosity was due to the fact that, although it seemed to have a β-lactam structure like

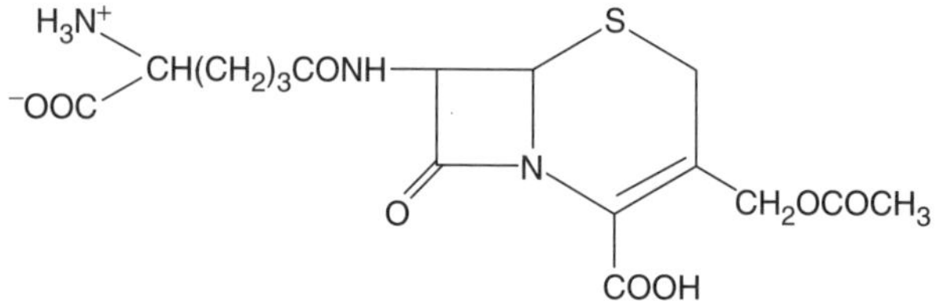

Fig. 4.4 Structure of cephalosporin C.

the penicillins, it was not inactivated by penicillinase, an enzyme responsible for penicillin resistance that Abraham and Chain had discovered as early as 1940 (76). By the 1950s some of the shine was wearing off penicillin because many of the staphylococci that were being isolated, especially in hospitals, were resistant to penicillin because of their ability to produce this enzyme.

Efforts to characterize cephalosporin C and examine its properties were hampered by the low yield from the producer mould, but in 1957, Brendan Kelly and colleagues at Clevedon obtained a mutant strain that produced sufficient cephalosporin C to allow the Oxford team to pursue their findings. By 1959 Abraham and Newton had worked out the structure of the new antibiotic and it was soon confirmed by Dorothy Hodgkin's team. It turned out to be a novel compound clearly related to penicillin, but with a β-lactam ring that was fused, not to a five-membered thiazolidine ring as in penicillin, but to a six-membered cyclical structure known to organic chemists as a dihydrothiazine ring (Fig. 4.4; cf. Fig. 4.3).

Lessons from the failure to protect by patent processes for the extraction and purification of penicillin had by this time been learned. In 1948 a body called the National Research Development Corporation (NRDC) had been established by an Act of Parliament, providing a mechanism for scientists in universities and government institutions to patent discoveries and inventions arising from their work.* Several patent applications in connection with investigations of the antibiotics found in Brotzu's mould were made by the workers at Oxford and Clevedon and assigned to the NRDC. Patents involving cephalosporin C were to prove the most profitable, earning around £125 million in royalties (77); a portion of this money was allocated to Abraham and Newton, enabling both of them to set up charitable trusts to support scientific research at Oxford. What Giuseppe Brotzu thought about this is not recorded. In the late 1960s he visited the Dunn School at Oxford, but communication was hampered by his lack of knowledge of English. No one in the school at that time spoke Italian, so Guy Newton had to resort to his imperfect French with hilarious results.[†]

---

* The NRDC was merged with the National Enterprise Board to form British Technology Group in 1981, 3 years before the last cephalosporin patent expired. It became a private company in 1992 through an employee and management buyout.

[†] I am indebted to Professor Jeremy Hamilton-Miller, who was an eye witness, for this anecdote.

The long journey of cephalosporin C from Brotzu's mould to a compound that might be developed for therapeutic use took nearly 12 years. After all this effort, it was never marketed. The problem of penicillin-resistant staphylococci was being solved in other ways, and cephalosporin C was too inactive to be a viable competitor. The effort had not, however, been in vain. Agreements were entered into, first with Glaxo Laboratories in Britain and Eli Lilly in the United States, and then with other companies, to develop derivatives of cephalosporin C. Meanwhile, progress was being made in developing new penicillins that improved in some ways on the original penicillin G. The era of semi-synthetic β-lactam antibiotics was beginning.

β-Lactam abundance

For all its phenomenal success, it was always realized that improvements could be made to penicillin G to overcome some of its perceived shortcomings: lack of stability in the acid conditions of the stomach, so that it could not be administered orally; extremely rapid excretion from the bloodstream by the kidneys (Howard Florey is said to have observed that maintaining an adequate concentration of penicillin in the body was like trying to fill a bath with the plug out); susceptibility to penicillinase; very poor activity against Gram-negative bacilli such as salmonellae, shigellae, and *Escherichia coli*; and a tendency to cause allergic reactions—ranging from mild rashes to rare, but potentially fatal anaphylaxis—in about 5 per cent of patients to whom it was administered.

Modifying penicillin

Penicillin V

The problem of oral administration was solved, albeit unwittingly, in the unlikely setting of a former brewery in the village of Kundl on the banks of the Inn in the Austrian Tyrol. After the end of the Second World War, Austria, like Germany, was divided into different sectors and the Tyrol region came under French control. One of the French officers was a chemist, Michel Rambaud—later Professor of Pharmaceutical Chemistry at the Sorbonne in Paris—who had briefly worked on penicillin production in England and was now in Austria with the French occupation forces. Rambaud suggested to the directors of the brewery company that owned the Kundl site, Österreichische Brau A. G. in Linz, that they should start penicillin production in the derelict, but intact brewery to help relieve the shortages of the drug in Austria. Since resuscitating the plant for its original purpose was not an immediate prospect in the conditions prevailing in post-war Austria, Brau A. G. agreed to the venture and in July 1946 a company given the name Biochemie (now part of Sandoz, the generics wing of Novartis) was founded in the former Kundl brewery. Rambaud scrounged a starter culture of the *Penicillium* mould from France. Small-scale investigations into the production and extraction of penicillin started under the supervision of a fermentation chemist from the brewing industry, Richard Brunner,* who, by

---

* Later (1962–72), professor in the Technischen Hochschule in Vienna.

chance, had already acquired a little experience of penicillin during the war. In 1942 Brunner had moved to Prague on the recommendation of Karl Josef Schröder an Austrian brewery director for whom he had previously worked and who was by then in Munich coordinating distribution of beer, malt, and hops throughout greater Germany. While in Prague, Brunner teamed up with the distinguished organic chemist, Konrad Bernhauer, who was leading the German war effort to produce penicillin (see p. 108), but by the end of 1944 it was clear that penicillin work in Czechoslovakia would have to be wound up. In March 1945 Schröder and Brunner met in Prague and discussed the possibility of Bernhauer's group returning to Austria to continue the penicillin work there. As a result of these discussions Brunner accompanied Bernhauer back to Austria with all his technical paraphernalia soon after the war ended. They successfully crossed the Austrian border, where the Russian authorities promptly confiscated all Schröder's equipment and prevented him from travelling further, but Brunner was able to proceed and eventually found a job with Brau A. G. He joined the incipient Biochemie project when it was set up in 1946 and set to work. With minimal knowledge of the specialized techniques required and a severe lack of apparatus and chemical supplies, Brunner's team nevertheless succeeded in producing a little impure penicillin at the Kundl plant in 1947. By November 1948 small supplies were being made available to Austrian doctors (78).

Production of high quality penicillin in the inadequate facilities of the old brewery was easier said than done and things did not go well. Numerous technical problems combined with the increasing availability of cheap American penicillin threatened to make the venture short-lived. By 1951, as a final throw of the dice, Brunner's erstwhile boss, Karl Schröder, was persuaded to join the ailing company to try to turn it round. Few believed that he would succeed, and without an amazing stroke of luck, it is unlikely that he would have done so.

Towards the end of 1951, the same year in which Schröder joined Biochemie, a company biologist, Ernst Brandl was charged with the task of solving persistent problems with contamination in the penicillin fermentation tanks. The difficulty was to inhibit growth of the contaminant micro-organisms without interfering with the *Penicillium* mould. Various conventional antibacterial substances were tested without success and with more hope than expectation, he tried adding phenoxyethanol to the fermentation broth. To his surprise, Brandl found that this stimulated an increased yield of penicillin. A young company colleague, the chemist Hans Margreiter was brought in to investigate the phenomenon. He discovered that the product of fermentation was not conventional benzylpenicillin since it was stable to hydrolysis by acids. He postulated that the alcohol Brandl had used was transformed to phenoxyacetic acid during the fermentation process and then incorporated into penicillin as it is synthesized by the mould. When the Austrian workers tried using phenoxyacetic acid in place of phenylacetic acid, the precursor normally used in benzylpenicillin manufacture, the product obtained was phenoxymethylpenicillin (79). Brandl and Margreiter realized that they had stumbled on something unexpected and possibly important: a form of penicillin that was not broken down in the acid conditions of the stomach and which could therefore be administered orally. The new penicillin became known in the company as penicillin V—'V' for vertraulich (confidential); it was soon interpreted more jubilantly as 'V' for victory. Tests in animals and man carried out with the help of their colleague Marco Giovannini indicated that the new formulation produced satisfactory blood levels when administered by mouth (80).

Further clinical studies by Karl Spitzy in Vienna confirmed the efficacy and safety of administering penicillin V by the oral route and in April 1952 Schröder presented a patent application on the new penicillin in Austria. To his dismay he learnt that Eli Lilly in the United States had already obtained a patent on a number of variant molecules obtained by fermentation, including the potassium salt of phenoxymethylpenicillin—Biochemie's penicillin V. Fortunately, Schröder successfully argued that the free acid produced by Biochemie differed from the potassium salt patented by Lilly. In October 1953 a cross-licensing agreement was negotiated with Lilly and by the following year Schröder was involved in discussing manufacturing rights with Bayer and other big pharmaceutical firms.

Over 100 different penicillins have been synthesized by presenting the producer mould with various side chain precursors in the fermentation broth—Otto Karl Behrens and his team at Eli Lilly had made phenoxymethylpenicillin by this means as early as 1948 (81)—but only penicillin G and penicillin V have found their way into therapeutic use. Phenoxymethylpenicillin is still widely used as a substitute for benzylpenicillin when the oral route is preferred.

Long-acting penicillins

Another early innovation, the injection of penicillin into muscle in a mixture of peanut oil and beeswax, was introduced by Monroe Romansky and his technician, George Rittman of the US Army Medical Corps in 1944 (82). Administering penicillin in this way delayed its absorption, thereby prolonging the presence of a therapeutic concentration in the body. The preparation allowed the cure of gonorrhoea by a single injection, thus fulfilling Ehrlich's ideal of a *therapia sterilisans magna*. This tactic was later refined by the development of an insoluble salt of penicillin, procaine penicillin, formulated as an oily suspension; like the earlier concoction, the preparation slowly releases penicillin into the bloodstream from the intramuscular injection site (83). Salts that are even less soluble, such as benzathine penicillin, benethamine penicillin, and clemizole penicillin were also developed, but are now seldom used. An alternative approach was (and is) to co-administer penicillin with another drug, probenecid—normally used in the control of gout—which competes with the renal excretion sites, effectively delaying elimination of the antibiotic by the kidneys.

Important though these modifications were, they merely represented ways of overcoming the poor oral absorption and rapid excretion of penicillin; the activity of the antibiotic remained unaltered. The development of penicillins with new antibacterial properties had to await the isolation of 6-aminopenicillanic acid: the basic skeleton of penicillin consisting of the fused ring structure with a modifiable amino (NH_2) group on the β-lactam ring.

Semi-synthetic penicillins

The race to produce semi-synthetic antibiotics produced by chemical manipulation of fermentation products was won by Beecham Research Laboratories, a company that evolved in 1943 from the business originally founded by Thomas Beecham, peddler of Beecham's Pills* (*'Worth a guinea a box. One trial will convince you that Beecham Pills are the best in the world for bilious and nervous disorders, wind and pain of the stomach, headache, giddiness, fullness and swelling after meals, drowsiness, cold chills, loss of appetite, shortness of breath etc. etc.'* (84)) At the end of the Second World War the Beecham organization was a small group of firms selling not only Beecham's Pills and Powders, but a mixed portfolio of over-the-counter medicines and other products such as Maclean's toothpaste, Brylcreem, the hair cream famously advertised by the cricketer Denis Compton, and the 'energy' drink aimed at invalids, Lucozade. Though the range of goods was well established, profits started to decline in the post-war climate of austerity. The fortunes of the company were turned round, not by a scientist, but by an accountant, Leslie Lazell, who boosted sales of its core products, but more importantly bought Brockham Park, a country house near Dorking in Surrey and staffed it with a team of research workers.

The road to 6-APA

Lazell, who was to become Chairman of the Beecham Group in 1951, clearly saw antibiotics as the future, a commitment symbolized by getting Alexander Fleming to open the new research laboratories in 1947, and later given practical weight by the appointment—after tortuous negotiations with his lawyers—of Ernst Chain as a consultant to the company. Chain's name was suggested in 1954 by the biochemist, Sir Charles Dodds, who was a consultant to the Beecham company and a friend of Chain's. Lazell lost no time in travelling to Rome to meet Chain and they took an instant liking to one another (85). Once Chain was on board, he started to attend research strategy meetings advising on the way forward and the means necessary to achieve their aims. Chain's view was that the best route to new penicillins was to get the *Penicillium* mould to produce penicillin with an amino grouping on the benzene ring, which could then be modified in various ways by chemical means. There were no facilities for this at Brockham Park, so two newly recruited young scientists, George Rolinson, who had been working on penicillin for the Boots Company in Nottingham, and Ralph Batchelor, a Cambridge graduate from the Water Pollution Research Laboratories in Surrey, were despatched to Rome in January 1956 to use Chain's own pilot plant (86).

The desired substance, *para*-aminobenzylpenicillin was duly produced by the known manoeuvre of adding *p*-aminophenylacetic acid as a side chain precursor in the fermentation broth, and Rolinson and Batchelor set about measuring the yield. Two methods were used: a chemical assay that simply recognized compounds with a β-lactam ring; and a biological assay that measured antibacterial activity. Both assays gave comparable

---

* And grandfather of the famous conductor of the same name.

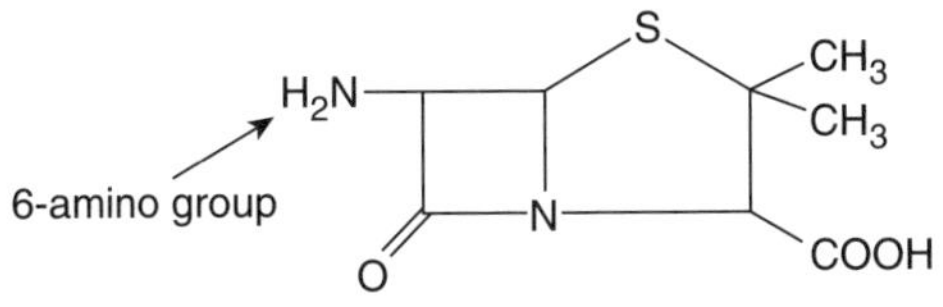

6-amino group

Fig. 4.5 Structure of 6-aminopenicillanic acid.

results for the p-aminophenylacetic acid-containing broth, but a control fermentation in which the precursor had been omitted gave widely discrepant results. When word finally got back to the chemists, Peter Doyle and John Nayler at Brockham Park, it was shown that the discrepancy was due to 6-aminopenicillanic acid (universally known as 6-APA; Fig. 4.5), a compound which is devoid of useful antibacterial activity, but contains the reactive amino group that offered a simple route to the addition of new side chains (87). They were able to crystallize 6-APA late in 1957 and immediately started to look for useful derivatives (88).

Beecham's at that time had few facilities for developing antibiotics and none for marketing them. They entered into an agreement with the American firm of Bristol Laboratories, who helped them to build a factory at Worthing in return for access to Beecham patents. Meanwhile, in 1959, the Beecham workers (89) and Bayer in Germany (90) almost simultaneously found a way of making 6-APA from penicillin G by removing the side chain enzymically. Unfortunately for Beecham, the Bayer discovery, patented by W. Kaufmann and K. Bauer (91) was more efficient and had priority and they approached the British firm with a deal to divulge details of their process, again in exchange for manufacturing rights. Patent rights on 6-APA were to be a source of acrimonious litigation for many years, especially between Beecham and John Sheehan in the United States, who was a consultant to Bristol Laboratories and had produced 6-APA and certain derivatives in the course of his efforts to synthesize penicillin (92).

The enzymic process for the production of 6-APA is an efficient way of making the molecule available in large quantities and the way was now open for the chemists to devise semi-synthetic penicillins with improved properties. The first compound to be produced by this route, phenethicillin was a joint development between Beecham's and Bristol. It is very similar in structure and properties to penicillin V, but is better absorbed after oral administration. Similar oral compounds were later developed, including, propicillin, phenbenicillin, and azidocillin, but none has superseded penicillin V as the preferred oral substitute for penicillin G.

Antistaphylococcal penicillins

More interesting compounds were now in the pipeline at Brockham Park. Just like Edward Abraham and Guy Newton in their pursuit of cephalosporin C, the Beecham team were stimulated by the problems that were emerging in hospitals with penicillinase-producing staphylococci that were resistant to penicillins G and V. As soon as 6-APA was crystallized, Peter Doyle and John Nayler started to experiment with adding bulky side chains that prevented penicillinase from interacting with the β-lactam ring—a process known as steric hindrance. By May 1959 they had made a compound that became known as methicillin*, which was not susceptible to penicillinase and retained adequate activity against staphylococci, though, like penicillin G, it had to be given by injection. In those days licensing regulations were much more lax than they are today—the thalidomide tragedy that was to have a major impact on safety testing was still 2 years away—and methicillin was on the market in less than 18 months. Beecham marketed methicillin through its subsidiary, CL Bencard, a company specializing in allergy products, originally founded in Devon in 1934. Lazell had acquired Bencard for Beecham in 1949[†] as part of his ambitions to expand the firm's pharmaceutical portfolio; methicillin was given the trade name 'Celbenin', reflecting the Bencard connection.

Within 2 years the Beecham research team had improved on methicillin with the synthesis of two derivatives, cloxacillin and oxacillin, which were more active and could be administered orally. Cloxacillin was deemed to be the better of the two and was developed commercially by Beecham, while oxacillin was favoured by Bristol Laboratories and was marketed in the United States. These penicillinase-stable penicillins belong to a group known tongue-twistingly as isoxazolylpenicillins. Two minor modifications, flucloxacillin (preferred in the United Kingdom) and dicloxacillin (used mainly in the United States), achieve better concentrations in the bloodstream after oral administration and have largely superseded the earlier congeners. Other solutions were sought to the problem of penicillin resistance in staphylococci in the 1960s: quinacillin, was developed by the Boots Company in Nottingham, while in the United States diphenicillin (ancillin) emerged from Smith, Kline, and French and nafcillin from Wyeth. However, the oral absorption of each of these derivatives is erratic and only nafcillin survived to go into therapeutic use, and that mainly in the United States.

Broad-spectrum penicillins

Beecham Research Laboratories were now on the way to becoming a world-class business, an aspiration that was to be given a boost in 1960 by the appointment of Graham ('Bob') Wilkins as managing director, and in 1961 by the marketing of another blockbuster drug, ampicillin. Although this compound was not immune to staphylococcal penicillinase, the antibacterial spectrum of penicillin G was considerably expanded to include many important Gram-negative pathogens, such as salmonellae, shigellae, *Escherichia coli*, and *Haemophilus influenzae* (93). This improvement was achieved, no doubt to everyone's surprise, by the simple expedient of introducing an amino group into the side chain of benzylpenicillin. Ampicillin, which was marketed under the nationalistic trade name 'Penbritin' (just as Bayer had given their antitrypanosomal drug,

---

* Methicillin was discontinued in 1993, but the name has survived in the term 'methicillin-resistant *Staphylococcus aureus*'—MRSA: bacteria that owe their resistance not to penicillinase, but to changes in the drug target. They are resistant, not just to methicillin, but to all presently available β-lactam antibiotics.

† Bencard remained part of Beecham until 1998, when it split off to form Allergy Therapeutics. In 1959 it assimilated the Wright-Fleming Institute's inoculation department business. The firm still trades as Bencard Allergie in Germany.

suramin, the name 'Germanin' in the 1920s; see p. 276), was an instant success. It became the treatment of choice for many urinary and respiratory tract infections, and was also widely used in bacterial meningitis (for which it offered cover for the three principal causes and some less common ones), shigellosis, and much else besides. Compounds with properties resembling those of ampicillin, notably epicillin and ciclacillin, were later marketed in some countries but they offer little therapeutic advantage and were not received with much enthusiasm.

A feature of ampicillin that contributed to its success was that it could be given by mouth, but in fact only about 30 per cent of the dose was absorbed after oral administration and it often caused diarrhoea by upsetting the normal intestinal flora. Ways were therefore sought of improving the oral absorption. The most effective solution was to form an ester with the free carboxyl group to produce compounds that are much better absorbed. Compounds of this type, known as ampicillin pro-drugs, include bacampicillin, lenampicillin, pivampicillin, and talampicillin, each of which has found regional use in various parts of the world. Paradoxically, the modification deprives the molecule of antibiotic activity, but fortuitously tissue esterases present in the intestinal mucosa release ampicillin during the transportation process in the gut. These esters are therefore a way of smuggling ampicillin into the bloodstream. A much less successful tactic is to create condensation products of ampicillin that hydrolyse in the bloodstream after oral absorption. Two such compounds have been devised, hetacillin (a condensation product with acetone) and metampicillin (a condensate with formaldehyde), but there has been little support for their use.

With impeccable timing, just as the patent on ampicillin was due to expire and just as the ampicillin pro-drugs were threatening to undermine its popularity, the Beecham chemists revealed a new version of their money-spinner in which a hydroxyl group had been added to the benzene ring on the ampicillin side chain. Despite its close resemblance to ampicillin, this compound, amoxicillin,* turned out, to everyone's surprise, to be much better absorbed when given by mouth and it became the preferred penicillin for oral administration, upstaging the ampicillin esters.

Antipseudomonal penicillins

Meanwhile, penicillins were being sought that might have some effect on a common environmental organism, Pseudomonas aeruginosa, a bacterium that causes little mischief in healthy individuals, but is very resistant to antibiotics and is responsible for many life-threatening opportunistic infections in seriously ill patients in hospital. It had been thought that the properties of Pseudomonas aeruginosa rendered it immune to the effects of β-lactam antibiotics, but the Beecham team again delivered the goods in 1967 with another very simple modification: by replacing the α-amino group of ampicillin with a carboxyl function, COOH, a compound called carbenicillin was produced that displayed unexceptional but clear-cut activity against Pseudomonas aeruginosa (94). Although the

---

* Originally spelt amoxycillin; amoxicillin is the international non-proprietary name.

potency is very weak—the activity of carbenicillin against pseudomonas is only about one thousandth of that of penicillin G against streptococci—the margin of safety of penicillins is such that it could be given in sufficiently high doses to achieve cures in many patients. However, the additional carboxyl group receives an extra sodium atom during production of the salt used for injection and this disodium formulation has sometimes been responsible for producing sodium overload in patients given the very high doses required.

Attempts were made to produce pro-drug formulations of carbenicillin to be given orally; two such preparations, carfecillin and carindacillin, were marketed, but were received with widespread scepticism. In 1970, the Beecham chemists came up with another injectable derivative, ticarcillin, which had somewhat improved activity, while in 1977 chemists at Bayer produced two compounds based on a different structural approach, mezlocillin and azlocillin, which exhibited even greater potency against pseudomonas. A similar derivative, piperacillin, was developed by the Toyama Chemical Company in Japan in 1976 and marketed by Lederle in the United States.* Other attempts by the Japanese pharmaceutical industry to interest the prescriber in antipseudomonal penicillins yielded apalcillin, aspoxicillin, and sulbenicillin, but these antibiotics offer little advantage and, as with the carbenicillin esters, such exhortations have largely fallen on deaf ears.

End of an era

Penicillins have now largely run their course and it is unlikely that we will see new derivatives to replace the older compounds that are well established and, despite the incursions of resistant bacterial strains, broadly still effective. The main unanswered threat, resistance in Gram-negative bacilli, has been, as we shall see, successfully counteracted in other ways. Indeed, one marketed penicillin that is active against amoxicillin-resistant Gram-negative bacilli, temocillin, has met with little commercial success, partly because of its very restricted spectrum of activity and the requirement for it to be given by injection. Another very unusual penicillin, mecillinam (known as amdinocillin in the United States), produced by the chemist Franz Lund of the Danish firm Leo Laboratories in 1972, also suffered from similar perceived shortcomings. Unlike other penicillins, the side chain of mecillinam is joined to 6-APA through an amidino linkage (CH=N) and it turns out that this modification reduces the range of cell wall targets that penicillins normally attack. The antibiotic has therefore been very helpful in unravelling the mode of action of penicillins, but it has not been much used in treatment. The only therapeutic application of note has been in urinary tract infection in which an orally administered pro-drug form, pivmecillinam, has achieved modest success.

---

* Originally the Lederle Antitoxin Company, founded by Ernst Lederle, formerly health commissioner in New York, in 1906. The firm specialized in pneumococcal vaccines and other biologicals. It was bought by the American Cyanamid Company (see footnote, p. 76) in 1930 and was subsequently acquired by Wyeth in 1994.

Semi-synthetic cephalosporins

Early attempts by Edward Abraham and his colleagues in Oxford to make chemically modified derivatives of cephalosporin C produced little of value. The future of the cephalosporins as a group lay with the drug firms that had negotiated licensing agreements with the National Research and Development Council in the United Kingdom. Most prominent were Eli Lilly in the United States, and Glaxo Laboratories in the United Kingdom who agreed to a deal that contained the provision that each firm should allow the others access to its results (77).

Both Lilly and Glaxo were old established companies. A Civil War veteran, Colonel Eli Lilly, had founded the firm that bears his name in Indianapolis in 1876. He had formerly been an assistant in a drug store and saw the need to produce traditional medicines to high standard. The business he founded with his son Josiah remained in family hands and developed from small beginnings to become a major player—notably under Josiah's son, also called Eli Lilly—in the market for human and veterinary medicines and agricultural products.

Glaxo had equally humble roots. The name was originally given to a dried milk product developed by Joseph Nathan a London-born emigrant to Australia, who moved on to New Zealand as a general trader. Among his enterprises he bought up several creameries and was soon looking for a use for skimmed milk generated as a by-product of butter making. Anticipating the advice of the cartoonist, Scott Adams: 'when life gives you lemon, make lemonade' Nathan saw the potential of a dried milk product that would be easy to handle and store. The first dried milk factory was built at Bunnythorpe, on New Zealand's north island and he started exporting the product to Britain and selling it there as 'Glaxo', a baby food ('Glaxo builds bonnie babies' was a favourite slogan) that was also recommended for invalids and the elderly (95). Profits rose when it was used as a convenient way of supplying milk to the armed forces during the First World War and success of the company was consolidated after a vitamin D-enriched form was successfully marketed as 'sunshine milk', later renamed 'Ostermilk', in 1923. Glaxo Laboratories was adopted as the name of the company in 1935 when vitamins and vaccines began to feature prominently in the company's portfolio and Harry Jephcott, who had been recruited as a research scientist in 1919, took over as managing director. As it grew Glaxo was involved in several mergers and takeovers, most famously taking over the Wellcome Foundation in 1995 before fulfilling a long held ambition to merge with Beecham (by this time SmithKline Beecham) to form GlaxoSmithKline at the end of 2000.

The transformation of cephalosporin C into a useful antimicrobial agent presented quite a challenge to the drug firms. Unlike penicillin, cephalosporin C has two side chains, one at the 7-amino position at the left hand side of the molecule and the other on the extra carbon atom (called C-3 in the international numbering system) on the right hand side (see Fig. 4.4). Theoretically, this allowed the chemists to make alterations at either end of the molecule in their efforts to make improvements, but producing a compound with the right properties was not easy. Modification of the C-3 end was relatively simple, but it soon became clear that the effect of altering this part of the molecule generally had little impact on the intrinsic antibacterial activity, although the pharmacological properties of the drug (for example oral absorption) might be profoundly affected. Alteration at the other end of the molecule required the isolation of 7-aminocephalosporanic acid (7-ACA), the cephalosporin analogue of 6-APA, but this proved to be more difficult than it had been with penicillin. Abraham's team had produced small amounts of 7-ACA by acid hydrolysis of cephalosporin C, but this was an inefficient process that also tended to affect other parts of the molecule. The problem of obtaining 7-ACA in acceptably high yield was eventually solved in 1962 by Edwin Flynn and his colleagues at Eli Lilly (96) and this opened the way for the development of therapeutically useful compounds. Later a method was devised of expanding the thiazolidine ring of penicillin by introduction of an extra carbon atom—as happens in nature in the biosynthesis of cephalosporin C.

The first fruits of research into new cephalosporins, cephalothin* and cephalexin, developed by Eli Lilly, and cephaloridine, developed by Glaxo, were marketed by both companies in 1964–65. Cephalothin and cephaloridine had to be administered by injection, but Flynn's group at Lilly discovered that linking the side chain found in Beecham's ampicillin at the 7-amino position allowed modest oral absorption. The first compound of this type was called cephaloglycin. Two of the chemists involved in this work, Robert Morin and Bill Jackson then discovered that conversion of the side chain at the other end of cephaloglycin to a simple methyl group further improved its absorption and stability. This derivative—cephalexin—is structurally the exact cephalosporin analogue of ampicillin, and very surprisingly is almost entirely absorbed when given by mouth.[†] Despite the obvious inferiority of cephaloglycin, Lilly went ahead with the marketing of the antibiotic in the United States in 1970.

Prospects for the cephalosporins at this time were far from secure. True, they offered some theoretical advantages over the early penicillins—stability to staphylococcal penicillinase and an extended spectrum of activity—but by the time the first semi-synthetic cephalosporins were marketed these properties seemed less important and the only distinct benefit of cephalosporins was that they could usually be administered safely in patients who were allergic to penicillins. In fact the reception received by the first cephalosporins in the United Kingdom was conspicuously lukewarm since they appeared to have no distinctive clinical role, though the persuasive powers of the pharmaceutical industry generated greater enthusiasm in some other countries.

* The compound originally known as cephalothin was subsequently given the recommended international non-proprietary name (rINN) cefalotin. Many later compounds adopted the American 'cef-' convention from the start. All cephalosporins are now spelt with an 'f' rather than a 'ph', but the original spelling is used here to retain the historical context. The correct modern spelling is shown in Table 4.1 (p. 130).

† An Italian firm, Sigma-Tau marketed an esterified version of cephalexin, pivalexin, in the late 1970s. Esterification is generally aimed at improving oral absorption (see p. 125), which is scarcely possible with cephalexin. Such are the enigmas of drug marketing!

Cephalexin, although in truth a fairly mundane compound, was particularly successful on the world market and gave rise to several copycat products—often called 'me-too' compounds, since commercial firms seeing profits being made elsewhere usually say 'I want some too'. Sales of one such compound, cephradine, actually overtook those of cephalexin at one point although it is practically identical in all its properties. It was produced by Squibb, a firm that had been founded in Brooklyn in 1856 by Edward Robinson Squibb* and which had been prominent in the early manufacture of penicillin. The big selling point of cephradine was that an injectable form was made available so that doctors could start treatment with an injection and then move to oral therapy as the patient improved—though why anyone would want to commence parenteral therapy with a cephalosporin that was manifestly less active than many others was never explained.

Me-too-ism was to be a recurrent theme with the cephalosporin family. In fact, there have been few really substantial advances in the 50-year history of this widely used family of antibiotics. Among the small number of cephalosporins that can authentically claim improved properties are cefuroxime, developed by Glaxo (97), and cefotaxime, from Hoechst-Roussel (98), both of which appeared in the mid-1970s. Cefuroxime was the first cephalosporin to exhibit genuine stability to the wide (and still growing) range of β-lactamase enzymes in Gram-negative bacilli that were uncovered following the introduction of ampicillin; cefotaxime succeeded in combining the β-lactamase stability of cefuroxime with an impressive increase in intrinsic antibacterial activity. A further improvement came from the Glaxo stable in the early 1980s with the appearance of ceftazidime, the first cephalosporin to show good activity against the opportunist pathogen, *Pseudomonas aeruginosa* (99). Most of the other cephalosporins that have been marketed throughout the world (Table 4.1) are chiefly blatant 'me-too' compounds, often based on the cephalexin or cefotaxime templates. A few offer sufficient pharmacological advantages—such as a long serum half-life allowing less frequent administration, or the property of absorption after oral administration, commonly achieved by esterification—to give the advertising copy writers and indefatigable sales staff of the drug companies something to get their teeth into. In fact, intense competition for market share in cephalosporins contributed to the transition from the rather sedate promotional practices of the immediate post-war period to the sometimes unseemly courting of 'opinion formers' and machiavellian marketing techniques that now prevail.

Variations on a theme

The two β-lactam antibiotics produced by the moulds that Fleming and Brotzu had fortuitously discovered generated such a rich harvest of therapeutically useful derivatives

---

* It is now part of Bristol-Myers Squibb after the merger in 1989 with Bristol-Myers, the business that William McLaren Bristol and John Ripley Myers formed in 1887 after buying the struggling Clinton Pharmaceutical Company in New York.

Table 4.1 Categorization of most important cephalosporins in clinical use

Injectable			Oral		
Cefalotin	Cefamandole	Ceforanide	Cefalexin[a]	Cefaloglycin	Cefroxadine
Cefaloridine	Cefacetrile	Cefonicid	Cefradine[a]	Cefadroxil[a]	Cefatrizine
Cefazolin	Cefapirin		Cefaclor[a]	Cefprozil[a]	
Improved β-lactamase stability			**Improved β-lactamase stability**		
Cefuroxime[a]	Cefmetazole	Cefotiam	**Non-esterified**		**Esterified**
Cefoxitin	Cefotetan	Cefminox	Cefixime[a]		Cefuroxime axetil
Improved intrinsic activity and β-lactamase stability			Ceftibuten		Cefpodoxime proxetil[a]
			Cefdinir		Cefetamet pivoxil
Cefotaxime[a]	Cefodizime	Cefmenoxime			Cefteram pivoxil
Ceftriaxone[a]	Ceftizoxime				Cefotiam hexetil
					Cefditoren pivoxil
Compounds distinguished by activity against *Pseudomonas aeruginosa*					
Broad	**Medium**	**Narrow**			
Ceftazidime[a]	Cefoperazone	Cefsulodin			
Cefpirome[a]	Cefpimizole				
Cefepime	Cefpiramide				

From Greenwood D, Finch RG, Davey PG, Wilcox MH. *Antimicrobial Chemotherapy*, 5th edn. Oxford University Press, Oxford. 2007. The spelling is that of the international non-proprietary name decreed by the World Health Organization.

[a] Compounds available in the United Kingdom (2006).

that expecting the natural world to yield further variations on the β-lactam theme might seem a supererogatory demand. But, ever fruitful, Mother Nature still had more β-lactam tricks up her voluminous sleeves. The first surprise she had in store in the 1970s was that β-lactam-containing molecules were to be found not only as products of moulds, but were also elaborated by species of bacteria, including the soil-inhabiting *Streptomyces* genus (100). Many different compounds with unusual β-lactam structures were subsequently unearthed (almost literally) and four types received particular attention because of their unusual properties: cephamycins, clavams, carbapenems, and monobactams (101).

Cephamycins

The cephamycins (102) differ from conventional cephalosporins in carrying a methoxy (CH_3–O–) grouping on the β-lactam ring. They were first discovered in the early 1970s as natural products of several species of *Streptomyces*, including *Streptomyces clavuligerus* and *Streptomyces lactamdurans*, through screening programmes at Lilly and Merck in the United States. Chemists had postulated that introduction of various groupings on the C-7 carbon might usefully alter the properties of cephalosporins, but none had been found to exhibit useful antibacterial activity. It therefore came as a surprise to find that natural cephamycins not only remained active, but the additional methoxy group stabilized the β-lactam ring allowing it to withstand hydrolysis by β-lactamase enzymes that would otherwise abolish the antibacterial activity. The first compound to be marketed with this

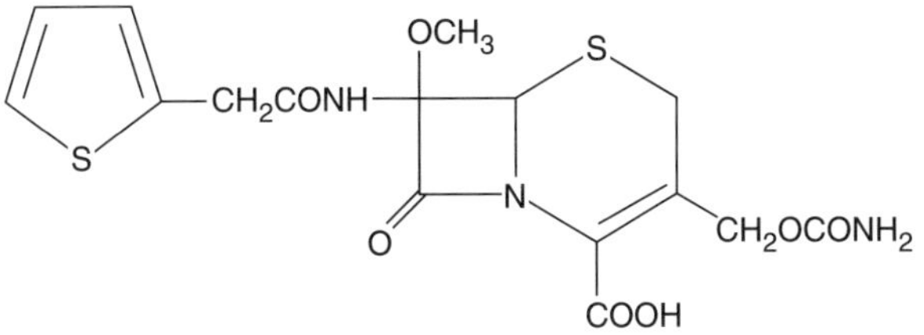

Fig. 4.6 Structure of cefoxitin (a cephamycin).

property, by Merck and Company in the United States*, was a semi-synthetic derivative of cephamycin C, cefoxitin (Fig. 4.6). Although its intrinsic antibacterial activity is modest, the β-lactamase resistance extended the spectrum of cephalosporins to include the important anaerobe *Bacteroides fragilis*, which often causes problems of infection, especially after abdominal or gynaecological surgery. It became popular as a prophylactic drug among surgeons performing such operations. Several other cephamycins, including cefotetan, cefbuperazone, cefmetazole, and cefminox have subsequently been marketed in some countries, but offer no real advantages.

Clavulanic acid

The clavams, of which there is only one really important example, clavulanic acid, display an even more extraordinary structure with no side chain on the β-lactam ring and oxygen replacing sulphur in the fused ring (Fig. 4.7).

Martin Cole and his colleagues at the Beecham Research Laboratories discovered clavulanic acid in 1977 (103). They had been screening a large collection of β-lactam compounds with the aim of finding an inhibitor of the β-lactamase enzymes that were causing increasing problems in clinical medicine. The thinking was that such a compound—which need not have any antibacterial activity in its own right—could be used in a protective role by combining it with a penicillin or cephalosporin that would otherwise be destroyed.

The notion of inhibitors of β-lactamases had been mooted many years before in the days when the enzymes were still called penicillinases (104). In fact several early β-lactam

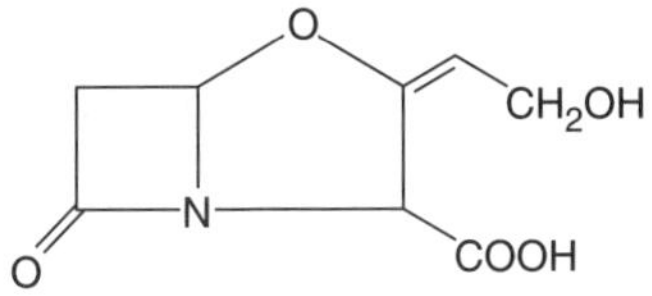

Fig. 4.7 Structure of clavulanic acid (a clavam).

* Merck was founded by Heinrich Emanuel Merck out of the family's retail pharmacy in Darmstadt, and still trades under the family name in Germany. The American firm was originally an affiliated company started by Emanuel Merck's grandson, Georg Merck, in 1889 and became independent when the German parent firm lost many of its overseas affiliates after the First World War. Georg Merck's son took over the business in 1925 and was instrumental in turning it into a major player in the United States chemical and pharmaceutical industry. The American business merged with Sharp and Dohme in 1953 in order to boost its research base and worldwide marketing potential. It is known as Merck, Sharp and Dohme (MSD) in most of the world outside the United States.

antibiotics, including cephalosporin C and cloxacillin were known to have weak inhibitory activity, but none was sufficiently potent to allow reliable use in treatment. During their investigations Cole and his colleagues found a substance produced by a strain of *Streptomyces* that was a potent β-lactamase inhibitor, but also very unstable. Under the mistaken belief that the substance might be one of the new cephamycins that had recently been described (it turned out later to belong to another class of novel β-lactam antibiotics, the olivanic acids), they decided to investigate the original cephamycin-producing strain of *Streptomyces clavuligerus*, presumably because the drugs themselves were not readily available at that time. Scientists at Lilly had deposited the producer strain in the American Collection of Type Cultures and the Beecham workers were able to purchase a culture in the normal way.

The decision to test *Streptomyces clavuligerus* proved to be a fortunate one: Cole and his co-workers discovered that this strain did indeed produce an extremely potent β-lactamase inhibitor, but when they fractionated the antimicrobially active products the inhibitor proved not to be a cephamycin, but an antibiotic with an even more novel structure, which they named clavulanic acid (105). Their good fortune was not at an end: extensive testing of the new compound showed that it was safe to use and that it possessed pharmacological properties (including absorption when given by mouth) that made it the ideal partner for their lead antibiotic, amoxicillin, which was under threat from the emergence of resistant strains of bacteria. Under the trade name Augmentin, the combination of amoxicillin and clavulanic acid has been enormously successful and became one of the top selling pharmaceutical products in the world. Other firms naturally wanted a share of the cake and alternative types of β-lactamase inhibitor, including the penicillanic acid sulphones, sulbactam (in combination with ampicillin) and tazobactam (combined with piperacillin) have been marketed with claims of marginal improvements.

Carbapenems

Clavulanic acid and other β-lactamase inhibitors possess little or no useful antibacterial activity of their own, but this is certainly not true of the carbapenems, the first of which, imipenem, came into clinical use in 1987. The original carbapenem, thienamycin, was isolated in 1976 by scientists at Merck (106) from a strain of *Streptomyces cattleya*—so named because the colour of cultures resembles that of some cattleya orchids. This unusual molecule differs from other β-lactam antibiotics in several ways, not least in having a carbon atom replacing sulphur in the fused ring structure. The natural antibiotic was too unstable to be developed commercially, but the Merck chemists produced an N-formimidoyl derivative (Fig. 4.8) that overcame this shortcoming. The ability to say

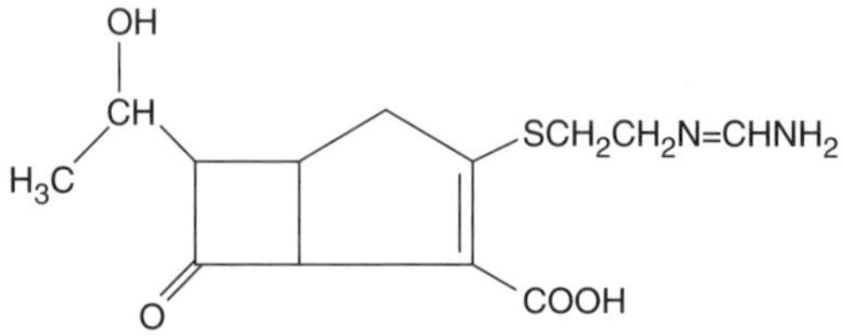

Fig. 4.8 Structure of imipenem (a carbapenem).

'N-formimidoylthienamycin' became something of a shibboleth among aficionados of antimicrobial chemotherapy, and there was relief all round at the decision to change the generic name to the more manageable 'imipenem'.

Imipenem was found not only to possess exceptionally good intrinsic antibacterial activity, but also stability to most of the prevalent β-lactamase enzymes. Furthermore, its spectrum, which includes organisms such as *Streptococcus faecalis*, and *Bacteroides fragilis* (against which conventional cephalosporins have no useful activity) as well as the opportunist pathogen, *Pseudomonas aeruginosa*, exceeds that of any available β-lactam compound. It is not absorbed when given by mouth, but this was not of crucial importance in such a broad-spectrum agent, the natural role of which was to be for the treatment of sepsis of uncertain aetiology in seriously ill patients.

Merck were clearly on to a winner, but nature still had one trick up her sleeve: despite the impressive stability to bacterial β-lactamases, it turned out that the β-lactam ring of imipenem was hydrolysed by an enzyme—dehydropeptidase I—naturally found in the mammalian kidney so that it was rapidly broken down in the body. The problem was solved with commendable speed by devising an inhibitor of dehydropeptidase, cilastatin, which fortunately proved to be a suitable, non-toxic partner for imipenem. Consequently, when imipenem was launched in the late 1980s as a new 'monotherapy' for serious sepsis, it was in fact a combination product of imipenem and cilastatin in a 1:1 ratio.

The properties of imipenem-cilastatin distinguished it from any β-lactam compound on the market, so it is unsurprising that other drug firms began to take an interest. A similar combination, panipenem-betamipron was marketed in Japan by the Sankyo company in 1993, but is virtually unknown elsewhere. An obvious challenge was to find a carbapenem that did not have the disadvantage of susceptibility to renal dehydropeptidase. Chemists at Merck discovered that methylation of the C-1 carbon had the desired effect, but it was the Japanese firm Sumitomo Pharmaceuticals that first brought a molecule with this feature to market when they launched meropenem in 1995.* Merck, not to be outdone, fought back with the development of ertapenem, which is excreted less quickly allowing less frequent administration; it became available in the United States and elsewhere in 2002. The search is now on for a carbapenem antibiotic that can be given by mouth, though whether there is a real need for such a product is far from certain.

Monobactams

The final β-lactam surprise that nature had in store in the 1970s was a group of compounds produced by bacteria in which the β-lactam ring had no accompanying fused ring structure at all—an arrangement that had been thought unlikely, if not impossible. Workers at the Fujisawa Pharmaceutical Company in Tokyo described the first monocyclic β-lactam compounds, the nocardicins, in 1976 (107). They were viewed largely as curiosities, since their antibacterial activity was poor, though some interest was generated

---

* Although meropenem was developed by Sumitomo it is marketed in most of the world by AstraZeneca, a firm formed in 1999 by a merger between Astra AB in Sweden and Zeneca, a British firm established in 1993 by a demerger from ICI.

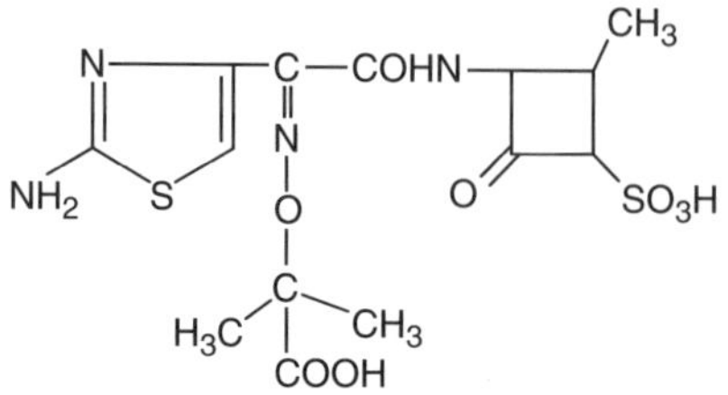

Fig. 4.9 Structure of aztreonam (a monobactam).

when nocardicin A was found to possess a modest ability to stimulate immune defences. Later another group of monocyclic compounds, the sulfazecins, produced by species of *Pseudomonas* were described from Takeda Chemical Industries in Japan.

Around the same time as the reports from Japan a monocyclic β-lactam antibiotic was discovered in the United States at the Squibb pharmaceutical company in New Jersey. The antibiotic was produced by an acid-tolerant strain of *Chromobacter violaceum* that had been isolated from the local Pine Barrens (now known as the Pinelands National Reserve) by one of their scientists, Jennie Hunter-Cevera. In 1979 Squibb recruited Richard Sykes, Glaxo's Head of Antibiotic Research,* and in his new role he enthusiastically promoted research into monocyclic β-lactam antibiotics as potential therapeutic agents first describing their properties, and giving them the class name by which they are now known, monobactam, in 1981 (108). The most important fruit of this research was a semi-synthetic monobactam called aztreonam (originally spelt azthreonam). It can have been no coincidence that the molecule (Fig. 4.9) has a side chain identical to that of ceftazidime, the antipseudomonal cephalosporin that Sykes had earlier helped to develop at Glaxo.

Some natural monobactams are similar to cephamycins in having a stabilizing methoxy group on the β-lactam ring, but although aztreonam lacks this feature, it is nevertheless, unaffected by many β-lactamases. Like ceftazidime, aztreonam is active against *Pseudomonas aeruginosa* and many other Gram-negative bacilli, but it is totally devoid of activity against common Gram-positive cocci such as staphylococci and streptococci, as well as anaerobic pathogens. This feature enabled Squibb to promote aztreonam as a narrow-spectrum targeted drug which would spare members of the bacterial flora that were innocent bystanders in the infectious process. Microbiologists have always passionately preached this therapeutic philosophy, but it proved to be aztreonam's downfall: although targeted treatment is certainly a desirable therapeutic ideal, the sort of patients who are gravely ill with infections caused by *Pseudomonas aeruginosa* or other Gram-negative bacilli also require adequate cover for more virulent Gram-positive cocci that may be lurking in the background. Consequently, if treatment with aztreonam was contemplated, it was usually deemed necessary to add an antibiotic able to deal with Gram-positive pathogens as well, defeating the object of the exercise.

---

* Richard Sykes returned to Glaxo in 1987 and subsequently became chairman and chief executive of Glaxo Group and, subsequently, GlaxoSmithKline. He was appointed rector of Imperial College, London in 2001 and relinquished his role at GlaxoSmithKline.

Several other monobactams made a brief appearance. One, carumonam, is still available in Japan. Squibb themselves briefly flirted with an orally absorbed version, tigemonan, but nothing more was heard of this compound once it was clear that aztreonam was not going to be a marketing success.

Oxacephems

The ingenuity of nature in creating novel β-lactam structures has not been matched by human beings, though many efforts have been made. True, chemists have been very successful in generating semi-synthetic derivatives of natural products. They have also made considerable progress in understanding how alterations in structure relate to activity, but even here theory has not always translated into practice as the Beecham scientists discovered when adding a cephamycin-like methoxy group to the antipseudomonal penicillin, ticarcillin. The result was the compound, temocillin, which was certainly very stable to β-lactamases, but at the expense of all trace of activity against *Pseudomonas aeruginosa* and Gram-positive cocci.

The most celebrated foray into wholly synthetic β-lactam antibiotics was the compound latamoxef (known by its original name, moxalactam, in the United States) an oxacephem, synthesized by Shionogi and Company in Japan in 1978 and subsequently marketed in most countries by Eli Lilly. If a camel is a horse designed by a committee, as Alec Issigonis the designer of the Morris mini motor car is said to have quipped, latamoxef is the antimicrobial equivalent. The structure (Fig. 4.10) features not only the novel substitution of oxygen for sulphur in the basic cephalosporin ring system, but also adds the stabilizing methoxy group of the cephamycins, the side chain carboxyl that gives carbenicillin its antipseudomonal activity, and the hydroxyl substitution on the benzene ring that had given amoxicillin the edge over ampicillin. It also carries an extraordinarily nitrogen-rich side chain at the C-3 position, a feature borrowed from cephamandole and several other cephalosporins, and this proved to be its undoing.

Latamoxef was launched onto the market around the same time as cefotaxime and with much the same credentials: an injectable compound with potent broad-spectrum activity and stability to β-lactamases. Comparatively poor efficacy against streptococci and staphylococci was compensated by activity against anaerobic bacteria and *Pseudomonas aeruginosa*. However, in therapeutic trials the complex C-3 side chain was found to be associated with postoperative bleeding caused by an effect on platelets—blood components involved in clotting—and with an unwanted interaction with alcohol.

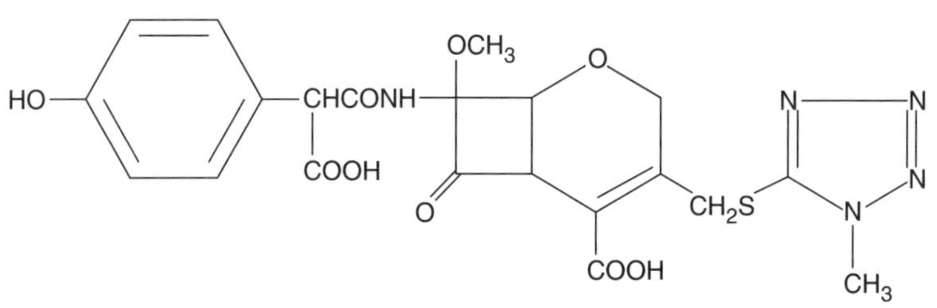

Fig. 4.10 Structure of latamoxef (an oxacephem).

These side effects could both be avoided, the first by co-administration of vitamin K and the second by abstinence from alcohol, but in the competitive world of drug marketing, the 'give a dog a bad name' principle often affects prescribing habits and latamoxef was largely shunned. It is no longer available in most countries and another oxacephem, flomoxef, which was designed in Japan to overcome the problems of latamoxef, has not been marketed in Europe or the United States.

Are the glory days of β-lactam antibiotics now at an end? In therapeutic terms, certainly not: they are sill among the most widely used agents and even the original benzylpenicillin still retains an important place in antimicrobial chemotherapy. In terms of new developments, all the signs are that the 50-year bonanza is well and truly over. Even in Japan, where new β-lactam compounds with dubiously improved properties continued to be described—and occasionally marketed—until very recently, fascination with these drugs seems to have finally waned. In the rest of the world, interest has for some time been muted by the realization that any improvements over existing β-lactam antibiotics is likely to be so marginal that the chance of recouping the investment in the necessary research and development would be extremely uncertain.

References

1. Hare R (1982). New light on penicillin. *Med Hist* **26**, 1–24.
2. Wyn Jones E, Wyn Jones RG (2002). Merlin Pryce (1902–1976) and penicillin: an abiding mystery. *Vesalius—Acta Int Historiae Medicinae* **7**, 6–25.
3. Fleming A (1929). On the antibacterial action of cultures of a penicillium, with special reference to their use in the isolation of *B. influenzae*. *Br J Exp Pathol* **10**, 226–36.
4. Malkin J (1981). *Sir Alexander Fleming. Man of penicillin*. Alloway Publishing, Ayrshire.
5. Macfarlane G (1984). *Alexander Fleming. The man and the myth*, pp. 18–26. The Hogarth Press, London.
6. Masters D (1946). *Miracle drug. The inner history of penicillin*, p. 20. Eyre & Spottiswoode, London.
7. Fleming A, Allison VD (1922). Observations on a bacteriolytic substance ("lysozyme") found in secretions and tissues. *Br J Exp Pathol* **3**, 252–60.
8. Fleming A (1929). The staphylococci. In: *A system of bacteriology in relation to medicine*, pp. 11–26. Medical Research Council, London.
9. Brunel J (1951). Antibiosis from Pasteur to Fleming. *J Hist Med* **6**, 287–301; Selwyn S (1980). The beta lactam antibiotics. *Penicillins and cephalosporins in perspective*, pp. 4–16. Hodder and Stoughton, London; Duckett S (1999). Ernest Duchesne and the concept of fungal antibiotic therapy. *Lancet* **354**, 2068–71.
10. Hare R (1970). *The birth of penicillin and the disarming of microbes*, pp. 81–7. George Allen and Unwin, London.
11. Hare R (1970). *The birth of penicillin and the disarming of microbes*, pp. 54–80. George Allen and Unwin, London.
12. Root-Bernstein RS (1989). *Discovering*. Harvard University Press, Cambridge.
13. Bentley R (2005). The development of penicillin. Genesis of a famous antibiotic. *Perspect Biol Med* **48**, 444–52.
14. Lax E (2004). *The mould in Dr. Florey's coat. The remarkable true story of the penicillin miracle*. Little Brown, London.
15. Fleming A (1944). *The discovery of penicillin*. In: *Penicillin 1929–1943* (British Council). *Br Med Bull* **2**, 4–5.

16. Macfarlane G (1984). *Alexander Fleming. The man and the myth*, p. 133. The Hogarth Press, London.

17. Wright AE (1927). A discourse on Ehrlich's "chemotherapy" and on certain general principles which require to be brought into application in all treatment of bacterial disease. *Lancet* **2**, 1327–34.

18. Fleming A (1928). The bactericidal power of human blood and some methods of altering it. *Proc R Soc Med* **21**, 859–67.

19. Rossiter P (2005). Keith Bernard Rogers (Obituary). *BMJ* **331**, 579.

20. Wainwright M, Swan HT (1986). C.G Paine and the earliest surviving records of penicillin therapy. *Med Hist* **30**, 42–56.

21. Wainwright M (1996). Roger Reid's early contribution to the study of penicillin. *J Med Biog* **4**, 14–7.

22. Pennsylvania State University libraries catalogue. http://cat.libraries.psu.edu/

23. Hobby GL (1985). *Penicillin. Meeting the challenge*, p. 46. Yale University Press, New Haven.

24. Reid RD (1935). Some properties of a bacterial-inhibitory substance produced by a mold. *J Bacteriol* **29**, 215–21.

25. Hare R (15 February 1979). Penicillin—setting the record straight. *New Sci* 466–8.

26. MRC Dunn Human Nutrition Unit (2000). History of the MRC Dunn Human Nutrition Unit. www.mrc-dunn.cam.ac.uk/about/history.html

27. Macfarlane G (1979). *Howard Florey The making of a great scientist*, pp. 226–50. Oxford University Press, Oxford.

28. Abraham E (1983). Ernst Boris Chain. *Biog Memoirs Fellows Roy Soc* **29**, 43–91.

29. Medical Research Council archives, London, file No. 1752, Vol. 1. Cited by Macfarlane G (1979). *Howard Florey The making of a great scientist*, p. 299. Oxford University Press, Oxford.

30. Macfarlane G (1979). *Howard Florey The making of a great scientist*, p. 300. Oxford University Press, Oxford.

31. Heatley NG (1990). Penicillin and luck. In: Moberg CL, Cohn ZA, eds. *Launching the antibiotic era*, pp. 31–41. Rockefeller University Press, New York.

32. Harris H (1998). Howard Florey and the Development of Penicillin. Florey Centenary Lecture given at the Sir William Dunn School of Pathology, Oxford, 29 September 1998. Reprinted in: *Notes and Records of the Royal Society of London* (1999) **53**, 243–52.

33. Chain E, Florey HW, Gardner AD, *et al.* (1940). Penicillin as a chemotherapeutic agent. *Lancet* **2**, 226–8.

34. Annotation (1940). Penicillin. *Lancet* **2**, 236.

35. Fletcher C (1984). First clinical use of penicillin. *BMJ* **289**, 1721–3.

36. Hobby G (1985). *Penicillin: meeting the challenge*, pp. 69–80. Yale University Press, New Haven.

37. Abraham EP, Chain E, Fletcher CM, *et al.* (1941). Further observations on penicillin. *Lancet* **2**, 177–89.

38. Editorial (1941). Penicillin in action. *Lancet* **2**, 191–2.

39. Florey ME, Florey HW (1943). General and local administration of penicillin. *Lancet* **1**, 387–97.

40. Fleming A (1943). Streptococcal meningitis treated with penicillin. Measurement of bacteristatic power of blood and cerebrospinal fluid. *Lancet* **2**, 434–8.

41. Liebenau J (1987). The British success with penicillin. *Soc Stud Sci* **17**, 69–86.

42. Brown, K (2004). *Penicillin man. Alexander Fleming and the antibiotic revolution*, pp. 127–8. Sutton Publishing, Stroud; Masters D (1946). *Miracle drug. The inner history of penicillin*, pp. 165–6. Eyre & Spottiswoode, London.

43. Garrod LP (1943). The treatment of war wounds with penicillin. *BMJ* **2**, 755–6; Jeffrey JS, Thomson S (1944). Penicillin in battle casualties. *BMJ* **2**, 1–4.

44. Editorial (1943). The penicillin position. *BMJ* **2**, 269. Reprinted in: Waterworth PM ed. (1985). LP Garrod on antibiotics. *J Antimicrob Chemother* **15** (Suppl. B), 15–16; Editorial (1944). The wider distribution of penicillin *BMJ* **2**, 118, reprinted in Waterworth PM ed. (1985). LP Garrod on antibiotics. *J Antimicrob Chemother* **15** (Suppl. B), 20–21.

45. Richards AN (1964). Production of penicillin in the United States (1941–1946). *Nature* **201**, 441–5.

46. Lax E (2004). The mould in Dr. Florey's coat. *The remarkable true story of the penicillin miracle*, pp. 1–3. Little Brown, London; Curtis J (1999) Fulton penicillin and chance. http://info.med.yale.edu/external/pubs/ym_fw9900/capsule.html

47. Sheehan JC (1984). *The enchanted ring*, pp. 123–60. MIT Press, Cambridge, Mass.

48. Digger History: an unofficial history of the Australian and New Zealand Armed Forces. Percival Landon Bazeley; Australia's WW2 penicillin hero. http://www.diggerhistory.info/pages-heroes/bazeley.htm

49. Bickel L (1972). *Rise up to Life. A biography of Howard Walter Florey who gave penicillin to the world*, pp. 208–15. Angus and Robertson, London.

50. Burns M, Bennett JW, van Dijck WM (2003). Code name bacinol. *Microbe Magazine*. American Society of Microbiology, Washington. Available at: http://www.asm.org/microbe/index.asp?bid=11780

51. Hobby GL (1985). *Penicillin: meeting the challenge*, pp.202–4. Yale University Press, New Haven.

52. Shama G (2003). Pilzkrieg: the German wartime quest for penicillin. *Microbiol Today* **30**, 120–3.

53. Bickel L (1972). *Rise up to life. A Biography of Harold Walter Florey who made penicillin and gave it to the world*, pp. 295–301. Angus and Robertson, London.

54. Bud R (2007). *Penicillin. Triumph and tragedy*, pp. 75–9. Oxford University Press, Oxford; Schneider WG, Valenta Z (1991). Karel František Wiesner 25 November 1919–28 November 1986. *Biog Memoirs Fellows Roy Soc* **37**, 463–90.

55. Yagisawa Y (1980). Early history of antibiotics in Japan. In: Parascandola J, ed. *The history of antibiotics. A symposium*, pp. 69–90. American Institute of the History of Pharmacy, Madison, Wisconsin.

56. Kumazawa J, Yagisawa M (2002). The history of antibiotics: the Japanese story. *J Infect Chemother* **8**, 125–33.

57. Pfizer Inc (2002). Exploring our history. http://www.pfizer.com/pfizer/history/1941.jsp

58. Editorial (1944). Penicillin in venereal disease. *BMJ* **1**, 428. Reprinted in: Waterworth PM ed. (1985). LP Garrod on antibiotics. *J Antimicrob Chemother* **15** (Suppl. B), 18–19.

59. Parascandola J (2001). John Mahoney and the introduction of penicillin to treat syphilis. *Pharm Hist* **43**, 1–13.

60. Enoch HE, Wallersteiner WKS (1944). A standardized antibacterial pyrogen-free metabolite preparation containing living *Penicillium notatum*. *Nature* **153**, 380–1.

61. Wright A. (31 August 1942). Letter. *The Times*.

62. Bankoff G (1946). *The conquest of disease. The story of penicillin*, pp. 175–6. Macdonald & Co, London.

63. Medical Research Council Patulin Clinical Trials Committee (1944). Clinical trials of patulin in the common cold. *Lancet* **2**, 373–5.

64. D'Arcy Hart P (1999). A change in scientific approach: from alternation to randomised allocation in clinical trials in the 1940s. *BMJ* **319**, 572–3.

65. Cornaglia G (2000). To the memory of an angel.. *Clin Microbiol Infect* **6** (Suppl. 3), 1.

66. Scarpa B (2000). Homage from one Sardinian to another. *Clin Microbiol Infect* **6** (Suppl. 3), 3–5.

67. Brotzu G (1948). Ricerche su di un nuovo antibiotico. *Lavori dell'Istituto di Igiene di Cagliari*.

68. Abraham EP (1979). A glimpse of the early history of the cephalosporins. *Rev Infect Dis* **1**, 99–105.

69. Bo G (2000). Giuseppe Brotzu and the discovery of cephalosporins. *Clin Microbiol Infect* **6** (Suppl. 3), 6–8.

70. Sarawak, Malaysia. Brief history. www.almanach.be/search/m/mal_sarawak.html

71. Obituary (1971). Charles Owen Swithin Blyth Brooke. *Lancet* **2**, 988–9; Obituary (1971). C.O.S. Blyth Brooke. *BMJ* **4**, 11.

72. Williams TI (1984) Howard Florey. *Penicillin and after*, pp. 219–93. Oxford University Press, Oxford.

73. Carlile M (2004). A strange episode in the history of antibiotics. *Microbiol Today* **31**, 9.

74. Crawford K, Heatley NG, Boyd PF, *et al.* (1952). Antibiotic production by a species of *Cephalosporium*. *J Gen Microbiol* **6**, 47–59.

75. Abraham EP, Loder PB (1972). Cephalosporin C. In: Flynn EH, ed. *Cephalosporins and penicillins. Chemistry and biology*, pp. 1–26. Academic Press, New York.

76. Abraham EP, Chain EB (1940). An enzyme from bacteria able to destroy penicillin. *Nature* **146**, 837.

77. Bard B (2000). In: Tansey EM, Reynolds LA, eds. *Post penicillin antibiotics: from acceptance to resistance? (A witness seminar held at the Wellcome Institute for the History of Medicine)*, pp. 39–40. The Wellcome Trust, London. Also available at: http://www.ucl.ac.uk/histmed/PDFS/Publications/Witness/wit6.pdf.

78. Koenig J (1984). *Die Penicillin-V Story. Eine Erfindung aus Tirol als Segen für die Welt.* Haymon Verlag, Innsbruck.

79. Brandl E (1983). β-Lactames: from biosynthesis to semisynthesis. In: Spitzy KH, Karrer K, eds. *Proceedings of the 13th International Congress of Chemotherapy*, Main lecture 3, 1/11–1/29.

80. Brandl E, Giovannini M, Margreiter H (1953). Untersuchung über das säurestabile, oral wirksame Phenoxymethylpenicillin (Penicillin V). *Wiener Medizinische Wochenschrift* **103**, 602–7.

81. Behrens OK, Corse J, Edwards JP, *et al.* (1948). Biosynthesis of penicillins IV. New crystalline biosynthetic penicillins. *J Biol Chem* **175**, 793–809.

82. Romansky MJ, Rittman GE (1944). A method of prolonging the action of penicillin. *Science* **100**, 196–8.

83. Sullivan NP, Symmes AT, Miller HC, Rhodehamel HW (1948). A new penicillin for prolonged blood levels. *Science* **107**, 169–70.

84. Anderson S, Homan P (2000). "Best for me, best for you"—a history of Beecham's Pills 1842–1998. *Pharm J* **269**, 921–4.

85. Lazell HG (1975). From pills to penicillin. *The Beecham story*, pp. 135–50. Heinemann, London.

86. Doyle P, Batchelor R (2000). In: Tansey EM, Reynolds LA, eds. *Post penicillin antibiotics: from acceptance to resistance? (A witness seminar held at the Wellcome Institute for the History of Medicine)*, pp. 25–31. The Wellcome Trust, London. Also available at: http://www.ucl.ac.uk/histmed/PDFS/Publications/Witness/wit6.pdf

87. Batchelor FR, Doyle FP, Nayler JHC, Rolinson GN (1959). Synthesis of penicillin: 6-aminopenicillanic acid in penicillin fermentations. *Nature* **183**, 257–8.

88. Rolinson GN (1998). Forty years of β-lactam research. *J Antimicrob Chemother* **41**, 589–603.

89. Rolinson GN, Batchelor FR, Butterworth D, *et al.* (1960). Formation of 6-aminopenicillanic acid from penicillin by enzymic hydrolysis. *Nature* **187**, 236–7.

90. Kaufmann W, Bauer K (1960). Enzymatische spaltung und resynthese von Penicillin. *Naturwissenschaften* **47**, 474–5.

91. Kallenberg AI, van Rantwijk F, Sheldon RA (2005). Immobilization of penicillin G acylase: the key to optimum performance. *Adv Synth Catal* **347**, 905–26.

92. Sheehan JC (1984). *The enchanted ring*, pp.161–97. MIT Press, Cambridge, Mass.

93. Rolinson GN, Stevens S (1961). Microbiological studies on a new broad-spectrum penicillin "Penbritin". *BMJ* **2**, 191–6.

94. Knudsen ET, Rolinson GN, Sutherland R (1967). Carbenicillin: a new semisynthetic penicillin active against Pseudomonas aeruginosa. *BMJ* **3**, 75–8.

95. Passey D. *Joseph Edward Nathan. Glaxo founder.* http://www.nzedge.com/heroes/nathan.html.

96. Huber FM, Chauvette RR, Jackson BG (1972). Preparative methods for 7-aminocephalosporanic acid and 6-aminopenicillanic acid. In: Flynn EH, ed. *Cephalosporins and penicillins. Chemistry and biology*, pp. 27–73. Academic Press, New York.

97. O'Callaghan CH, Sykes RB, Griffiths, Thornton JE (1976). Cefuroxime, a new cephalosporin antibiotic: activity in vitro. *Antimicrob Agents Chemother* **9**, 511–9.

98. Heymès R, Lutz A, Schrinner E (1977). Experimental evaluation of HR 756, a new cephalosporin derivative: pre-clinical study. *Infection* **5**, 259–60.

99. O'Callaghan CH, Acred P, Harper PB, Ryan DM, Kirby SM, Harding SM (1980). GR 20263, a new broad-spectrum cephalosporin with antipseudomonal activity. *Antimicrob Agents Chemother* **17**, 876–83.

100. Nagarajan R, Boeck LD, Gorman M, *et al.* (1971). β-lactam antibiotics from *Streptomyces. J Am Chem Soc* **93**, 2308–10.

101. Demain AL, Elander RP (1999). The β-lactam antibiotics: past, present and future. *Antonie van Leeuwenhoek* **75**, 5–19.

102. Stapley EO, Jackson M, Hernandez S, *et al.* (1972). Cephamycins, a new family of β-lactam antibiotics. 1. Production by actinomycetes, including *Streptomyces lactamdurans* sp. N. *Antimicrob Agents Chemother* **2**, 122–31.

103. Reading C, Cole M (1977). Clavulanic acid: a beta-lactamase-inhibiting beta-lactam from *Streptomyces clavuligerus. Antimicrob Agents Chemother* **11**, 852–7.

104. Behrens OK, Garrison L (1950). Inhibitors for penicillinase. *Arch Biochem* **27**, 94–8.

105. Cole M (2000). In: Tansey EM, Reynolds LA, eds. *Post penicillin antibiotics: from acceptance to resistance? (A witness seminar held at the Wellcome Institute for the History of Medicine)*, pp. 50–2. The Wellcome Trust, London. Also available at: http://www.ucl.ac.uk/histmed/PDFS/Publications/Witness/wit6.pdf

106. Kahan JS, Kahan FM, Goegelman R, *et al.* (1979). Thienamycin, a new β-lactam antibiotic. 1. Discovery, taxonomy, isolation and physical properties. *J Antibiot* **32**, 1–12.

107. Hashimoto M, Komori TA, Kamiya T (1976). Nocardicin A and B, novel monocyclic beta-lactam antibiotics from a *Nocardia* species. *J Am Chem Soc* **98**, 3023–5.

108. Sykes RB, Cimarusti CM, Bonner DP, *et al.* (1981). Monocyclic β-lactam antibiotics produced by bacteria. *Nature* **291**, 489–91.

Chapter 5

The taming of tuberculosis and leprosy

I've known over thirty men that found out how to cure consumption. Why do people go on dying of it, Colly? Devilment, I suppose. There was my father's old friend George Boddington of Sutton Coldfield. He discovered the open-air cure in eighteen-forty. He was ruined and driven out of his practice for only opening the windows; and now we wont let a consumptive patient have as much as a roof over his head.

George Bernard Shaw, 1906, *The Doctor's Dilemma Act 1.*

There are various kinds of infection caused by mycobacteria, but two types loom large in human history: the terrible afflictions designated within the Latin names of their causative organisms, *Mycobacterium leprae* and *Mycobacterium tuberculosis*. Leprosy is a truly horrific condition, especially in its most florid form, and one from which, historically, individuals and communities have recoiled in terror. But without diminishing the seriousness of that disease, it is tuberculosis—the white plague—that far outstrips it in importance among the major microbial enemies of humankind.

Infection with *Mycobacterium tuberculosis*—often called 'the tubercle bacillus'—can take many forms. Skin, bone, joints, intestine, indeed almost any part of the body can be affected; generalized infection—miliary tuberculosis*—is a devastating and not uncommon manifestation of the disease. Tuberculous meningitis often strikes children and can kill within days of the onset of symptoms. Jane Austen probably died from tuberculosis of the adrenal cortex. Samuel Johnson suffered from scrofula, an infection of the cervical lymph nodes, which was then called the king's evil because it was thought to be curable by the royal touch. He was touched by Queen Anne, but evidently Queens do not have the same knack for it did not succeed.

Most common of all, and most infectious, is pulmonary tuberculosis, frequently leading to progressive weight loss and inevitable death: the 'galloping consumption' of popular Victorian parlance, more usually called phthisis by their classically educated physicians. Attention has been drawn many times to the long list of artists, writers, composers, and

---

* Literally 'like millet seed'. Ludwig von Buhl, professor of pathology in Munich during the nineteenth century, popularized the term to describe rapidly spreading disseminated tuberculosis in a classic work: *Lungenentzündung, Tuberkulose und Schwindsucht*. Oldenbourg, München, 1872.

other celebrities who succumbed, often in the prime of life, before reliable treatment became available, but millions of unknown men, women, and children, rich and poor alike, have also been victims. Even today, it is estimated that one-third of the world's population harbour the tubercle bacillus and it is thought to be responsible annually for 8 million new cases and at least 2 million deaths (1).

The pathos of tuberculosis has been captured many times in art, most famously in the portrait of the dying poet John Keats by his friend Joseph Severn; but perhaps most poignantly by the Norwegian Edvard Munch, who had observed at close quarters the death of his sister Sophie at the age of just 16. The fear in which tuberculosis was universally held was vividly captured by Charles Dickens in describing the illness of the abused young man Smike in *Nicholas Nickleby*:

> There is a dread disease which so prepares its victim, as it were, for death; which so refines it of its grosser aspect, and throws around familiar looks unearthly indications of the coming change; a dread disease, in which the struggle between soul and body is so gradual, quiet, and solemn, and the result so sure, that day by day, and grain by grain, the mortal part wastes and withers away, so that the spirit grows light and sanguine with its lightening load, and, feeling immortality at hand, deems it but a new term of mortal life; a disease in which death and life are so strangely blended, that death takes the glow and hue of life, and life the gaunt and grisly form of death; a disease which medicine never cured, wealth never warded off, or poverty could boast exemption from; which sometimes moves in giant strides, and sometimes at a tardy sluggish pace, but, slow or quick, is ever sure and certain (2).

Fighting tuberculosis without drugs

Tuberculosis in Western countries was in decline long before effective drugs for the condition were discovered. There are many reasons for this including the slow, but progressive rise in general living conditions during the twentieth century, improved hygiene (including the outlawing of spitting in public places), campaigns of public education,* and the segregation of infected persons in sanatoria, which were built outside the main urban areas not just to provide an environment conducive to recovery, but also to lessen the chance of spread to the general population.

The availability of an effective vaccine also played an important part. Starting in 1908, the French medical bacteriologist Albert Calmette and the veterinarian Camille Guérin spent over 10 years trying to devise a safe antituberculosis vaccine based on a strain of *Mycobacterium bovis* that had been isolated from the udder of a sick cow by Guérin's former teacher Edmond Nocard. Calmette and Guérin had fortuitously observed in 1908 that the strain lost some of its virulence for laboratory animals when cultured on a growth medium of potato starch and glycerinated ox bile. Repeated subculture further attenuated its virulence, raising the prospect that it might be used to induce immunity without causing actual disease in man.

---

* I still possess a book presented to my mother, then a 12-year-old pupil of SS Peter and Paul's School, Bolton, as first prize for an essay on the Bolton Tuberculosis Exhibition of 1910.

The development of the vaccine was not without its problems and personal events were not to help. In March 1914, Henriette Caillaux, wife of Joseph Caillaux, a controversial pacifist politician, killed Calmette's brother, Gaston, who was the Editor of *Le Figaro*, in a crime passionelle (3). Incensed over revelations about the private life of her husband, Mme Caillaux confronted Gaston Calmette in his office, drew a pistol from her fur muff and shot him at point-blank range. In court she convinced the jury that the event was a tragic accident and she was acquitted.

During the Great War, Lille, where Calmette and Guérin worked, came under German military control and the two scientists were virtual prisoners in the Pasteur Institute there. To add insult to injury, Calmette's wife was deported to Germany and kept under arrest for 6 months (4). Guérin's wife died of tuberculous meningitis just before the signing of the armistice in 1918.

Despite these difficulties, work continued on the vaccine and by 1921 it was decided to embark on an experimental vaccination programme by oral administration to young children. Safety was not thought to be a major issue since the bovine bacillus, *Mycobacterium bovis*, was mistakenly thought to have a very limited capacity to infect human beings. The reasoning may have been faulty, but the bacille Calmette–Guérin (BCG) was shown to work. The vaccine appeared vindicated, but troubles were not at an end. Prospects for BCG received a severe setback in 1930 by an event that became known as 'the Lübeck disaster'. In the North German city of Lübeck BCG vaccine supplied by the Pasteur Institute in Paris, but prepared for use by a local laboratory, was administered orally to 250 newborn babies; 72 infants died within a year, and a further 135 became infected. The scandal caused enormous shock waves as accusations and counter-accusations flew between France and Germany, neighbours with a long history of mutual suspicion. Extreme political factions used the event to stir up antagonism against the Weimar Republic, which was already in economic crisis. An enquiry into the events found that the Pasteur vaccine was not to blame, but that it had been accidentally contaminated with virulent tubercle bacilli in the Lübeck laboratories. Three local doctors and a nurse were brought to trial and two received prison sentences. Though Albert Calmette himself was not accused, he was badly affected and the affair probably hastened his premature death a few years later.

The Lübeck affair nearly scuppered the chances of introducing BCG vaccine throughout the world. Fortunately, clinical investigations continued in some countries, notably in Scandinavia. It eventually became clear that the vaccine was generally safe and effective, and intracutaneous injection was established as the preferred route of administration. Nevertheless suspicions remained and it took a large Medical Research Council trial undertaken among young people in 1950 to convince the medical authorities in the United Kingdom of its efficacy. This evaluation of BCG was coordinated by the Director of the Medical Research Council's Tuberculosis Research Unit, Philip D'Arcy Hart, who was also responsible for organizing the streptomycin trial in the United Kingdom after the war (see p. 162–4). Hart was a pioneer of controlled clinical trials, who had been appointed as a staff scientist at the Medical Research Council's National Institute for

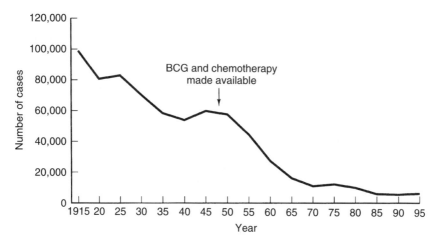

Figure 5.1 Notifications of tuberculosis in England, Wales, and Scotland, 1915–95. From: Reid D. Epidemiology and control of community infections. In: *Medical Microbiology* 17th edn. (Greenwood D, Slack R. C. B., Peutherer J. F., Barer M., eds.) Churchill Livingstone, Edinburgh, 2007. Reproduced with permission from Elsevier.

Medical Research (NIMR) in 1937, initially to study lung disease in Welsh miners.* He lived to the ripe age of 106 and was still an active, if unpaid, member of the Institute 50 years after carrying out his work on BCG, publishing his last scientific paper with Joe Colston (who died in 2003 at little over half D'Arcy Hart's age) in 2004 (5).

Even with convincing evidence of its effectiveness, arguments as to the true value of the BCG vaccine and the most appropriate strategy to deliver maximum benefits continued for many years (6). To add to the confusion, BCG proved ineffective in some countries of the world, notably parts of India and the United States, although paradoxically it seemed to confer some protection against leprosy in communities in which the disease was endemic. The marked variation in efficacy among different communities has never been satisfactorily explained, but may be due to genetic diversity, or the compromise of the immune response caused by prior exposure to environmental mycobacteria.

Between 1915 and 1939 notifications of tuberculosis in Great Britain declined from around 100,000 to 55,000 per year. During the Second World War the figure rose once more, but went into steep decline once the war had ended (Fig. 5.1). Introduction of mass vaccination and mass X-ray campaigns were to play their part in this spectacular fall, but it was the discovery of three potent antituberculosis agents—streptomycin, *para*-aminosalicylic acid (PAS), and isoniazid—in the decade between 1943 and 1952 that made the most impact by offering for the first time the possibility of a radical and reliable cure.

---

* The study established that miners were suffering from an occupational disease, pneumoconiosis. Hart, a lifelong socialist campaigned successfully for affected mineworkers to receive compensation.

Antituberculosis agents

Empirical therapy and false dawns

Early attempts to treat tuberculosis with drugs were admirably reviewed by Philip D'Arcy Hart in the Mitchell Lecture, delivered at the Royal College of Physicians, London on 9 July 1946 (7), just as streptomycin was arousing widespread interest in the medical community. Among traditional drugs that were used empirically in tuberculosis from ancient times, and may conceivably have conferred some slight benefit, were inorganic arsenical compounds, tannin, seaweed (rich in iodides), powdered crayfish (rich in calcium), mercury, and gold. Other widely used remedies included large doses of cod-liver oil or creosote, compounds that were thought to aid the body's fight against the disease and which remained popular well into the twentieth century. Chaulmoogra oil, a traditional remedy for leprosy (see p. 190f), was briefly investigated, but without success.

More outrageous nostrums that enjoyed widespread credence included drinking asses' milk and inhaling the salubrious air of a cowshed. Adolphe Sax, the Belgian inventor of the saxophone, promoted the lung-strengthening benefits of playing wind instruments (8). Pills, powders, potions, and panaceas (accompanied by glowing endorsements from satisfied customers) offering a certain cure for consumption were, unsurprisingly, a rich source of profit for charlatans and the self-styled 'eclectic physicians' of Victorian times, playing on the fear of this dreaded disease, which carried off so many young people and breadwinners. Needless to say, none of these quack remedies provided any reliable benefit and most reputable doctors preferred to recommend the harmless triad of fresh air, rest, and diet—experienced, if one could afford it, in a sanatorium idyllically situated in the Swiss Alps, as immortalized in Thomas Mann's celebrated novel *Der Zauberberg* (*The Magic Mountain*).

Genuine hopes of a reliable cure were not raised until after Robert Koch's discovery of the bacterial cause of tuberculosis in 1882; an event that cemented his reputation as the foremost bacteriologist in Germany and the rival, if not the equal, of Pasteur. Koch was a naturally cautious man, who always liked to be sure of his facts before publicizing them. Thus, his announcement at the 10th International Congress of Medicine in Berlin in August 1890 that he had discovered a substance that offered a possible cure for tuberculosis on the basis of preliminary experiments in guinea pigs was uncharacteristic. Indeed, there are strong suspicions that his superiors pressurized him into making the revelation prematurely (9). Although the announcement was couched in cautious terms the reaction of the medical profession and the public was little short of hysterical. Trials were undertaken with great enthusiasm and public acclaim turned to ashes as it soon became clear that the remedy was useless and even dangerous.

The 'cure', the nature of which was at first kept secret, turned out to be an extract of killed tubercle bacteria harvested from guinea pigs, later called 'old tuberculin'. The spurious claims for the efficacy of this substance arose from an intense reaction of the body's cellular immune system to the antigenic stimulus. Undeterred, Koch went on to develop a 'new tuberculin', but results with this were equally disappointing. All was not lost, however; the Austrian paediatrician and pioneer of allergy studies, Clemens von Pirquet, later used Koch's tuberculin as a diagnostic skin test to determine the likelihood of prior exposure to tuberculosis. In due course, Florence Seibert, a biochemist at the Henry Phipps Institute,* Philadelphia, refined the test in the 1930s by developing a pyrogen-free extract that became known as 'purified protein derivative' or more simply PPD (10). PPD was accepted as the national standard in the United States in 1941 and was adopted by the World Health Organization as the international standard at a meeting in Geneva in early December 1951. It is still widely used as a diagnostic test of susceptibility to tuberculosis.

Koch's reputation suffered badly from the tuberculin affair and was not helped when he sought solace from his disappointments in the arms of a 17-year-old art student, Hedwig Freiberg. In 1893, he divorced his wife of 27 years, Emmy, and married his paramour. Despite public disapproval of these events, Koch's scientific contributions, now concentrated largely in the field of tropical medicine, continued unabated and his rehabilitation was complete when, in 1905, he was awarded the Nobel Prize in Physiology or Medicine.

A second false dawn in the therapeutic history of tuberculosis was to emerge in the 1920s when gold therapy became the rage. Gold salts had, of course, long been favoured by those of a Paracelsian bent, and interest had been revived by a gold compound called Krysolgan, marketed in Germany in 1917 by Schering in Berlin. Interest in gold salts in tuberculosis has been traced to another remark made by Robert Koch in his Berlin conference address in August 1890, when he announced that gold cyanide (!) was much the most active of various dyes and other compounds that he had tested on laboratory cultures (11). Although Koch tempered enthusiasm by stating that gold cyanide did not appear to have any effect in laboratory animals, two researchers in Breslau, C. Bruch and A. Glück, working in the laboratory of Albert Neisser (discoverer of the gonococcus, now known as *Neisseria gonorrhoeae*) titrated the toxicity of the compound in rabbits as a prelude to treating 20 hapless patients suffering from skin tuberculosis. The results were unremarkable, but fortunately no serious toxic effects were reported.

The popularity of Krysolgan and several similar remedies was short-lived, but one compound, Sanocrysin, the double thiosulphite of gold and sodium, introduced in 1924 by Holger Møllgaard in Denmark, was to have a longer lasting appeal. Møllgaard had claimed on the most tenuous evidence that Sanocrysin was a true chemotherapeutic agent in Ehrlich's sense. He was enthusiastically supported by his Danish colleagues Knud Secher and Knud Faber who had applied the drug clinically. Despite the lack of convincing evidence, use of Sanocrysin briefly became fashionable. It took the discouraging

---

* The Henry Phipps Institute for the Study Treatment and Prevention of Tuberculosis was founded in 1903 by a Philadelphia doctor, Lawrence Flick, with money provided by Henry Phipps a steel magnate and partner of the Scottish-American industrialist and philanthropist Andrew Carnegie. In 1965 the institute was subsumed into the University of Pennsylvania's Department of Genetics under the chairmanship of the British immunologist Rupert Everett Billingham.

results of several clinical trials and, as with Koch's tuberculin, reports of serious side effects, including some fatalities, to shake confidence in the remedy. In one of these early trials, conducted in 1931 by J. Burns Anderson and his colleagues at the Detroit Municipal Tuberculosis Hospital in Northfield, Michigan, patients were allocated to Sanocrysin treatment or normal care by the toss of a coin, one of the earliest attempts at true randomization in clinical trials (12). By 1935 reports of toxicity were too persistent to be ignored and gold therapy went into decline, though it was not completely abandoned for another decade.

Meanwhile, optimists who hoped that a miracle cure might yet be found were given renewed hope as first Prontosil and other sulphonamides, then penicillin, emerged as genuine chemotherapeutic agents with activity against bacterial pathogens. In the event, none of these compounds was to prove effective, though some sulphonamides did seem to show a very feeble effect on experimental tuberculosis in the laboratory and Karl Folkers, a pharmaceutical chemist with Merck, was still pursuing sulphonamide derivatives as possible antituberculosis agents in the mid-1940s. Predictably, sulphonamides were also the starting point for research on tuberculostatic compounds that Gerhard Domagk and his colleagues instigated at the start of the Second World War (see p. 170).

More promising than the sulphonamides themselves were a group of related compounds, the sulphones. These included dapsone (diaminodiphenylsulphone; a by-product of sulphanilamide production), Promin (the didextrosesulphonate of dapsone; called Promanide in Britain), Diasone (sulfoxone; the disodium sulphoxylate derivative of dapsone), Sulphetrone (solapsone) and the somewhat better tolerated Promizole (thiazosulphone). Animal tests of these compounds and small clinical trials were started in the early 1940s and gave modestly encouraging results (13). Promin, a sulphone synthesized by Parke, Davis and Company in Detroit,* was the subject of a clinical trial at the Mayo Clinic in 1941; Promizole, another Parke, Davis product, was briefly used by Edith Lincoln a paediatrician working in the children's chest clinic at New York's Bellevue Hospital. Unfortunately haematological toxicity militated against the acceptance of the sulphones. All would have been consigned to the dustbin of history when they were overshadowed by the developments of the next 10 years had they not also shown to be effective in the treatment of leprosy (see p. 194–7). The seminal event for the treatment of tuberculosis was the discovery of streptomycin in 1943. It was the work of a talented Frenchman, René Dubos, at the Rockefeller Institute in New York that was to provide the initial momentum for the breakthrough.

---

* Parke, Davis & Co., once the largest maker of drugs in the world, had its roots in a small business started by Samuel P. Duffield in 1862. In 1866 he formed a partnership with Hervey C. Parke. A salesman, George S. Davis, joined the firm in 1867 and was made a partner in 1869 when Duffield's successor, A. F. Jennings retired. In 1970 Parke, Davis & Co. was acquired by Warner-Lambert (itself formed in 1955 from the firms created in the nineteenth century by William R. Warner in Philadelphia and Jordan Wheat Lambert in St Louis) and the business merged with Pfizer in 2000.

Antibiotics from the soil

The investigation that eventually yielded streptomycin, the first successful treatment for tuberculosis, was not originally aimed specifically at finding a cure for that disease, but was the result of a random search for metabolites of soil micro-organisms that might exhibit antimicrobial activity. The unlikely location of the discovery was the New Jersey Agricultural Experiment Station founded in 1880 as a State research institution addressing issues relating to agriculture and natural resources. The research station was (and is) part of Rutgers, a college with university status in New Brunswick (since 1945 New Jersey's State University), named in honour of a revolutionary war veteran, Colonel Henry Rutgers, who was an early benefactor. The scientist who initiated the search for antibiotics—and popularized the term in the modern sense of a substance elaborated by living organisms that can inhibit or kill other micro-organisms—was a Russian émigré whose reputation at the time lay in the less glamorous study of humus, peat bogs, compost heaps, and manure. His name was Selman Abraham Waksman.

It is difficult to construct a convincing pen portrait of Selman Waksman. Although he had an interesting and varied life, no scholarly biography has ever been written and most of the details about his life that are available come from his autobiography, *My Life with the Microbes*, first published in the United States in 1954 (14). The book cannot be described as a work of great literature, but it offers much background information about Waksman's early life and revealing insights into his personality. Waksman presents himself to the world as a dedicated searcher after truth, blessed by providence and much honest sweat to emerge as a major benefactor of humankind. The impression one gets, rightly or wrongly, is of a rather patriarchal figure who never escaped (nor probably wished to) from his Russian–Jewish roots; somewhat solitary and humourless, but driven to work hard to exploit above average, but not exceptional talents. The fame and adulation that discovery of streptomycin brought him was received, not with the bemused pleasure that seemed to typify Alexander Fleming's attitude in similar circumstances, but with a rather solemn pride in an achievement that also conferred a duty (not entirely unwelcome) to bask in unaccustomed limelight.

Whatever the truth of these speculations, the bare facts of Waksman's life are these: he was born in Priluka, a small town in the Ukrainian steppes 200 miles from the regional capital Kiev. Situated in an agricultural region it suffered badly during the early Soviet era and was finally destroyed by the German army in the Second World War. Finding little opportunity for advancement in the immediate area of his home town, the 20-year-old Waksman travelled in 1908 to the city of Odessa on the Black Sea, where he studied at one of the five gymnasiums and succeeded in obtaining his matriculation diploma. Soon afterwards his mother died and, at the urging of cousins in the United States, he decided, like many others, to seek his fortune by emigrating. He arrived in America in 1910 with $40 in his pocket and little knowledge of the language. His cousin, Molki had married a farmer, Mendel Kornblatt, who had left Priluka some 20 years earlier and they gave Waksman a home and work on the farm, which was only a few miles from Rutgers College. The head of the department of bacteriology at Rutgers at this time was Jacob

Lipman, another Russian immigrant with whom Waksman felt an immediate affinity. Spurning an opportunity to read medicine in New York (which would have meant a much larger financial burden), he applied for, and obtained, a scholarship to study at Rutgers. In his final year he specialized in soil bacteriology and graduated in 1915 with a thesis on bacteria and protozoa in the soil. A research assistantship in soil microbiology in Lipman's department allowed him to obtain a master's degree in the following year, but, feeling the need to expand his biochemical training, he then crossed to the west coast, spending 2 years as a research fellow at the University of California, Berkeley.

Waksman returned to Rutgers in 1918 at the invitation of Lipman, who offered him the dual post of lecturer in soil microbiology and microbiologist at the research station, but the need to earn more money (he was now married to his childhood sweetheart, Bobili Mitnik, who had joined him in America and their only son, Byron,* was on the way) meant that he had to find other work to supplement his income. He obtained a job in a chemical laboratory that had been established in Clifton, New Jersey, by a Japanese enzyme chemist, Jokichi Takamine. The work there provided Waksman with his first insight into a chemotherapeutic agent, for one of the firm's products was Salvarsan and one of his tasks was to investigate its toxicity. He was still able to spend 1 day a week at Rutgers and eventually, when the financial situation improved, he returned there full time.

At Rutgers Waksman dedicated himself single-mindedly to the study of microbes in the natural environment and particularly to a group of bacteria called actinomycetes, which are largely responsible for giving soil its characteristic earthy smell. Over the following years he established a formidable reputation in this field, publishing numerous papers and several books including the definitive *Principles of Soil Microbiology*, which appeared in 1927, with a revised edition in 1932 (15).

In 1924 Waksman sailed to Europe to attend the International Conference on Soil Science in Rome, taking the opportunity to visit England, France, and Switzerland on the way to Italy, and to include a nostalgic return to Priluka on the return leg. Among the people he visited in France was the famous Russian soil microbiologist, Sergei Winogradsky, who had settled in France after escaping from Russia during the revolution.

While at the Rome conference Waksman met René Dubos, a footloose young French microbiologist, who had also been influenced by Winogradsky's ideas. Dubos had decided to travel to the United States after the Rome meeting to further his career, and on boarding the ship, the *Rochambeau*, fortuitously found that Waksman was also on board. Discovering that the young man had no definite plans in America, and impressed with his microbiological ambitions, Waksman offered him the possibility of studying at Rutgers, where he was to spend the next 3 years, earning a PhD with a study of the decomposition of cellulose by soil bacteria.

In 1927, Dubos applied to the National Research Council for a fellowship, but was refused because he was not a United States citizen. Appended to the rejection letter was a

---

* Their son was not named after the famous poet, but after one of Waksman's teachers at Rutgers, Byron Halsted.

handwritten note advising him to consult fellow Frenchman, Alexis Carrel. Dubos wrote to Carrel and arranged to meet him at the Rockefeller Institute. Although Carrel was sympathetic he was unable to help,* but at lunch Dubos found himself sitting by chance next to the Canadian medical bacteriologist and pioneer molecular biologist, Oswald Avery,[†] in the Welch Hall dining room of the Institute (16). Avery, was interested to hear about the work Dubos had done for his PhD, since he had a related interest in finding a substance that would decompose the capsule of pneumococci and render the bacteria innocuous. With the brash confidence of Gallic youth, the 26-year-old Frenchman boldly asserted that the techniques he had developed at Rutgers could solve Avery's problem. To his astonishment, Avery wrote to Waksman asking if he could recommend the young man and, on being assured that he could, offered him a job studying the decomposition of the polysaccharide capsule of virulent pneumococci by soil microbes. Except for a brief sojourn at Harvard Medical School between 1942 and 1944 Dubos remained at the Rockefeller for the rest of his working life establishing a formidable reputation as researcher, prolific author, popularizer of science, and commentator on all things medical and environmental.

Within 3 years of arriving at the Rockefeller Dubos amply confirmed Avery's hunch in his ability by isolating an enzyme from a bacillus found in a New Jersey cranberry bog that dissolved the capsular polysaccharide of virulent pneumococci and cured mice infected with the organism. The discovery was greeted with great enthusiasm, but turning an enzyme into a useful therapeutic product was problematical. When, a few years later the unprecedented activity of Prontosil and the sulphonamides was announced work on the enzyme all but ceased.

Avery reacted to the success of the sulphonamides badly, thinking that most of his work had been in vain, but Dubos responded differently. The gradual realization that the sulpha drugs represented a major breakthrough served to reinforce his interest in the interactions between microbes in the soil and their ability to produce substances that helped to ensure their chance of survival in a highly competitive environment. In 1937 he started experiments in which he introduced suspensions of Gram-positive bacteria into samples of soil in order to investigate, by a laborious process of progressive enrichment, whether indigenous microbes present in the soil could competitively destroy the intruders, feed off them and hence flourish at the expense of others. The most important outcome of this research was the discovery in 1939 of a Gram-positive bacillus, *Bacillus brevis*, which was able to use the proteins of streptococci and staphylococci as a food source and produced a substance, alcohol-soluble extracts of which were strongly inhibitory. The substance, which

---

* When Carrel left the Rockefeller in 1939 at the outbreak of war in Europe (he returned to France in 1941), Dubos and his colleague Rollin Hotchkiss were given research space that he had abandoned.

[†] In 1944, Avery, together with Colin MacLeod and Maclyn McCarty, established that DNA is the genetic material by showing that DNA from inactivated pneumococci possessing a polysaccharide capsule could restore capsule production and virulence to avirulent, non-capsulate variants—a process they called 'transformation'.

unlike his previous discovery was clearly not an enzyme, was given the name tyrothricin, apparently because of a probable relationship to *Tyrothrix* (17) an obsolete name coined by Emile Duclaux (a colleague of Louis Pasteur) for filamentous spore-forming bacteria found in cheese (Greek: *turos* = cheese, *thrix* = thread).

Dubos lost no time in writing up the work on tyrothricin in a series of papers in 1939, but perhaps more importantly, he unveiled the compound with great panache at the Third International Congress of Microbiology at the Waldorf-Astoria Hotel in New York, which opened on 2 September 1939, the day before England and France declared war on Germany (18). Among the delegates at the Congress, were Howard Florey, Alexander Fleming, and Selman Waksman. Dubos showed the audience a bottle containing 500 g of tyrothricin, announcing that it was sufficient to protect 5 trillion mice against strepto-coccal blood poisoning. The presentation came on the last day of the 7-day meeting and Florey may have missed the dramatic display, as he hurried back to England when the news of war came through. Fleming appears to have been unmoved by Dubos's claims, but Waksman took quiet pride in the achievements of his former pupil and began to make plans of his own.

Dubos's colleague at the Rockefeller, the organic chemist Rollin Hotchkiss, working alone as he preferred to do, and without the sanction of the institute's authorities, soon discovered that crude extracts of *Bacillus brevis* could be fractionated into two separate antibacterial components, which he was able to crystallize. The two products were named tyrocidine (retaining the *Tyrothrix* connection) and gramicidin (not, as has sometimes been suggested, to honour the discovered of the eponymous Gram stain, but simply to reflect the activity against Gram-positive bacteria) (17). A cyclic peptide antibi-otic with properties similar to that of gramicidin (which is a linear peptide) and called gramicidin S (Soviet) was discovered in the former Soviet Union in 1944 by Georgii Frantsevich Gauze.

Tyrocidine and gramicidin were soon found to be too toxic for systemic use in man, although gramicidin, which turned out to be more active and somewhat less toxic than tyrocidine, was tentatively tried at the Mayo clinic in Rochester, Minnesota* by the infec-tious disease physician Wallace Herrell in collaboration with his bacteriologist colleague, Dorothy Heilman (19). Aware of the toxicity of the compound, the drug was cautiously used chiefly to treat skin conditions and superficial abscesses, but administration by instillation into nasal sinuses and the bladder was also tried. Results were mixed and gramicidin therapy never really caught on. It was successfully used for a time in bovine mastitis and is still found in some topical preparations for human use, such as eye drops and ointments. A more lasting legacy of Dubos's discovery is its likely influence on Howard Florey's decision to investigate the therapeutic potential of penicillin (see p. 97) and Selman Waksman's equally momentous decision to undertake a systematic study of antibiotic products of his beloved soil micro-organisms.

---

* The Mayo Clinic developed from the pioneering group medical practice in Rochester, Minnesota founded by and English-born physician, William Worrall Mayo and his two sons, William James Mayo and Charles Horace Mayo.

Dubos himself became disillusioned with antibiotic research and did no more work in the field after 1942, when he sought new challenges by accepting the George Fabyan Chair of Comparative Pathology and Tropical Medicine at Harvard—a post that was offered to him unconditionally notwithstanding the fact that he had neither a medical degree nor tropical experience! The decision to renounce antibiotic research was strange for one who had been so enthusiastic only a few years earlier. A clue may lie in a personal tragedy that enveloped him in the early 1940s. His wife, Marie-Louise suffered a recrudescence of childhood tuberculosis, perhaps exacerbated by the stressful news of the German invasion of France and fears about the fate of friends and relations. Her illness ran a stormy course and she died 9 days after her husband accepted the Harvard post. A book on tuberculosis, *The White Plague* (20), which Dubos wrote in 1952 in collaboration with his second wife, Jean, reflects his disenchantment with the new wonder drugs. The short account of antituberculosis chemotherapy is curiously muted and unenthusiastic, despite the fact that evidence of its effectiveness was accumulating daily; most remarkably, the book contains no mention whatsoever of the contribution of Waksman, though the two men appeared to have remained on good terms.

The road to streptomycin

Waksman's search for antibiotics did not require a radical realignment of his research interests. He had long been interested in the ways in which bacteria interact with one another in the competitive environment of the soil, and he was familiar, through his knowledge of the language, with Russian literature describing the antibacterial activity of soil micro-organisms. Since November 1938 he had been a consultant on bacterial chemotherapeutic agents to Merck, the local pharmaceutical firm situated at Rahway less than 20 miles to the north-east of New Brunswick and one of the firms that was already showing an interest in Fleming's penicillin (see p. 104). But it was Dubos's discovery of tyrothricin that seems to have finally convinced him that the microbes to which he had devoted his professional life might be the source of products useful in human therapy. Like Florey with penicillin, his decision to embark on a systematic hunt for microbial products with antibiotic activity occurred in autumn 1939, coincidental with Dubos's enthusiastic account of tyrothricin at the New York Congress. During 1940 Waksman assembled his thoughts on the matter, encapsulating them in a comprehensive review of antagonistic relationships among micro-organisms, which appeared early the following year (21). The review incorporated a section devoted to what was known about products that might be useful in disease control, with discussion of Fleming's penicillin, the newly described work of Florey's team, and Dubos's gramicidin.

Waksman's approach differed from that of Dubos. He rejected his former pupil's enrichment techniques, which could take months, and developed simple plate cultivation methods that enabled the numerous soil micro-organisms to be randomly screened for antibiotic activity. Bernard Davis, a colleague of Dubos's who developed tuberculosis while working in his laboratory and who himself became eminent, not least for extensive studies of the definitive mode of action of streptomycin (which has proved elusive) contrasted Dubos's restless energy with Waksman's dogged persistence:

[Waksman's] really important discovery was not streptomycin: it was the principle that a patient, systematic search for useful antibiotics will eventually pay off (22).

Not surprisingly, Waksman concentrated his efforts on the actinomycetes that had occupied so much of his professional attention. Success was not long in coming. In 1940, in collaboration with his graduate student Boyd Woodruff, he was able to describe several antibiotic substances, including one, actinomycin (23), which was sufficiently interesting to convince scientists at Merck to take out a patent on the substance and follow-up the work. Woodruff later joined the staff of Merck and was closely involved in a number of other important antibiotic discoveries during 40 years spent with the company.

Actinomycin was to prove a great disappointment. Like tyrothricin it was found to have serious side effects, though it was later shown to belong to a family of related antibiotics, one of which, actinomycin D (dactinomycin) is used in cancer chemotherapy, where the severity of the disease and lack of safe alternatives often override limitations of toxicity. Undeterred, the screening project continued, and in 1942 several antibiotics that were less toxic than actinomycin—including fumigacin and clavicin—created transient interest. Most exciting was streptothricin, a product of *Streptomyces lavendulae* that seemed to be non-toxic in preliminary animal tests. Merck, who by this time were already engaged in producing penicillin for the first American trials,* once more took up the challenge of taking the antibiotic forward. To Waksman's dismay, further tests revealed delayed renal toxicity and planned human trials of streptothricin had to be abandoned.

One of the graduate students who briefly played a part in the investigations in 1942 was a young man from Norwich, Connecticut, Albert Schatz, who, like Waksman, was of Russian–Jewish parentage. Following his graduation from Rutgers in 1942, Schatz had been recruited to Waksman's team on the antibiotic project, but his work was interrupted when he joined the US Air Force. Discharged with a back problem in June 1943, he returned to Waksman's laboratory and resumed research towards his PhD. By October that year he had discovered the antibiotic that was to transform his life.

According to Schatz, streptomycin was discovered at around 2 p.m. on Tuesday 19 October 1943, though what precise event this records is unclear.† The discovery was described in a paper authored by Schatz with another graduate student, Elizabeth Bugie, and Waksman (24). The organism that produced the new antibiotic was *Streptomyces* (formerly *Actinomyces*) *griseus*, which had only recently been reclassified by Waksman; it was, ironically, a species that he had worked on as early as 1915. Although this original isolate was still maintained in the laboratory culture collection it was not the source of streptomycin. In fact it was later shown not to produce streptomycin, perhaps having lost the ability, as often occurs, through numerous subcultures. Schatz had found the antibiotic in two different strains of *Streptomyces griseus*: one isolated from heavily manured soil; the

---

* Norman Heatley was at Merck helping on the penicillin project from 16 December 1941 until 25 June 1942 and probably met Woodruff, who had been seconded there to complete his PhD studies.

† In *My life with the microbes* Waksman gives the date of discovery as 23 August 1943.

other (a less active producer of the antibiotic) grown from the throat of a chicken by a fellow graduate student, Doris Jones (later Ralston), who was working on potential antiviral antibiotics in the adjacent laboratory with the poultry pathologist Fred Robert Beaudette.

Streptomycin led to a classic dispute, which was to end up in the courts, as to who deserves the true credit for the discovery: the bench worker in the laboratory, or his chief, who initiated the project, employed the worker, and provided the research facilities. Of course, at the time of the discovery of streptomycin none of those involved could have had much inkling of the vast importance of the finding; it was simply another antibiotic with interesting properties that may or may not have been worth progressing further. Previous experience with actinomycin, streptothricin, and other antibiotics had not been encouraging. Moreover, though it was the revolutionary activity of streptomycin in tuberculosis that was to ensure its fame, the importance of this property does not appear to have been appreciated at first. The first published description of streptomycin presents the chief property of the antibiotic—distinguishing it from penicillin—as activity against Gram-negative bacilli; *Mycobacterium tuberculosis* is not mentioned in the main text of the original paper, appearing only in a table listing the activity of the antibiotic against various Gram-positive and Gram-negative bacteria (25).

Albert Schatz always strenuously maintained (26) that it was his drive and energy that led to the discovery of streptomycin and that Waksman cynically underplayed his role when it became clear that the antibiotic was going to represent an important breakthrough in the treatment of tuberculosis. Schatz contended that he alone was responsible for the work with *Mycobacterium tuberculosis*, claiming that Waksman was (with justification) fearful of having such a dangerous organism in the laboratory.

While this may be true, Waksman was certainly not unaware of the potential for soil organisms to inhibit tubercle bacilli. In 1932 he had received a grant from the National Tuberculosis Association to study the fate of tubercle bacilli in natural environments. In the course of these studies, one of his students, Chester E. Rhines, working with avian strains of *Mycobacteria*, showed that certain fungi could suppress the growth of the bacilli, especially in manured soil (27), but the time was not ripe for the connection to be made with therapy in a laboratory dedicated to the fundamentals of soil research and the observation was not followed up. On 2 April 1940, after Dubos's discovery of tyrothricin had been published, the Committee on Medical Research of the National Tuberculosis Association convened a special meeting on micro-organisms in soil at the request of Merck and the firm of Sharp and Dohme,* a company that, together with Parke, Davis, had a longstanding interest in tuberculosis, particularly in the development of tuberculin testing. The meeting was attended by a small group of delegates, including Selman Waksman and representatives of the two pharmaceutical companies. The first item on the agenda was 'The possibility of there being micro-organisms in the soil that are antagonistic to the tubercle bacillus or give rise to antigenic substances in the animal body of

---

* Sharp and Dohme merged with Merck & Co. in 1953. Outside the United States they trade as Merck, Sharp, and Dohme to prevent confusion with the German firm of Merck (see footnote p. 131).

value in changing the disease process.' Comments, recorded in the minutes, of the Chairman of the group, William Charles White, medical director of the Tuberculosis League of Pittsburgh, Pennsylvania, are revealing. Noting that Dubos's tyrothricin was active against Gram-positive bacteria, White stated:

> Since the tubercle bacillus is also Gram-positive there is a faint possibility that a similar effect might be exerted on the acid-fast* bacilli . . .If the Dubos substance has no effect on the acid-fact group, there is a possibility that other soil micro-organisms, fungi, coccidia, et cetera, might exercise such an antagonistic function on the acid-fast group (27).

Three years later, an additional incentive to looking more closely at the effect of antibiotics on tubercle bacilli was provided by a timely visit to Waksman on 16 November 1943—after the discovery of streptomycin, but before publication of the finding—by a researcher from the Graduate School of the Mayo Clinic, William Feldman.

William Feldman was born William Gunn in Glasgow, but after his father died he was taken to America by his mother at the age of two. He took the name of his stepfather when his mother remarried. Feldman was not a medical doctor, but a veterinarian. He had studied veterinary science at Colorado State College (later Colorado State University). After graduation in 1917 he joined the college teaching staff, supplementing his income by playing trumpet in a local dance band. Like many of his college contemporaries, he tried to enlist in the army Veterinary Corps, but was rejected on the grounds that he was not a United States citizen—an oversight that was remedied in 1922. In November 1918 he became a victim of the pandemic of 'Spanish' influenza, but survived. Feldman joined the Institute of Experimental Medicine at the Mayo Clinic in 1927, rising to become probably the top veterinary pathologist in the country, notably in the fields of bovine and avian tuberculosis (28).

After a chance meeting on the return journey from a tuberculosis conference in St Paul, Minnesota, Feldman formed a close collaboration with a chest physician from the Mayo Clinic, Corwin Hinshaw. Hinshaw was born to a Quaker family in Iowa Falls, Iowa and had studied zoology and bacteriology to doctoral level before accepting a position teaching parasitology and bacteriology at the American University in Beirut. Returning to the United States in 1931, he was awarded a medical degree at the University of Pennsylvania in 1933 and joined the Mayo Clinic, where he developed a special interest in lung diseases (29).

Feldman and Hinshaw's first foray into chemotherapy was in tests of the effect of sulfapyridine on experimental tuberculosis in guinea pigs. Later they tested Parke, Davis's Promin, which produced some encouraging results in guinea pigs and was briefly tried in human patients (30). The trial met with only moderate success and revealed serious side effects. Nevertheless, Promin gave the first glimmer of hope that drug treatment of tuberculosis might eventually be possible and encouraged Feldman and Hinshaw to continue to explore the chemotherapeutic approach. Another sulphone from Parke, Davis,

---

* The term 'acid-fast' refers to the fact that tubercle bacilli, once stained, are subsequently resistant to decolorization by mineral acids (see p. 6).

Promizole, which was thought to be safer than Promin, was still in trial when their attention turned to the results emanating from Waksman's laboratory.

Feldman had followed with interest Waksman's publications on actinomycin and streptothricin. The purpose of his visit in November 1943 was to pick Waksman's brains about antibiotics that might be useful in tuberculosis; to encourage him to include *Mycobacterium tuberculosis* in the screening tests; and to let him (Feldman) know if anything promising turned up. Whether streptomycin was discussed during the meeting is unclear, but on 1 March 1944, soon after the streptomycin paper was safely in print, Waksman wrote to Feldman asking whether he would test the drug for antituberculosis activity in his guinea pig model. A 10 g quantity, sufficient to treat four animals, was laboriously accumulated by Schatz, and sent to the Mayo workers. The experiment was as rudimentary as the one Florey had used to investigate the curative effect of penicillin in mice (see p. 99), but the results were sufficiently encouraging for Waksman and Feldman to approach Merck, who agreed to scale up production of streptomycin. Under the leadership of their inspirational chemist Max Tishler the promise was quickly fulfilled. With the greater resources available to them in July 1944, Feldman and Hinshaw set-up a more ambitious experiment using guinea pigs that they had optimistically infected for the purpose even before they knew that an additional supply of drug would be forthcoming. The two researchers personally injected, every 6 h round the clock for up to 61 days, 25 guinea pigs with established tuberculosis, comparing the results with those of 24 control animals (31). The results (Fig. 5.2) exceeded their wildest expectations, indicating unequivocally the beneficial effect and apparent safety of the new compound.

The work of Feldman and Hinshaw convinced everyone that streptomycin had real potential. Merck held the patent rights on the antibiotic—eventually signed on 31 January 1945—according to the longstanding contract with Rutgers that gave the college 2.5 per cent of revenue on any sales (32). Schatz and Waksman were named as co-inventors as American patent law required; Elizabeth Bugie agreed not to be named, partly because her contribution was a minor one, but also because at that time, as a woman destined to become a wife and mother, it was accepted that she did not need such recognition to further her career prospects (33).

Waksman was dissatisfied with the arrangement that gave Merck exclusive rights to develop and market streptomycin. He successfully argued that the drug was too important to be bound by patent restrictions and should be made available to other manufacturers in order to allow free competition and maximize humanitarian benefit. In an altruistic gesture that can have had few commercial precedents, George Merck himself agreed to forego the exclusive marketing rights and relinquished the patent to the Rutgers Research and Endowment Foundation in 1948. This was not the first time that George Merck had put public spirit before profit. In a telegram to Alfred Newton Richards, Chairman of the Committee on Medical Research of the National Defense Research Committee (see p. 105) dated 26 July 1941, when Richards was seeking help in the wartime production of penicillin, he had stated 'Command me and my associates . . . if you think we can help you' (34).

At first no one questioned the arrangements between Waksman and Merck, but by 1950 it had become clear that big money was involved. Schatz, who had left Rutgers in

CONTROLS

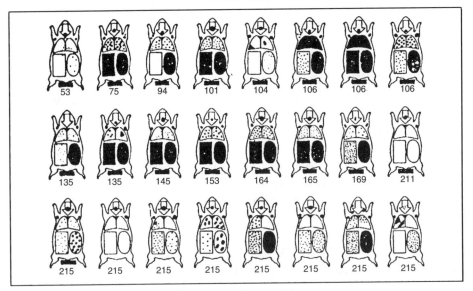

STREPTOMYCIN SERIES

TREATED AFTER 49 DAYS

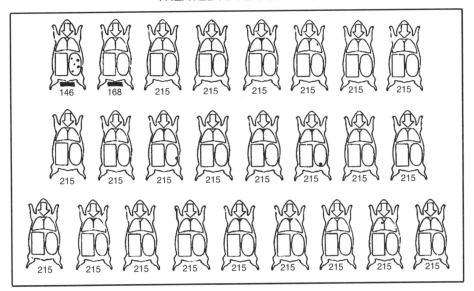

Figure 5.2 Feldman and Hinshaw's representation of the results of their initial experiments with streptomycin in guinea pigs. The various boxes and symbols represent the progress of disease in different organs. The numbers below each animal indicate the days for which each animal survived, a black bar signifying that the animal died. From Feldman W. H., Hinshaw H. C., Mann F. C. Streptomycin in experimental tuberculosis. *American Review of Tuberculosis* 1945; 52: 269–298.

1946 to work in New York (where he was involved with another antibiotic, the antifungal agent, nystatin; see p. 350) before moving on to California, believed that Waksman was benefiting personally and that suspicions that his part in the discovery had been systematically misrepresented, had been vindicated. Without more ado, Schatz sued his former chief.

Waksman felt betrayed and was thunderstruck. In his benign paternalistic way he regarded his researchers as his apprentices; scientific wards with himself as guardian and protector. He had even advanced Schatz money from the streptomycin royalties to help him move to California. Moreover, although the foundation had awarded Waksman 20 per cent of the streptomycin royalties, he always maintained that this was mainly used to further the cause of microbiology in various ways. In fact, half of it was dedicated to setting up the Institute of Microbiology at Rutgers (renamed the Waksman Institute after his death in 1973); in 1951, a further tranche was used to establish a Foundation for Microbiology (known since 2001 as the Waksman Foundation).

At first, supported by Rutgers, Waksman contested the lawsuit, but when the action became drawn out and attracted wide publicity, he caved in and agreed to an out of court settlement that granted Schatz 3 per cent of the royalties paid to the Rutgers Foundation. Waksman was awarded 17 per cent, of which 7 per cent was shared among all members of his laboratory staff, including Elizabeth Bugie.

Many young researchers would have been satisfied with this outcome, but Albert Schatz could not rid himself of a festering resentment. No doubt he was justified in seeking to defend his role in the discovery of streptomycin and as a struggling young scientist he can scarcely be blamed for attempting to get his hands on a share of the financial rewards. However, he carried the matter much further. He had now moved on to the National Agricultural College in Pennsylvania and in 1952, when the Nobel Prize was awarded to Waksman, Schatz, with the support of his new employers, formally protested to the Nobel Committee. He even sent a personal letter of complaint to King Gustav VI of Sweden—an astonishingly audacious attempt to influence an independent organization. Schatz publicly challenged Waksman's integrity and attempted to enlist the support of eminent scientists around the world in his campaign for recognition. Not surprisingly, he found himself shunned by the scientific establishment in the United States. In 1962 he left the country for a post in the University of Chile, before returning in 1965 to become Professor of Education at the Washington University Graduate Institute in St Louis. Throughout a long and peripatetic life as scientist, educationalist, and guru of 'alternative' therapies, he received many awards, including, in 1994, the Rutgers University Medal, a recognition that must have afforded him a great personal satisfaction and a feeling of vindication. None of this seems to have lessened his sense of grievance; he continued to protest the legitimacy of his claim and to question Waksman's behaviour long after his former chief was around to defend himself.

The proving of streptomycin

Once their guinea pig experiments had unequivocally demonstrated streptomycin's potential, William Feldman and Corwin Hinshaw lost no time in seeking to confirm the results in human beings. They enlisted the support of Dr Karl H. Pfuetze, Medical Director of the

Mineral Springs Sanatorium at Cannon Falls, Minnesota about 70 miles North of Rochester, close to St Paul. The first patient to be successfully treated,* a 21-year-old woman—named simply as 'Patricia' in most accounts, but called Patty Thomas in an article in the Rochester Post-Bulletin in 1994 (35)—was in the late stages of pulmonary tuberculosis. She had been given surgical treatment at the Mayo Clinic, but the infection was spreading and her condition was deteriorating. Therapy with streptomycin was commenced on 20 November 1944. After five 10–18 day courses of the drug over a 6-month period, she was sufficiently improved to be fit for further surgical treatment. In 1946 she was discharged from the sanatorium, married, and became a mother of three children. Another very early recipient of the drug was Pfuetze's assistant at Mineral Springs Sanatorium, Marjorie Pyle who had developed tuberculosis as a young physician. She was successfully treated with the new drug in 1944 and stayed on at Mineral Springs to complete a postdoctoral study analysing the results of treatment (36), before moving on to become director of the State of Illinois Tuberculosis Sanatorium. She later wrote a book for lay people, *Help Yourself Get Well; a Guide for TB Patients and their Families*, published in 1951.

By 1946, case reports of 100 treated patients had been accumulated and described in cautious terms (37). The results showed unequivocal benefit from streptomycin in checking the inexorable course of the disease, but not always in effecting a cure. Aware of the public reaction that premature and over-optimistic reporting of the findings might engender, Hinshaw and Feldman placed an embargo on giving personal interviews to the press. Despite these precautions, accounts of the unexpected breakthrough in the treatment of tuberculosis inevitably found their way into newspapers, magazines, and radio stations. News of 'miracle cures' spread like wildfire and anyone thought able to provide a supply of the precious drug was soon fending off desperate demands from around the world that were impossible to fulfil.

Caution was well founded. Tuberculosis was a disease with a notoriously unpredictable course. Moreover, although pharmacokinetic information assembled at the Mayo Clinic by Hinshaw's colleagues, the bacteriological husband and wife team of Dorothy and Fordyce Heilman (38) allowed better control of dosage regimens, it rapidly became clear that two problems faced use of the drug: frequent relapse caused by the emergence of streptomycin-resistant bacilli; and toxicity, mainly to the ear, causing dizziness, vertigo, and in extreme cases deafness.

Waksman's foresight in arguing the case for allowing abrogation of Merck's exclusive patent rights was now vindicated as additional supplies came on stream; at least six companies—Abbott Research Laboratories,[†] Lilly, Merck, Pfizer, Squibb, and The Upjohn Company[‡]—were manufacturing streptomycin by 1946 and Merck had built

----

* There were at least two earlier patients, virtually hopeless cases that were given short courses of streptomycin and showed some improvement, but did not survive.

† Founded in Chicago in 1892 by Dr Wallace Calvin Abbott.

‡ Founded in 1886 by Dr William E Upjohn and his three brothers in Kalamazoo, Michigan. It merged with the Swedish firm, Pharmacia AB in 1995 and eventually became part of Pfizer after their acquisition of Pharmacia in 2003.

a new factory for production of the drug at Elkton, in the Shenandoah Valley, Virginia. Control of the manufacture of streptomycin and allocation of supplies was in the hands of the Civilian Production Administration, a federal body charged with regulating the production and distribution of essential goods that had taken over from the War Production Board in 1945. Such was the global clamour for streptomycin that demand remained far in excess of supply and the drug was one of the few products that remained restricted in 1947 when most emergency controls were lifted. Despite the restrictions, limited quantities became available outside the United States, some for compassionate use, some in the form of small export quotas; as usual, some found its way on to the black market.

The first co-operative trial of the value of streptomycin in tuberculosis was conducted in the United States under the auspices of the American Trudeau Society, named to commemorate Dr Edward Livingston Trudeau a sanatorium pioneer who had attributed his own survival from tuberculosis to diet and exercise in the healthy air of the Adirondacks in Northern New York State. After his unexpected recovery—though he was never completely cured—he founded a sanatorium at Saranac Lake, starting with a small building known as the 'little red cottage' in 1884. The community into which this developed became the model for similar institutions throughout the United States. The Scottish author and indefatigable traveller, Robert Louis Stevenson was briefly under Trudeau's care during a visit to Saranac Lake in the winter of 1887–88. The writer had gone there to recuperate from an attack of tuberculosis, a disease he had probably suffered from since childhood. The Trudeau Society evolved in 1938 from the American Sanatorium Association, originally founded in 1905 as an offshoot of the National Association for the Study and Prevention of Tuberculosis, which Trudeau had helped to form in the previous year; it further metamorphosed into the American Thoracic Society in 1960.

In the autumn of 1946 the American Trudeau Society was approached by a consortium of manufacturers of streptomycin, who offered, with the approval of the Civilian Production Administration, to provide more than a million dollars worth of the drug to carry out definitive clinical studies. The Society agreed with alacrity and eight clinical researchers—J. Burns Amberson, Emil Bogen, Corwin Hinshaw, Kirby Smith Howlett, Walsh McDermott, Edward Newman Packard, H. McLeod Riggins, and Henry Stuart Willis—leaders of their profession at the time, but mostly now long forgotten, were invited to participate in and coordinate the trial (39).

Meanwhile, a similar co-operative trial was being planned by the Veterans' Administration and the medical services of the United States army and navy to investigate the role of streptomycin in the treatment of tuberculosis in troops returning from the war. The study was initially meant to involve seven hospitals, but was soon expanded so that eventually 46 Veterans' Administration hospitals, an army hospital, and a navy hospital participated. It seemed sensible to harmonize this trial with that of the American Trudeau Association, if only to share information and coordinate the findings. In 1947 a Tuberculosis Study Section, representing the various bodies involved, was set-up by

Thomas Parran, Surgeon General of the United States Public Health Service. A mutually acceptable arrangement was agreed, with the National Institutes of Health providing some financial assistance to both trials.

The Trudeau study got underway in November 1946, but was soon criticized for its lack of a control group. The Veterans' Administration study was larger and better planned. Patients with pulmonary tuberculosis were admitted to the trial only if they conformed to standard case definitions; a common treatment regimen—decided by guesswork since there was little hard evidence of the best dose and duration of therapy—was administered according to agreed protocols. Radiological assessment of progress was made 'blind' without knowledge of the treatment given. It was originally planned that there should be an untreated control group, but because of the difficulty of finding sufficient cases that fitted the exacting entry criteria for the trial it was decided to treat all eligible patients. In the absence of untreated controls, patients were observed for 2 months without treatment and then for a further 4 months on streptomycin therapy—each patient effectively acting as his own control (40). By 1947, barely 3 years after the publication of the first paper on streptomycin from Waksman's laboratory, the two trials and other smaller investigations—notably one conducted by Walsh McDermott and his colleagues at the New York Hospital–Cornell Medical Center on tuberculous meningitis and disseminated tuberculosis—had firmly established the benefits of streptomycin treatment; alas, they also amply confirmed the twin problems of treatment failure or relapse caused by drug resistance, and toxicity, mainly, but not exclusively to the functions of the ear (41).

Concurrently with the trials in tuberculosis, studies of the efficacy of streptomycin in other infections were proceeding under the supervision of Chester Keefer in his role as Chairman of the Committee on Medical Research of the Office of Scientific Research and Development. These studies confirmed the complementary spectrum of activity of streptomycin *vis-à-vis* penicillin: good activity against most Gram-negative bacilli, but feeble potency against streptococci and anaerobes.*

William Feldman and Corwin Hinshaw were nominated for the 1952 Nobel Prize alongside Selman Waksman, but in the end it went to Waksman alone. The justice of this decision has often been debated—Hinshaw himself was of the opinion that he and Feldman had been ruled out because of failure of their superiors to support their nomination (42)—but the prize committees' verdicts have regularly been criticized. All awards, from knighthoods to Oscars, are made by fallible groups charged with difficult decisions; the lucky recipients should enjoy their rewards, and those who are overlooked do well to keep their disappointment under wraps. The magnanimity of Peter Medawar, who in 1960 shared his prize money with his former student and colleague, Rupert Billingham, was a truly noble gesture, but not one that is likely to be often repeated.

....

* The poor activity against streptococci and anaerobes was later shown to be due to the fact that streptomycin is actively transported into bacterial cells by an aerobic mechanism that streptococci and anaerobes lack.

The first British trial

The ethical considerations that ruled out a placebo-controlled study of the efficacy of streptomycin in the United States were not a barrier in Britain, since supply of the drug was strictly limited. Pilot plants for the production of streptomycin were already being set-up by 1946, notably by The Boots Company in Nottingham,* Glaxo Laboratories in Greenford, and Distillers (Biochemicals) Ltd. at Speke on Merseyside (see, p. 109), but none was yet available for domestic use. In November 1946 the British government bought 50 kg of the drug on behalf of the Medical Research Council at a cost of $320,000 (about £70,000 at the prevailing exchange rate) (43). Some of the streptomycin was set aside for the treatment of miliary tuberculosis and tuberculous meningitis, conditions with a uniformly grave prognosis, but most of the purchase was used by the Council to set-up a streptomycin trial that was to become a benchmark for the conduct of randomized clinical trials.

There were 15 members on the committee that oversaw the trial, but the mastermind behind the randomization method that was adopted was the statistician Austin Bradford Hill. Bradford Hill had planned to study medicine, but was frustrated in his ambition by contracting tuberculosis during the First World War, when he served as a pilot in the fledgling Royal Navy Air Service. Discharged from active service and not expected to survive, he took up the study of statistics under the wing of Major Greenwood, the foremost medical statistician of his day. Bradford Hill took to statistics like a fish to water. During a long career at the Medical Research Council and later as an inspirational lecturer at the London School of Hygiene and Tropical Medicine (where Major Greenwood had also worked), he made many important contributions to the application of statistics to medical epidemiology, most famously collaborating with Richard Doll in the pioneering studies that established the link between smoking and lung cancer (44).

Aware of the numerous pitfalls that awaited any therapeutic trial in a disease as capricious in its progress as tuberculosis, and acutely conscious of the exaggerated claims that had been made for Sanocrysin before the war, the Streptomycin Clinical Trials Committee was determined to design a trial that would provide convincing evidence with the limited resources that were available. The committee took great pains in the selection of patients with a similar type of disease, which should conform to an agreed definition: 'acute progressive bilateral pulmonary tuberculosis of presumably recent origin, bacteriologically proved, unsuitable for collapse therapy, age group 15 to 25 (later extended to 30)' (45). Patients were recruited into three hospitals in the Metropolitan area: The Brompton Hospital, Colindale Hospital, and Harefield Hospital. However, it was soon realized that in order to find enough patients who met the inclusion criteria it would be necessary to

* The Company formed in 1883 by Jesse Boot from the herbalist shop in Goose Gate, Nottingham founded in 1849 by his parents. By the turn of the century, Jesse Boot was selling his products in over 250 'Boots Cash Chemists' shops throughout Britain. The company was one of those funded by the Ministry of Supply during the Second World War to produce penicillin.

extend the trial and four other centres were invited to participate: The Northern Hospital (London); Sully Hospital, a sanatorium in the Vale of Glamorgan; Bangour Hospital in West Lothian (where patients from a sanatorium situated in a disused aerodrome at East Fortune, 22 miles East of Edinburgh, had been transferred when the site was requisitioned by the Royal Air Force in 1941); and Killingbeck sanatorium, a former smallpox hospital in Leeds. Recruitment was started in January 1947 and ended in September 1947. By then 109 patients had been accepted, but two died before entering the trial, leaving 107 patients that could be evaluated.

Patients entering the trial were chosen by a selection panel, which ensured that they conformed to the agreed entry criteria. The scheme adopted for randomization was carefully designed to eliminate any possible bias in the allocation of treatment:

> Determination of whether a patient would be treated by streptomycin and bed-rest (S case) or by bed-rest alone (C case) was made by reference to a statistical series based on random sampling numbers drawn up for each sex at each centre by Professor Bradford Hill; the details of the series were unknown to any of the investigators or to the co-ordinator and were contained in a set of sealed envelopes, each bearing on the outside only the name of the hospital and a number. After acceptance of a patient by the panel, and before admission to the streptomycin centre, the appropriate numbered envelope was opened at the central office; the card inside told if the patient was to be an S or a C case, and this information was then given to the medical officer of the centre. Patients were not told before admission that they were to get special treatment. C patients did not know throughout their stay in hospital that they were control patients in a special study; they were in fact treated as they would have been in the past, the sole difference being that they had been admitted to the centre more rapidly than was normal. Usually they were not in the same wards as S patients, but the same regime was maintained (45).

Randomization in clinical trials had, of course, often been used before the streptomycin trial, usually by strict alternation of treatments (as in the patulin trial of 1943–44; see p. 113) or by the toss of a coin as in the trial of Sanocrysin (p. 147). Randomization itself was not the issue. As Guy Scadding, a member of the original streptomycin committee, recalled many years later (46), a system of strict alternation would have been statistically acceptable. The difficulty was that, because of the nature of the trial, treatment could not be allocated blind as it had been in the earlier patulin trial. There was no true placebo in the sense of a dummy injection of an indistinguishable substance in those not receiving streptomycin—which would have made the trial 'double blind': treatment unknown to both doctor and patient—since this would have been impracticable. The control group received the normal care that any patient with tuberculosis could expect. Bradford Hill's sealed envelope method, supervised centrally, excluded the possibility of local selection bias such as may have occurred if the attending physicians had allocated the treatment categories themselves. The method additionally guaranteed that the trial remained focussed on answering the primary question—was streptomycin truly effective in a disease of unpredictable course?—by ensuring strict comparability between groups within the trial, for example those with disease of differing severity.

Patients' progress was assessed monthly by X-ray, by standard laboratory tests, and by various criteria of well-being, such as weight gain or loss. Radiological assessment was carried out blindly by a local radiologist and centrally by a radiologist and a clinician who had no knowledge of the cases. The results, published in October 1948 amidst the tensions of the nascent National Health Service, demonstrated the ability of streptomycin to influence the course of tuberculosis as convincingly as the studies carried out in America. They were also equally disturbing in revealing that early improvement in the patient's condition was often followed by relapse of infection that no longer responded to treatment. It soon became clear that within the large masses of tubercle bacilli harboured by infected patients, a few resistant variants—less than one in a million of the bacterial population—survived and re-established the infection.*

The committee that oversaw the American trials and the Streptomycin Committee in Britain both realized that what was needed was a second drug that could deal with the relatively small number of bacteria that were unresponsive to streptomycin. Indeed, Promin or Promizole were sometimes used with this in mind, at least in the United States. However, unknown practically to everyone, a much better drug had been in the process of development in Sweden since 1943.

Para-aminosalicylic acid (PAS)

There was something in the air that was changing attitudes to antimicrobial chemotherapy as war approached in the late 1930s. The work of Dubos at the Rockefeller, of Florey's team in Oxford and of Waksman's group in New Jersey all had their roots in this remarkably productive period. Of course, Dubos's work almost certainly influenced the other two to some extent, but there was also something else going on: a sea change in the way in which antibacterial agents were viewed. Perhaps it was the success of sulphonamides; perhaps it was the impending war itself that was concentrating minds. Most likely, it was a combination of the two: sulphonamides had changed the sceptical intellectual climate that had prevailed only a few years before to the extent that it was now conceivable that something could be done about the ghastly effects of bacterial contamination of wounds that had caused such suffering and death in the 1914–18 conflict.

Certainly thoughts of war were very much to the forefront of minds, as several of the protagonists have affirmed in recalling events of the time. Few believed, however, that tuberculosis, which always increased in times of war, would become easily treatable, if only because of the impermeable waxy coat that surrounds mycobacteria (see p. 6) and the nature of the thick cheesy lesions formed by the organisms in the body. Two investigators were not deterred by these considerations—perhaps because neither were bacteriologists or pathologists—Frederick Bernheim in the United States and Jörgen Lehmann in Sweden.

Frederick Bernheim, like his wife Mary (Molly), an Englishwoman whom he had met while they were each pursuing doctoral studies at Cambridge in 1926, was a biochemist. In 1930, after a stint at the Johns Hopkins University School of Medicine in Baltimore,

---

* In tuberculous meningitis the bacterial burden is smaller and many seemingly miraculous cures of this condition were achieved in the early days of streptomycin therapy.

they were offered positions at the newly founded Duke University School of Medicine in North Carolina, where they both had long and distinguished careers in teaching and research (47). Frederick Bernheim's appointment at Duke was to head the pharmacology programme and, not surprisingly, he concentrated his efforts on biochemical aspects of the subject.

In 1939, motivated, according to an account he gave to the pharmacologist and physiologist Julius Comroe, by the desire to find something that would mitigate the problem of infection that war would inevitably bring (31), he turned his attention to tuberculosis. Bernheim had no experience of bacteriology and, although he used a bovine strain of tubercle bacilli for his experiments, his readiness to have such a difficult-to-handle and virulent organism in his laboratory suggests a certain naïvety. Certainly, his description of how the organism was handled without the benefit of modern safety cabinets (48), though not uncommon at the time, would terrify most present day microbiologists. But what Bernheim lacked in bacteriological expertise, he more than made up for in biochemical know-how. Frustrated by finding that the organisms were biochemically inert when fed conventional substrates, he searched round for a substance that would encourage them into showing signs of metabolic life. To his surprise he found that salicylic acid (Fig. 5.3), the substance from which aspirin had been derived (see p. 48), strongly stimulated uptake of oxygen by the organisms, indicating that they were probably using it for metabolic purposes. Bernheim promptly wrote up the findings in a short paper in the journal *Science* (48).

The prevailing (and correct) view of the action of sulphonamides at this time was that they inhibited bacterial growth by blocking an essential metabolic function, tentatively identified by Paul Fildes and Donald woods at the Medical Research Council's Department of Bacterial Chemistry at the Middlesex Hospital, London, as resulting from competitive inhibition of *para*-aminobenzoic acid (49). Paul Fildes, director of the department had championed the view that research in chemotherapy should be aimed at finding similar compounds that competed for 'growth factors': essential metabolites that the organism could not manufacture for itself (50).

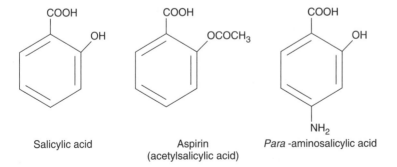

| Salicylic acid | Aspirin (acetylsalicylic acid) | *Para*-aminosalicylic acid |

Figure 5.3 Molecular structures of: salicylic acid (2-hydroxybenzoic acid); aspirin (2-acetyloxybenzoic acid); and para-aminosalicylic acid (4-amino-2-hydroxybenzoic acid).

As a biochemist, Bernheim heartily endorsed this view. He set about trying to find analogues of salicylic acid that would block the uptake of oxygen by tubercle bacilli by competitive inhibition. Dozens of analogues were tried and several found to fit the bill, but all proved disappointingly toxic and his efforts were ultimately fruitless. Significantly, PAS (Fig. 5.3) did not feature among the compounds that he tested. However, Bernheim had the foresight in 1940 to send a copy of his paper on salicylic acid to Jörgen Lehmann in Sweden. The two had become friends in 1935 when Lehmann was a visiting worker at the Rockefeller Institute in New York, where he had fortuitously met Dr Alice Bernheim and discovered that she was the mother of a biochemist with whom he had previously corresponded.

Outside Scandinavia, Jörgen Lehmann is one of the forgotten men of antimicrobial chemotherapy. He is widely acknowledged as the discoverer of the antituberculosis activity of PAS, but until Frank Ryan conducted a series of revealing interviews with Lehmann's family, friends, and colleagues for his book *Tuberculosis: The Greatest Story Never Told* (33), little had been written about his life and the circumstances surrounding the discovery.

Lehmann was born in Denmark, son of a professor of theological history. His mother was a sculptor and close friend of Mette Gauguin, the Danish wife of the artist Paul Gauguin. The Lehmann family moved to Berlin while Jörgen was still a child, but at the beginning of the First World War they moved again to Lund in Sweden, where Jörgen became a medical student and developed an interest in enzyme chemistry. In 1935–36 he spent 18 months at the Rockefeller Institute in New York, working with the Nobel laureate-to-be Herbert Gasser on the physiology of nerve cell conductivity. An invitation to accept the post of professor of biochemistry in Aarhus, Denmark lured him back to Europe and he started work in the currently fashionable topic of vitamins. During this period he established what was to prove a valuable contact with a small local pharmaceutical firm, Ferrosan,* who were later to provide him with PAS.

The move to Aarhus was not a success and in 1938 Lehmann accepted a position as chief of chemical pathology at Sahlgrenska Hospital, Gothenburg. Here he got down to some serious research, initially on the newly described vitamin K and the effect of coumarin derivatives. This work brought him into renewed contact with Ferrosan, and with its chief chemist in Malmö, Karl-Gustav Rosdahl. In 1940, he received Frederick Bernheim's paper on the effect of salicylates on tubercle bacilli, but, busy with the coumarin work, he did nothing at the time to follow it up. He did, however, keep track of Bernheim's subsequent papers on the subject and decided to pursue some ideas of his own in early 1943.

In considering the various derivatives of salicylic acid and related compounds that Bernheim had tested, Lehmann had the inspired hunch that a compound that had not been included, 4-aminosalicylic acid—otherwise known as PAS†—might be the one to go for. On 3 March 1943 he wrote to Ferrosan suggesting that salicylates might have antibacterial activity and requesting samples of promising compounds, including the

---

* Ferrosan was a small family firm that was later swallowed up by Kabi. Through a series of mergers, Kabi metamorphosed into Pharmacia and eventually (2003) became part of Pfizer.

† 'Para-amino' refers to the position of the amino (NH_2) group diametrically opposite the carboxyl (COOH) group on the six-membered benzene ring.

4-amino version. Curiously, there seemed to be no record that this compound had ever been made, although a method was described in a standard reference work.

The explanation for the mystery of the missing PAS, as Rosdahl soon discovered, was that the synthesis was extremely difficult. None the less, he persevered and eventually succeeded where others had failed by devising a complex process that yielded small quantities of the substance. By early December 1943, Rosdahl was able to supply 13 g of PAS, which Lehmann immediately used to test against the avirulent BCG strain (see p. 142–3) of *Mycobacterium bovis*. The hunch that he had proved triumphantly correct: even in high dilution PAS completely inhibited growth of the organism.

Rudimentary tests in laboratory animals with the very limited supplies that slowly became available seemed to indicate that there were no serious problems of toxicity and in January 1944, the first therapeutic tests of PAS in guinea pigs infected with a virulent strain of *Mycobacterium tuberculosis* were begun. The results were encouraging, but inconclusive. In March 1944, Lehmann persuaded a colleague at Gothenburg's children's hospital to try dressings soaked in PAS on wounds discharging tuberculous pus. The lesions showed sufficient improvement to convince Lehmann that he should seek a more extensive trial. With more faith than evidence he approached Gylfe Vallentin, director of Gothenburg's Renstroemska sanatorium to ask him to test the new compound on his patients. Vallentin was unenthusiastic, but tentatively agreed to use PAS in patients in whom he would be draining pus from the chest wall; in effect replacing the pus with dilute drug. Once again there seemed to be some beneficial effect and Lehmann persuaded his colleague to extend the test by giving PAS by mouth to patients with pulmonary tuberculosis.

The first patient, known to us only as Sigrid, was a 24-year-old woman who had developed tuberculosis following a pregnancy and whose condition was rapidly declining. Treatment with PAS began 20 October 1944—3 weeks before the first recorded case of treatment with streptomycin in far-away Minnesota (see p. 159). She received three 1-week courses of 10 g PAS daily over a period of 2 months; astonishingly she recovered sufficiently to be fit for subsequent surgery that offered the prospect of a complete cure (51).

Further successes followed and under normal circumstances, the results would have been published without delay, but Ferrosan were having trouble obtaining a patent and did not want details of the compound in the public domain. It was not until January 1946 that the preliminary description of PAS, with two illustrative clinical cases (one of which was the young woman) was reported in *The Lancet* in the first issue of the year.

At the time that the *Lancet* paper appeared nothing remotely resembling a controlled clinical trial of PAS had been attempted. Fewer than 50 patients had received the drug, either by instillation into the chest cavity or by the oral route. Results had been mixed, but encouraging given the uncertainties that surrounded PAS: it was still in short supply; the purity of the compound was doubtful; and the correct dosage was unknown. Ferrosan were still having trouble producing the substance economically and the cost to the small company, both financially and in manpower terms, were beginning to tell; the future for PAS was by no means secure.

Against this background, Lehmann, Vallentin, and Olof Sievers, a bacteriologist from Helsinki, Finland, who had moved with his Swedish wife to the Sahlgrenska Hospital and had taken over the laboratory work, decided to present their findings to the meeting of Nordic tuberculosis physicians that was held in Gothenburg in June 1946. Mindful of the response that adverse publicity might bring, they took the precaution of issuing a press release, couched in very cautious terms, before the meeting. Needless to say, it did not prevent Scandinavian papers from running headlines announcing a breakthrough in a Swedish hospital.

The clinical results that Gylfe Vallentin was able to present to the Gothenburg meeting were unavoidably very mixed and the assembled delegates were far from convinced. Spontaneous remission in tuberculosis was too well known and the resemblance of the new drug to aspirin inevitably brought the criticism that apparent improvement might simply be due to an antipyretic effect. Moreover, memories of the earlier débâcles with Koch's tuberculin and Møllgaard's Sanocrysin (which had been a poor advertisement for Scandinavian clinical research) were still too fresh for a new therapy to be easily accepted by sceptical physicians struggling with the daily tragedy of tuberculosis.

The directors of Ferrosan were also unconvinced of the future of the drug. Development had cost the company a lot of money; manufacture of PAS was labour intensive and putting a great strain on the finances of this small firm. Lehmann was not to be put off and, in any case, PAS had now become unstoppable after the clamour that followed the *Lancet* paper and the press reports. A few doctors were sufficiently convinced to want to try the drug and when Ferrosan announced that they were unable to continue supplying it free of charge, Lehmann and Vallentin had to raise cash from supporters and grateful patients for trials to continue. Just when it seemed that manufacture of PAS might have to be abandoned, putting the whole future of the drug under threat, a young assistant of Rosdahl's at Ferrosan, Sven Carlsten, devised an efficient method of synthesizing the drug, making production much simpler and securing the continuation of supplies.

In April 1947 a group of Swedish doctors, including Lehmann and Vallentin, got together to design a controlled trial that would, like the British Medical Research Council's streptomycin trial, compare PAS with conventional bed rest, but with the important addition that the control group also received a placebo mimicking PAS in appearance, smell, and taste. Although streptomycin was by then available in Sweden in limited quantity, it was reserved for the treatment of miliary tuberculosis and tuberculous meningitis and such patients were excluded from the trial. The Swedish study, carried out in five of the country's sanatoria, provided statistically significant evidence of benefit from the use of PAS, but the study design was less than ideal. Treatment was assigned randomly, but the suitability of a patient for admission to the trial was left to the individual physicians. Moreover, the important question of the emergence of resistance was not addressed and there appears to have been no systematic monitoring of side effects (52).

Meanwhile, the British Medical Research Council was designing a new study that would address the problem of whether resistance to streptomycin could be prevented by the simultaneous administration of PAS. The trial in patients with pulmonary tuberculosis was designed with the same attention to detail as the earlier streptomycin trial. It was plainly no longer ethical to include an untreated group. Instead, there were now to be three arms to the study: one group of patients receiving streptomycin alone; another receiving PAS alone; and a third cohort receiving both drugs. The early results were so striking that it was felt necessary to issue a preliminary report in the *British Medical Journal* on New Year's Eve 1949 while the trial was still under way:

> The trial is not yet completed, but certain results already obtained are of such importance that the joint committee responsible for guiding the trial has decided to issue the following preliminary statement . . . the trial has demonstrated unequivocally that the combination of PAS with streptomycin reduced considerably the risk of development of streptomycin-resistant strains of tubercle bacilli during the six months following the start of treatment (53).

The full results of the Medical Research Council trial were published just over 10 months later in November 1950 (54). The findings established that PAS was considerably less effective than streptomycin and confirmed that combination treatment significantly reduced, but did not entirely prevent, the incidence of treatment failure associated with the development of resistance to streptomycin. In fact, it transpired that the suppression of resistance worked both ways; the streptomycin also prevented the emergence of resistance to PAS, although the evidence adduced was weaker because of the difficulty of accurate testing the susceptibility of *Mycobacterium tuberculosis* to PAS. The mutual effect is based on simple mathematics: if mutation to each drug occurs independently, then the probability of a double mutation developing is the product of multiplying the mutation frequencies. Thus, if a mutation to resistance to either streptomycin or PAS occurred independently in (say) one in every million (1 in 10^6) bacteria, the chance of a double mutation becomes one in a million million (1 in 10^{12}). If the frequency of mutation is lower, the odds become progressively longer. This is certainly not beyond the bounds of possibility in a heavily infected person, but treatment failure due to relapse with resistant organisms becomes much less likely.

The British findings were quickly confirmed in the United States, and a new era of combined treatment for tuberculosis was ushered in. In a fine example of the way poetic justice can sometimes operate benignly, one of the first to benefit from combination therapy was William Feldman. A routine chest X-ray taken late in 1948 revealed a worrying shadow in Feldman's lung and tubercle bacilli were found by examination of his sputum. The infection had been undoubtedly acquired during his long association with the disease in his laboratory. Feldman made a full recovery after treatment with streptomycin, PAS, and Promin, two of which drugs he had helped to develop. As his collaborator and friend, Corwin Hinshaw commented: 'It must be a rare circumstance in medical history that a scientist is stricken as a result of his experiments and is also rescued by his own hand'(55).

In retrospect, it can be seen that neither streptomycin nor PAS was the perfect answer to the problem of chemotherapy of tuberculosis. Streptomycin and its analogue dihydrostreptomycin (which appeared in1948 with promises of lower ototoxicity that failed to stand up to subsequent scrutiny) have to be administered by regular injections; both suffer from problems of adverse reactions that can be severe. Problems of resistance meant that neither drug could be reliably used alone. PAS is given by mouth, but its activity against *Mycobacterium tuberculosis* is quite modest: it must be given in large doses (10–15 g daily) that commonly cause nausea and other side effects that make compliance problematic. PAS is also extensively metabolized in the liver to inactive products and is rapidly excreted by the kidneys so that doses have to be given frequently.

Once the molecular structure of streptomycin, which is quite complex, had been worked out it was found to belong to a family of compounds, some of which have proved very useful in diseases other than tuberculosis (see Chapter 6, p. 229f). In the case of PAS, efforts were made to find analogues with improved properties, but disappointingly, other salicylic acid and benzoic acid derivatives were found to have little or no activity against *Mycobacterium tuberculosis* and none was found that improved on the substance that Lehmann had intuitively backed in 1943.

Sixty years on, streptomycin is still used in the treatment of tuberculosis and, occasionally, some other diseases, but it is no longer a natural first choice in any type of infection. Unlike streptomycin, PAS has no useful activity against organisms other than *Mycobacterium tuberculosis*. Its use gradually declined during the 1970s as experience with other antimycobacterial compounds accumulated. It is now rarely used, unless problems of multidrug resistance render alternative therapies unreliable.

Isoniazid

The combined use of streptomycin and PAS effectively reduced the incidence of treatment failure due to the emergence of resistance, but relapses still occurred in some cases. In patients in whom streptomycin or PAS resistance had already developed, combination therapy was, of course, no different from using a single active drug. A third drug was needed to make the reliability of treatment more secure. Promin and other sulphones were too toxic and unreliable to provide the answer. Fortunately other drugs were soon to become available and, one of them turned out to be, so to speak, just what the doctor ordered. That drug was isonicotinic acid hydrazide, more usually called isoniazid, or INH. The initial lead was provided by Gerhard Domagk and his colleagues, who continued to investigate sulphonamide derivatives in the Bayer laboratories of IG Farben* throughout the Second World War.

Domagk had included basic screening tests of activity against *Mycobacterium tuberculosis* in the investigations that led up to the discovery of Prontosil in 1932 and finding a compound with antituberculosis activity remained a high priority. As early as 1940 it was realized that, among sulphonamides, sulphathiazole and its close relatives were the only ones that showed feeble, but convincing activity against tubercle bacilli. A chemist, Robert Behnisch, who had been recruited by IG Farben as a young graduate in 1933, joined the old hands, Fritz Mietszch and Hans Schmidt—both had been at Elberfeld since the 1920s—in investigating derivatives that might show enhanced tuberculostatic

---

* Although Bayer was part of IG Farben, research and production remained largely independent and the Bayer name and logo was still used on the products.

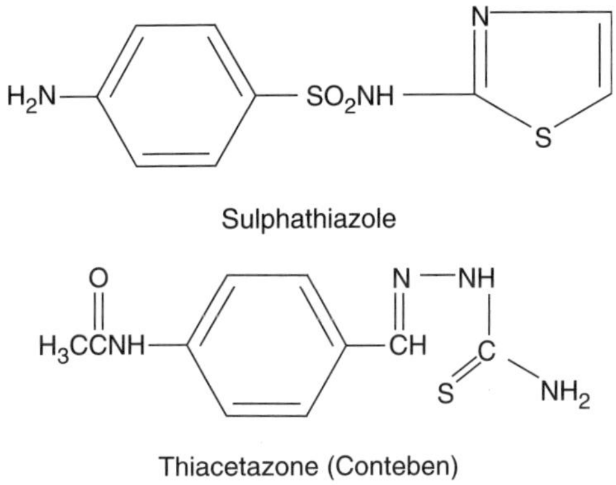

Sulphathiazole

Thiacetazone (Conteben)

Figure 5.4 Molecular structures of sulphathiazole and thiacetazone (Conteben) a
thiosemicarbazone.

activity. Sulphathiazole derivatives were prepared from organic sulphur-containing
chemicals known as thiosemicarbazones, linear molecules that could be transformed
into thiazoles (cyclic molecules containing sulphur and nitrogen atoms) by joining the
ends together to form a five-membered ring structure of the appropriate form (Fig. 5.4).

Behnisch realized that, since sulphonamides other than the thiazole derivatives showed
little ability to inhibit tubercle bacilli, it was likely to be the thiazole part of the molecule
that was responsible for the activity against tubercle bacilli. Moreover, since thiazoles
were derived from thiosemicarbazones it was logical to assume that the latter may also
possess some useful activity. Consequently in late 1941 Behnisch synthesized benzaldehyde thiosemicarbazone as an intermediate step in the formation of sulphathiazole and
passed it to Domagk for laboratory testing. The hunch turned out to be correct: the
thiosemicarbazone was found to exhibit promising activity against tubercle bacilli in laboratory tests (56).

As the war progressed research work became ever more difficult. The whole of the
Ruhr valley was subjected to almost nightly bombardment from the air. Only a handful
of staff remained in the Elberfeld works and production naturally took precedence.
Remarkably, some research on the thiosemicarbazones continued until early 1944 but
was finally brought to a halt by the impossible working conditions. Ironically, Hans
Schmidt had just come up with a thiosemicarbazone called Tb I/698—later given the
name Conteben (Fig. 5.4)—that showed vastly superior activity against tubercle bacilli in
the test tube.

The years 1945–47 were years of hardship, deprivation, and hunger throughout
Germany. The cities and towns were in ruins, the infrastructure to a large extent
destroyed and the demoralized population, much of it homeless or displaced, was living
on its wits. The old Reichsmark was worthless and it was not until monetary reform in
1948 that things began to improve. Elberfeld, the town in which Bayer's research and
production facility was concentrated, was almost totally destroyed; the factory itself was
badly damaged, but retained sufficient capacity for some work to continue. After the war
IG Farben was put under the control of the Allied forces and its assets confiscated, but

from October 1945 essential production was allowed to resume under the supervision of Ulrich Haberland, a chemist who had been manager of the Leverkusen site since 1943. Farbenfabriken Bayer was not re-established as an independent firm until December 1951.

The sense of isolation under which German researchers laboured in the immediate post-war period may perhaps be gauged from the fact the even in December 1947, when he was eventually able to travel to Sweden to collect his Nobel diploma, Domagk refrained from comment in his Nobel lecture, entitled *Further Progress in Chemotherapy of Bacterial Infections*, on the properties of streptomycin (57). The textbook on chemotherapy that he was writing at this time is equally silent (58), though an aside in the paper in *Die Naturwissenschaften* describing the antituberculous activity of thiosemi-carbazones, written in February 1946, showed that he was at least aware of streptomycin's existence (56).

Cautious trials of Conteben were carried out in 1947 and 1948 in Germany, where the post-war famine had exacerbated the problem of tuberculosis. Favourable results were reported, especially in skin tuberculosis. The news soon reached America, and in autumn 1949 Corwin Hinshaw and Walsh McDermott were despatched to Germany to investigate the claims. They visited various places where Conteben had been used and reported back to their colleagues in the United States that it seemed to have activity similar to that of PAS, but to be rather more liable to cause side effects (59). Conteben—by now given the generic name thiacetazone—was marketed by Imperial Chemical Industries (ICI) in the United Kingdom in the 1950s as 'Berculon' A. It is occasionally still used in developing countries as a cheap component of antituberculosis regimens, but its activity is relatively poor and side effects are common. A closely related compound synthesized by Behnisch, Tb III/1374, briefly aroused some interest in Germany and Britain, but problems of toxicity led to its abandonment.

The road from Conteben (thiacetazone) to isoniazid was not direct. Equally important was the observation made by a team of scientists led by Yellapragada SubbaRow, an Indian physician who had originally gone to the United States in 1923 with the support of a small scholarship to study at Harvard. He stayed to become head of research at the Lederle laboratories division of the American Cyanamid Company in Pearl River, New York. In 1948, shortly before SubbaRow died, Sam Kushner and his colleagues discovered that nicotinamide (the amide of nicotinic acid: niacin, one of the B-complex vitamins; Fig. 5.5) had an inhibitory effect on mycobacteria *in vitro* and in infected mice (60). In fact, the Lederle researchers had stumbled on a phenomenon that had already been described 3 years earlier in newly liberated France, where two French scientists—Vitaly Chorine,* a researcher in the field of tropical diseases, and Ernest Huant, a doctor specializing in the radiotherapy of tumours—independently, serendipitously and almost simultaneously noted the effect of nicotinic acid on mycobacteria.

---

* Chorine's paper gives his first name as Vital, but all other sources name him as Vitaly.

Chorine was studying the effect of various vitamins in rat leprosy, a disease caused by *Mycobacterium lepraemurium*. In carrying out an autopsy on rats infected on 21 July 1944—just before the liberation of Paris on 25 August—he noticed that, in animals that had been given nicotinic acid, the mycobacteria had failed to cause infection and those remaining at the injection site appeared to be damaged. Intrigued by this result, he repeated the test in guinea pigs infected with a human strain of tubercle bacilli and obtained a similar effect; *in vitro* studies confirmed the antituberculous effect (61). Chorine's findings were reported at a session of l'Académie des Sciences in Paris on 15 January 1945 and Huant, whose paper appeared in print on 15 August 1945 (62), seems to have been unaware of the results. His observations were also first made in 1944; he had been investigating nicotinic acid as an alternative to colchicine, which was used at that time as an adjunct to radiotherapy of tumours, in the hope of protecting tissues from unwanted harmful effects. In treating a 45-year-old woman with breast cancer, Huant noticed that subsequent X-rays showed regression of a tuberculous lesion in the woman's lungs. He went on to carry out some preliminary studies of high doses of nicotinic acid in patients with tuberculosis, and obtained a clear or limited effect in about half the cases.

Neither of the French reports seems to have aroused any interest (understandably, given the state of scientific communication in those difficult days), and when SubbaRow's team rediscovered the effect in 1948 it was thought to be novel. The Lederle scientists tested about 30 compounds related to nicotinamide and came to the erroneous conclusion that tuberculostatic and vitamin activity went hand in hand. When this finding was investigated by Herbert Fox from the research laboratories of Hoffmann–La Roche* in America, he at first confirmed the interrelationship, but then found that two analogues that had not featured in the Lederle investigation, 3-aminoisonicotinic acid and its methyl ester, retained tuberculostatic activity, but had no effect as vitamins. As Fox explained at a meeting of the New York Academy of Sciences in April 1953, this led him to widen his investigation to thiosemicarbazone derivatives of nicotinic acid and it was through manipulations of these compounds that isoniazid (Fig. 5.5) eventually emerged as a compound with unprecedented activity against *Mycobacterium tuberculosis* (63).

The conclusions that the scientists at Lederle had reached took their research in a different direction and in 1952 they described a nicotinamide derivative, pyrazinamide (Fig. 5.5), which also showed enhanced activity against tubercle bacilli and has become a useful agent in the fight against tuberculosis. The activity of pyrazinamide is highly dependent on the acidity or alkalinity (pH) of the surrounding milieu; it is most effective in acidic conditions and is almost inactive at a neutral pH. When it was first evaluated clinically was thought to be too toxic and unreliable to be used in antituberculosis regimens. However, Walsh McDermott and his colleagues at Cornell showed that it possessed the important property of killing, rather than just inhibiting growth of tubercle bacilli in

---

* Founded in Basel in 1896 by Fritz Hoffmann, from the firm Hoffmann, Traub & Co. that he had established with Carl Traub in 1892. He married Adèle La Roche in 1895 and gave the new company the name Hoffmann–La Roche. The firm soon expanded into several countries including the United States (in 1905) and the United Kingdom (in 1908).

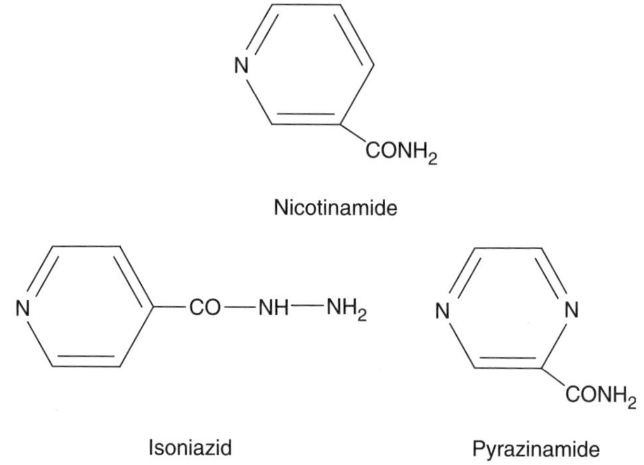

Figure 5.5 The molecular structures of nicotinamide, isoniazid, and pyrazinamide.

experimental infections of mice (64). More importantly, unlike streptomycin or isoniazid, which also kill tubercle bacilli, it was found to retain this bactericidal activity against dormant bacilli within the acidic environment of tuberculous lesions. It was later shown that the propensity to cause side effects could be largely prevented by controlling the size and frequency of the dose. In due course, these properties established pyrazinamide in its present position as a component of short-course antituberculosis regimens (see p. 185–7). Two further nicotinamide derivatives, ethionamide and protionamide emerged in the late 1950s after Noël Rist and his colleagues obtained encouraging results in a trial at the Hôpital Cochin in Paris. These drugs exhibit a broader antimycobacterial spectrum than pyrazinamide or isoniazid, with some activity against *Mycobacterium leprae*, but are not sufficiently reliable to be used as first-line therapy in either tuberculosis or leprosy.

By early 1951 animal tests on Roche's isoniazid were under way. They were also investigating the isopropyl derivative of isoniazid, iproniazid. In June 1951 a trial of both compounds began in patients with tuberculosis at the Sea View Hospital, a sanatorium on Staten Island, New York. Unbeknown to Roche and the clinical investigators, animal tests of isoniazid were also progressing at the Squibb Institute for Medical Research in New Brunswick, not far from Rutgers where streptomycin had been discovered. Harry L. Yale and his colleagues at the Squibb Institute under the direction of James A. Shannon had also been investigating the tuberculostatic activity of nicotinic acid derivatives and had independently come up with isoniazid. They were soon approaching Walsh McDermott, influential head of the division of infectious diseases at the New York Hospital–Cornell Medical Center to carry out clinical studies. McDermott had himself contracted tuberculosis in 1935, while still a resident medical officer learning his trade, and had spent some time at Trudeau's Saranac Lake sanatorium. Although he was eventually treated with the various chemotherapeutic agents as they became available, the illness continued to dog him throughout his distinguished career and he was one of the first to benefit from treatment with isoniazid during and after extensive chest surgery that he underwent in 1951.

While the American studies were in progress, scientists at the Wellcome Research Laboratories in Beckenham, Kent were also investigating antituberculosis agents and were concentrating their attention of a group known as phenanthridine hydrazides. According to the eyewitness account of the Wellcome chemist, John Henry Gorvin, isoniazid was one of the compounds synthesized in the period between 1949 and 1952 by Gordon Caldwell, who led this research (65). The compound was inexplicably found to be inactive by the Beckenham researchers and a chance to upstage the American discoveries was lost.

To add to the coincidence of simultaneous discovery, Domagk and his colleagues in the newly re-established Bayer organization in Germany had been busy following their own line of investigation. By 1951 they had reached the stage of being almost ready for the triumphant unveiling of their latest chemotherapeutic brainchild, which they called Neoteben. It was the most active drug against tubercle bacilli that they had yet discovered, and would surely help to revive the fortunes of the German drug industry. It was not to be. Although the Bayer team had no inkling of it at the time, Roche and Squibb were investigating the same substance in the United States.

Ironically, Gerhard Domagk came within touching distance of discovering the truth during a visit to America in 1951. In September of that year he travelled to New York for the 12th International Congress of Pure and Applied Chemistry. Roche's isoniazid and iproniazid were already in trial at the nearby Sea View hospital and Walsh McDermott at Cornell was testing Squibb's version of isoniazid. Domagk had met McDermott in Germany during his fact-finding mission with Corwin Hinshaw and while in New York he took the opportunity to renew his acquaintanceship with this important colleague. McDermott later described the pantomime that ensued:

> . . . we had a considerable discussion of antituberculous therapy in general and thiosemicar-
> bazones in particular. Neither of us mentioned the exciting promise of isoniazid, which each of us
> thought he alone knew. I feel certain that each of us walked away from our warm friendly parting
> with the thought, "Isn't *he* in for a surprise" (59).

In the event, it was McDermott who was first to be surprised. On new year's eve 1951, Elmer Sevringhaus, medical director of Hoffmann–La Roche came to visit him to ask if would take part in trials of Roche's new antituberculosis agents. He disclosed that they were isonicotinic acid derivatives, and one of them was isoniazid—the very drug that McDermott was already testing for Squibb.

Once it emerged that both Roche and Squibb had isonicotinic acid derivatives in clinical trial representatives of the two companies agreed to release laboratory information about the new drugs in papers to be published simultaneously in the *American Review of Tuberculosis* in April 1952 (66). Details of trials in man were to be restricted to a cautiously worded preliminary report from Sea View Hospital, for fear of fuelling the sort of public reaction that had accompanied the news of streptomycin in 1946. Regrettably the press had already got wind of 'miraculous' cures being achieved at Sea View. Even before the *American Review of Tuberculosis* papers had appeared reporters were descending on the hospital. Marcus Kogel, the Austrian-born Commissioner of

Hospitals for New York City (and soon to become Founder Dean of the Albert Einstein College of Medicine in the Bronx) hastily called a news conference to play down the story, but it was to no avail. On 21 February 1952 banner headlines in the *New York Post* and the *Washington Evening Star* proclaimed spectacular cures of patients dying of tuberculosis; the influential *Time* magazine joined the fun in early March. Unedifying pictures of ecstatic patients dancing in the wards fuelled the hysteria and the sensational media reports rapidly circulated round the world.

While all these events were proceeding, there was still the question of patent rights to be settled. Who had precedence for the discovery of isoniazid, Roche, Squibb, or Bayer? The answer turned out to be none of the three. In a replay of the sulphanilamide saga nearly 20 years before, isonicotinic acid hydrazide was a chemical that had been synthesized many years before. It had been described in Prague in 1912 by Hans Meyer and Josef Mally, who seem to have created it for no better reason than that it formed part of a doctoral research project. Freed of patent restrictions, production of isoniazid started in England in 1951 at a small company in Welwyn Garden City called Herts Pharmaceuticals Ltd.,* which was producing thiosemicarbazones and related compounds for Howard Florey in Oxford (67). Florey was at that time following a different lead in the search for antituberculosis agents with a young PhD student, George Mackaness, who was later recruited (no doubt on Florey's recommendation) by the John Curtin School of Medical Research in Australia, before moving to the United States in 1965 to become director of the Trudeau Institute and then president of the Squibb Institute for Medical Research.

Even as the media frenzy continued, clinical researchers in the United States, Great Britain, Germany, and elsewhere set about the task of evaluating isoniazid in controlled trials with material from Roche, Squibb, and Herts (68). In Britain it was once again the Medical Research Council that coordinated a trial, which started with admirable speed in March 1952, comparing isoniazid with what had become the standard chemotherapeutic regimen: streptomycin plus PAS. By October 1952, the remarkable efficacy of isoniazid was clear, but so was the old problem of drug resistance. In 1953, the trial was reorganized to compare three combination regimens: PAS plus isoniazid, isoniazid plus streptomycin, and streptomycin plus PAS.

These trials, and others elsewhere, established isoniazid as an important breakthrough in the chemotherapy of tuberculosis. It was relatively cheap to produce, could be given orally, and was also more active than either streptomycin or PAS; it was also less likely to cause side effects, although liver damage and occasionally, neurotoxicity were soon recognized. Resistance precluded administration of the drug alone, but combinations with streptomycin or PAS were effective in preventing relapse in patients harbouring tubercle bacilli initially susceptible to both drugs of either combination. A minor complication of the use of isoniazid was that a proportion of persons were found to have a genetic predisposition to metabolize the drug rapidly, necessitating adjustment of dosage.

---

* Makers of Nivea cream. The firm was acquired in 1951 by the surgical dressing company Smith and Nephew to provide them with a research base.

By the mid-1950s, tuberculosis, confounding the predictions of the pre-war experts, had become a curable disease. In 1959, John Crofton, professor of respiratory diseases and tuberculosis at the University of Edinburgh, and pioneer of chemotherapy studies in tuberculosis, was able to start his address to a meeting of the British Medical Association in Birmingham with the encouraging statement:

> The right use of modern methods of chemotherapy now makes it possible to aim at 100% success in the treatment of pulmonary tuberculosis (69).

The words 'the right use of' were carefully chosen. He went on to stress that success presupposed that the organisms were sensitive to the standard drugs and that recommended treatment regimens were strictly adhered to:

> Unfortunately, such results are attainable only by exercising the greatest care in prescribing the right combination of drugs, by handling the patient so that he continues to take his chemotherapy conscientiously over long periods of time, during which he is feeling perfectly well, and by carrying out the most careful drug resistance tests in those in whom there is any reason to suspect that resistance may have occurred

Crofton also championed the view that, with adequate chemotherapy, recourse to the extensive surgery to which tuberculosis sufferers were commonly subjected could safely be abandoned. The results confirmed this belief, but the message took some time to sink in with colleagues reluctant to abandon established practice.

The medical consensus, heavily influenced by Crofton's tireless work to perfect what became known as 'the Edinburgh method', eventually became convinced that triple therapy with streptomycin, PAS, and isoniazid was the most reliable regimen for the treatment of pulmonary tuberculosis. Although the early trials had generally concentrated on observing the results of 3 months of treatment, it rapidly became plain that a much longer course of therapy—up to 2 years, sometimes more—was necessary if success was to be assured. Since combination therapy rapidly rendered the patient non-infectious confinement in hospital for long periods became unnecessary. Sanatoria gradually altered their character by admitting patients with other pulmonary conditions such as lung cancer or the epidemic disease of industrial pollution, chronic bronchitis; some became general hospitals or closed down entirely. Edward Trudeau's pioneering Saranac Lake sanatorium was one of the first to go in America, closing its doors in 1954.*

As with PAS, much research was done on congeners of isoniazid, but none was found to possess properties superior to that of the parent compound. In 1953 Gladys Hobby (who had formerly worked at The College of Physicians and Surgeons, Columbia University, on the first clinical use of penicillin; see p. 100–101) and her colleagues at Pfizer produced a condensate of streptomycin and isoniazid, streptomycyclidene isonicotinoyl hydrazide (70). The intention was to combine the properties of the two active compounds, which *in vitro* studies had indicated acted synergically, to blunt the toxic side effects of streptomycin

---

* It survives as the Trudeau Institute, inaugurated by Edward Trudeau's grandson, Francis B. Trudeau (d. 1995) in 1964 as a centre for immunological research.

and to prevent the emergence of resistance. The product was briefly subjected to clinical trial, but soon abandoned.

An intriguing variant of this approach was pursued in the laboratories of the Irish Medical Research Council at Trinity College, Dublin by Vincent Barry, who is better known for his synthesis of the antileprosy drug, clofazimine (see p. 199–201). In 1954 he developed a compound called hinconstarch, which was conceived as a product that would combine the properties of isoniazid and thiosemicarbazones in the treatment of tuberculosis. As Barry explained to a symposium on antibiotics held at University College, Dublin on 1 February 1955 (71), he had been trained as a carbohydrate chemist and starch suggested itself as an ideal non-toxic vehicle for delivering isoniazid and a thiosemicarbazone to their site of action. He therefore synthesized two condensation products, hinstarch (with isoniazid) and constarch (with the thiosemicarazone, amithiazone). After demonstrating their activity and safety in experimental animals he went on to produce hinconstarch, in which the condensation product was prepared from an equimolar mixture of the two drugs. The compound was tested in several Irish hospitals and sanatoria with encouraging results and remarkable lack of toxicity, although 'an odd case has not done as well as we think it might have done (71)'. Hinconstarch briefly aroused some interest, but was soon discarded. It probably owed its efficacy to breakdown in the body to the component compounds.

Roche went ahead with the marketing of the isopropyl analogue, iproniazid (perhaps because, unlike isoniazid, it was a novel structural entity that could be patented), despite the fact that its activity against *Mycobacterium tuberculosis* was considerably poorer than that of the parent compound and its toxicity greater. Although it was never widely accepted as a component of antituberculosis regimens, it joined the remarkably long list of pharmacologically active compounds that have serendipitously found a use in conditions for which they were never intended.

In the early days of the use of isoniazid some patients had noted that the drug enhanced their sense of well-being. The effect might easily have been attributed to the improvement in the patients' general condition, except that the isopropyl congener, iproniazid, marketed under the name Marsilid, seemed to have an even greater effect in transforming the mental outlook of severely depressed patients. The phenomenon was first noted in 1952 by David Bosworth, an orthopaedic surgeon who was testing iproniazid on patients with painful bone and joint tuberculosis at the Sea View Hospital. On 4 July 1952 in an address to a joint meeting of the Orthopaedics Association in London, Bosworth observed:

> Pain relief has been universal and marked. Within a week or ten days narcotics have usually been discarded if previously used. With the relief of pain, euphoria has gradually developed. After three or four weeks the euphoria has decreased and the patient has been left with a normally optimistic instead of a depressed attitude. Occasionally the euphoria has been of such extent and its effect so prolonged that the patient's state has resembled that of mild narcotism . . . The above observations suggested to us the use of this chemical in conditions other than tuberculosis (72).

Around 1956, the psychopharmacologist Nathan Kline of the Rockland Psychiatric Center (now the Nathan Kline Institute) in Orangeburg, New York State started to use iproniazid as a mood-elevating drug in psychiatric patients. Examination of the pharmacological action of the drug had already found in 1952 that it achieved its effect by inhibiting monoamine oxidase, an enzyme that decomposes amines thought to function as neurotransmitters in the brain. Use of iproniazid was discontinued in the 1980s because of a high incidence of liver toxicity, which was much more common than with isoniazid, but the discovery gave rise to the investigation and, in due course, use of other monoamine oxidase inhibitors in depression.

The enzyme that was eventually given the name monoamine oxidase was discovered in 1928 by a 26-year-old postgraduate biochemistry student at Oxford, Mary Hare (73). In the same year she married a fellow biochemist, the American Frederick Bernheim, who was to carry out the initial research that led Jörgen Lehmann to PAS (see p. 164). Such are the interconnections in chemotherapeutic research.

The icing on the cake

The success of streptomycin, PAS and isoniazid encouraged the pharmaceutical houses to invest in research on drugs targeted at tubercle bacilli. Despite the success of the antibiotic streptomycin, synthetic chemicals at first seemed to offer the most productive route to compounds with therapeutically useful activity. As well as pyrazinamide and other nicotinamide derivatives (see above), a variety of novel substances offering activity against *Mycobacterium tuberculosis* began to appear. Some, like the thiocarbanalides (thioureas), which appeared in the mid-1950s, were short-lived. The only compound of this type to arouse much interest was, thiambutosine (*para*-butoxy-diphenylthiourea), produced by the Swiss firm CIBA (Gesellschaft für Chemische Industrie, Basel) a company, founded in 1874, which merged in 1971 with JR Geigy to form CIBA-Geigy.* Even this drug was not incorporated into antituberculosis regimens: it owed its survival to its status as a reserve drug in the treatment of leprosy (see p. 198).

More successful was ethambutol, one of the large series of ethylenediamine derivatives synthesized by Robert G. Shepherd, Raymond G. Wilkinson, and their colleagues at Lederle Laboratories, Pearl River. The activity of ethylenediamines against *Mycobacterium tuberculosis* had been discovered during screening of randomly selected compounds (74). Ethambutol was chosen as the compound with the most attractive pharmacological properties and was first described in 1961 (75). It exhibits excellent tuberculostatic activity, but a propensity to cause optic neuritis has limited its usefulness to the early intensive phase of modern antituberculosis regimens.

As the worldwide pharmaceutical industry started to turn its attention to naturally occurring antibiotics after the Second World War (see Chapter 6) inclusion of *Mycobacterium tuberculosis* in screening procedures began to yield various compounds with potentially useful activity. Already in 1949, Waksman and his colleague Hubert

---

* J. R. Geigy had been established in Basel in 1758 by Johann Rudolf Geigy-Gemuseus. In 1996 CIBA–Geigy joined up with Sandoz to form Novartis. Sandoz was originally a dyestuff company founded in 1886 as Kern & Sandoz by Alfred Kern and Edouard Sandoz.

Lechevalier, had described a new antibiotic, neomycin, isolated from *Streptomyces fradiae*, which seemed destined to repeat his earlier success with streptomycin. Like many antibiotics, neomycin turned out later to be a mixture of compounds displaying minor variations of a common basic structure and very similar, but not identical properties. The antibacterial spectrum of neomycin mirrored that of streptomycin, with good activity against *Mycobacterium tuberculosis* and a variety of other organisms; unfortunately, its toxicity to the ear and kidney proved to be much greater than that of streptomycin. Systemic therapy with neomycin was, nevertheless, sometimes used, faute de mieux, though seldom in tuberculosis. The distinguished microbiologist Lawrence Paul Garrod and his faithful assistant Pamela Waterworth at St Bartholomew's Hospital in London once published a report of a patient with streptococcal endocarditis who had been treated with neomycin and penicillin after therapy with streptomycin and penicillin had failed. The paper bore the stark title *Deaf or Dead?* (76) Neomycin remains available today in topical preparations, but it has few advantages over other antibacterial agents and is not much favoured. Framycetin, an antibiotic produced by a strain of *Streptomyces lavendulae* isolated in 1947 by L. J. Decaris from a damp patch on the wall of his home in Paris,* proved to be identical to neomycin B, one of the components of the original antibiotic complex. It was developed by the French firm, Roussel and is still found as an ingredient of topical preparations, such as ear and eye ointments.

Scientists from Parke, Davis, and Pfizer in the United States independently described, in 1951, an antibiotic that was at first thought to be related to streptomycin and neomycin (77). The producer organism found by Pfizer was named *Streptomyces puniceus* because of the violet colour of the colonies (Latin puniceus = purplish-red) and the colour violet gave the antibiotic its name, viomycin. Parke, Davis more prosaically named their organism *Streptomyces floridae*, presumably from the location in which it was found. Viomycin was eventually shown to have a complex cyclic structure based on six linked amino acids (hexapeptide). It has many properties in common with those of streptomycin and neomycin and shares the tendency of those compounds to cause damage to the ear and the kidney. Initially hailed as a promising addition to the list of drugs useful in combating tuberculosis, it soon yielded to the appearance of less toxic compounds, such as PAS and isoniazid. A related antibiotic, capreomycin, was described from the Lilly Research Laboratories in Indianapolis in 1962 as a product of a newly described species, *Streptomyces capreolus* (78). Ototoxicity, nephrotoxicity, and other side effects also militated against the routine use of this agent in antituberculosis regimens. Viomycin and capreomycin have both long been relegated to the role of reserve drugs for use when all else fails.

Scarcely less toxic, but this time exhibiting a high incidence of neurotoxic symptoms, including convulsions, is cycloserine. According to a comprehensive review published in 1966, this naturally occurring compound, a simple analogue of the amino acid D-alanine,

---

* The findings were not published until 1953: Decaris L. J. A strain of *Streptomyces lavendulae*, producer of a new antibiotic. *Annales Pharmaceutiques Française* 1953; 11: 44–46. (See also: Barber M., Garrod L. P. *Antibiotic and Chemotherapy*. E & S Livingstone, Edinburgh, 1963, pp. 104–105).

was discovered independently in 1954 by scientists from three commercial laboratories in the United States and by the Kayaku Antibiotic Research Company in Japan (79).* Two of the American companies involved were Merck and Pfizer, but the version of cycloserine that came to be most widely used, Seromycin, was developed and marketed by Eli Lilly. It was, however, not a Lilly discovery; the antibiotic was actually found by Roger L. Harned and his colleagues at the Commercial Solvents Corporation (80) (now part of Schering-Plough Animal Health), a chemical company established in1919 in Terrre Haute, Indiana, not far from Lilly's Indianapolis headquarters. The company had been involved in the American drive to produce penicillin during the Second World War and was one of the first to use deep fermentation technology (see p. 110). It had originally made its mark through the production of acetone by a process licensed from the Russian-born chemist, Chaim Weizmann, who in 1948 was destined to become the first president of Israel. Weizmann had developed and patented the fermentation process[†] in 1915 as a lecturer at Owen's College, Manchester (now the University of Manchester), where, coincidentally, his chief was Professor William Perkin, son of the discoverer of the first aniline dye (see p. 49–51).

The antibiotic discovered by the Commercial Solvents Corporation was originally obtained as a product of *Streptomyces orchidaceus* obtained from a local soil sample. The Merck compound (Oxamycin) was isolated from *Streptomyces garyphalus*; the Pfizer version (known only as PA-94) from *Streptomyces lavendulae*; and the Japanese product (Orientamycin) from *Streptomyces roseochromogenus*. Within a year of the initial discovery Karl Folkers and his colleagues at Merck had devised a process that allowed cycloserine to be manufactured economically by chemical synthesis. A related compound, O-carbamyl-D-serine—also a product of *Streptomyces* species—was isolated in France in 1955, but did not survive early evaluations (79).

The first clinical studies of cycloserine in human pulmonary tuberculosis were carried out on behalf of Eli Lilly at the New York Metropolitan Hospital in 1954. The drug was provided by Michael G. Mulinos, medical director of the Commercial Solvents Corporation, who also held the position of associate professor of pharmacology at New York Medical College. The trial of cycloserine (81) seems to have been carried out with unseemly haste; there was little hard evidence of its activity against mycobacteria as an acerbic editorial in the *British Medical Journal* observed (82). In fact, animal tests had failed to confirm the activity (itself erratic) revealed by *in vitro* tests and it had been expected that large doses (justified by an apparent lack of toxicity in animals) would be necessary in human tuberculosis. In the event, the more modest doses that were prudently given in the first trial proved to be adequate to achieve an effect, but it soon became evident that the safety of the drug had been seriously underestimated. Neurological effects of cycloserine were sufficiently severe to lead to discontinuation of

* The Nippon Kayaku Company was established in Japan in 1916, initially as a manufacturer of dyestuffs and explosives.

† Acetone, which was needed for the production of cordite was in short supply during the First World War. The process Weizmann devised involves use of the anaerobic bacterium *Clostridium acetylbutylicum*, which produces acetone from starch as a metabolic product.

treatment in 11 per cent of the patients. Nonetheless, many of the patients had previously failed to respond to standard triple therapy with streptomycin, PAS and isoniazid and the clinical results were considered dramatic enough for the authors to claim that another potent antituberculosis antibiotic had been found.

The neurotoxicity of cycloserine militated against its widespread acceptance in antituberculosis regimens, but against all odds, it has remained in the pharmacopoeia. It is still used as a second- or third-line choice in tuberculosis caused by bacilli resistant to the front-line drugs. Its survival was partly due to a lingering hope that it might be of value in infections other than tuberculosis. From the start it was claimed that cycloserine displayed a broad antibacterial spectrum, though, in truth, the activity against most bacteria is feeble by the standards of most clinically useful antibiotics. It is excreted in the urine in sufficient quantity to have encouraged hope that it might be of value in urinary tract infection. It enjoyed a brief and mystifying popularity in certain quarters as a treatment for uncomplicated cystitis, though it is doubtful that the benefits outweighed the risks in this condition.

It was no doubt the neuropsychiatric side effects of cycloserine that alerted researchers to the possibility that it might join the ranks of those drugs that find a use for which they were not originally intended. Experiments in rats have revealed that it displays some activity as a so-called 'cognitive enhancer'. The results have led to small-scale human trials of cycloserine in such conditions as schizophrenia, phobias, and Alzheimer's disease. Whether these investigations will lead to anything useful is still under investigation, but a Cochrane review* has found no evidence of a meaningful clinical effect in published reports describing the use of cycloserine in Alzheimer's disease (83).

The jewel in the crown

Despite all the efforts to find alternative antituberculosis agents, streptomycin, PAS, and isoniazid ruled supreme for over a decade. The situation was not to change until a powerful new drug, rifampicin (known in North America as rifampin), was introduced into the therapy of tuberculosis in 1968.

Many people bring back souvenirs of their holiday. At the height of the antibiotic boom in the 1950s employees of pharmaceutical companies were often encouraged to bring back samples of soil, especially if they had been to exotic places. In 1957 Piero Sensi, a scientist working for Lepetit Research Laboratories, a small pharmaceutical firm in Milan,† went no further than St Raphaël on the Côte d'Azur for his vacation, but true to form he returned with local soil samples. Back home in Milan a new species of actinomycete was

---

* The Cochrane Collaboration is an international non-profit organization, founded in 1993, which produces independent assessments of treatment in various clinical conditions, based on systematic reviews of clinical trials and other published evidence. It is named in honour of the distinguished Scottish epidemiologist, Archie Cochrane.

† Lepetit joined up with Dow Corning in 1968, and was eventually swallowed up in the series of mergers that led to the creation of Aventis in 1999. The Lepetit research laboratories, which moved to Gerenzano, Varese in the 1980s, survived through a management buyout as Biosearch Italia. In 2003 it merged with Versicor Inc., King of Prussia, Pennsylvania, to form Vicuron Pharmaceuticals.

isolated from the soil; the new organism appeared to be a member of the *Streptomyces* genus and in recognition of its origin it was given the name *Streptomyces mediterranei* (since twice reclassified; first as *Nocardia mediterranei*, then as *Amycolatopsis mediterranei*). Random isolates of this type generally yield nothing of interest, but this one was different: routine screening tests of the crude extract from fermentation broths showed antibiotic activity with high potency against many common Gram-positive pathogens, including *Mycobacterium tuberculosis*.

There cannot be many drugs that have taken their name from a gangster movie, but the scientists at Lepetit had a predilection for whimsical names. The antibiotic substances produced by the newly discovered micro-organism were called rifomycins (later changed to rifamycins), a name suggested by the 1955 French movie *Du rififi chez les hommes* (*Rififi* in the English version) (84). The film became famous for a 25-min long robbery sequence during which there is no dialogue. Whether Sensi had spent a similar length of time silently capturing his prize during his holiday in the South of France is not recorded.

Streptomyces mediterranei produced a complex of five antibiotics, designated rifamycins A–E according to the order in which they were separated by the technique of chromatography. They were found to be large heterocyclic molecules, a characteristic feature of which is a large chain-like bridging structure, the 'ansa' chain (Latin ansa = handle), which gave rise to the generic name sometimes used to describe these compounds, ansamycins.

The individual components of the rifamycin complex proved difficult to isolate because of their instability; the only one that could be easily obtained in a pure, crystalline form was rifamycin B. This component exhibited poor antibacterial activity and could easily have been discarded but for the fact that it was found to degrade spontaneously in aerated aqueous solution to a much more active substance, rifamycin S (85). This in turn could be easily manipulated chemically to yield a stable form, designated rifamycin SV, which is very active against mycobacteria and many Gram-positive cocci.

Rifamycin SV was tentatively introduced into therapy in 1963, but it is not absorbed when given by mouth and the performance of the drug in early clinical trials did not match expectations. Rifamycin SV was nevertheless marketed in various formulations in some parts of Europe; it was never widely used, although it is still available in certain countries finding its main use as a topical application, for example to wounds and bedsores.

It was clear that the rifamycins had great potential, but further development was needed and this required greater resources than Lepetit were able to provide. Consequently, a collaborative research agreement was signed with the CIBA company in Basel. The objective of the joint venture was to establish which parts of the rifamycin structure were amenable to alteration without loss of activity and to prepare and test semi-synthetic analogues that might overcome some of the shortcomings of the naturally occurring compounds and their immediate derivatives. The chief problems with rifamycin SV were that it was poorly absorbed by the oral route and rapidly excreted in the bile—features that it was hoped to modify by chemical manipulation of the basic structure. Once the minimum requirements for potent antibacterial activity were established, numerous semi-synthetic rifamycins were produced, but the first derivative to find its way into therapeutic use in

1965, the diethylamide of rifamycin B, rifamide, turned out to have drawbacks similar to those of rifamycin SV.

Persistence paid off with the discovery that introduction at the appropriate position of a methyl (CH_3) substituted piperazine ring (a cyclic structure composed of four carbon and two nitrogen atoms) provided a compound that was not only highly active against mycobacteria and Gram-positive cocci, but was also well absorbed after oral administration and appeared safe in toxicological tests. This substance, called rifampicin, but given the name rifampin by the United States Adopted Name Council, was unveiled at the sixth Interscience Conference on Antimicrobial Agents and Chemotherapy (an international congress convened each year by the American Society for Microbiology; see p. 211) held in Philadelphia in October 1966 (86).

Rifampicin transformed the treatment of tuberculosis and the other major mycobacterial disease, leprosy. Easy to administer, extremely active, and generally free from serious side effects, it outshone anything that had previously been used. Sadly, it suffered from the curse of antituberculosis drugs: high rates of mutation to resistance among bacteria within its spectrum of activity. Consequently, it had to be used in combination with other antituberculosis drugs, but it soon supplanted streptomycin as the preferred workhorse—at least in countries in which it could be afforded—of antituberculosis regimens.

Rifampicin is not only highly active against *Mycobacterium tuberculosis* and *Mycobacterium leprae*; it also exhibits unrivalled potency against staphylococci and good activity against streptococci. However, the drug has been used very sparingly in the treatment of conditions other than tuberculosis and leprosy because of the fear—exaggerated in the view if some authorities—of inadvertently encouraging resistance in persons harbouring mycobacterial pathogens. Considerable excitement was aroused when rifampicin was found to display some antiviral activity, notably against poxviruses, but it soon transpired that this was insufficient to offer any realistic hope of therapeutic use.

The general safety of rifampicin, even in long-term use, is widely acknowledged, but the idea of a completely safe drug is a pharmacological fantasy and rifampicin is certainly no exception. Many adverse reactions—most importantly disturbances of liver function—are recognized; some, notably a 'flu syndrome', are more common when the drug is given intermittently. There are a few other problems: in common with other rifamycins, rifampicin is pigmented and in patients taking the drug bodily secretions such as urine, tears, and sweat, turn an alarming orange–red colour; soft contact lenses may be permanently damaged. More importantly the drug is a potent inducer of liver enzymes and may affect the handling of other drugs that are being taken; oral contraceptives are among compounds that are affected and in women unwanted pregnancy may result.

Various other rifamycins have been described over the years, but none has been found with properties as attractive as those of rifampicin. Rifabutin, a semi-synthetic derivative of rifamycin S introduced in the late 1980s, is most widely used. It has found particular use in the treatment of infection with organisms of the *Mycobacterium avium* complex—environmental mycobacteria of normally low human pathogenicity, which are prone to infect patients who are severely immunocompromised, including those with AIDS.

Around the same time, rifapentine was introduced in some countries as an improved version of rifampicin, which it closely resembles. Although it is retained in the body for longer than rifampicin it seems to have no other advantages and is not commonly used. Rifaximin, a drug that is very poorly absorbed when taken orally has been used chiefly for gastro-intestinal complaints. Some success has been claimed in the treatment of Crohn's disease, an inflammatory condition usually affecting the lower small intestine.

Short-course therapy

As John Crofton had emphasized in his address in Birmingham in 1959 (see p. 177) complete conformity to the full course of treatment was important if a successful cure of tuberculosis was to be achieved. The requirements of the original triple therapy regimen were formidable: up to 2 years of treatment with streptomycin (requiring daily injections and with the risk of problems with balance or hearing), PAS (given in a dose of 5 g or more three times a day and likely to cause constant nausea) and isoniazid (better tolerated, but prone to neurological side effects, especially in patients with a genetic predisposition to acetylate the drug slowly). Within a very short time of starting treatment, patients began to feel completely well and needed every persuasion to continue with the medication. Even in developed countries with good medical services and well-motivated patients, compliance was a constant problem. In communities already burdened with social deprivation, the difficulty of delivering effective treatment meant that much of the population remained untreated, and among those that were fortunate enough to receive therapy, resistance became a problem because of failure of adequate compliance.

The first priority was clearly to reduce the need for daily injections. A commonly adopted solution for pulmonary tuberculosis was to discontinue streptomycin once tubercle bacilli were no longer detectable in the sputum, provided the causative organism had been shown to be susceptible to isoniazid and PAS. A trial by the British Medical Research Council in the early 1960s put this on a firm scientific footing by showing that daily streptomycin could be dropped from the triple therapy regimen after 6 weeks without seriously affecting the outcome. Simple, effective treatment became even more secure—and more expensive—in 1968 when rifampicin appeared on the market as an effective oral replacement for streptomycin and when careful adjustment of the dosage of ethambutol or pyrazinamide allowed them to replace the widely disliked PAS. Despite opposition from physicians who regarded it as a dangerous drug, the ability of pyrazinamide to kill dormant bacteria within tuberculous lesions (see p. 173–4) eventually led to its adoption as an important ingredient of truncated antituberculosis regimens.

Much of the early progress in defining optimum drug regimens chiefly benefited affluent countries with well-developed health care systems and reliable radiological and laboratory facilities. For the poorer nations, the cost alone was prohibitive and the logistics of delivering adequate long-term treatment, especially to rural communities, all but impossible. In 1956, a major collaborative project between the Indian Council of Medical Research, the Madras State Government, the World Health Organization, and the British

Medical Research Council set out to tackle this problem. Following a visit to India in 1955 by a Medical Research Council delegation consisting of Guy Scadding, Philip D'Arcy Hart, and Wallace Fox, a Tuberculosis Chemotherapy Centre was set-up in Madras (Chennai), South India. Wallace Fox, a member of the scientific staff of the Medical Research Council's Tuberculosis and Chest Disease Unit at the Brompton Hospital, London, was temporarily seconded to the World Health Organization to set-up the scheme.

The first trial, a classic project that has become known in the annals of mycobacteriology as 'the Madras Experiment', aimed to compare 1 year of treatment (the maximum feasible in a country with extremely limited resources) with PAS and isoniazid in two groups of patients: those fortunate enough to be cared for in the small number of sanatorium beds available; and those treated at home, often in the poorest parts of Madras. The results were startling: both groups did equally well, with around 90 per cent yielding negative sputum cultures during a 5-year follow-up period (87). The results paved the way for the general adoption of domiciliary treatment, especially as the study produced two other important findings: the tuberculosis sufferers treated in the community did not seem to pose a threat to close family contacts; and their inevitably poorer diet had had no effect on the outcome.

The success of the Madras experiment allowed the Centre to extend its work—which continues to this day—with backing from the World Health Organization and the British Medical Research Council. Wallace Fox returned to the Medical Research Council's Tuberculosis and Chest Disease Unit at the Brompton Hospital in 1961, eventually becoming Director in 1965. Hugh ('Bill') Stott, an Indian-born doctor with experience of working in rural Kenya, took over as Senior Medical Officer in Madras, although Fox continued to take a close interest in the centre and paid frequent visits. Like others they quickly discovered that supervised treatment was essential; simply distributing the drugs and leaving the patient to take the medication in the correct manner invited failures of compliance that compromised the effectiveness of therapy and encouraged the emergence of resistance. One course of action that was tried by the Madras team, and which seemed to offer encouraging results, was to administer the drugs in appropriate dosage twice a week instead of every day. This policy of supervised intermittent therapy considerably lessened the burden on the health care teams responsible for delivering treatment in the community.

Encouraged by the Madras results Fox turned his attention to the heretical notion that, if suitable regimens could be devised, a reduction in the length of therapy might be possible without compromising its effectiveness. Ably abetted by Denny Mitchison, head of the experimental tuberculosis unit at the Royal Postgraduate Medical School, Hammersmith Hospital and scion of the outrageously talented and seemingly indestructible Haldane family, Fox set about organizing collaborative studies throughout the world in which short-course regimens were devised and subjected to rigorous trial in comparison with standard 1-year therapy.

Exhaustive (and no doubt exhausting) studies in East Africa in the early 1970s established that a 6-month regimen of daily treatment of newly diagnosed severe pulmonary tuberculosis with streptomycin, isoniazid, and rifampicin was as effective as 18 months of standard therapy. Results obtained with a 6-month regimen in which pyrazinamide was substituted for the more expensive rifampicin were almost as good.

Various other trials were carried out around the world with the support of bodies such as the World Health Organization, the International Union Against Tuberculosis (an organization established at a conference in Paris in 1920), and the British Medical Research Council. As well as the continuing work in Madras and East Africa, important studies were done in Hong Kong, Singapore, Brazil, and many other countries.

Further refinements of treatment eventually led to the recommendation, at least for uncomplicated cases of pulmonary tuberculosis, of a 6-month regimen, consisting of a 2-month intensive phase with daily administration of three or four drugs—usually rifampicin, isoniazid, and pyrazinamide, often with ethambutol or streptomycin as a cover for the possibility of resistance—followed by a 4-month continuation phase in which rifampicin and isoniazid alone are given. Intermittent therapy (doses given two or three times a week) is often used during the continuation phase, particularly if 'directly observed therapy'—popularly known as DOTS—is used. DOTS, in which health care and community workers observe and record that the drugs have been properly taken is successful in 95 per cent of cases, even in the most disadvantaged communities, and is now part of the official policy of the World Health Organization in its continuing fight against tuberculosis.

The perils of complacency

In the affluent nations of the world, tuberculosis had, by the 1970s, become a relatively rare disease, chiefly associated in the minds of medical practitioners with immigration, vagrancy and, in the case of bovine tuberculosis, cattle. Research into tuberculosis was no longer considered a priority, not least in the pharmaceutical industry, where drugs specifically aimed at *Mycobacterium tuberculosis* were not considered commercially viable. Organizations dedicated to the study of the disease began to change their character. In America the Trudeau Society had altered its name to the American Thoracic Society as early as 1960. The International Union Against Tuberculosis added 'and Lung Diseases' to its name in 1986; their official journal *Tubercle* followed suit in 1992. To its credit, the British Medical Research Council, which had originally been setup (initially as the Medical Research Committee) in 1913 at the recommendation of a Royal Commission on tuberculosis, continued to give strong support to the disease as the work on short-course therapy bears eloquent witness.

Of course, tuberculosis had never gone away. It had simply become a disease predominantly affecting poor people in far away places, albeit one that killed around 3 million of them every year. Two events towards the end of the twentieth century altered that complacent view: the pandemic of disease caused by the human immunodeficiency virus (HIV), which formed a sinister partnership with tuberculosis; and the emergence of strains of *Mycobacterium tuberculosis* that were resistant to rifampicin and isoniazid, earning them the epithet 'multidrug-resistant', though they usually remained susceptible to the less active antituberculosis agents (see p. 399).

The trigger for concern was the occurrence in the United States of several outbreaks of multidrug-resistant tuberculosis in hospitals and prisons (euphemistically named 'correctional facilities'), notably in Florida and New York. Most of the disease was in patients or inmates with HIV and mortality was high; infection was transmitted to at least nine health care workers and prison guards and five died, prompting the formation of a task force to formulate a national action plan (88).

Despite these events there have been few signs of a resurgence of interest in the development of new antituberculosis drugs. A small number of possible alternatives have been found among the general-purpose antibacterial agents that have emerged over the years: certain aminoglycosides related to streptomycin, such as amikacin and kanamycin, retain activity against streptomycin-resistant strains of tubercle bacilli (see pp. 230, 233), but are otherwise unremarkable; some quinolones (p. 256f) display sufficient antimycobacterial activity to allow their use if resistance to the older drugs is present. Fortunately, standard well-tried therapeutic regimens remain highly effective in the vast majority of cases. Provided the resistance threat can be contained—and this is certainly attainable if treatment guidelines are adhered to—the future should be relatively secure. Crucial to this on a global scale is the World Health Organization's 'DOTS-plus' strategy, which is aimed at extending the successful DOTS scheme to the more difficult task of longer treatment with more toxic drugs in areas in which multidrug-resistance is prevalent.

Antileprosy agents

It is likely that the lepers described in the bible and other ancient texts suffered from a variety of skin diseases of which that caused by *Mycobacterium leprae* is just one example. True leprosy was, however, certainly widespread throughout the ancient world, including most of Europe, from where it mysteriously declined and eventually disappeared—perhaps influenced by an upsurge in tuberculosis which confers some cross-immunity—over a period of many centuries. The last known person to have acquired the disease in Great Britain died in the Shetland Islands in 1798. It is still widespread throughout the tropics, particularly in the Indian subcontinent, Myanmar (Burma), Brazil, and parts of Africa. The causative bacillus was discovered in 1873—well before Koch's description of the related tubercle bacillus—by Armauer Hansen a physician working with leprosy patients in Bergen, Norway.

Although *Mycobacterium leprae* and *Mycobacterium tuberculosis* are closely related and share many characteristics, the diseases they cause are quite different. Leprosy is not normally fatal, but it causes disfigurement and disability on a truly horrific scale. The bacilli target cells surrounding neurons causing failure to respond to stimuli (leading to accidental injury), muscle paralysis, and destructive changes in the skin and associated tissues. Blindness is common if the disease remains untreated. Not all sufferers are equally affected. There is a well-described spectrum of disease ranging from the condition known as tuberculoid leprosy, in which an intense immunological response leads to severe nerve damage, but few bacilli are present, to lepromatous leprosy, in which the immune reaction is muted and numerous bacilli are found. Various intermediate states are recognized. Contrary to popular belief the condition is not highly contagious: many dedicated people have worked for years among leprosy patients without acquiring the disease.

Research into leprosy, including that aimed at chemotherapy of the disease, has always been hampered by the failure to develop an artificial culture medium in which *Mycobacterium leprae* could be reliably grown outside the body. Laboratory animals are also refractory to infection, so that early research had to rely on the use of mice infected with *Mycobacterium lepraemurium*—a notoriously unreliable model of human leprosy— or human volunteers with all the associated ethical difficulties. Chapman H. Binford, Medical Director of the Leonard Wood Memorial* (American Leprosy Foundation) postulated in 1956 that the failure to infect laboratory animals might be related to their body temperature, since leprosy bacilli prosper in superficial parts of the body in which the temperature is reduced. Indeed, in America in the 1930s attempts had been made to exploit this feature of leprosy by subjecting some patients to 'fever therapy' involving 5-h sessions in sauna-like conditions at 60–70° C. The technique proved ineffective and was soon abandoned.

Working on Binford's theory, Charles C. Shepard, head of leprosy and rickettsial research at the Unites States Public Health Service's Communicable Disease Center in Montgomery, Alabama and Chairman of the United States Leprosy Panel, obtained limited multiplication of the bacilli after inoculation into mouse footpads (89). In 1976 Joe Colston and Dick Hilson of St George's Hospital, London improved Shepard's technique—which Hilson had seen at first hand during a sabbatical spent in Shepard's laboratory in 1963—by the use of congenitally athymic ('nude') mice, which are more susceptible because of their impaired immune system (90).

A more important breakthrough had occurred in 1970, when it was discovered that *Dasypus novemcinctus*, the nine-banded armadillo, could be successfully infected with *Mycobacterium leprae*. Around 1968, an American biologist, Eleanor E. Storrs working at the Gulf South Research Institute†, a private foundation in New Iberia, Louisiana, proposed that, since armadillos—animals on which she had earlier worked for her PhD— have a relatively low body temperature similar to that of the superficial tissues in which the organism thrives, and since they are sufficiently long-lived to allow time for the disease to develop, they might provide a suitable model for leprosy studies. In order to obtain a grant to pursue the idea, she sought the collaboration of Waldemar F. Kirchheimer, a German-born microbiologist in the nearby United States Public Health Service leprosarium in Carville, Louisiana (see p. 194), a fateful decision which was to lead to an acrimonious dispute over priority. In 1970, after several failures with material supplied by Kirchheimer, Storr successfully inoculated several armadillos with lepromatous tissue

---

* An organization named to commemorate Leonard Wood, an army surgeon who rose to become chief of staff of the United States Army during the First World War. He was later appointed Governor-General of the Philippines and campaigned for the improvement of treatment facilities for leprosy, which was a major problem on the islands.

† Where her husband, Harry P. Burchfield had recently been appointed Scientific Director.

obtained from Chapman Binford, but Kirchheimer maintained that he had provided the crucial expertise and used his influence to ensure that a paper describing the results was published with his name as senior author (91). A paper outlining the use of armadillos as a leprosy model that Storrs submitted at the same time was relegated to second place (92). Further animosity was generated when leprosy was later discovered in wild armadillos in Louisiana and unsubstantiated allegations were made that the Gulf South Institute staff had negligently allowed leprosy to escape into the wild. The dispute flared into accusations and counter-accusations of scientific misconduct, incompetence, fraud, and defamation that have never been satisfactorily resolved (93).

The mouse footpad and armadillo models enabled the production of sufficient material for standardized skin test reagents—lepromins and leprosins—which are used in the diagnosis and epidemiology of leprosy. Efforts to produce a vaccine have been unavailing, though some protection seems to be afforded by BCG (see p. 144). Animal models were also quickly employed to test susceptibility to many antimicrobial agents, including all those used in tuberculosis, but few were found to be of much value. In fact, the present day treatment of leprosy relies largely on just three compounds: dapsone, rifampicin, and clofazimine.

More than any other condition, the care and treatment of leprosy sufferers has inevitably taken place largely outside mainstream medicine, since the victims themselves were shunned by society and often forced to live in isolated communities. Much heroic work has been performed by medical missionaries. Some became famous—who has not heard of Albert Schweitzer of Lambaréné, doctor, theologian, pastor, and organ scholar, and Mother Teresa of Calcutta (Agnes Bonxha Bojaxhiu) both of who founded leprosaria in their mission hospitals; or of Father Damien of Molokai (Joseph de Veuster). But many others have worked in dedicated anonymity.

Consequently trials of drugs aimed at alleviating the scourge of leprosy have mostly taken place outside the glare of publicity. A large debt of gratitude is owed to many selfless and unsung medical missionaries who undertook these studies (often on their own initiative) and carefully recorded the results.

The rise and fall of an ancient remedy

Curiously a treatment for leprosy that seems to have had some limited efficacy existed well before the antimicrobial revolution of the twentieth century. The substance was chaulmoogra oil (later called hydnocarpus oil in the British Pharmacopoeia) obtained from the seeds of the fruit of various tropical trees that have been used since ancient times for the treatment of leprosy in India, China, and other countries of the Far East (94). There are many fanciful tales of how the efficacy of chaulmoogra oil came to be known. One story from India recounts how the god-king Rama contracted leprosy and was cured after eating the fruit of the Kalaw tree. He went on to use the fruit to cure an Indian princess, Piya, who had been banished to the forests after being branded a leper. The pair returned joyfully to the holy city of Benares (Varanasi) and spread the word of their discovery.

However unlikely this tale may be, use of chaulmoogra oil was widespread in India in the nineteenth century. Its introduction to western medicine is credited to Frederic John Mouat an English doctor who entered the Indian Medical Service in 1840 and rose to become professor of medicine at Bengal Medical College Hospital. He had always been interested in exploiting local remedies and in 1853 a friend, known only as Mr Jones, headmaster of the local Hindu College, recommended chaulmoogra oil to him as a specific for leprosy. Mouat's first patient is said to have been a drunk brought to the hospital by the police and subsequently diagnosed with leprosy. Pulped chaulmoogra seeds given orally and daily dressings of the ulcers with the oil improved the patients condition so remarkably—before he absconded after 2 months' treatment—that Mouat was persuaded to write up the findings and to recommend the treatment to fellow physicians as far afield as China and Mauritius (95).

Administration of the oil by mouth was not for the faint-hearted; its effect was so nauseating that many leprosy sufferers refused the treatment. Topical use, besides being messy, needed great persistence, and was of dubious efficacy. Injections of chaulmoogra oil into the affected areas seemed an obvious alternative. Introduction of the technique of hypodermic injection through a hollow needle is usually described as a dead heat between the Edinburgh Physician Alexander Wood and the French surgeon, Charles Pravaz of Lyons. Both described the method in 1853, but a Dublin surgeon, Francis Rynd used a similar device in 1844 and has a credible claim to precedence (96). Whatever the provenance, it became a popular way of administering certain drugs (notably narcotics) in the second half of the nineteenth century. The first person to adopt the technique for the treatment of leprosy was an Egyptian, Tortoulis Bey, private physician to Sultan Hussein Kamel. He had been using subcutaneous injections of creosote in patients with tuberculosis and in 1894, decided to try similar injections of chaulmoogra oil in a 35-year-old Egyptian Copt who had been unable to tolerate oral treatment. After an astonishing 584 injections administered over a 6-year period, the patient was declared cured (94). Later, Victor Heiser an American doctor in Manila and his house physician, Elidoro Mercado, introduced injections of a mixture of chaulmoogra oil with camphor and resorcin (97). This preparation reduced the nausea, but the injections were extremely painful and liable to cause tissue damage.

The solution to parenteral administration lay in the production of a purified derivative of the active constituents of the seeds. Fractionation of the complex mixture of natural oils was accomplished by Frederick B. Power, an American pharmacist and analytical chemist working at the Wellcome Chemical Research Laboratories,* which Henry Wellcome had established in London—with Power as director—after the premature death of his partner, Silas Burroughs. Power was an old and trusted friend of Wellcome's; they had met when they were both impoverished young men working in Chicago drug

---

* Eventually subsumed, together with the Wellcome Physiological Research Laboratories (established 1899) and the Wellcome Laboratories of Tropical Medicine (1946), into the Wellcome Research Laboratories at Beckenham in Kent.

stores. He was to have an important influence in establishing the research capability of Burroughs Wellcome and Company and its successor, the Wellcome Foundation, set-up in 1924 to unite the disparate activities of Henry Wellcome's empire (98).* Power's analysis of chaulmoogra oil from *Hydnocarpus anthelminthica*, *Hydnocarpus wightiana*, and *Taraktogenos kurzii* revealed two closely related long-chain fatty acids, which he called chaulmoogric acid and hydnocarpus acid. He also confirmed that seeds of *Gynocardia odorata*, sometimes recommended as an alternative source of chaulmoogra oil, did not contain the characteristic fatty acids of the other species.

Production of ethyl esters of the fatty acids, which were to become the basis of a standardized formulation, is often attributed to Arthur Dean, head of the chemistry department in the College of Hawaii. Dean was following up work commenced by one of his postgraduate students, Alice Ball an African–American whose career was cut short at the tragically early age of 24. In the year before her death she had become the first woman to graduate with a master's degree in science from the College of Hawaii (97).

The Hawaiian scientists were not, however, the first to hit upon the idea of esterification. A commercial formulation of the esters had already been patented and marketed a decade earlier in Germany. Franz Engel-Bey a German physician who had emigrated from Berlin to Egypt in 1879 for health reasons (99), had approached Bayer in Elberfeld to ask if they could produce a purified preparation of chaulmoogra oil that was free from the injurious side effects of the natural product. Felix Hoffmann and his colleagues took up the challenge. Following up Power's work at the Wellcome Chemical Research Laboratories, they produced a formulation containing the mixed esters of the total fatty acids of chaulmoogra oil that was suitable for injection. It was introduced commercially by Bayer in 1908 as 'Antileprol'. Even earlier, in 1891, Merck of Darmstadt had marketed a product containing the sodium salts of the fatty acids of the commercial oil. This substance was confusingly called sodium gynocardate, reflecting the erroneous belief that the seeds of *Gynocardia odorata* were a source of chaulmoogra oil. Around 1920, Burroughs Wellcome themselves launched a product similar to Bayer's Antileprol, which they branded as 'Moogrol'.

The celebrated Indian Medical Service physician, Leonard Rogers used injections of Merck's sodium gynocardate for the treatment of leprosy and also for tuberculosis. Rogers was a very influential member of the Service who had long been interested in leprosy and helped to found the British Empire Leprosy Relief Association (BELRA; now LEPRA) in 1924. Earlier he had been instrumental in setting up the School of Tropical Medicine in Calcutta in 1921, with the Ulsterman, John Megaw as the first director. When supplies of Merck's gynocardate became unavailable during the First World War, Rogers experimented with alternative formulations of the oil made for him in the chemistry department of Calcutta Medical College by Professor Chuni Lal Bose. He additionally introduced a locally

---

* The Wellcome Foundation became a subsidiary of Wellcome plc in 1986, and was later acquired by Glaxo to form Glaxo-Wellcome (now GlaxoSmithKline). Non-commercial activities had earlier been hived off into the Wellcome Trust, one of the world's most important medical charities.

made salt of cod-liver oil, which he called sodium morrhuate (from the Latin name for cod, *Gadus morrhua*), which was used in the belief that it acted on the waxy coat characteristic of acid-fast bacilli.

Rogers was one of the Indian Medical Service's most distinguished sons. He was well known for pursuing his aims with boundless energy and contributed to many fields of tropical medicine. He was nominated several times for a Nobel Prize, but the honour always eluded him. Not all his work was of unimpeachable quality, but such was his eminence that he wielded considerable influence. Thomas Henry, Director of the Wellcome Chemical Research Laboratories in King Street in the City of London, worked closely with Rogers and in 1926 was persuaded to prepare sodium salts of selected fractions of hydnocarpus oil according to Rogers' preferred 'gynocardate' formula. The compound was first used by Rogers on behalf of BELRA in India in 1926 and 1927 and was later sold by Burroughs Wellcome under the trade name 'Alepol'. The preparation could be given by the subcutaneous, intramuscular, and intravenous routes, though the manufacturers admitted that the intravenous administration might be hazardous (94).

In 1926 the chemist, Thomas Marvel Sharp, working under Henry at the Wellcome laboratories, also devised a formulation of mercury in hydnocarpus oil, marketed as Avenyl, intended to treat leprosy complicated by syphilis. An Avenyl–Moogrol compound followed. They additionally experimented with preparations of Rogers' sodium morrhuate and other oils such as soya and linseed, but none of these found their way on to the Wellcome list.*

Just how effective chaulmoogra oil and its derivatives were is hard to judge. All reports from reliable sources suggest that it had a definite alleviatory effect, but that relapses were common, even usual. The difficulty of establishing the true benefit of any treatment of leprosy is compounded by the fact that progression of the disease is slow and the prognosis uncertain. Even advanced cases with gross deformities can undergo apparent spontaneous cure: the so-called 'burnt-out case'.

Leonard Rogers was in no doubt of the drug's efficacy—or of his role in its development, which he trumpeted in 1948 in a paper reprinted from one he had written 30 years earlier with the preposterously vainglorious title *Conquest of the Leprosy Scourge. How I Found a Cure for the World's Most Dreaded Disease* (100).[†] Writing in 1933, the Scottish medical missionary Ernest Muir, one of the most distinguished leprologists of his day, had been more cautious. He regarded chaulmoogra and its derivatives more highly than any of the numerous other preparations that had been proposed for the treatment of the disease, but counselled against over-optimistic claims of its benefits (101). Others were even more sceptical. The difficulties of administration of chaulmoogra coupled with doubts about its effectiveness were already leading to a waning popularity for the treatment by the 1940s

---

* I am indebted to Dr Tilli Tansey of the Wellcome Trust Centre for the History of Medicine for information on Wellcome's antileprosy products in the 1920s.

† Rogers does graciously pay tribute to the crucial part played in the enterprise by his wife, Una Elsie (née North), formerly Sister North of the London Hospital.

when new drugs, the sulphones, began to offer sufferers from leprosy a realistic prospect of reliable and permanent cure without the pain and nausea of the only treatment that had previously been on offer.

Sulphones: exploiting the antituberculosis rejects

Much of the early work on chaulmoogra oil and its derivatives in America was carried out at Carville hospital, the United States national leprosarium. The hospital was founded in 1894 on a remote and run-down estate known as Indian Camp Plantation by the Mississippi river in Louisiana, 85 miles upriver from New Orleans and 2 miles from the small village of Carville. On 30 November 1894, the first patients, five men and two women, previously housed in what was known as 'Dr Beard's Hagan Avenue Pesthole'— close to Storyville in New Orleans, where the first stirrings of jazz, were being heard— were taken to their new home in a coal barge towed by the tug *Ellen Andrews*. Provisions and 80 beds donated by a New Orleans charity hospital were carried on the barge. The Indian Camp estate, a typical southern plantation, boasted an imposing but dilapidated mansion and seven former slave cabins in the largest of which the new arrivals were housed. John Smith Kendall, a cub reporter for a local newspaper the *Daily Picayune*,* recorded the event for posterity (102).

It was Dr Isadore Dyer, a dermatologist from Tulane University, New Orleans, who had first floated the idea of a hospital dedicated to patients with leprosy. He had originally wanted it to be sited near the university, where he later became Dean of the Medical School, but local opposition forced him to look elsewhere. In 1894 a lease was obtained on the Carville site on the pretext that it was to be used as an ostrich farm. Dr L. A. Wailes, a former Mississippi cavalry officer, was appointed as resident physician. In 1896 four nuns[†], Daughters of Charity of St Vincent de Paul, arrived to share the patients' meagre existence and to provide what care they could. Gradually, new buildings were constructed with help from the state and in 1921 Carville hospital was established as the national leprosarium under the auspices of the United States Public Health Service. It was later named the Gillis W. Long Hansen's Disease Center after Gillis Long, who had briefly been a Louisiana State representative of the United States Congress in the 1960s (103). If chaulmoogra oil was held in high esteem by the medical staff at Carville, the long-suffering recipients did not share their view. The American medical historian John Parascandola cites the memoirs of one long-term resident, Stanley Stein (Sidney Maurice Levyson):

> Whether I was to take the oil externally, internally, or—as someone once said—eternally, was up to me. The oral doses were nauseously given out in the cafeteria at mealtime. The injections were administered in what to me was a distressingly public manner . . . the after effects were sometimes frightful—painful suppurating abscesses which would generate on the patient's backside (104).

---

* Kendall later became a professor at Tulane University and in 1922 wrote a history of New Orleans.

[†] Patrick Feeny, in his book *The fight against leprosy* (95) names them as Sisters Beatrice Hart, Mary Thomas Stockum, Annie Costello, and Cyril Coupe.

In the circumstances it is not surprising that sulphones, when they became available, were welcomed as a major breakthrough, despite their evident toxicity.

In 1940, the chief medical officer at Carville was Guy Faget, a physician who had previous experience of treating tuberculosis. On hearing of the work of William Feldman and Corwin Hinshaw at the Mayo Clinic (see p. 155), Faget wrote to Elwood Sharp, director of the Department of Clinical Investigation at Parke, Davis in Detroit, where Promin had been synthesized in 1938, expressing an interest in the sulphone. Further encouraged by results obtained in the treatment of rat leprosy by Edmund Cowdry, a pathologist at Washington University in St Louis, Faget began treating volunteers with Promin in March 1941. To monitor the effect of treatment photographs of the patients were taken at intervals, by Sister Hilary Ross, a remarkable nun who was also the hospital's pharmacist, laboratory technician, and research biochemist (105). The results were encouraging, but the drug had to be given by intravenous injection and toxicity was a serious problem, especially as prolonged treatment was needed.

Promin had been developed as a more soluble version of diaminodiphenylsulphone (see p. 147)—a compound related to the sulphonamides, which was later given the generic name dapsone and is often known as DDS (Fig. 5.6). It also had the advantage of being patentable. Like sulphanilamide, dapsone's antibacterial potential had lurked unsuspected in the chemical literature: Emil Fromm, professor of chemistry in the Medical Faculty of the ancient Albert-Ludwig's university (founded 1457) in Freiburg im Breisgau, Germany, had described its preparation, buried deep within a scholarly paper on various *para*-nitrothiophenol derivatives, in 1908 (106). Coincidentally, it was the same year in which Paul Gelmo in Vienna described sulphanilamide (see p. 64).

Realizing its relationship to the sulphonamides, Gladwin Buttle and his colleagues at Burroughs Wellcome and Ernest Fourneau's team at the Institut Pasteur in Paris had investigated dapsone for antistreptococcal activity. The two groups were on friendly terms and it is probably no coincidence that their results were publicized within 2 days of one another: Buttle's in a paper in *The Lancet* on 5 June 1937 (107); Fourneau's at a session of l'Académie des Sciences held on 7 June 1937 (108). Both reports concluded that the sulphone was more active than sulphanilamide, but much more toxic to mice.

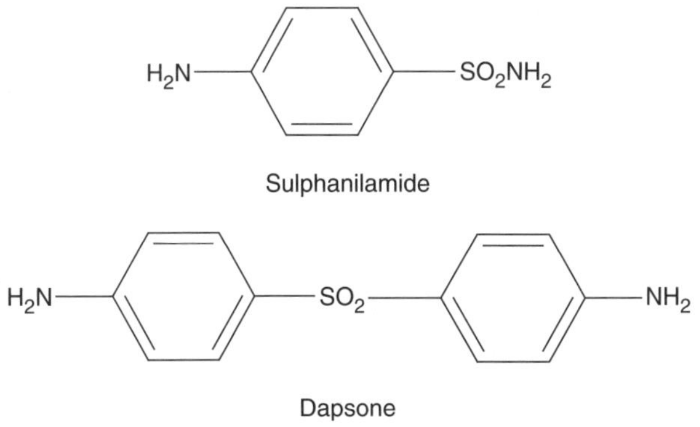

Sulphanilamide

Dapsone

Figure 5.6 Structures of sulphanilamide (a sulphonamide) and dapsone (a sulphone).

In Promin the two amino groups of dapsone were substituted with complex, but symmetrical chemical groupings. Various pharmaceutical companies joined in the hunt for further sulphone derivatives with improved properties. William Herbert Gray, a long-serving chemist at the Wellcome Chemical Research Laboratories in London who had earlier worked on antimony compounds and Salvarsan derivatives in the 1920s, synthesized Sulphetrone (solapsone) in 1938; Abbott Laboratories in America produced Diasone (sulfoxone), like solapsone a variation on the Promin theme, while Parke, Davis developed Promizole (thiazosulphone), in which only one of the amino groups is substituted. Solapsone and Diasone had the advantage of being absorbed when given by mouth; Promizole was promoted for a supposedly reduced propensity to cause side effects. ICI, a firm that were anxious to expand their drug portfolio, having launched a pharmaceutical division—Imperial Chemical (Pharmaceuticals) Ltd.—in 1942 (109),* marketed their own variety of dapsone, Avlosulfon, initially as a veterinary product for the treatment of streptococcal mastitis in cattle. Several other compounds were described offering variations on these themes, including a long-acting depot preparation of dapsone, acedapsone, which achieved some popularity, especially in India.

Although some trials of the American products Diasone and Promizole were probably carried out at Carville, among the first workers to examine systematically the effectiveness of sulphones, including Diasone, Sulphetrone and, later, dapsone, in field conditions were the Methodist medical missionaries Frank Davey and John Lowe working for the Nigeria Leprosy Service in Uzuakoli, Eastern Nigeria. Encouraged by Ernest Muir, by then medical secretary of the British Empire Leprosy Relief Association, Davey initiated studies of sulphones in March 1946, with Lowe taking over the work from the end of 1947. Abbott, Burroughs Wellcome and ICI supplied the drugs free of charge (110).

Meanwhile, Robert Cochrane had started to use the parent substance, dapsone, at Chingleput Leper Settlement, Madras (later the Lady Willingdon Leprosy Sanatorium and Madras Central Leprosy Teaching and Research Institute). Born in China of missionary parents, Cochrane Graduated from Glasgow University Medical School in 1924. After brief spells at St Bartholomew's Hospital in London and the London School of Tropical Medicine and Hygiene, he sailed for India in late 1924 as medical secretary for the Mission to Lepers (now the Leprosy Mission) an organization founded by the Irishman, Wellesley Bailey in 1874. Cochrane's first mentor in the leprosy field was no less an authority than Ernest Muir in Calcutta, who had worked on leprosy in India since 1908. Cochrane left India in 1927 critical of the work of the Mission to Lepers, but returned to the country as medical and general secretary of the British Empire Leprosy Relief Association in 1929, eventually becoming director of the Christian Medical College in Vellore, Madras. There he was instrumental in recruiting the famous orthopaedic surgeon, Paul Brand who specialized in the prevention and treatment of the limb and facial

---

* According to Reader (reference 109), ICI (Pharmaceuticals) Ltd. was set-up as a sales company, mainly for tax purposes. A Pharmaceuticals Division followed in 1944, but remained at first dependent on the Dyestuffs Division, which controlled the research laboratories.

deformities of leprosy. After a spell in London from 1951–65 as director of research and training at the Leprosy Study Centre (which he founded) Cochrane returned to India before moving again to Tanzania working as medical superintendent in leprosaria (111).

Cochrane learned that dapsone was being used to treat streptococcal mastitis in cows during a fund-raising trip to England in December 1945, not long after the end of the Second World War. He contacted ICI at their Alderley Park headquarters in Wilmslow, Cheshire, and was given a free supply of the drug to try in his leprosy patients. The first patients were treated in 1947, a year of euphoric celebration and turmoil in India as it gained its independence and a separate state of Pakistan was created, partitioned into West and East Pakistan (now Bangladesh).

Although dapsone is well absorbed when given orally, Cochrane used twice-weekly injections, apparently because the patients believed that jabs were more effective than pills (110). Results were impressive, but the doses used caused unacceptable side effects. The following year Frank Davey's team in Nigeria started using oral dapsone at the suggestion of Ernest Muir. By varying the dosage they were able to establish a twice-weekly escalating dosage regimen that was effective and well tolerated. Around the same time and independently, Hervé Floch and his colleague Pierre Destombes at the Pasteur Institute in French Guiana, and Lauro de Souza Lima in Brazil were carrying out similar trials of dapsone.

These pioneering studies established that Diasone, Sulphetrone, and dapsone had similar efficacy, Sulphetrone being rather less toxic, but also less well absorbed when given by mouth—properties that were probably related. Despite the fact that Diasone and Sulphetrone were thought to exert their effect after being metabolized in the body to dapsone, it had been widely expected that toxicity of the parent compound would preclude human use. But dapsone had one clear advantage over its rivals: the price. Lowe and Davey calculated that the cost of 1 year's treatment with Diasone or Sulphetrone was £15–20 per patient; the corresponding cost of dapsone treatment was 14 shillings (70 pence) a year. The figure could be further reduced to 10 shillings (50 pence) or less as it became clear that lower and less frequent dosage than that originally considered necessary was effective (110).

Since cost was of overriding importance in parts of the world where treatment of considerable numbers of poor people was most urgently required, it was an unequal contest. Dapsone, cheap, effective, easy to administer and—once a truncated regimen had been shown to work—acceptably safe, rapidly became the drug of choice for the treatment of all forms of leprosy. By 1950 it was clear that it represented, in the words of Lowe and Davey 'a revolution in the treatment of leprosy'.

What of other antituberculosis drugs? Streptomycin was tried and seemed to have some effect, but the need for repeated injections over a very long period, and the risk of toxicity at the doses required, made it a virtual non-starter. PAS and isoniazid were disappointingly found to have little or no influence on the course of leprosy. The inactivity of isoniazid was particularly disappointing since Vitaly Chorine had discovered the activity of nicotinamide, the precursor of isoniazid (see p. 172–3), in experiments on rat leprosy—underlining the unreliability of infection with *Mycobacterium lepraemurium* as a model of the human disease.

Interest was also shown in other tuberculosis rejects: thiambutosine, thiacetazone, ethionamide, and its congener, protionamide. All have some effect against *Mycobacterium leprae*; thiambutosine (under its manufacturer's code, CIBA 1906) was briefly tried in 1964 by the Baptist medical missionary, Stanley Browne. Browne was a much-celebrated and much-travelled tropical disease expert who had taken over in 1959 the directorship of the Leprosy Research Unit at Uzuakoli in Eastern Nigeria (where he was known as 'Mr Leprosy' or 'Bonganga'). Thiambutosine is less toxic than dapsone, but resistance develops more readily. Thiacetazone also fell victim to rapid development of resistance. Ethionamide and the somewhat better tolerated protionamide remain, as in tuberculosis, as rather unsatisfactory reserve drugs for use when all else fails.

Other drugs appeared on the scene in the late 1950s. The Swiss firm of Edward Geistlich and sons, originally founded in the nineteenth century to make glue, branched out into pharmaceutical products in 1943. In 1958 the firm produced a compound called Vadrine (and later Neovadrine), which came to the attention of the leprologist William Jopling, Director of the Jordan Hospital in Earlswood near Redhill, Surrey, which was opened in 1950 to accommodate leprosy patients from the Hospital for Tropical Diseases in St Pancras, London.* Jopling, together with his colleague at the Hospital for Tropical Diseases, the Histopathologist Dennis Ridley, found Vadrine to be similar in potency to the sulphones (112), but early hopes were not fulfilled and use of the drug quickly lapsed.

Another short-lived drug that became available for the topical treatment of leprosy around 1959—and was investigated by, among others, Frank Davey and Stanley Browne in Nigeria—was ditophal, developed and marketed by ICI as Etisul. It is a mercaptan compound (having a sulphydryl [–SH] group linked to carbon), several of which had been examined as potential antituberculosis compounds in the late 1940s and early 1950s (113). As anyone who has handled mercaptans knows, they have an unpleasant, penetrating, and persistent smell. Etisul was sometimes formulated with fragrances intended to mask the odour, but long-term use was precluded by resistance both in the bacteria and in patients who understandably objected to the distasteful stench. It remained available into the 1970s, but was then abandoned.

Multidrug therapy

Dapsone reigned supreme for 25 years. Amazingly, resistance did not seem to be a major problem despite the fact that low-dose intermittent therapy regimens that were widely used provided seemingly optimal conditions for the emergence of resistant mutants. Warning bells first began to ring in 1964, with a well-substantiated report of the development of sulphone resistance from John Pettit of the Sungei Buloh Leprosarium, Selangor, Malaysia in collaboration with Dick Rees at the National Institute for Medical Research, Mill Hill, London (114). Pettit selected seven patients from 2500 residing in the leprosarium who still had active lepromatous leprosy despite

---

* The Jordan Hospital closed in 1967.

treatment with Sulphetrone or dapsone for 13–15 years. Rees was able to show that three of the seven harboured leprosy bacilli refractory to sulphone action in mouse footpad infections.

Despite this scare, primary resistance in previously untreated patients still appeared to be rare and dapsone monotherapy remained standard until the late 1970s, when it became clear that the problem of resistance could no longer be ignored. Plainly, combination therapy, similar to that which was by now standard in the treatment of tuberculosis, would also be needed in leprosy. Fortunately, by this time two new drugs were available: the antituberculosis wonder drug, rifampicin (see p. 182–5), which had shown itself just as effective in leprosy; and clofazimine, developed by the Irish organic chemist, Vincent Barry, not as an antileprosy compound, but as an antituberculosis agent.

Clofazimine

Vincent Barry, originally from Cork, graduated in chemistry at University College, Dublin and took a job in the chemistry department of University College, Galway, working on polysaccharide chemistry. In 1943, the Irish government, concerned about the continuing rise of tuberculosis, and no doubt cognizant of developments that were occurring elsewhere in chemotherapy, provided funds for the Medical Research Council of Ireland to fund a Fellowship to investigate antituberculosis compounds. Barry was appointed to the Fellowship and took up his position in the chemistry department at University College, Dublin the following year. Searching round for leads, he discovered that predecessors in the chemistry department had left behind substances obtained from their studies of lichens, one of which was the organochlorine compound, diploicin, obtained in Ireland from the lichen, *Buellia canescens*. Barry found that a simple modification of this compound exhibited tuberculostatic activity, prompting examination of similar substances (115). Pursuing this line of enquiry, Barry's team found in 1948 a phenazine compound, which they called B 283 (the 'B' stands for 'Barry') that displayed impressive antituberculosis activity and, astonishingly, increased in potency over time as it spontaneously oxidized; as the activity increased the colour of the compound turned from pink to deep red. B 283, already known to chemists as anilinoaposafranine, was briefly tested in renal tuberculosis. It was also used in a few cases of leprosy by the Irish doctor, Joseph Barnes, at a Missionary Hospital run by the Irish Medical Missionaries of Mary in Ogoja, Nigeria which he had helped to set-up in 1944 (116). Unfortunately this substance and its close relatives proved highly toxic and were overtaken by other drugs that were becoming available, but the observation pointed the way to the investigation of further phenazine derivatives that might retain activity against tubercle bacilli, but be less toxic (117).

In 1951, the chemotherapy research unit moved from University College to better accommodation at their old rival, Trinity College, Dublin with Vincent Barry as Director. The occasion was celebrated by the organization of a Colloquium on the chemotherapy of tuberculosis to which Barry and his colleagues managed to attract delegates from the United Kingdom and continental Europe, and an eminent panel of speakers, including Gerhard Domagk, William Feldman, and the Austrian biochemist Edgar Lederer, then working at the Centre Nationale de la Recherche Scientifique in Paris*—quite a coup for a small group of Irish scientists at a time when Europe was still recovering from war.

During the 1950s, Barry was briefly deflected from his research with phenazines by the prospect of developing an improved isoniazid formulation, hinconstarch (see p. 178), but ramifications of the earlier project were still being explored. By 1954 related molecules known as iminophenazines were being investigated. In collaboration with the Swiss drug firm, Geigy, a series of iminophenazines were synthesized in which substitutions were added to the imino (NH–) group† and one of the first ones to be made, originally given the laboratory code B663 (and the Geigy code, G30320), turned out to have two highly desirable characteristics: it was very active *in vitro* against tubercle bacilli; and it was taken up and deposited as crystals within macrophage cells of the reticuloendothelial system—cells in which tubercle bacilli multiply (115).

The discovery of B663—subsequently called clofazimine—was trumpeted at the Fourteenth International Tuberculosis Conference in New Delhi in 1957, but celebrations were premature. Studies of experimental tuberculosis in guinea pigs and monkeys failed to confirm the in-vitro activity against *Mycobacterium tuberculosis*. A small trial on sanatorium patients at Davos in Switzerland similarly showed no effect. It later transpired that this was due to poor oral absorption, which could be improved by reformulating the drug, but the damage was done. Interest in clofazimine, which, outside Dublin, had never been great, waned further. Truth to tell, its credentials did not look promising: it was a bright red phenazine dye—a thoroughly old-fashioned and discredited concept for an antimicrobial agent in 1957—and was expensive to produce. Moreover, Ireland, though celebrated for many things, including outstanding contributions to world literature, was not at the forefront of medical research; the track record of earlier phenazines and hinconstarch from Barry's department was scarcely persuasive. Clofazimine was shelved.

There was relief among Geigy's scientists at the decision to abandon clofazimine, since everything with which it came into contact was stained red and it was difficult to handle. Their relief was short-lived. Late in 1959, Y. T. Chang of the National Institutes of Health in America, with whom Barry had earlier collaborated, found that clofazimine was active in murine leprosy and, although this is a poor model for the human disease, the finding was sufficient to keep interest in the compound alive. In 1960, Wolfgang Vischer of Geigy met Vincent Barry and Robert Cochrane at the Leprosy Study Centre in London and Cochrane offered to ask Stanley Browne, who had just taken over as director of research at the leprosy unit in Uzuakoli, if he would carry out a clinical trial (118). The trial started in Nigeria later the same year, but despite favourable results, the verdict was not encouraging: the drug appeared to be slower in its action than dapsone and there was a

---

* Lederer had been instrumental in developing the important technique of chromatography while working at the University of Heidelberg in 1932. While at Heidelberg he met and married a French woman, Hélène Fréchet, and went to live in France when Hitler came to power in 1933.

† The letter 'R' is conventionally used to collectively designate substitutions made to a particular part of a molecule; with this in mind Barry coined the term 'rimino' compounds for his imino derivatives.

suspicion (not substantiated by later studies) that resistance might easily develop. Since the manufacture of clofazimine was problematic and the cost likely to be prohibitive, development was again halted.

Fortunately, Browne still had sufficient clofazimine to continue with his clinical studies. Further investigation disclosed that the drug was not only effective, but that it also had an anti-inflammatory action that reduced the frequency and severity of erythema nodosum leprosum, a painful complication of the disease.* The finding coincided with the first reports of dapsone resistance and Browne successfully urged Geigy not to abandon development of clofazimine. Further trials confirmed the value of the compound and it was finally marketed under the name Lamprene in 1969. Rarely can a useful drug have been twice rescued from the brink of obscurity before finding its place in therapy.

The availability of clofazimine and rifampicin forestalled in the nick of time the threat of widespread dapsone resistance and ushered in a new era in the treatment of leprosy. The introduction of rifampicin was especially significant, allowing leprosy patients to be rendered non-infectious within a few days of starting therapy. The World Health Organization enthusiastically promoted multidrug regimens with great success. Twelve months of therapy with monthly rifampicin together with daily dapsone and clofazimine was found to be highly effective even in aggressive lepromatous leprosy.

Although leprosy is now a curable disease, chemotherapy still rests on relatively insecure foundations: dapsone is potentially toxic; clofazimine causes skin discoloration and dryness, which some patients find objectionable; and rifampicin, though very effective, is prone to the development of resistance. As with tuberculosis, ensuring compliance is of paramount importance. Apart from ethionamide, protionamide, thiacetazone, and thiambutosine, all of which have been largely abandoned, only a handful of alternative drugs have useful activity against *Mycobacterium leprae*. The oldest is the tetracycline derivative, minocycline (see p. 228), but newer agents such as the fluoroquinolone ofloxacin (p. 259) and the macrolide clarithromycin (p. 239) are also proving useful. In the less aggressive forms of the disease, single-dose therapy with rifampicin, minocycline, and ofloxacin may sometimes be effective if used early before multiple lesions develop (119).

There has been a dramatic reduction in the prevalence of leprosy since multidrug therapy was instituted as World Health Organization policy in 1982, with the number of countries in which the disease is endemic reduced from 122 to 24 in 1999 and to just 12 in 2002 (120). In that time it is estimated that around 8 million patients have been successfully treated—albeit retaining irreversible disability and disfigurement in many cases. Nevertheless, there are still around half a million known sufferers, mostly in India and other parts of south-east Asia, and many people in the Third World have no access to the drugs that would cure them. In 1999 the World Health Organization, in partnership with the Nippon Foundation of Japan, the pharmaceutical giant, Novartis (formerly CIBA-Geigy), the Danish International Development Assistance Agency, and governments of

* The same claim was later made for thalidomide but has since been discredited.

the countries in which the disease is still endemic, launched a Global Alliance for the Elimination of Leprosy (121). The goal is to free the world completely of the disease and drugs are being provided free of charge. It will not be easy, but success would mean a great burden has been lifted from humankind.

References

1. World Health Organization. http://www.who.int/mediacentre/factsheets/who104/en/index.html

2. Dickens C. *The life and adventures of Nicholas Nickleby,* Chapter 49. http://www.dickens-literature.com/Nicholas_Nickleby/index.html

3. Larané A. Jours d'histoire. 16 Mars 1914. Mme Caillaux tire sur Gaston Calmette. http://www.herodote.net/histoire03161.htm

4. Sakula A (1983). BCG: who were Calmette and Guérin? *Thorax* **38**, 806–12.

5. Richmond C (2006). Philip D'Arcy Hart (obituary). *BMJ* **333**, 449.

6. Heaf FRG (1955). BCG vaccination. *Lancet* **1**, 315–20.

7. D'Arcy Hart P (1946). Chemotherapy of tuberculosis. Research during the past 100 years. *BMJ* **2**, 805–12 and 849–55.

8. Dubos R, Dubos J (1953). *The white plague. Tuberculosis, man and society*. Little Brown & Co., Boston, 1952; Gollancz, London.

9. Brock TD (1988). *Robert Koch. A lifetime in medicine and bacteriology*, pp. 195–213. Science Tech Publishers, Madison.

10. Seibert FB (1941). History of the development of purified protein derivative tuberculin. *Am Rev Tuber* **44**, 1–8.

11. Benedek TG (2004). The history of gold therapy for tuberculosis. *J Hist Med Allied Sci* **59**, 50–89.

12. Amberson JB, McMahon BT, Pinner M (1931). A clinical trial of sanocrysin in pulmonary tuberculosis. *Am Rev Tuber* **24**, 401–35; Diaz M, Neuhauser D. James Burns Amberson (1890–1979). *The James Lind Library* (www.jameslindlibrary.org)

13. Tytler WH (1944). Sulphone compounds in the chemotherapy of tuberculosis: a review of experimental results and pharmacological data. *Tubercle* **25**, 95–104 and 1945; **26**, 23–8.

14. Waksman SA (1954). *My life with the microbes*. Simon and Schuster, New York. UK edition, Robert Hale, London, 1958.

15. Waksman SA (1927). *Principles of soil microbiology*, 2nd edn. Williams & Wilkins, Baltimore.

16. Moberg CL (1990). Friend of the good earth: René Dubos (1901–1982). In: Moberg CL, Cohn ZA, eds. *Launching the antibiotic era*, pp. 85–97. The Rockefeller University Press, New York.

17. Hotchkiss RD (1990). From microbes to medicine: gramicidin, René Dubos, and the Rockefeller. In: Moberg CL, Cohn ZA, eds. *Launching the antibiotic era*, pp. 1–18. The Rockefeller University Press, New York.

18. Cooper JE. A brief romance with magic bullets: René Dubos at the dawn of the antibiotic era. http://www.nyam.org/library/historical/hist99_4.html

19. Herrell WE, Heilman D (1941). Experimental and clinical studies on gramicidin. *J Clin Invest* **20**, 583–91.

20. Dubos R, Dubos J (1952). *The white plague. Tuberculosis, man and society*. Little Brown & Co, Boston; Gollancz, London, 1953.

21. Waksman SA (1941). Antagonistic relations of microörganisms. *Bacteriol Rev* **5**, 231–91.

22. Davis BD (1990). Two perspectives: on René Dubos, and on antibiotic actions. In: Moberg CL, Cohn ZA, eds. *Launching the antibiotic era*, pp. 69–81. The Rockefeller University Press, New York.

23. Waksman S, Woodruff HB (1940). Bacteriostatic and bactericidal substances produced by soil Actinomyces. *Proc Soc Exp Biol Med* **45**, 609–614.

24. Schatz A, Bugie E, Waksman SA (1944). Streptomycin, a substance exhibiting antibiotic activity against gram-positive and gram-negative bacteria. *Proc Soc Exp Biol Med* **55**, 66–9.

25. Conroe JH (1978). Pay dirt: the story of streptomycin. Part I. From Waksman to Waksman. *Am Rev Res Dis* **117**, 773–81.

26. Schatz A (1965). Antibiotics and dentistry. Part I: Some personal reflections on the discovery of streptomycin. *Pakistan Dental Rev* **15**, 125–34; Schatz A. The true story of the discovery of strepto-mycin. Undated. http://www.oneearthherbs.com/Streptomycin.htm

27. Cameron V, Long ER (1959). *Tuberculosis medical research. National Tuberculosis Association 1904–1955*, pp. 38–9. National Tuberculosis Association, New York.

28. Myers JA (1961). William Hugh Feldman D.V.M., M.Sc., D.Sc. (Hon). *Lancet* **91**, 173–81.

29. The Hinshaw Family Association. *Horton Corwin Hinshaw*. http://www.rawbw.com/~hinshaw/cgi-bin/id?1375

30. Feldman WH, Hinshaw HC, Moses HE (1941). The treatment of experimental tuberculosis with Promin (sodium salt of *p,p'*-diamino-diphenyl-sulfone-*N,N'*-didextrose sulfonate): a preliminary report. *Proc Staff Meet Mayo Clinic* **16**, 187–90; Feldman WH, Hinshaw HC, Moses HE (1942). Promin in experimental tuberculosis. *Am Rev Tuber* **45**, 303–33.

31. Conroe JH (1978). Pay dirt: the story of streptomycin. Part II. Feldman and Hinshaw; Lehmann. *Am Rev Respir Dis* **117**, 957–68.

32. Lechevalier HA (1980). The search for antibiotics at Rutgers University. In: Parascandola J, ed. *The history of antibiotics—a symposium*, pp. 113–23. American Institute of the History of Pharmacy, Madison, WI.

33. Ryan F (1992). *Tuberculosis: the greatest story never told*. Swift Publishers, Bromsgrove, pp. 332–3; Snowbeck C (14 April 2001). Did McCandless woman get fair share for role in discovery of strepto-mycin? Pittsburgh Post-Gazette. Cited at http://fox.rollins.edu/~egregory/parent.html#article

34. Helfand WH, Woodruff HB, Coleman KMH, Cowen DL (1980). Wartime industrial development of penicillin in the United States. In: Parascandola J, ed. *The history of antibiotics—a symposium*, pp. 31–56. American Institute of the History of Pharmacy, Madison, WI.

35. Rochester Post-Bulletin (24 January 1994). *Mayo clinic helped test tuberculosis treatment*. Archive article retrieved from: http://news.postbulletin.com/

36. Cameron V, Long ER (1959). *Tuberculosis medical research. National Tuberculosis Association 1904–1955*, p. 112. National Tuberculosis Association, New York.

37. Hinshaw HC, Feldman WH, Pfuetze KH (1946). Treatment of tuberculosis with streptomycin: a summary of observations on one hundred cases. *J Am Med Assoc* **132**, 778–82.

38. Heilman D, Heilman F, Hinshaw H, *et al.* (1945). Streptomycin: absorption, diffusion, excretion and toxicity. *Am J Med Sci* **210**, 576–84.

39. Cameron V, Long ER (1959). *Tuberculosis medical research. National Tuberculosis Association 1904–1955*, p. 66. National Tuberculosis Association, New York.

40. Streptomycin Committee, Central Office, Veterans Administration (1947). The effect of strepto-mycin upon pulmonary tuberculosis. Preliminary report of a coöperative study of 223 patients by the Army, Navy, and Veterans Administration. *Am Rev Tuber* **56**, 485–507.

41. Riggins HM, Hinshaw HC (1947). The streptomycin–tuberculosis research project of the American Trudeau Society. *Am Rev Tuber* **56**, 168–73.

42. Ryan F (1992). *Tuberculosis: the greatest story never told*, pp. 366–7. Swift Publishers, Bromsgrove.

43. Yoshioka A (1998). Use of randomisation in the Medical Research Council's clinical trial of strepto-mycin in pulmonary tuberculosis in the 1940s. *BMJ* **317**, 1220–3. Also available at: http://bmj.bmjjournals.com/cgi/content/full/317/7167/1220

44. Wilkinson L (1997). Sir Austin Bradford Hill; medical statistics and the quantitative approach to the prevention of disease. *Addiction* **92**, 657–66.

45. Medical Research Council (1948). Streptomycin treatment of pulmonary tuberculosis. *BMJ* **2**, 769–82.

46. Scadding JG (1999). Memories of why allocation by random sampling numbers was used. *BMJ* **318**, 1352; Chalmers I, Clarke M. J Guy Scadding and the move from alternation to randomization. In: *The James Lind Library* (www.jameslindlibrary.org)

47. Gifford JF. The chemistry of life. In: Duke University, *The Faculty Forum 1998*, Vol. 9 http://www.duke.edu/web/FacultyForum/vol9/ffapr98.htm

48. Bernheim F (1940). The effect of salicylate on the oxygen uptake of the tubercle bacillus. *Science* **92**, 204.

49. Woods DD (1940). The relation of *p*-aminobenzoic acid to the mechanism of action of sulphanilamide. *Br J Exp Pathol* **21**, 74–90.

50. Fildes P (1940). A rational approach to research in chemotherapy. *Lancet* **1**, 955–7.

51. Lehmann J (1946). *Para*-aminosalicylic acid in the treatment of tuberculosis. *Lancet* **1**, 15–16.

52. The therapeutic trials committee of the Swedish National Association against tuberculosis (1950). Para-aminosalicylic acid treatment in pulmonary tuberculosis. Comparison between 94 treated and 82 untreated cases. *Am Rev Tuber* **61**, 597–612.

53. Medical Research Council (1949). Treatment of pulmonary tuberculosis with para-aminosalicylic acid. Preliminary report. *BMJ* **2**, 1521.

54. Medical Research Council (1950). Treatment of pulmonary tuberculosis with streptomycin and para-amino-salicylic acid. *BMJ* **2**, 1073–85.

55. American Philosophical Society (1925–1994). H. Corwin Hinshaw papers, http://www.amphilsoc.org/library/mole/h/hinshaw.htm

56. Domagk G, Behnisch R, Mietzsch F, Schmidt H (1946). Über eine neue, gegen Tuberkelbazillen in vitro wirksame Verbindungsklasse. *Naturwissenschaften* **33**, 315.

57. Domagk G (1947). Further progress in chemotherapy of bacterial infections. Nobel Lecture, December 12. http://www.nobel.se/medicine/laureates/1939/domagk-lecture.html

58. Domagk G (1947). *Pathologische Anatomie und Chemotherapie der Infektionskrankheiten.* Georg Thieme Verlag, Stuttgart.

59. McDermott W (1969). The story of INH. *J Infect Dis* **119**, 678–83. Also published as 'Early days of antimicrobial therapy.' In: Hobby G, ed. *Antimicrobial agents and chemotherapy—1968*, pp. 1–6. American Society for Microbiology, Bethesda, MD.

60. Kushner S, Dalalian H, Cassell RT, Sanjurjo JL, McKenzie D, Subbarow Y (1948). Experimental chemotherapy of tuberculosis. I. Substituted nicotinamides. *J Org Chem* **13**, 834–6; McKenzie D, Malone L, Kushner S, Oleson JJ, SubbaRow Y (1948). The effect of nicotinic acid amide on experimental tuberculosis of white mice. *J Lab Clin Med* **33**, 1249–53.

61. Chorine V (1945). Action de l'amide nicotinique sur les bacilles du genre Mycobacterium. *Comptes Rendu Hebdomadaires des Séances de l'Académie des Sciences* **220**, 150–1.

62. Huant E (1945). Note sur l'action de très fortes doses d'amide nicotinique dans les lésions bacillaires. *Gazette des Hôpitaux Civiles et Militaires* **118**, 259–60.

63. Fox HH (1953). The chemical attack on tuberculosis. *Trans NY Acad Sci* **15**, 234–42.

64. McCune RM, Tompsett R, McDermott W (1956). The fate of mycobacterium tuberculosis in mouse tissues as determined by the microbial enumeration technique. II. The conversion of tuberculous infection to the latent state by the administration of pyrazinamide and a companion drug. *J Exp Med*, **104**, 763–802.

65. Gorvin JH (1998). The development of chemical research in the Wellcome Laboratories (UK) 1896–1965. In: *Wellcome's legacies*, pp. 53–92. The Wellcome Trust, London.

66. Various authors and titles (1952). *Am Rev Tuber* **65**, 357–442.

67. Mackaness GB (1990). New remedies for an ancient infection: antibiotics and tuberculosis. In: Moberg CL, Cohn ZA, eds. *Launching the antibiotic era*, pp. 57–68. Rockefeller University Press, New York.

68. Christie DFA (2005). In Tansey EM, ed. *Short course therapy of tuberculosis*, p. 10. Witness Seminar No. 24. Wellcome Trust Centre for the history of medicine at University College London. Available at: http://www.ucl.ac.uk/histmed/PDFS/Publications/Witness/wit24.pdf

69. Crofton J (1959). Chemotherapy of tuberculosis. *BMJ* **1**, 1610–14.

70. Hobby GL, Lenert TF, Rivoirez C, Donikian M, Pikula D (1953). In vitro and in vivo activity of streptomycin and isoniazid singly and in combination. *Am Rev Tuber* **67**, 808–26.

71. Barry VC (1956). Hinconstarch: a new chemotherapeutic agent for tuberculosis. *J Irish Med Assoc* **38**, 68–71.

72. Bosworth DM, Wright HA, Fielding JW (1953). The treatment of bone and joint tuberculosis; the effect of 1-isonicotinyl-2-isopropylhydrazine: a preliminary report. *J Bone Joint Surg Am* **34**-A, 766–71.

73. Slotkin TA (1999). Mary Bernheim and the discovery of monoamine oxidase. *Brain Res Bull* **50**, 373.

74. Shepherd RG, Baughn C, Cantrall ML, Goodstein B, Thomas JP, Wilkinson RG (1966). Structure–activity studies leading to ethambutol, a new type of antituberculous compound. *Ann NY Acad Sci* **135**, 686–710.

75. Thomas JP, Baughn C0, Wilkinson RG, Shepherd RG (1961). A new synthetic compound with anti-tuberculous activity in mice: ethambutol (dextro-2,2′-(ethylenediimino)-di-l-butanol). *Am Rev Respir Dis* **83**, 891–3.

76. Havard DWH, Garrod LP, Waterworth PM (1959). Deaf or dead? A case of subacute bacterial endocarditis treated with penicillin and neomycin. *BMJ* **1**, 688–9.

77. Caltrider PG (1967). Viomycin. In: Gottlieb D, Shaw PD, eds. *Antibiotics I. Mechanism of action*, pp. 677–80. Springer Verlag, Berlin.

78. Stark WM, Higgens CE, Wolfe RN, Hoehn MM, McGuire JM (1963). Capreomycin, a new antimy-cobacterial agent produced by *Streptomyces capreolus* sp. n. In: Sylvester JC, ed. *Antimicrobial agents and chemotherapy—1962*, pp. 596–606. American Society for Microbiology, Ann Arbor, MI.

79. Neuhaus FC (1967). D-Cycloserine and O-carbamyl-D-serine. In: Gottlieb D, Shaw PD, eds. *Antibiotics I. Mechanism of action*, pp. 40–83. Springer Verlag, Berlin.

80. Mulinos MJ (1956). Cycloserine: an antibiotic paradox. In: Welch H, Marti-Ibañez F, eds. *Antibiotics annual 1955–1956*, pp. 131–5. Medical Encyclopedia Inc., New York.

81. Epstein IG, Nair KGS, Boyd LJ (1955). Cycloserine, a new antibiotic, in the treatment of human pulmonary tuberculosis: a preliminary report. *Antibiotic Med Clin Ther* **1**, 80–93.

82. Editorial (1955). Cycloserine. *BMJ* **1**, 1140–1.

83. Laake K, Oeksengaard AR (2003). D-Cycloserine for Alzheimer's disease (Cochrane review). The Cochrane Library, Issue 4. John Wiley & Sons, Chichester. Abstract available at: http://www.cochrane.org/cochrane/revabstr/ab003153.htm

84. Sensi P (1983). History of the development of rifampin. *Rev Infect Dis* **5** (Suppl. 3), S402–6.

85. Frontali L, Tecce G (1967). Rifamycins. In: Gottlieb D, Shaw PD, eds. *Antibiotics I. Mechanism of action*, pp. 415–26. Springer Verlag, Berlin.

86. Sensi P, Maggi N, Füresz S, Maffii G (1967). Chemical modifications and biological properties of rifamycins. In: Hobby GL, ed. *Antibiotics and chemotherapy—1966*, pp. 699–714. American Society for Microbiology, Ann Arbor, MI.

87. Dawson JJY, Devadatta S, Fox W, *et al.* (1966). A 5-year study of patients with pulmonary tuberculosis in a concurrent comparison of home and sanatorium treatment for one year with isoniazid plus PAS. *Bull World Health Organ* **34**, 533–51.

88. Report (1992). National action plan to combat multidrug-resistant tuberculosis. *Morbidity and Mortality Weekly Report*41 (RR-11): 1–48. Also available at: http://www.cdc.gov/mmwr/preview/mmwrhtml/00031159.htm

89. Shepard CC (1960). The experimental disease that follows the injection of human leprosy bacilli into foot-pads of mice. *J Exp Med* **112**, 445–54.

90. Colston MJ, Hilson GRF (1976). Growth of *Mycobacterium leprae* and *M. marinum* in congenitally athymic (nude) mice. *Nature* **262**, 399–401.

91. Kirchheimer WE, Storrs EE (1971). Attempts to establish the armadillo as a model for the study of leprosy. *Int J Lepr Other Mycobact Dis* **39**, 693–702.

92. Storrs EE (1971). The nine-banded armadillo: a model for leprosy and other biomedical research. *Int J Lepr Other Mycobact Dis* **39**, 703–14.

93. Burchfield H. Our story. http://pandoras-box.org/my02000.htm; Martin B. Armadillo–leprosy controversy. http://www.uow.edu.au/arts/sts/bmartin/dissent/documents/Burchfield/

94. Tomb JW (1933). Chaulmoogra oil and its derivatives in the treatment of leprosy. *J Trop Med Hyg* **36**, 170–8, 186–9 and 201–7.

95. Feeny P (1964). *The fight against leprosy*, pp. 105–15. Elek Books, London.

96. Coakley D (1992). *Irish masters of medicine*, pp. 99–105. Town House, Dublin.

97. Parascandola J (2003). Chaulmoogra oil and the treatment of leprosy. http://lhncbc.nlm.nih.gov/lhc/docs/published/2003/pub2003048.pdf

98. James RR (1994). *Henry Wellcome*. Hodder & Stoughton, London.

99. Dünschede H-B (1971). *Tropenmedizinische Forschung bei Bayer*, pp. 8 and 10–14. Michael Triltsch Verlag, Düsseldorf.

100. Rogers L (1948). Conquest of the leprosy scourge. How I found a cure for the world's most dreaded disease. *Lepr India* **20**, 153–7.

101. Muir E (1933). Treatment of leprosy. *Int J Lepr* **1**, 407–61.

102. The Daily Picayune (2 December 1894). Seven sufferers quietly removed from the local hospital at the close of the city's insufficient keeping and taken to a lovely home in Iberville parish where comforts will be provided and doctors and nurses placed in charge. Available at: http://bphc.hrsa.gov/nhdp/images/pdfs/THE_PICAYUNE_1894.pdf

103. A history of Carville (1973). Excerpted from: Furman B. *A Profile of the United States Public Health Service 1798–1948*, pp. 308–11. U S Government Printing Office, Washington, DC. Available at: http://fortyandeight.org/thestar/carville/carville_history.htm

104. Stein S (with Blochman LG) (1963). *Alone no longer: the story of a man who refused to be one of the living dead*, pp. 38–9. Funk and Wagnalls, New York. Cited in reference 97 above.

105. Gould CM. *Sister Hilary Ross and Carville. Her thirty-seven years struggle against Hansen's disease.* Master's degree thesis, University of New Orleans. Available at: http://fortyandeight.org/thestar/sisters/V50I5P6.htm

106. Fromm E, Wittmann J (1908). Derivitate des *p*-nitothiophenols. *Berichte der Deutschen Chemischen Gesellschaft* **41**, 2264–73.

107. Buttle GAH, Stephenson D, Smith S, Foster GE (1937). The treatment of streptococcal infections in mice with 4:4′diaminodiphenylsulphone. *Lancet* **1**, 1331–4.

108. Fourneau E, Tréfouël J, Nitti F, Bovet D, Tréfouël J (1937). Action antistreptococcique des derives sulfurés organiques. *Comptes Rendu Hebdomadaires des Séances de l'Académie des Sciences*, 1763–6.

109. Reader WJ (1975). *Imperial Chemical Industries. A history. Volume II. The first quarter century 1926–1952*, p. 459. Oxford University Press, London.

110. Lowe J, Davey TF (1951). Four years' experience of sulphone treatment of leprosy. *Trans R Soc Trop Med Hyg* **44**, 635–62.

111. Banerjee A (1996). Dr Robert Greenhill Cochrane CMG MD FRCP DTM & H: leprologist par excellence. *J Med Biog* **4**, 137–40.

112. Jopling WH, Ridley DS (1958). Vadrine (S. 131) in the treatment of lepromatous leprosy. *Lepr Rev* **29**, 143–7.

113. Barry VC (1964). The development of the chemotherapeutic agent for tuberculosis. In: Barry VC, ed. *Chemotherapy of tuberculosis*, pp. 46–64. Butterworth, London.

114. Pettit JHS, Rees RJW (1964). Sulphone resistance in leprosy. An experimental and clinical study. *Lancet* **2**, 673–74.

115. Barry VC (1969). Boyle Medal lecture. Synthetic phenazine derivatives and mycobacterial disease: a twenty year investigation. *Sci Proc R Dublin Soc*, Series A3, 153–70.

116. Allday EJ, Barnes J (1952). Treatment of leprosy with B. 283. *Ir J Med Sci*, 421–5.

117. Barry VC, Belton JG, Conalty ML, Twomey D (1948). Anti-tubercular activity of oxidation products of substituted *o*-phenylene diamines. *Nature* **162**, 622–3.

118. Yawalkar SJ. *Contributions of Novartis to the development of MDT for leprosy.* http://www.novartisfoundation.com/pdf/leprosy_medical_paramedical_18.pdf

119. Lockwood DNJ, Kumar B (2004). Treatment of leprosy. *BMJ* **328**, 1447–8.

120. Lockwood DNJ, Suneetha, S (2005). Leprosy: too complex a disease for a simple elimination paradigm. *Bull World Health Organ* **83**, 230–5.

121. World Health Organization. *Elimination of leprosy as a world problem.* http://www.who.int/lep/

Chapter 6

The golden years of pills and profits

'Holding out suppliant Petri dishes', as Florey picturesquely called it, soon gave way to soil surveys, on which the great pharmaceutical houses spent millions in the hope of hundredfold returns. A large and very profitable industry grew up, thanks to which and a few more chance discoveries we now have antibiotics to deal with almost any infection except those due to viruses.

Medicine's debt to Florey. *British Medical Journal,*
2 March 1968, p. 529[*]

The post-war bonanza

The 50 years that followed the end of the Second World War witnessed a seemingly endless flow of new antibacterial agents. Well over 250 individual compounds suitable for systemic use (i.e. excluding those restricted to topical application, which would include many antiseptics) found their way on to the market throughout the world and, although some were mere copycat products or novel compounds of dubious value, many proved to be of genuine benefit in helping to transform the treatment of infectious disease.

There is no dispute that it was the success of sulphonamides and penicillin that provided the impetus for pharmaceutical and chemical firms to invest in research into what clearly had the potential to be an extremely lucrative area. Streptomycin and other anti-tuberculosis and antileprosy agents further helped to point the way, but these drugs were not to be the really big money-spinners. After all, some of the most useful antimycobacterial compounds were not patentable and any profits to be made quickly evaporated as the drugs became victims of their own success; the bulk of the market was soon confined to the world's most impoverished communities. What these agents did do was to reinforce the view that twin approaches were likely to be rewarding: the hunt for naturally occurring antimicrobial products from the inexhaustible resources of Mother Nature; and the more difficult pursuit of synthetic chemicals that would specifically attack vulnerable targets in the bacteria cell. In the event it was antibiotics that led the way, but one of the most profitable avenues, once the major antibiotic families had been uncovered,

---

[*] See footnote, p. 85.

turned out to be the synthesis of semi-synthetic variants of these drugs with improved antibacterial or—more commonly—pharmacological properties.

The brilliant success in making penicillin generally available at an affordable price during and immediately after the war, thanks largely to the efforts of the American pharmaceutical industry, provided the evidence of what might be to come. There was renewed confidence in the ability of commercial scientists to deliver the goods, and such confidence was not misplaced. The pharmaceutical houses were right at the forefront of the antibiotic revolution and practically all the drugs that have helped to mitigate the impact of infection since the end of the Second World War have resulted from their efforts. The input of academia and government agencies has been marginal while scientists in totalitarian regimes have been singularly unproductive. Of course, some of the less edifying practices of the drug industry have rightly attracted censure, but it would be churlish not to acknowledge the positive side of their activities. If their energies have been amply rewarded, human health has also benefited immeasurably.

For the pharmaceutical industry the antibiotic revolution occurred at a crucial time just after the Second World War. The profits made by the most successful compounds were enormous. Antibiotics vastly improved the prospects of firms like Beecham, Glaxo, and Lilly and many other pharmaceutical firms—notably in the United States, Britain, continental Europe, and Japan—profited to a greater or lesser degree during the antimicrobial boom years. Moreover, by providing large returns that could be ploughed back into more general research in much expanded and well-resourced facilities, the antimicrobial goose laid golden eggs in many other therapeutic areas.

The dominance of the pharmaceutical industry makes the task of identifying the brains behind the post-war advances difficult. The brilliance of individual scientists was submerged in the teamwork that business efficiency demanded. Detailed descriptions of how discoveries were made became commercially sensitive information; much was hidden in company archives unavailable outside the firm. Public disclosure was often delayed to protect patent rights so that the date when a particular antibiotic was discovered can be difficult to pin down. When information was finally published, the wording was circumspect and sometimes unrevealing in important details. In many of the early studies, compounds are often identified by laboratory codes that have long fallen into disuse. Piecing together the sequence of events and attributing credit many years after the event is at best problematical and at worst impossible. The main sources of evidence remaining in the public arena, aside from the occasionally revealing memoirs of the chief protagonists, are the proceedings of scientific conferences and the mass of other published literature that flourished in the palmy days of antibiotic discovery.

Getting the message across

After the Second World War books on antibiotics began to proliferate, among them Howard Florey's monumental two-volume *Antibiotics*, written with the other members of the original Oxford team and published by Oxford University Press in 1949 (1). The need for forums in which developments in the discovery and use of antimicrobial agents could be brought to the attention of the medical, scientific, and commercial communities also led to the formation of specialist periodicals and regular scientific meetings dedicated to the subject of antimicrobial chemotherapy.

Japan led the way with the *Journal of Antibiotics*, first published in 1947 as the *Journal of Penicillin* (the name was changed to the more familiar title the following year). It remains one of the chief repositories for much basic antibiotic research, especially that emanating from Japanese laboratories. In the United States, several symposia devoted specifically to antimicrobial agents were convened soon after the war and an abortive attempt was made to publish a new journal, also to be called *Journal of Antibiotics* under the editorship of Henry Welch, Director of the Division of Antibiotics of the Food and Drug Administration (FDA). The venture fell through, but Welch in partnership with Félix Martí-Ibáñez rescued the idea, setting up a business, Medical Encyclopedia Inc., to publish medical books and journals, predominantly on antibiotics. Many of the famous figures in the antibiotic world, including Ernst Chain and Howard Florey, were persuaded to act on their various editorial boards. Martí-Ibáñez was a Spanish psychiatrist who had found himself on the wrong side at the end of the Spanish civil war and fled to the United States where he eventually became Professor of the History of Medicine at New York Medical College. One of Welch and Martí-Ibáñez's joint projects was *Antibiotics Annual*, which documented the proceedings of an annual symposium sponsored by their company and the FDA, Welch's employer. It appeared each year from 1953 to 1960 briefly changing its name to the more accurate *Antimicrobial Agents Annual* for the final volume. Martí-Ibáñez was a prolific writer who fancied himself as a philosopher and social commentator. As well as providing a useful source of information on developments in antibiotics, *Antibiotics Annual* contains rambling essays expounding his often idiosyncratic views.

By the end of the 1950s Medical Encyclopedia's publications, particularly one called *Antibiotic Medicine and Clinical Therapy*, which had a short-lived British edition, but also including *Antibiotics Annual*, were being openly criticized by many doctors as being biased to particular company products and policies. Welch's extramural activities, which were clearly incompatible with his official job of overseeing antibiotic regulation, were at last being called into question at the FDA. They also came under scrutiny during a congressional enquiry into the pharmaceutical industry that was taking place at the time (see p. 227). Welch was forced to resign and the FDA was made to put its house in order (2).

The Welch affair led to *Antibiotics Annual* losing all credibility and there were calls for an independent non-commercial structure that would bring together representatives of the various disciplines involved in antimicrobial drug research. In 1960 the American Society for Microbiology agreed to assume responsibility for the organization of an annual symposium—to be called the *Interscience Conference on Antimicrobial Agents and Chemotherapy*—and to publish the proceedings. The first of these conferences was held in New York City from 31 October–2 November 1961 and was published in book form the following year. These annual volumes continued to be published until 1970, by which time it was clear that the deluge of information generated on the subject of antimicrobial agents necessitated publication of a monthly journal; thus, in 1972, *Antimicrobial Agents and Chemotherapy*, the most influential of the journals devoted to the subject, was born.

The annual conference—now known universally by its acronym, ICAAC—continued and remains hugely popular, attracting several thousand delegates from all over the world. It continues to be the major platform for the disclosure of new antimicrobial compounds; hundreds of novel agents—mostly now long forgotten—have been premièred at the annual autumn meetings. Unfortunately, since 1970 the proceedings are published only as abstracts which offer little opportunity for critical assessment.

1961 also saw the foundation of the International Society of Chemotherapy, which sponsors a large congress devoted to antimicrobial and anticancer agents in suitable locations throughout the world at 2-year intervals. Since 1991 it has published its own journal, the *International Journal of Antimicrobial Agents*. During the Seventh International Congress of Chemotherapy in Prague in 1971 the British Society for Antimicrobial Chemotherapy was founded at a meeting convened by David Williams, then at Dudley Road Hospital, Birmingham, but later (from 1974) Goldsmith Professor of Microbiology at the London Hospital Medical College in Whitechapel. He became the first General Secretary of the British Society and is generally credited with being its inspiration.* In 1975 he founded—and for 6 years edited—the *Journal of Antimicrobial Chemotherapy*, which has become one of the leading academic journals in the field.

International meetings devoted to chemotherapy have from the start been dominated (and largely funded) by the pharmaceutical industry, with large trade exhibitions associated with the events. Companies anxious to present their products in the best possible light sponsor many of the scientific sessions. Competition to wine and dine the most distinguished speakers is intense, while liberal hospitality and inducements are on offer to all but the most reticent of delegates. It is easy to be cynical about these events—not, of course, restricted to the world of antibiotics—but there is usually plenty of wheat to be found among the chaff for the discerning. While some meetings are outrageously commercialized, the best of them do provide a valuable arena for the interchange of ideas in congenial surroundings.

Antibiotics

Most of the antibiotics that were to emerge in the wake of penicillin and streptomycin were the products of the actinomycetes that abound in soil, but the *Bacillus* species on which Dubos had concentrated his efforts also provided two early—albeit relatively minor—advances: bacitracin and the polymyxins. Bacitracin was chronologically the first and notwithstanding the dominance of the pharmaceutical industry in productive antibiotic research in the post-war years, the discovery was made in a hospital laboratory in New York.

---

* David Williams was a serial meeting arranger and organization founder: as well as the British Society for Antimicrobial Chemotherapy, he was in the forefront of starting the Hospital Infection Society, the Association of Medical Microbiologists, and the Federation of Infection Societies in the United Kingdom. Among many international distinctions, he was for a time Secretary-General of the International Society for Chemotherapy and eventually became its President.

Dubos's legacy: antibiotics from *Bacillus* species*

Although Selman Waksman had confidence that his beloved actinomycetes would pro-vide the main source of therapeutically useful antibiotic compounds, it was by no means obvious in the 1940s that this would turn out to be the case. Penicillin had come from a fungus and Dubos's gramicidin and tyrocidine were products of a conventional bac-terium, *Bacillus brevis*. Indeed, it was soon obvious that species of *Bacillus* were almost as prolific as actinomycetes as producers of antibacterial agents.

Rod-shaped Gram-positive bacilli that are classified in the genus *Bacillus* are ubiqui-tous in the environment, where they are able to survive by the production of spores that are highly resistant to desiccation and other adverse conditions. They are generally harm-less to human beings. The most notable exception is *Bacillus anthracis*, the cause of anthrax, an animal infection that is occasionally transmitted to man, often through han-dling infected leather or wool. *Bacillus cereus* and, occasionally, other species produce toxins that can precipitate diarrhoea and vomiting; these organisms commonly contami-nate prepared food and may flourish in dishes such as lightly cooked rice to cause the 'Chinese restaurant syndrome'.

Numerous antimicrobial substances produced by species of *Bacillus* were described in the 1940s and 1950s. Some, such as subtilin and nisin† (both from *Bacillus subtilis*) belong to a class of compounds known as bacteriocins, chemicals produced by many bacteria, apparently as a protection mechanism targeted at related species. Others, among them licheniformin (from *Bacillus licheniformis*); circulin and polypeptin (both from *Bacillus circulans*); and edeine (from *Bacillus brevis*) are classified as antibiotics, though the distinction is not clear-cut. All these compounds are loosely related struc-turally insofar as they are polypeptides: chains of amino acids arranged linearly, as in subtilin and nisin, or in a cyclic fashion. Sadly, they all proved unsuitable for therapeutic use, although nisin, which is also produced by *Lactococcus* (*Streptococcus*) *lactis* is suffi-ciently safe when ingested to be used as an approved food preservative. Just four cyclic peptides isolated from *Bacillus* species have survived into the pharmacopoeia: Dubos' gramicidin; bacitracin; and two polymyxins, polymyxin B and colistin. Of these, only colistin is used systemically, and that only by default as a drug of last resort.

Bacitracin

The popular acclaim of Alexander Fleming as the discoverer of penicillin (see p. 111) was not confined to the general public. Bacteriologists all over the world harboured illusions of following in the great man's footsteps and laboratory cultures were scrutinized for antibiotic phenomena as never before. The organisms that were to provide the major source of antibiotics for the pharmaceutical firms—members of the *Streptomyces* genus

---

* Some species of *Bacillus* have since been reclassified; they are, however, taxonomically closely related and the original names will be used here.

† Nisin was recognized as a product of lactic acid fermentation as early as 1928, but was not isolated until 1947. The polypeptide chain contains lanthionine, an analogue of the amino acid, cystine, and nisin is sometimes called a lantibiotic.

and their actinomycete relatives—are not commonly encountered as laboratory contaminants, but ubiquitous environmental organisms such as fungi and bacteria belonging to the *Bacillus* genus certainly are. It came as no surprise, therefore, when, in October 1945, a group of workers in the departments of surgery and biochemistry of the College of Physicians and Surgeons, Columbia University, New York, described an antibiotic produced by an organism of the *Bacillus subtilis* group (3), later identified as *Bacillus licheniformis*.

A bacteriologist, Balbina Johnson, had made the discovery in June 1943 (4), at a time when conversation at the College must have been filled with tales of the new wonder drug, penicillin: successful trials of the compound in the treatment of bacterial endocarditis (formerly an inexorably fatal condition) were at the time underway under the wing of Henry Dawson and his colleagues at the Presbyterian Hospital, Columbia's University Hospital (5). Johnson worked in the surgical bacteriological laboratory established by Frank Meleney, one of a rare breed of surgeons to take a passionate interest in the role of infection in surgical practice. Meleney is better remembered for his work on an aggressive form of ulceration that sometimes complicates abdominal surgery, known as progressive bacterial synergistic gangrene, or more simply and eponymously as Meleney's gangrene.

In June 1943, a 7-year-old girl, Margaret Tracy had been involved in a road accident in New York and had been brought to the Presbyterian Hospital for treatment. She had suffered a compound fracture of the tibia, which became infected with *Staphylococcus aureus*. Plate cultures on blood agar yielded the offending pathogen accompanied by a contaminant *Bacillus* species, but in broth cultures the staphylococci did not survive. Meleney and Johnson were at the time carrying out a study on the bacterial flora of contaminated civilian wounds and had noted a similar phenomenon before, but the strain of *Bacillus* from Margaret Tracy's wound appeared particularly active when cell-free filtrates were tested against staphylococci and streptococci (3). A biochemist, Herbert Anker was enlisted to carry out a preliminary characterization of the antibiotic, which was found to differ from Dubos' gramicidin and similar substances. The new antibiotic was named bacitracin in acknowledgment of its origin from a species of *Bacillus* and the patient Margaret Tracy. It is not clear whether there was a direct intention to honour the young girl's name as the source of the organism: the isolate had been given the laboratory identifier 'Tracy I' to differentiate it from other investigational strains and the name suggested by precedent, 'subtilin', (the organism was at first thought to be *Bacillus subtilis*) was already in circulation to describe another antibiotic product of the species.

A few years after the fortuitous observation in New York, Edward Abraham and his colleagues in Oxford rediscovered bacitracin. The team were investigating the antibiotic activity of an isolate of *Bacillus licheniformis* brought to them in 1947 from Chile by a visitor, A. Arriagada. At home, Arriagada and his colleagues had demonstrated lytic activity of extracts of what they thought was *Bacillus subtilis*, but when the culture he brought to Oxford was examined it was found to be a mixture of *Bacillus subtilis* and *Bacillus licheniformis*. Both strains had antibiotic activity, but it was *Bacillus licheniformis* that seemed more interesting. The strain had been assigned the identification code A5 and when it was shown to produce a substance inhibitory to many Gram-positive and Gram-negative cocci, a laboratory wag gave the antibiotic the whimsical name 'ayfivin' (6). Subsequent investigation showed it to be virtually identical to bacitracin and the designation 'afyvin' was mercifully withdrawn (7). Biochemical work on bacitracin continued fitfully in Oxford well into the 1950s, but commercial development of the compound was left to companies in the States.

At the time the big players in the pharmaceutical industry were preoccupied with penicillin and seem to have taken little or no interest in bacitracin, but some of the smaller firms were persuaded to take up production. To the fore was Commercial Solvents Corporation in Terre Haute, Indiana, the same firm that was to discover cycloserine in 1954 (see p. 181). Also involved was Ben Venue Laboratories in Cleveland, Ohio (now part of the Boehringer Ingelheim Corporation), a small company founded in 1938 which had made its name during the war as a supplier of freeze-dried blood plasma to the United States armed forces. Both companies had also taken part in the American effort to produce penicillin during the Second World War.

The New York and Oxford strains both turned out to produce a complex of several closely related substances, not all of which displayed antibiotic activity; the major active constituent was called bacitracin A. Hopes were high that a useful new agent had been found. There were plainly problems with toxicity in animal studies, but early trials with doses deemed to be within safe limits offered some encouragement that systemic bacitracin might be of value, alone or together with another drug such as penicillin; attention began to focus on serious infections like bacterial endocarditis or meningitis. Sadly, initial optimism that bacitracin was safe proved wide of the mark: severe kidney damage precluded systemic treatment with the new agent. As late as 1953, 10 years after the original discovery, Frank Meleney, if no one else, still cherished hopes that a formulation or derivative suitable for injection might be found. It was not to be, but Meleney was reluctant to accept defeat. In 1956 he was still clinging to his belief that the antibiotic might have a useful place in medicine by recommending oral bacitracin in combination with neomycin—both drugs are very poorly absorbed in the intestinal tract—for gut sterilization prior to surgery (8).

Bacitracin was a disappointment in the treatment of human disease, but other uses ensured its survival. By the 1960s the growth enhancing properties of certain antibiotics in animals had been observed (see p. 403). Several firms, notably S. B. Penick and Co. in Jersey City, New Jersey,* were manufacturing formulations of bacitracin, principally as a complex with zinc, which improves the stability and eliminates the otherwise bitter taste. The product was marketed as a feed additive and became a popular growth stimulant in cattle pigs and poultry. Such use, along with that of other antibiotics has been banned in the European Union (see p. 405). Human use of bacitracin is now restricted to creams and ointments, generally in combination with other topical medications.

....

* Founded in Marion, North Carolina in 1914 to manufacture and sell drugs derived from plant products S. B. Penick flourished until 1967 when it was acquired by Corn Products Company. The assets were gradually sold off, the final part, Penick Pharmaceuticals, being bought by a private investor in 1988. The bacitracin business was sold to the generic drugs firm Alpharma in 1975. See: http://www.penickcorp.com/history.htm and http://www.alpharma.com/media/flash/animo.swf.

Bacitracin also proved a boon to medical bacteriologists. In 1952, Winston Maxted of the Streptococcal Reference Laboratory of the Public Health Laboratory Service laboratories at Colindale, North London, noticed that growth of haemolytic streptococci was inhibited in the vicinity of a contaminant organism that turned out to be *Bacillus licheniformis*. Preliminary enquiries indicated that the antibiotic was likely to be bacitracin and samples of purified bacitracin and licheniformin obtained from Edward Abraham and Philip D'Arcy Hart, respectively, indeed indicated that bacitracin was the likely active substance. Any initial illusions Maxted might have fostered that he had discovered another wonder drug were dashed, but as a laboratory scientist he chose to follow Alexander Fleming's example of investigating the value of the phenomenon in routine laboratory practice (see p. 91). Experiments showed that *Streptococcus pyogenes*— haemolytic streptococci belonging to group A in the scheme devised by the American microbiologist, Rebecca Lancefield—was much more sensitive to bacitracin than were haemolytic streptococci of other Lancefield groups (9). Maxted devised a simple disc diffusion test that, in the vast majority of cases, reliably distinguishes the important pathogen *Streptococcus pyogenes* from other haemolytic streptococci. The test became the standard method used in hospital bacteriology laboratories for the presumptive identification of Lancefield group A haemolytic streptococci.

Polymyxins

Given the frenzy of activity in the antibiotic world in the years following the end of the Second World War, it is perhaps not surprising that the polymyxins should have been discovered independently in several places. The first news of the findings came within a 4-month period in mid-1947 in the United States (twice) and in England; in 1950 a further report came from Japan. Initially there was some confusion about the interrelationships of the various substances, but this was soon resolved (10).

The first public announcement of the discovery of an antibiotic product of *Bacillus polymyxa* was made on 16 May 1947 by Robert G. Benedict and Asger Langlykke of the North Regional Research Laboratories in Peoria, Illinois, at a meeting of the Society of American Bacteriologists held in Philadelphia (11). In July 1947, Philip Stansly, Robert Shepherd, and Harold White of the Stamford Research Laboratories of the American Cyanamid Company at Stamford, Connecticut published in the *Bulletin of the Johns Hopkins Hospital* details of an antibiotic from the same bacterial species, which they called 'polymyxin' (12). The Stamford group claim to have begun their investigation in the summer of 1944 (13). On 19 May 1947 the British journal *Nature* received a short paper from the celebrated mycologist Geoffrey Ainsworth* and his colleagues, Annie Brown and George Brownlee of the Wellcome Research Laboratories in Beckenham, England, which was published in the issue of August 23 1947. The article described a new

---

* Geoffrey Clough Ainsworth, was born in Birmingham and studied at University College, Nottingham (now the University of Nottingham) obtaining first class honours in botany in 1930. He became a noted mycological scholar and historian of the subject, eventually becoming director of the Commonwealth Mycological Institute at Kew.

antibiotic from *Bacillus aerosporus* (later shown to be identical to *Bacillus polymyxa*), which they named 'aerosporin' (14). The Wellcome scientists had isolated the bacterium from soil of a market garden in Surrey in February 1946; similar antibiotic-producing strains of the bacterium were subsequently found in soil from Yorkshire and from an airborne strain of the bacillus.

The properties of all these agents turned out to be remarkably similar: they were plainly closely related chemically; they were much more active against Gram-negative bacilli than Gram-positive cocci (in marked contrast to gramicidin and bacitracin); and they were all nephrotoxic. In order to clarify the situation the Stamford and Wellcome scientists decided to exchange material to investigate the biological and chemical properties of the two compounds (13). When chromatographic analysis of Stansly's polymyxin and Ainsworth's aerosporin showed small differences in the amino acid composition it became apparent that the compounds represented closely related variants of an antibiotic family. In 1949, agreement was reached between Wellcome and American Cyanamid that the antibiotics should be given the generic name 'polymyxin'. Aerosporin was called polymyxin A, and the American compound became polymyxin D. Other variants discovered by the Wellcome scientists to be subtly different from the original compounds were designated polymyxins B, C, and E (15). When, in 1950, Yasuo Koyama and his colleagues in the Kobayashi Bacteriological Laboratory,* Japan, independently reported the discovery of a new antibiotic called colistin (or colimycin) produced by *Bacillus polymyxa* subspecies *colistinus* (16), it was discovered to be identical to polymyxin E. Further fractionation of polymyxins B and E showed that each probably consists of two or more subcomponents which are difficult to separate. In subsequent years at least 10 other polymyxins were discovered; none has received much attention, although polymyxin M, produced by a strain of *Bacillus polymyxa* isolated from soil in Moscow in 1958, was used in the former Soviet Union.

Given the uninspiring precedents of gramicidin and other antibacterial peptides isolated from *Bacillus* species, and their obvious nephrotoxic potential, the polymyxins could easily have been rejected as interesting, but commercially unprofitable molecules, but the bactericidal activity, apparent freedom from resistance problems, and above all, the extraordinary spectrum of activity kept hopes alive. It was soon realized that the peculiar spectrum was attributable to a structural feature not possessed by other peptide antibiotics. Scientists in American Cyanamid had found evidence that the peptide of polymyxin D was linked to a fatty acid chain and in 1949 Sam Wilkinson of the Wellcome Laboratories showed this to be methyloctanoic acid, a chain with eight carbon atoms (17). The fatty acid chain of polymyxins confers a detergent-like property, which allows them to disrupt lipid membranes. As well as a cytoplasmic membrane, Gram-negative bacilli have a lipopolysaccharide-rich outer membrane not present in Gram-positive bacteria; moreover, the inner membrane of Gram-positive organisms is protected by a thick cell wall, which lipids find hard to traverse. Unfortunately,

* This was probably the laboratory set up in 1907 by Tomijiro Kobayashi as part of his soap manufacturing company now known as the Lion Corporation.

mammalian cell membranes are not immune and much of the toxicity of polymyxins has been ascribed to binding to host cells.

It was the scientists at Wellcome that were most active in pursuing these compounds further and their interest soon focused on polymyxins B (for which Wellcome quickly registered the brand name Aerosporin) and E: polymyxin C was isolated only in small amounts and was never subjected to intense scrutiny; toxicity tests in animals showed that the renal damage caused by polymyxins A and D was too great for them to be considered for human use. At first there were hopes that polymyxins B and E might be used in a wide variety of serious infections caused by Gram-negative bacilli. There were some early trials in both Britain and United States, including some speculative forays by the paediatrician Peter Swift at Farnborough Hospital, Kent in diseases as diverse as whooping cough (18) and haemophilus meningitis (19), but general clinical experience of the efficacy and toxicity of polymyxin B was not encouraging. Attention was quickly directed to *Pseudomonas aeruginosa*, a common opportunist pathogen that rarely causes problems in healthy individuals, but frequently leads to life-threatening infection in seriously ill patients, particularly those with extensive burns, or impaired immune systems. In the early days of antimicrobial chemotherapy, infection with *Pseudomonas aeruginosa* was very bad news, since none of the other agents developed before the 1960s had much effect, whereas the polymyxins were almost universally active against the organism and few instances of resistance were reported.

One of the first indications of the value of polymyxin in *Pseudomonas aeruginosa* infection (then known as *Pseudomonas pyocyanea*) came from the Medical Research Council's Burns Research Unit at Birmingham Accident Hospital directed by the medical microbiologist and poet, Edward Lowbury (20). Following the introduction of penicillin and sulphonamides, pseudomonas had taken over from *Streptococcus pyogenes* as the scourge of burns units, and Lowbury obtained some impressive results with topical polymyxin E, provided by Wellcome, in preventing colonization of burns with this difficult organism. Effectiveness in established infection was less striking, but the drug clearly helped and was sometimes curative. It was not long before polymyxin was being used by injection to treat difficult urinary infections and serious systemic disease caused by *Pseudomonas aeruginosa*. Injections were painful and side effects commonplace, but use was justified by the lack of alternative therapies and the remarkable response that was sometimes obtained.

Among the unusual structural features of the polymyxins is the presence of five diaminobutyric acid residues within the amino acid chain. Treatment with sulphuric acid modifies the diaminobutyric acid molecules to produce the polymyxin sulphates that were first used clinically. In 1954, Japanese workers showed that if formaldehyde and sodium bisulphite is used instead of sulphuric acid, some or all of the diaminobutyric acids become converted to sulphomethyl derivatives. Although sulphomethyl polymyxins appear less active than the sulphates *in vitro*, they are less painful to inject and are associated with fewer side effects; furthermore, they spontaneously decay to the more active sulphates so that full potency is gradually restored. For these reasons, sulphomethyl polymyxins began to replace the sulphates during the 1960s. Sulphomethyl derivatives of both polymyxin B and colistin—which became the preferred name for polymyxin E—were marketed, but it was colistin sulphomethate that prevailed and is the only injectable form of polymyxin now available.

Polymyxins were a major advance in the treatment of infection with *Pseudomonas aeruginosa*, but by the time colistin sulphomethate became available things were beginning to change. Over the next 10 years, aminoglycosides (see p. 231) and penicillins (p. 125–6) with antipseudomonal activity began to appear, bolstered later by some other β-lactam antibiotics (p. 129 and 133–4) and fluoroquinolones (p. 258–9). Polymyxins went into decline and are now rarely used in systemic infection unless other options prove ineffective.

Waksman's legacy: antibiotics from the soil

The sensational impact of penicillin on the treatment of infection provided the first real clue to the untapped potential of naturally occurring antibiotics. Streptomycin focussed attention on the teeming micro-organisms found in soil and other parts of the environment. Soon the pharmaceutical industry was collecting soil samples by the hundred thousand from all over the world. Bacteria, especially the mould-like actinomycetes, were laboriously isolated and screened for antibiotic activity. The countless thousands of antibiotics that were discovered (and frequently rediscovered) by this means in the 20-year period between 1945 and 1965 must have exceeded even Selman Waksman's most optimistic predictions.

Of course, most proved to be useless: too toxic in preliminary animal experiments; too feeble in their activity; too unstable; or too difficult to isolate and purify. Still, a number of therapeutically useful compounds were uncovered in this way. Already by the mid-1950s representatives of most of the antibiotic families that formed the basis of the 'antibiotic revolution' were in clinical use. The first fruits of the revolution were chloramphenicol and the early tetracyclines, antibiotics that turned out to have an unprecedented breadth of spectrum.

Chloramphenicol

In 1943, no doubt alert to the work that Waksman was doing at Rutgers, but not yet wishing to commit company resources to an uncertain field of study, Parke, Davis and Co. in Detroit provided the funds for Paul Burkholder, Eaton professor of botany at Yale to screen samples of soil for micro-organisms producing substances with antibiotic activity (21). It was probably in 1945 that a culture of *Streptomyces* was isolated that seemed promising enough for John Ehrlich and his colleagues at Parke, Davis to investigate further. The soil sample yielding the organism had been taken from a mulched field near Caracas in Venezuela.

Publication of the finding in October 1947 (22) stimulated a group of scientists at the University of Illinois to report that they too were working on an antibiotic with identical properties. The Plant Pathologist David Gottlieb had discovered the antibiotic as a product of a species of *Streptomyces* isolated from composted soil from the horticultural farm of the Illinois Agricultural Experiment Station at Urbana (23); Gottlieb's colleague, the Professor of Chemistry, Herbert Carter, had crystallized the active principle. A collaborative study by

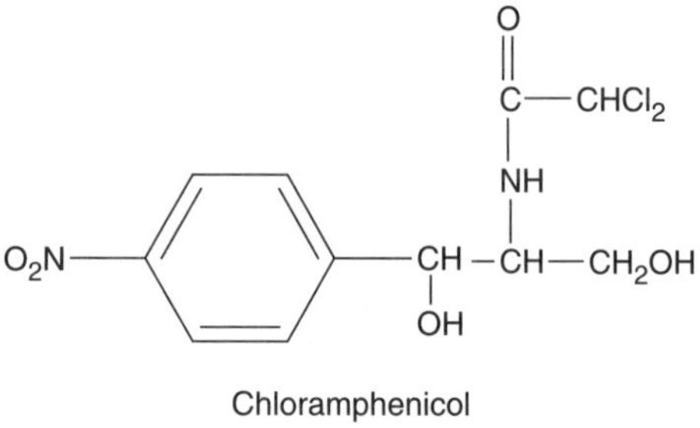

Fig. 6.1 The structure of chloramphenicol.

Chloramphenicol

Ehrlich, Gottlieb, and Burkholder subsequently concluded that the two producer organisms were identical and belonged to a new species, *Streptomyces venezuelae* (24); Burkholder's isolate was accepted as the type culture and the Illinois group gracefully withdrew.

The antibiotic produced by *Streptomyces venezuelae* was originally called chloromycetin, but this was adopted as the trade name and the non-proprietary name, chloramphenicol was agreed upon. The structure (Fig. 6.1) was quickly elucidated and then synthesized by Mildred Rebstock and her associates, John Controulis, and Harry Crooks at Parke, Davis (25). It is an unusually simple molecule for a naturally occurring antibiotic and chloramphenicol represents one of the few cases in which synthesis is cheaper than production by fermentation.

Although the original descriptions of chloramphenicol recognized the uncommonly broad spectrum of activity, most of the early interest centred on its activity against rickettsiae—obligate intracellular bacteria named after the American pathologist Howard Ricketts, who did much of the early work on these organisms. Rickettsiae are variously transmitted by lice, fleas, or ticks and cause a range of diseases such as typhus (from which Ricketts died, probably acquiring the infection from a louse in the course of his research) and Rocky Mountain Spotted Fever (on which Ricketts did much of the seminal research). Epidemic typhus, caused by *Rickettsia prowazeki*—the species name honours Stanislaus von Prowazek, another rickettsial pioneer, who died investigating the disease in a Russian prisoner of war camp—is one of the diseases that have shaped human history. Its impact is graphically described in the classic book, *Rats, lice and history*, written by the eminent American microbiologist, Hans Zinsser (26).*

Rickettsial diseases represented an unsolved problem in 1947, since they were unaffected by drugs then available and such vaccines as had been developed were unsatisfactory. The original description of chloramphenicol revealed that it showed marked activity against *Rickettsia prowazekii* in tests on infected chick embryos (22). Even before publication, Parke, Davis had made available samples of purified material to Joseph Smadel, chief of the Viral and Rickettsial Disease section of the Army Medical Center in

---

* Zinsser also wrote an autobiography: *As I remember him. The biography of R.S.* (1940). The curious title was chosen to conceal the fact that it was written after he had discovered that he was soon to die.

Washington.* He was able to establish that the drug displayed broad activity against rickettsiae and against the agent causing psittacosis (27)—then thought to be a virus, but now known to belong to a group of intracellular bacteria known as chlamydiae.

A successful small early trial of chloramphenicol carried out in Mexico by Joe Smadel and his assistant, Herbert Ley[†] on patients suffering from typhus encouraged further studies. In 1948, in the aftermath of the Second World War, Smadel organized a mission to Kuala Lumpur to investigate the treatment of scrub typhus—otherwise known as tsutsugamushi fever (Japanese, tsutsugamushi = insect disease)—a mite-borne infection caused by an organism originally called *Rickettsia orientalis*, but which has since been reclassified in the related *Orientia* genus as *Orientia tsutsugamushi*. One member of the team that went to Malaya was Theodore Woodward, who went on to become one of America's most distinguished infectious disease physicians and received a Nobel Prize nomination for his work on the clinical use of chloramphenicol. Woodward later wrote a colourful account of the scrub typhus mission (28).

The scrub typhus study was conducted from the Institute of Medical Research in Kuala Lumpur, where the director was Raymond Lewthwaite, a British typhus expert who had worked in Malaya since 1926 and was field director of the British Medical Research Council's scrub typhus campaign in south-east Asia in the latter years of the war; he eventually became director of colonial medical research at the Colonial Office. Lewthwaite met the aeroplane carrying Smadel's team at Singapore on Sunday 14 March 1948, drove them to Kuala Lumpur, and immediately took them to the bedside of a 26-year-old Malayan soldier, Mohammed Nook bin Osman. After laboratory tests confirmed the diagnosis of scrub typhus, the young soldier was treated with high doses of chloramphenicol for 12 days. He made a rapid and complete recovery. A second patient, a 19-year-old British corporal with classic scrub typhus similarly responded promptly and completely.

Additional testing of chloramphenicol quickly established the credentials of the new drug beyond doubt, a verdict endorsed by Howard Florey, who saw the impressive results during a stopover en route to London from Australia, where he was actively involved in setting up the new Australian National University. Flushed with success, Smadel extended the study to investigate the effectiveness of chloramphenicol in the prevention of scrub typhus by exposing volunteers, including himself, 8 h a day for 10 days in a notoriously mite-infected plantation close to Kuala Lumpur.

Further, unexpected success emerged from the mission. On Saturday 3 April 1948, two patients suspected of scrub typhus were admitted for treatment; both were actually suffering from the unrelated condition, typhoid fever, caused by the bacterium *Salmonella*

----

* Founded in 1893 by the distinguished United States Army surgeon, General George Sternberg. Since 1953, known as the Walter Reed Army Institute for Research, in honour of the equally eminent Army bacteriologist, Walter Reed.

† A Harvard graduate, Ley went on to become, in 1966, Director of the FDA's Bureau of Medicine. He left the Bureau in controversial circumstances in December 1969.

typhi (now more correctly called *Salmonella enterica* serotype Typhi) and the diagnosis was proven by culture of the organism from one of the two men. Chloramphenicol was effective in each case, though the proven typhoid victim had a stormy recovery with relapse that subsequently responded to renewed treatment with the drug. By the time the scrub typhus mission left in June 1948, firm evidence had been accumulated that two formerly untreatable diseases were susceptible to oral treatment with chloramphenicol and considerable progress had been made on establishing optimal dosage regimens. Later the scrub typhus results were extended to other rickettsial diseases. The finding that chloramphenicol was highly effective in typhoid fever was particularly important, since the disease is much more widespread than typhus or other rickettsial diseases in many countries.

As experience with chloramphenicol increased it became plain that the properties of the new agent were close to ideal: potent, exceptionally broad-spectrum antibacterial activity; almost complete absorption when given by mouth (it is extremely bitter, but this can be mitigated by formulation as an ester); free diffusion into tissues; and relative freedom from serious side effects. It also turned out to be one of the few antibiotics that penetrate well into the cerebrospinal fluid, making it extremely useful in meningitis. But soon after Parke, Davis marketed the drug in 1949 an unexpected cloud appeared on the horizon. Reports began to surface of a rare, but frequently fatal side effect, aplastic anaemia, in which the bone marrow ceases to produce red blood cells. By 1952, an investigation by the United States FDA had uncovered nearly 180 cases, many of them fatal, associated with the use of chloramphenicol.

The reason for this unfortunate effect is far from clear. A non-life-threatening reversible depression of bone marrow function occurs quite commonly during chloramphenicol therapy and is dose related. In contrast, aplastic anaemia is not related to dosage (there have even been reports after use of chloramphenicol eye drops, though this is extremely rare), can occur weeks after treatment has ended, and is seen only in around one in 25,000–40,000 courses of treatment (29). It is possible that there is a genetic predisposition that makes certain persons susceptible to the side effect, but, if so, it has so far eluded formal identification.

The news that chloramphenicol caused aplastic anaemia was a bombshell. Was such a side effect to be revealed in a new antibiotic today, it would almost certainly lead to withdrawal of the licence to market the drug. The climate of the 1950s allowed Parke, Davis to continue to promote the product. Controversy raged over the balance to be struck between the degree of risk—rare fatalities from anaphylactic reactions also occurred with that paragon of safety, penicillin—and the clinical benefit of an exceptionally effective antibiotic. Sales of chloramphenicol briefly plummeted reaching a nadir in 1954, but quickly recovered as reassurance about the rarity of fatalities convinced many doctors that the benefits outweighed the dangers (30).

The use of chloramphenicol eventually declined again as controversy continued and doctors became persuaded of the reality of the risks, but not before many people had died, some after receiving the drug for trivial infections. Meanwhile, another life-threatening hazard was uncovered in infants who have not yet developed an efficient mechanism for excreting the drug: a condition known as 'grey baby syndrome'. Prominent among the advocates of banning or severely restricting the use of chloramphenicol were doctors who had personal experience of deaths, sometimes occurring in small clusters, that were directly attributable to the drug. As Mary Barber* and Paul Garrod put it in their influential book *Antibiotic and Chemotherapy*, first published in 1963:

> Apparently the profession is divided into those who, perhaps having seen chloramphenicol cause marrow aplasia, fear this effect and rarely use the drug, and a large number who ignore this possibility because it seems too remote and prescribe chloramphenicol freely (31).

Garrod had himself observed three cases of aplastic anaemia, two of them fatal, among 1200 patients treated at St Bartholomew's Hospital, London up to 1952. In the following 7 years the annual consumption of the drug in the hospital fell from 5900 to 290 g (32). Certainly, seeing patients die unnecessarily because of their decisions is one of the most potent incentives for doctors to change prescribing habits. Equally potent, no doubt, in influencing use of toxic drugs like chloramphenicol were increasingly common accusations of malpractice.

Debate over the safety of chloramphenicol may have raged in affluent western nations, but because it was cheap, effective, easy to administer and chemically stable in tropical temperatures, it rapidly became a favoured drug throughout the poorer countries of the world. Even today, it can be commonly found openly on sale for self-medication in local markets in many countries, often for trivial or wholly inappropriate conditions. One can only guess at the number of deaths that have followed its unrestricted use. In countries with better regulation of prescription drugs recommended indications became restricted to just a handful of life-threatening infections—notably typhoid fever and many forms of bacterial meningitis. With the availability of safer alternatives chloramphenicol eventually fell into disuse even in these cases. It is now seldom used at all in developed countries, except in topical ophthalmic preparations, where the risk is held to be negligible.

Manipulation of the chloramphenicol molecule to produce congeners with a better safety profile was energetically pursued, but turned out to be singularly unsuccessful, since alterations to the molecule generally result in a considerable reduction in activity. Most interest centred on thiamphenicol, a compound in which a sulphomethyl (SO_2CH_3) substituent replaces the nitro (NO_2) group of chloramphenicol. It is said to be free of the problem of aplastic anaemia, but reversible bone marrow toxicity is more common and the compound is less active than the parent drug. It is available in some countries of continental Europe and elsewhere, but is not widely used. A fluorinated derivative of thiamphenicol, florfenicol, has been developed, but only for veterinary use.

....

* Mary Barber, Professor of Clinical Bacteriology at the Royal Postgraduate Medical School, Hammersmith Hospital, was an authority on antibiotics and a pioneer of agreed policies of antibiotic use in hospitals. She died in a road accident in September 1965. Her place as co-author of *Antibiotic and Chemotherapy* was taken by Francis O' Grady.

Tetracyclines

Did the ancient inhabitants of the Nile valley know about tetracycline? This fascinating question was raised in 1980, when evidence of the presence of the drug was reported in human bone excavated from a cemetery in Sudanese Nubia dating from AD 350–500 (33). Later reports documented the presence of tetracycline in bones from the Roman period excavated from the Dakhleh oasis, 250 km West of Luxor, in Egypt (34) and in Nubian bones from a cemetery used up to the mid-fifteenth century (35). The discovery was made by detection of the distinctive tetracycline pigment, which has a characteristic appearance when examined under a fluorescence microscope. All antibiotics of the tetracycline family are yellow coloured compounds that readily bind to calcium and hence are deposited in calcium-rich tissues like teeth and bones. The pattern of deposition of the pigment indicated periodic, seasonal ingestion of the antibiotic and the most likely explanation is that it represents accidental intake of the drug with stored grain that had become contaminated with tetracycline-producing streptomycetes. In some cases, the degree of fluorescence present indicates therapeutically active concentrations and there is some intriguing evidence that it may have contributed to lower than expected levels of infections in the affected communities (34).

While it is a mistake to underestimate the skill and perspicacity of ancient healers, it is extremely unlikely that these early populations could meaningfully exploit the therapeutic benefits of contaminated grain in preventing infection. For sure, there are numerous tales of the use of mouldy or decomposing foods among folk remedies throughout history, but what is known about the distribution of antibiotic-producing organisms in nature, and the conditions under which the active substances are formed, make it highly improbable that any useful effect could have been reliably achieved.

Discovery of the first of the tetracyclines, chlortetracycline, in the twentieth century was made in the Lederle Laboratories division of the American Cyanamid Company in Pearl River, near New York City by Benjamin Duggar, a retired plant pathologist. There can have been few important medical discoveries made by persons in their eighth decade of life, but Duggar's was one of them.

Benjamin Duggar was born in the village of Gallion, Alabama, about 100 miles West of Montgomery in 1872. Before the end of the century he had been awarded a master's degree from Harvard and a doctorate from Cornell. He became professor of Botany at the University of Missouri in 1902 at the age of 30 and in 1909 published the first ever book to be written on plant pathology *Fungus diseases of plants*. After a peripatetic life as a plant physiologist in various American institutions he retired at the statutory age of 70. Finding retirement insufficiently challenging, and wishing to contribute to a nation at war, he accepted, in 1944, an offer from Lederle Laboratories—a former PhD student had suggested his name—to identify a species of rhododendron known to be used in China in the treatment of malaria. Having successfully hunted down the correct species and established cuttings in the greenhouse of a wealthy neighbour, he was asked by Dr Wilbur 'weed' Malcolm,* director of research at Lederle, to advise on whether the

---

* The nickname was earned during his teenage years when he suddenly shot up to 6′ 3″.

company should seek a licence to produce streptomycin, the potential of which was just becoming clear. Duggar's response was that vast potential of the soil had hardly been touched and better antibiotics remained to be discovered. With the two female assistants that had been allocated to him he set out to find one (36).

Soil specimens were solicited from colleagues and friends and Duggar himself collected many samples on his travels. In 1945 he was sent a soil sample from his old stamping ground in the University of Missouri, which was labelled 'Columbia plot No. 23, Timothy field, unfertilized, swamp ground, University of Missouri (37).' The specimen was given the laboratory number A377 and from it Duggar isolated a new species of *Streptomyces* that exhibited strong inhibitory activity towards various bacteria in screening tests. The producer organism sported a rich golden colour, so it was named *Streptomyces aureofaciens* and since the active principle was also pigmented, it was called Aureomycin. Satisfactory animal experiments were completed the following year and the antibiotic was first given to patients in January 1948.* Within 6 months impressive results had been obtained in a wide variety of infections in several prestigious centres in the United States and Lederle knew they were on to a winner.

Aureomycin was unveiled at a symposium sponsored by the New York Academy of Sciences on 21 July 1948, the first occasion on which Duggar was publicly able to disclose his discovery (38). The spectrum of activity was at least as great as that of chloramphenicol, for which only preliminary results had by then been published, and no serious toxicity had yet come to light. The drug was approved by the FDA with astonishing speed on 20 October 1948 (3 months ahead of chloramphenicol) and marketed on 1 December the same year.

Meanwhile, scientists at Pfizer had embarked on their own ambitious research programme involving tens of thousands of soil samples from around the world:

> By enlisting the aid of foreign correspondents, explorers, travelers, and friends, soils from a multitude of locations on the various continents were obtained. From Alaska to Australia, from the banks of the Amazon to the shores of the Ganges, from the swamps of Florida and from the Swiss Alps, collectors scraped up small portions of earth for mycological studies (39).

The tone might be flamboyant and heroic, but it conveys something of the intense excitement of the time. Comparable programmes were being duplicated in pharmaceutical company laboratories all over the world.

The Pfizer effort was certainly enormous: by the late 1940s it was claimed that they had examined around 100,000 soil samples, culminating in 1949 with the isolation of an actinomycete, *Streptomyces rimosus*—the name derives from the cracked appearance of the colonies; Latin rimosus = full of cracks)—from which a highly active yellow pigmented antibiotic was obtained in crystalline form by the chemists, Peter Regna and I. A. Solomons. Pfizer called their new antibiotic Terramycin—an antibiotic from the earth. Gladys Hobby and her microbiological colleagues at Pfizer soon established the spectrum

---

* Louis T. Wright a black American physician and surgeon working at New York's Harlem Hospital, is often credited with the first clinical use of Aureomycin, but the exact facts are now difficult to verify.

of activity of the compound, which bore a remarkable similarity to that of Lederle's Aureomycin. The discovery was made public in a short paper in *Science* on 27 January 1950 (40). There can be no better example of how teamwork had taken over since Fleming's solo effort in 1929: the Pfizer paper, which occupies less than a page of print has 11 authors.

With Aureomycin already on the market, frantic efforts were already underway to prove the value of the new drug. In an unprecedented operation, sufficient Terramycin was rapidly manufactured and distributed to physicians to allow adequate information on the activity and safety to be accumulated for the issue of a licence. With a speed that would be impossible in the regulatory climate that prevails today, Pfizer were able to put the drug on sale in the United States as soon as approval was given on 15 March 1950. At a conference dedicated to Terramycin, held in New York on 16 and 17 June 1950, about 1000 case reports were presented (41).

The success of Aureomycin and Terramycin was undisputed, but the precise structure of both compounds was a puzzle that eluded the chemists. The problem was solved in 1952 by the brilliant Harvard chemist, Robert Woodward, who went on to receive a Nobel Prize in 1965. From the conflicting evidence that had been presented he deduced the complex tetracyclic structure of Terramycin (42) and went on, with his associates, to formally establish the molecular architecture (43). It quickly became clear that Aureomycin and Terramycin not only shared close similarities in their antibacterial and pharmacological properties, but they were, in fact, extremely closely related (Fig. 6.2).

The four-ring arrangement naturally suggested the generic name tetracycline for this class of antibiotics and by 1953 this name was in common use. The chlorine-containing molecule (Aureomycin) was called chlortetracycline and the hydroxyl variant (Terramycin), oxytetracycline; Aureomycin and Terramycin were retained as the trade names. The revelation that, although the two compounds were nearly identical, they were sufficiently different to be regarded a distinct chemical entities, no doubt came as a great relief to both companies. Establishment of the structure also allowed the chemists to set to work modifying the molecule with a view to altering its properties.

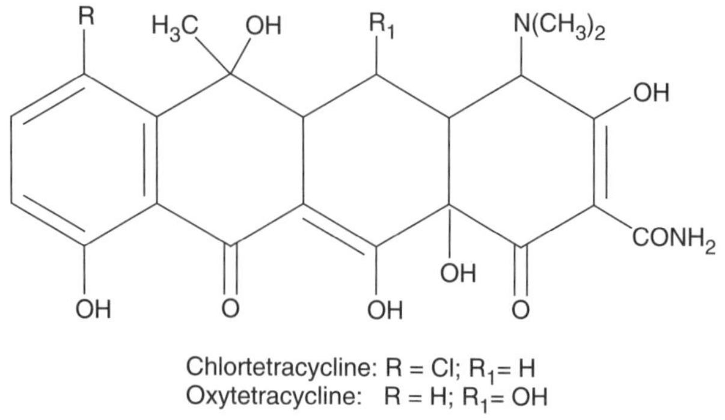

Fig. 6.2 Molecular structures of chlortetracycline (Aureomycin) and oxytetracycline (Terramycin).

Chlortetracycline: R = Cl; R_1 = H
Oxytetracycline: R = H; R_1 = OH

Pfizer had taken some of the shine off Lederle's achievement by their aggressive promotion of oxytetracycline and Lederle retaliated in November 1953 by a high-profile launch, backed by a massive promotional budget, of a new chemically modified derivative, Achromycin, which was claimed to be safer and more stable than its predecessors. Achromycin lacked both the chlorine of chlortetracycline and the hydroxyl group of oxytetracycline, giving it the simple generic name, 'tetracycline'. Bristol, Squibb, and Upjohn also had their eye on the profits to be made from broad-spectrum antibiotics and were already planning to market their own formulations of tetracycline.

To further complicate matters, a naturally occurring version of tetracycline was discovered in 1952 as a product of an unidentified *Streptomyces* species found in soil from Texas. The discovery was made by Paul Minieri and his colleagues (44) at the now defunct Heyden Chemical Corporation, Princeton, New Jersey, which was originally established before the First World War as a branch of the German firm that produced salicylic acid (see p. 48). With the help of Clark Bricker from the Department of Chemistry at the local Princeton University the antibiotic was purified; it was soon realized that it was identical to the product obtained by removal of chlorine from chlortetracycline. Although Dr Sol Katz chief of pulmonary medicine at the Gallinger Municipal Hospital, Washington (since 1953, the District of Columbia General Hospital) carried out tolerance studies on behalf of Heyden, further development was in the hands of Lederle, which bought the antibiotics division of Heyden in December 1953, and acquired with it the Minieri patent.

Unfortunately for Lederle and other companies hoping to profit from the new molecule, a patent application for tetracycline had already been submitted in October 1953 by the chemist Lloyd Conover of Pfizer; the full patent was eventually granted on 11 January 1955. After prolonged argument and bitter litigation, the United States Federal Trade Commission sanctioned a complex patent sharing and licensing agreement in 1958. Lederle, Pfizer, and Bristol were given the right to manufacture and sell the drug; Squibb and Upjohn were allowed to sell drug manufactured under contract by Bristol. This did not prevent further courtroom battles, which continued until a final judicial ruling was made in 1982.

A lot was at stake. Antibiotics were beginning to be used with great abandon and huge profits were there to be made. Among the drug firms the gloves were off. Allegations of market rigging, overpricing, and irresponsible promotion of antibiotics, together with safety fears over chloramphenicol, prompted a United States federal enquiry into the drug industry in 1960. During the enquiry, led by Senator Estes Kefauver, news began to filter from Europe on birth defects caused by thalidomide, more than 2 million tablets of which had already been distributed in the United States for investigational use. A Canadian-born pharmacologist, Frances Kelsey, working for the FDA, had blocked approval of the drug because of suspicions about its safety. When these were found to be well founded, supplies were rapidly seized, avoiding a major drug catastrophe in the United States (45).* These events led Kefauver to sponsor a bill seeking more effective

---

* Only 17 birth defects occurred in the United States compared with several thousand in Europe. In 1962 Frances Kelsey was awarded the Distinguished Federal Civilian Service Award for her efforts to prevent a greater tragedy.

drug regulation, which was signed into law by President John F. Kennedy in 1962. The bill, known as the Kefauver–Harris amendments, gave the FDA greater powers to regulate investigational studies and marketing practices and required drug manufacturers to prove the efficacy and safety of their products before marketing them.

In the meantime the tetracyclines were enjoying great success. Their broad-spectrum activity (including not only most conventional bacterial pathogens, but also rickettsiae, mycoplasmas, and even some protozoa, such as malaria parasites and *Entamoeba histolytica*, the cause of amoebic dysentery), relative safety and ease of oral administration recommended them to use in a wide variety of infections. They quickly took over from chloramphenicol as the treatment of choice in rickettsial and chlamydial infections of all kinds. By 1956, there were nearly 4000 publications detailing clinical and laboratory studies of tetracyclines (46) and annual production of broad-spectrum antibiotics in the United States (including chloramphenicol, which was in decline because of the doubts about its safety) was approaching 400,000 kg.

In 1957 scientists at Lederle found a new tetracycline derivative, produced by a mutant strain of *Streptomyces aureofaciens*. The novel molecule lacked a methyl group in the chlortetracycline structure and was therefore called demethylchlortetracycline, soon shortened to demeclocycline. Surprisingly, this molecule proved to be more stable, better absorbed and somewhat more active than earlier derivatives. Although such factors do not necessarily translate into clinical benefit, they are seized on by pharmaceutical manufacturers, who are able to exploit these features in making extravagant claims of 'improvements' in their new and inevitably more expensive products. The dilemma for manufacturers is well exemplified by the tetracyclines, since all exhibit similar antibacterial activity and the most notable differences are in the pharmacological handling of the various congeners. Over the next decade many semi-synthetic derivatives of tetracyclines were described and some, notably methacycline, doxycycline, and minocycline, found their way on to the market, each offering new and ostensibly superior properties.

The most compelling reason why prescribers might be persuaded to switch to a new compound is a promise of greater safety. Although early use of tetracyclines revealed few side effects other than a propensity to cause diarrhoea, cases of nephrotoxicity and liver damage gradually emerged, especially when the drugs were used in high dosage in patients with pre-existing kidney or liver disease. Certain tetracyclines may have some advantages in this regard: for example, doxycycline is generally free from nephrotoxicity as it is preferentially excreted by the liver. Permanent staining of teeth when the tetracyclines were given to children in whom the dentition was developing emerged as a problem in the early 1960s.

Tetracyclines are still quite popular antibiotics, but widespread resistance has diminished their usefulness in many types of infection. Reports of reduced susceptibility of bacteria to tetracyclines began to emerge shortly after the drugs became widely used in the 1950s and became increasingly frequent during the next decade. It was soon recognized that the genetic information for resistance was carried on extrachromosomal pieces of DNA (plasmids) that moved easily from one bacterial cell to another by a quasi-sexual process called conjugation (see p. 405). To further aid the rapid spread of the resistance trait, the genes were often found located on transposons—so-called 'jumping genes'—fragments of DNA that can migrate between different plasmids, or even to the bacterial chromosome.

A contributory factor in the dissemination of tetracycline-resistant organisms was strongly suspected to be the use of tetracyclines in animal feeds as growth promoters (see p. 403–4). Chlortetracycline and oxytetracycline in particular have been among the most widely used agents for growth promotion. How antibiotics increase growth yield in animals is uncertain. Experiments comparing the growth rate of conventional animals with that of animals raised from birth in conditions that render them germ free, suggest that an effect on the bacterial flora may be part of the answer. However, many other theories have been put forward as to why antibiotics may enhance the efficiency of feed conversion and the effect seems likely to involve the interplay of several factors (47).

Circumstantial evidence linking animal use to tetracycline-resistance in organisms of the shared bacterial flora, such as *Escherichia coli* and salmonellae is strong, but is much less compelling for many other common human pathogens. Whatever the role of animals, tetracycline-resistance is certainly common, though slowly declining as the drugs become less frequently prescribed. Unfortunately, resistance affects virtually all members of the tetracycline family, although exceptions occur, especially with minocycline. Attempts to find tetracycline derivatives that retain activity against bacteria resistant to other members of the group have focused on semi-synthetic derivatives in which substituted glycine residues have been introduced—a group given the tongue-twisting name, glycylcyclines. The most promising of these is tigecycline, which was developed by Wyeth in the United States and is now available for intravenous administration in certain serious infections.

Aminoglycosides

The earliest aminoglycoside antibiotics, streptomycin (see p. 153), and neomycin (see p. 179–80), had been found in Waksman's laboratory, but other examples of what was to become an important antibiotic family were to arrive on the scene in due course elsewhere. The first noteworthy development, the discovery of kanamycin in 1956, signalled the entry of Japanese scientists as important players on the antibiotic scene. They were to have increasing influence as the century progressed. Japan has been keen to foster its science base since the nineteenth century, when Yukichi Fukuzawa founded the University of Keio (in 1867) with the aim of opening up Japan to western learning, and pioneers like Shibasaburo Kitasato travelled to Europe to sit at the feet of such famous figures as Robert Koch, Emil Behring, Paul Ehrlich, and Louis Pasteur (see p. 54).

It was appropriate that the first impact should be made with an aminoglycoside, since Waksman had travelled with his wife to Japan immediately after the Nobel Prize ceremony in 1952. There he was honoured with an audience with the Emperor, who awarded him the Japanese Order of Merit of the Rising Sun. Waksman was also given an honorary degree, appropriately from the University of Keio. Later Japan became one of the beneficiaries of royalties from streptomycin when the Waksman Foundation of Japan was set-up.

Kanamycin was discovered by a team at the Institute of Microbial Chemistry in Tokyo led by Hamao Umezawa. Umezawa was born in Obama, a fishing port on the Sea of Japan. He completed his medical studies in 1937 and was involved, with his elder brother and lifelong collaborator Sumio Umezawa, in Japan's penicillin programme at the end of the Second World War, preluding a long and productive career in the development of natural products as antimicrobial and anticancer agents.* In 1949 Umezawa and his colleagues discovered an antibiotic produced by *Streptomyces fradiae*, which they called fradiomycin. Although it turned out to be identical to Waksman's neomycin it was marketed in Japan, where it is still known as fradiomycin. Kanamycin was found in 1956 as a product of a previously undescribed streptomycete, *Streptomyces kanamyceticus*, grown from soil collected in the Nagano Prefecture. The paper describing the antibiotic was published the following year (48) and by 1958 it was on the market in Japan and the United States. As commonly occurs with natural products, the antibiotic turned out to be a complex of several closely related substances: a major component, kanamycin A, and two minor variants, kanamycins B and C. Kanamycin B was later developed as a separate antibiotic, marketed in Japan in 1969 with the name, bekanamycin.

The chief attraction of kanamycin was that it retained activity against streptomycin-resistant bacteria, including *Mycobacterium tuberculosis*. Its general spectrum of activity mirrors that of streptomycin and it is somewhat less ototoxic, though more damaging to the kidneys. Like streptomycin and other aminoglycosides it has to be administered by injection. Kanamycin never achieved much favour as an antituberculosis agent, but it was widely used in hospitals for several years, particularly in serious infections caused by Gram-negative bacilli. In the 1960s it was replaced by aminoglycosides with more attractive properties. It remains available, but its use is no longer recommended.

Umezawa's group went on to discover another aminoglycoside antibiotic, kasugamycin, produced by *Streptomyces kasugaensis*, a species isolated from soil collected at Kasuga-Taisha, a Shinto shrine established in 768 AD in Nara City. Kasugamycin, first described in 1965 (49), was found during a research programme aimed at finding a way to control rice blast disease, a serious fungal infection caused by *Pyricularia oryzae*, which is a major problem in Japan's very important rice agriculture. The antibiotic was discovered by spraying culture filtrates of various streptomycetes on to young infected rice plants, but puzzlingly could be shown to have an effect on the fungus in conventional laboratory tests only when extracts of rice plant leaves were included in the culture medium. It is now widely used in rice crop protection, but has no place in human medicine.

Kanamycin was dislodged from its perch as the aminoglycoside of choice in serious infection by gentamicin, discovered around 1961 by Marvin Weinstein, George Luedeman and their colleagues at the Schering Corporation in Bloomfield New Jersey. Schering had a chequered history in the United States and was a relative newcomer to the antibiotic field. Originally formed as an offshoot of the German firm, Schering AG, founded by the Berlin

---

* Among anticancer antibiotics developed in Umezawa's laboratory are sarkomycin discovered in 1953 as a product of *Streptomyces erythrochromogenes*, and bleomycin found in 1966 to be produced by *Streptomyces verticillus*.

pharmacist Ernst Schering in 1851, the American subsidiary was taken into public ownership during the Second World War and re-emerged as a private company in 1952 with the Schering name, but independent of the German parent company. In 1971 it merged with Plough, a consumer products manufacturer, to form Schering-Plough.

The organisms producing gentamicin are not streptomycetes, but belong to the *Micromonospora* genus, a fact signalled by 'i' rather than 'y' in the spelling. The antibiotic complex was isolated from two *Micromonospora* cultures among a collection provided by Americo Woyciesjes (50), a soil microbiologist from Syracuse, New York also known in his early career for his exploits as a particularly aggressive amateur boxer (51). One of the producer organisms, *Micromonospora purpurea*, was originally grown from a soil specimen taken from a park in Syracuse; the other, *Micromonospora echinospora* from a mud sample from Jamesville, New York (52). The two species are now thought to be closely related, if not identical, with *echinospora* as the preferred species name. Like other aminoglycosides the natural product is a complex of closely related molecules. The preparation developed commercially contains three variants of gentamicin C: gentamicin C_1, C_{1a}, and C_2.

Gentamicin shares the general pharmacological properties and toxicity profile of kanamycin, but offers two crucial advantages: it displays potent bactericidal activity against the important opportunist pathogen, *Pseudomonas aeruginosa*; and the activity against most other bacterial species within the spectrum (with the exception of *Mycobacterium tuberculosis* against which it has no useful activity) is at least four-fold greater than that of kanamycin. At the time of the discovery of gentamicin, polymyxin, and colistin—both highly toxic compounds (see p. 218–19)—were the only drugs available for the treatment of pseudomonal infections, and a new safer option for the treatment of seriously ill patients was greeted with open arms. Moreover, aminoglycoside resistance in other organisms was beginning to appear and many kanamycin-resistant strains remained susceptible to gentamicin.

Gentamicin was first given to patients in March 1962 by the eminent American infectious disease physician, George Gee Jackson and an infectious disease trainee from the Philippines, Rodolfo Jao (later a naturalized American citizen), at the University of Illinois College of Medicine, Chicago (53). Speaking at a symposium on gentamicin held at the College in 1969, Jackson recalled that the first patient was a woman with pseudomonas septicaemia following extensive burns. Three other patients quickly followed: two men with proteus septicaemia; and a woman with polycystic kidney disease complicated by pseudomonas infection, who was cured at the expense of damage to the inner ear (54).

After its launch in 1967, gentamicin soon became an essential drug in serious hospital infections, especially in patients at risk of infection with *Pseudomonas aeruginosa*. The main drawback, as with all aminoglycosides, is the twin problem of renal and ototoxicity, but this can be mitigated to a large extent by close laboratory monitoring of the concentrations of drug achieved in the bloodstream during treatment.

In the hope of building on their success with gentamicin Weinstein and his colleagues at Schering went on to develop related aminoglycosides. In 1970 they described sisomicin, a close relative of gentamicin C_{1a}, produced by *Micromonospora inyoensis*, isolated not in Japan as the species name might suggest, but from soil from the Inyo National Forest in the Eastern Sierra of California. Later they produced the N-ethyl derivative of sisomicin, which they named netilmicin. Neither drug achieved the success of gentamicin, despite a vigorous promotional campaign in favour of netilmicin, based on tenuous evidence of improved safety. In 1975 John Wright and Peter Daniels from Scherico, Schering's Swiss subsidiary applied for a patent on isepamicin, a gentamicin B derivative that was marketed in Japan in 1988, but has elicited little interest elsewhere.

It was in the research laboratories of Eli Lilly that an aminoglycoside antibiotic to rival gentamicin was found and, surprisingly, it turned out to be a close relative of kanamycin B. In 1968, the Lilly team described a strain of *Streptomyces tenebrarius*—the name indicated that the organism was sensitive to light—isolated from a soil sample collected in Hermisillo in north-west Mexico not far from the border with Arizona. The organism produced a complex of at least seven components, collectively called nebramycins, two of which, factors 2 and 6 displayed activity similar to that of gentamicin and seemed less toxic in animal tests. Nebramycin factor 2 became apramycin, which is used is veterinary medicine; factor 6, which proved to be identical to kanamycin B save for the loss of an atom of oxygen, was originally given the generic name of ebbramycin but is now known as tobramycin.

Tobramycin was introduced into clinical medicine in the mid-1970s and made an immediate impact. In truth, its properties are so similar to those of gentamicin that it is difficult to see where it has any clear advantage, but much was made of modestly improved activity against *Pseudomonas aeruginosa* (balanced by slightly reduced potency against some other bacterial species), and differential susceptibility to some of the bacterial enzymes commonly involved in resistance to gentamicin.

Resistance to aminoglycosides was a hot topic at the time tobramycin was marketed and this probably acted in its favour. It had long been known that resistance to streptomycin and its close analogues was caused by a simple mutation that alters a single amino acid in a ribosomal protein. This is the site at which streptomycin acts and the antibiotic is unable to bind to ribosomes of organisms carrying the mutation. Later aminoglycosides such as neomycin, kanamycin and the rest act in a different way and are unaffected by this change, but differential resistance to these compounds arises nonetheless. Investigations in Japan (initially by Hamao Umezawa's group), United States, and Europe in the late 1960s and early 1970s revealed that bacteria may produce one or more of a family of enzymes (there are more than 20 of them) that are able to modify exposed amino or hydroxyl groups in aminoglycoside molecules (Fig. 6.3); the modified antibiotic is then unable to penetrate to the intracellular site of action. If a particular aminoglycoside lacks a potentially vulnerable amino or hydroxyl group the susceptibility to individual enzymes is altered and this is the basis for differential resistance patterns that are observed.

One way of overcoming enzymic resistance to aminoglycosides was obviously to remove by chemical means target amino or hydroxyl groups from existing compounds. This approach did not have much success, although in 1971 Umezawa's group described

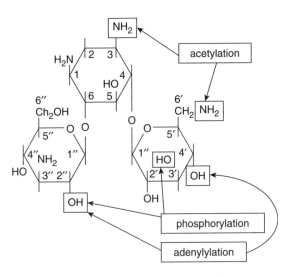

Fig. 6.3 Structure of kanamycin A, showing the numbering system used to define each carbon atom and the sites at which bacterial enzymes can modify the molecule by the addition of acetyl, phosphoryl, or adenyl groups. The enzymes are named according to the target amino or hydroxyl group. Thus an enzyme able to phosphorylate the hydroxyl group at the 2″ carbon is called aminoglycoside phosphorylase 2″ (APH 2″). From Greenwood D., Finch R. G., Davey P. G., Wilcox M. H. *Antimicrobial Chemotherapy* 5th edn. Oxford University Press, Oxford, 2007.

such a compound, dideoxykanamycin B (i.e. tobramycin with a second oxygen atom removed), which was later called dibekacin and marketed in Japan and some other countries. In 1972, Hiroshi Kawaguchi and his colleagues at the Bristol-Banyu Research Institute in Tokyo found a novel way of creating an antibacterially active, but enzyme-resistant aminoglycoside from kanamycin A.

Kawaguchi's team had been investigating an antibiotic complex produced by a bacterium grown from a soil sample collected in Taiwan. Although the producer organism was not an actinomycete, but a conventional bacterium, the antibiotic appeared to be an aminoglycoside with unusual properties, including susceptibility to kanamycin- and neomycin-resistant bacteria. While the researches were underway, Parke, Davis were granted a United States patent for two compounds, butirosin A and butirosin B produced by *Bacillus circulans*, which turned out not only to be identical to the compounds being studied in Japan, but to be very closely related to another Japanese antibiotic, ribostamycin, described in 1970 by Takashi Shomura and associates from Meiji Seika Kaisha, Ltd. (a firm renowned in Japan as much for its chocolates as for its antibiotics) as a product of *Streptomyces ribosidificus*. The major difference between the butirosins and ribostamycin is the presence in the former compounds of an unusual amino acid, aminohydroxybutyric acid and Kawaguchi postulated that adding this grouping to an existing aminoglycoside might favourably alter its characteristics. In this way amikacin—aminohydroxybutyryl kanamycin A—was born (55). The compound proved to be more active than kanamycin against many bacterial species, including *Mycobacterium tuberculosis* and *Pseudomonas aeruginosa*, and to retain its activity against most resistant strains. The latter property was surprising, since amikacin still possessed the amino and hydroxyl groups ostensibly susceptible to enzymic attack. Evidently, the addition of aminohydroxybutyric acid altered the steric configuration of the molecule sufficiently to protect the vulnerable groups, fortunately without affecting antibacterial activity.

Amikacin was marketed in 1977 and became very popular in units troubled by gentamicin resistance. There have been few noteworthy developments in aminoglycosides since that time. Some interest was generated by a compound called arbekacin when reports surfaced in Japan of its successful use against *Staphylococcus aureus* strains showing reduced susceptibility to vancomycin (see p. 241 and 396). Shinichi Kondo and his colleagues at Meiji first described this semi-synthetic aminoglycoside in 1973, but it was not marketed in Japan until 1990. It is very similar to amikacin, except that the aminohydroxybutyric acid group has been linked to dibekacin rather than to kanamycin A.

Dozens of other aminoglycosides have been described. A few have found their way on to the apparently insatiable Japanese market: as well as isepamicin, ribostamycin, and arbekacin—antibiotics scarcely known elsewhere—micronomicin (sagamicin, gentamicin C_{2b}; first described in 1974), and astromicin (fortimicin A; 1976), both from natural products developed by the Kyowa Hakko Kogyo Company, are available in Japan. In addition, there have been brief flirtations with several substances that failed to make the grade, such as bluensomycin (glebomycin; Banyu Pharmaceutical Company, 1962) and lividomycin (Kowa Company, Japan, 1971).

Two other aminoglycosides deserve mention: paromomycin and spectinomycin. Paromomycin—also known as aminosidine and catenulin among sundry other names—is an extraordinary substance that has no place in antibacterial therapy, but has been recommended at various times in the therapy of protozoal infections as diverse as amoebic dysentery (see p. 312) and leishmaniasis (see p. 309–10). Even more remarkably, it has been proposed as an effective drug against several types of human tapeworms, although there were precedents for this: hygromycin B, from *Streptomyces hygroscopicus* (discovered in the Lilly Research Laboratories, Indianapolis, in the1950s) and destomycin A, an aminoglycoside discovered as a product of *Streptomyces rimofaciens* in 1965 by Shinichi Kondo's team at Meiji, have both been used as veterinary anthelminthic compounds in some countries.

Paromomycins I and II are closely related products of a variant form of *Streptomyces rimosus*, first found in soil from Columbia as early as 1958 by John Ehrlich's group at Parke, Davis in Detroit. Paromomycin is related to neomycin and, although some preliminary human pharmacological studies were carried out it was soon clear that it was too toxic to be administered by injection. In common with other aminoglycosides almost all of an oral dose remains in the gut and it was proposed as an oral alternative to neomycin for the purpose of reducing the bacterial flora of the intestinal tract before gut surgery, and as an agent for use in bacillary dysentery, salmonellosis, and other forms of enteritis. None of these uses caught on, but successful use in another intestinal infection, amoebic dysentery, served to prolong interest in the drug. Activity against amoebae had come to light early on through studies on laboratory cultures by the parasitologist Paul Thompson, who was Director of Parasitology at Parke, Davis for over 20 years before moving to the University of Georgia in 1968. At first it was thought that the effect was due to antibacterial action, since in-vitro culture of *Entamoeba histolytica*, the causative agent of amoebiasis is dependent on the addition of bacteria as a food source, but the findings were confirmed in experiments in animals. A successful worldwide trial of oral paromomycin in patients with amoebic dysentery was carried out in 1960.

Strenuous efforts were made to find other uses for paromomycin. Attempts to exploit weak in-vitro activity against other protozoa, including *Giardia lamblia*, a common cause of chronic diarrhoea, and the vaginal pathogen, *Trichomonas vaginalis*, did not provide encouraging results. Marketing of an antibiotic in a disease largely confined to the poorer countries of the tropical world is unlikely to cause much of an impression on a drug company's profits and it is surprising that the drug has remained available for so long.

The longevity of spectinomycin (originally known as actinospectacin) is equally surprising. It was first discovered in 1959 as a product of *Streptomyces spectabilis* in the laboratories of the Upjohn Company (56) and independently found soon afterwards as a product of *Streptomyces flavopersicus* by workers at Abbott Laboratories in Chicago (57). Strictly speaking, spectinomycin is not an aminoglycoside, since the molecule does not include an amino sugar. The structure contains an aminocyclitol group, which is also a characteristic feature of aminoglycosides (the upper ring in Fig. 6.3) and, for want of somewhere better to classify it, spectinomycin usually finds a place among that rather diverse family of compounds. Its properties differ from those of the true aminoglycosides in that it generally inhibits rather than kills bacteria within its spectrum and it probably acts in a different way. It has found its main use in veterinary practice, often in combination with lincomycin (see p. 241–3), but for many years retained a niche in human medicine as an effective agent in the treatment of gonorrhoea that fails to respond to penicillin. Although its antibacterial activity is relatively modest, it has the advantage over other aminoglycosides in that it can be given safely and effectively in a single high intramuscular dose. It has since been overtaken by a variety of more suitable treatments and no longer features in the British National Formulary. However it remains available in some countries and is still occasionally used in patients in whom other drugs are contraindicated.

Narrowing the spectrum

The amazing cures achieved by sulphonamides, penicillin, and streptomycin, followed by the equally spectacular success of tetracyclines and chloramphenicol in diseases as diverse as typhus and typhoid fever, helped to fuel the opinion widely held in the 1950s—sometimes by those who should have known better—that infectious disease was on the way out. By the 1950s it was clear to anyone monitoring such trends that one of the consequences of unrestrained prescribing of antibiotics was inevitably the development of bacterial resistance (see Chapter 9). For the pharmaceutical industry, riding high on their early successes, resistance merely offered an opportunity to prove that they had plenty more tricks up their sleeves.

Although breadth of spectrum remained a top priority for firms looking for new agents that would make an impact in the marketplace, compounds with the extraordinarily wide range of chloramphenicol and the tetracyclines proved surprisingly elusive. Consequently, when antibiotic screening programmes in the 1950s and early 1960s turned up a variety of narrow-spectrum agents that offered a potential solution to the ever-increasing threat of staphylococci resistant to penicillin and tetracycline, they were viewed with renewed interest. The diversity of molecules with such properties turned out to be astonishing. It included vastly dissimilar molecules such as those that came to be known chemically as macrolides, lincosamides, glycopeptides, and streptogramins as well as the steroid antibiotic fusidic acid, and the coumarin-like compound, novobiocin. Although each has its own idiosyncrasies of spectrum, it was their antistaphylococcal activity that attracted most attention.

Macrolides The macrolide group of antibiotics are naturally occurring or semi-synthetic compounds characterized by a chain of up to 15 carbon atoms (more in some of the more obscure compounds) formed into a large ring through an oxygen atom; one or more unusual sugars are usually joined to the main structure. Chemically the molecules are described as macrocyclic lactones, but they are universally known by the generic term macrolide, proposed by the distinguished chemist Robert Woodward in 1957. As with aminoglycosides and many other antibiotics, the natural products are mixtures of closely related substances.

The first macrolide to be described—though not recognized as such at the time—was a compound called proactinomycin discovered in 1942 by Gardner and Chain in the heady days of penicillin research at the Sir William Dunn School in Oxford (58). The organism found to produce the antibiotic was sent to Waksman for identification and originally declared to be a species of *Proactinomyces*, but later given the name *Streptomyces gardneri*. Since the antibiotic exhibited bacteristatic activity directed against bacteria similar to those affected by penicillin, while being less potent and more toxic, it was not progressed further. A similar, and possibly identical antibiotic, picromycin, was described in Germany in 1950 and subjected to limited clinical trial as a topical agent in skin infections.

At least 100 naturally occurring macrolide antibiotics have subsequently been discovered, but only a few have found their way into therapeutic use in human medicine. Some, like tylosin and its derivative tilmicosin are exclusively used in veterinary medicine. By far the most important macrolide is erythromycin A, the most active member of a complex of antibiotics produced by *Saccharopolyspora erythraea* (formerly *Streptomyces erythreus*). Erythromycin A has little activity against most Gram-negative bacilli, since it penetrates with difficulty through the outer membrane characteristic of those organisms and is unable to reach the target site on the bacterial ribosome. In essence the spectrum resembles that of benzylpenicillin and the antibiotic attracted immediate attention because of its activity against strains of staphylococci resistant to penicillin and tetracyclines.

The producer organism was isolated from a sample of soil obtained in 1949 by a Filipino doctor, Abelardo Aguilar in the province of Ilo-Ilo in the central Philippines (59). Aguilar had been acting as a local sales representative for Eli Lilly and he sent the specimen to the company in United States in October 1950. Whether he had himself in the meantime investigated the sample for antibiotic activity is unclear. Once a potentially useful antibiotic had been identified, Lilly acknowledged the origin of the gift in their registered trade name Ilotycin (and later Ilosone; erythromycin estolate), but neither Aguilar, nor the local community saw any of the eventual profits.

Whatever the validity of Aguilar's claim to have discovered Erythromycin, the antibiotic was undoubtedly developed and brought to market by Lilly. Robert Bunch and James McGuire were named as co-inventors in a patent application on behalf of the company submitted on 14 April 1952 and granted in September the following year (60). But surprisingly the antibiotic was also marketed in 1952 under the name Erythrocin (erythromycin stearate) by the firm of Abbott in Chicago. According to *The Abbott Almanac*, published in 1988 for the company's centenary, research on erythromycin had been shared by Lilly, Abbott, and Upjohn, though the latter firm did not register a trade name for the product (61). It seems extraordinary that this should have happened. The massive soil-screening programmes carried out in many drug company laboratories in the post-war period had not been particularly productive in terms of substances that survived preliminary tests of activity and safety; one would imagine that a saleable product would have been regarded as hot property.*

It was the Abbott formulation that was used in a landmark study by George Gee Jackson and his colleagues at the University of Illinois and the Municipal Contagious Disease Hospital, Chicago, which was to set the trend for the way erythromycin was used in the following decades. With admirable foresight, Jackson saw the opportunity to track the development of resistance to a new antibiotic in a population that had never been exposed to it. During the last week of September 1952, just before erythromycin was introduced into the wards of the Contagious Disease Hospital, nose and throat swabs were taken from all patients and staff concerned with patient care. On 28 September 1952, immediately after the survey, use of erythromycin was started. Penicillin usage was greatly curtailed and the only other antibiotic used during the course of the study was chlortetracycline. Erythromycin was found to be very effective in treating staphylococcal infection and in reducing colonization in patients undergoing tracheostomies. However, over the 5-month period of the study the proportion of strains resistant to erythromycin (not inhibited by a concentration of 100 μg/ml) increased from zero to 95 per cent in staphylococci colonizing patients with tracheostomies and from zero to 75 per cent in hospital personnel who were carriers of staphylococci. As resistance increased, the effectiveness of erythromycin fell (62).

The evident ease with which resistance to erythromycin occurred led to calls for restrictions on its use, especially within hospitals. The advice from infectious disease experts—not always heeded—was to keep the drug in reserve for use against resistant strains and for patients allergic to the preferred drug, penicillin. As newer antistaphylococcal agents appeared, the weight of this advice diminished, but erythromycin became accepted as an antibiotic to be held in reserve and it never quite achieved the rank of a first-choice agent.

----

* There is, however, an earlier precedent for collaboration between James McGuire of Lilly and scientists from Abbott and Upjohn. See: Loo Y. H., Skell P. S., Thornberry H. H., Ehrlich J., McGuire J. M., Savage G. M., Sylvester J. C. Assay of streptomycin by the paper-disc plate method. *Journal of Bacteriology* 1945; 50:701-709.

Hard on the heels of erythromycin came several other macrolides. Scientists at Pfizer described carbomycin as a product of *Streptomyces halstedii* in 1952; it was subjected to clinical trial by Maxwell Finland in Boston, but soon rejected as inferior to erythromycin. Pfizer tried again in 1954 with oleandomycin, isolated from *Streptomyces antibioticus* and, in due course with a better-absorbed derivative, triacetyloleandomycin (troleandomycin). The compounds survived early investigations that failed to reveal any properties of particular note and soon reached the marketplace. In an effort to boost the fortune of oleandomycin it was marketed in a fixed-dose combination with tetracycline despite lack of evidence of any convincing synergic interaction or other benefit. Oleandomycin, with or without tetracycline has long disappeared, but remarkably, troleandomycin is still available in the United States, though it has little to recommend it over erythromycin.

In 1954, a new macrolide antibiotic, spiramycin, was described by Sylvie Pinnert (known as Pinnert-Sindico at the time of the discovery) and her colleagues in the research laboratories of Rhône-Poulenc (now part of Aventis) in France (63). The producer organism, a previously unrecognized species of *Streptomyces*, was isolated from soil collected near Péronne—a town on the River Somme whose soil had been bitterly fought over during the First World War. The new species was found to produce two different antibiotics, spiramycin and one identified as congocidine,* which had previously been described 2 years earlier in the same laboratory (64); it was thus given the name *Streptomyces ambofaciens*: 'maker of both'. The name 'spiramycin' refers to the characteristic spirals, seen under the microscope that helped to differentiate the producer organism from a closely related species, *Streptomyces griseolus*.

The new antibiotic was quickly recognized to belong to the erythromycin group of compounds. As usual it proved to be a mixture of several closely related molecules, of which spiramycin 1 is the major component. Compared with erythromycin, its activity was unremarkable, but claims were made for improved results in animal experiments attributed to peculiarities of distribution and persistence in tissues. Human studies confirmed its efficacy and lack of side effects associated with other macrolides (65). It remains popular in France and has achieved a particular niche for itself because of its idiosyncratic activity against the protozoan parasite *Toxoplasma gondii*, the cause of toxoplasmosis.

Meanwhile, in 1953, Japan had joined the hunt for new macrolides with leucomycin (later called kitasamycin) isolated at the Kitasato Institute by Toju Hata (son-in-law of Sahachiro Hata† of Salvarsan fame; see p. 58) from a soil organism inevitably given the name *Streptomyces kitasatoensis*. Similar compounds followed: josamycin, a product of *Streptomyces narbonensis* subspecies *josamyceticus* from the Yamanouchi Pharmaceutical Company in 1967; and midecamycin, a product of *Streptomyces mycarofaciens* from Meiji

---

* Originally investigated as an antitrypanosomal agent, Cogocidine was later shown to possess antipoxvirus activity, but was never brought into use. See: Becker Y., Asher Y., Zakay-Rones Z. Congocidine and distamycin A, antipoxvirus antibiotics. *Antimicrobial Agents and Chemotherapy* 1972; 1: 483–488.

† According to Japanese custom if a distinguished man has a daughter but no son, the man who marries the daughter takes her family name.

in 1971. Miokamycin and rokitamycin, derivatives of midecamycin A_1 and leucomycin A_5 respectively, also appeared in due course. None has made much impact in human medicine, though several of these compounds remain on the Japanese market and, more surprisingly, that of some European countries.

The flagging fortunes of the macrolides received a boost during the 1980s, when a rash of semi-synthetic derivatives of erythromycin A were described. These newer macrolides—azithromycin, clarithromycin, dirithromycin, flurithromycin, and rox-ithromycin—claimed pharmacological advantages over earlier compounds, including better tissue distribution and reduced side effects. Azithromycin has attracted most attention, though clarithromycin has also been enormously successful, more due to skilful marketing than to any inherently outstanding properties.

Azithromycin was synthesized in 1980 by Gabrijela Kobrehel and Slobodan Djokić in the laboratories of the Croatian Company, Pliva,* where Djokić was Director of Research. It was licensed in 1986 to Pfizer in the United States, a company which, ironically, had already discovered and patented the same compound almost simultaneously. The patent applications were submitted independently and both were erroneously allowed owing to confusion over the way the structures were presented, which made them appear to be different compounds. The Pfizer patent was actually issued first, in October 1984, more than 7 months before the one granted to Pliva, but the Croatian company had submitted their application in March 1980, a year and a half ahead of the American giant. When the two substances were found to be identical, they were awarded priority and Pfizer were forced to negotiate terms to benefit from their own discovery (66).

In azithromycin a nitrogen atom has been inserted into the macrocyclic lactone ring of erythromycin and the drug is often referred to as an azalide, rather than a macrolide. This feature gives it exceptional persistence in the body, and it has been successfully used in the single-dose treatment of chlamydial infections, including the eye infection trachoma—a common cause of blindness in many developing countries—and sexually transmitted chlamydial disease. Single-dose therapy has long been used for the treatment of gonorrhoea in clinics dealing with sexually transmitted infections, and similar therapy for chlamydial disease is welcomed since the clients do not always comply with longer treatment courses. Clarithromycin was developed in Japan around 1980 by Yoshiaki Watanabe and his colleagues at the Taisho Pharmaceutical Company† and marketed elsewhere by Abbott.

The renaissance of macrolides continued with telithromycin, described in 1997 by scientists at Hoechst Marion Roussel (since 1999, Aventis). Telithromycin is another semi-synthetic derivative of erythromycin A in which one of the associated sugar groups has been removed and a substituted ketone (C=O) function introduced on to the lactone ring. Because of the latter feature it is often called a ketolide. The strongest selling point of telithromycin is that it retains activity against many strains of staphylococci that are

---

* Pliva, originally so named in 1941 as the State Institute for Production of Medicines and Vaccines, was formed from a firm called Kastel in Zagreb, which in 1936 had recruited the chemist and future Nobel laureate, Vladimir Prolog to synthesize sulphanilamide. Prolog emigrated to Switzerland in 1941.

† Taisho was founded in Tokyo in 1912 to manufacture and sell non-prescription medicines.

resistant to erythromycin and other macrolides. Since its launch in Europe (in 2001) and the United States (2004) it has been dogged by problems of toxicity and its place in therapy remains under scrutiny.

Novobiocin The antibiotic eventually given the name novobiocin may hold the record for multiple discovery: it was originally described independently in 1955 under the names cathomycin (Cathocin, Merck) and streptonivicin (Albamycin,* Upjohn); a Pfizer investigational compound, PA93, was also found to be identical with the two drugs and the generic name novobiocin was approved in 1956. A few months later, an antibiotic isolated by scientists at Lepetit from a streptomycete discovered in a soil sample from Rome also turned out to be novobiocin. In 1958, evidence emerged from Japan that a previously uncharacterized antibiotic, griseoflavin, described in 1953 from Tohoku University in Sendai, Japan as a product of *Streptomyces griseoflavus*, was the same substance (67).

The Merck compound was a product of *Streptomyces spheroides*, isolated from pasture soil in Vermont by Boyd Woodruff's group; Upjohn's antibiotic came from *Streptomyces niveus*, an organism with a snow-white colonial morphology isolated by the actinomycete expert, Alma Dietz and her colleagues. Novobiocin attracted attention because of high activity against staphylococci and exceptionally good absorption when given by mouth. Another attractive feature was that it had a novel structure related to the coumarins—anticoagulants extracted from tonka beans (locally called cumaru in Suriname)—so that bacteria resistant to other agents remained sensitive. Early trials revealed that resistance developed readily and a variety of troublesome side effects were reported. It was used for a time, often in combination with other agents (a combination with tetracycline was marketed by Upjohn), but it was quickly overtaken by the antistaphylococcal penicillins and gradually disappeared from view, though it remained available in some countries for many years for human and veterinary use. An unexpected effect in enhancing the potency of certain anticancer drugs may yet see the life of novobiocin further extended and provide yet another example of an antimicrobial agent fulfilling a purpose quite different from the one originally envisaged.

Glycopeptides Within a few years of the appearance of erythromycin Lilly and Abbott again found themselves in intense rivalry over two novel antibiotics—vancomycin (Lilly) and ristocetin (Abbott)—with a very similar spectrum directed mainly against staphylococci and streptococci. Both compounds were found to be toxic, but the rapid development of resistance did not seem to be a problem and the need for reliable antistaphylococcal agents encouraged the companies to pursue them.

Vancomycin (the name was intended to convey its ability to vanquish the staphylococcus) was first obtained in 1956 from an organism grown from a soil sample sent by a missionary from the interior of Borneo; the same organism was later found in two strains from India (68). The organism was consequently given the name *Streptomyces orientalis*,

---

* To add to the confusion over novobiocin derivatives, an unrelated antibiotic, albomycin, was described from the Soviet Union in the early 1950s (See Gause GF. Recent studies on albomycin, a new antibiotic. *British Medical Journal* 1995; 2: 1177.

but was reclassified first as *Nocardia orientalis* and then as *Amycolatopsis orientalis* subspecies *orientalis*. Ristocetin is a mixture of two similar antibiotics found a year later as a product of a soil actinomycete, *Nocardia lurida* (now *Amycolatopsis orientalis* subspecies *lurida*) (69). The soil sample yielding the antibiotic had been taken from the Garden of the Gods, a scenic area of rock formations in Colorado Springs Parks, south of Denver, Colorado.

It soon became clear that ristocetin was too unsafe for human use and Abbott withdrew it in the early 1960s. Vancomycin continued to be used in difficult staphylococcal infections, but gained a reputation for toxicity and was quickly left behind by newer antistaphylococcal agents, including some penicillins (see p. 123–4). Some of the adverse side effects encountered in the early days of vancomycin were undoubtedly caused by impurities in the commercial preparations. The antibiotic was difficult to extract and purify and early lots were contaminated with fermentation broth, earning the drug the nickname 'Mississippi mud' (70). In the course of time, improved purification techniques produced a much cleaner and safer product and vancomycin lived to fight another day. Towards the end of the century it rose to prominence as a reliable drug for the treatment of infections caused by multiresistant staphylococci. Ristocetin was also given a new lease of life when it was discovered to act, in a way that has not been fully elucidated, as a useful reagent in the diagnosis of von Willebrand's disease, an inherited defect of blood clotting.

The structure of vancomycin is large and intricate and took some time to unravel; the molecule eventually turned out to be formed from an unusual tricyclic arrangement of seven amino acids linked to a disaccharide, giving it the generic name glycopeptide. Numerous antibiotics of this general type have been discovered, including avoparcin, from *Streptomyces candidus* and actaplanin, from *Actinoplanes missouriensis* found in barnyard soil in Hamilton, Missouri; these agents are designed for use as growth promoters in animal husbandry, though they are now banned in Europe along with other agents (see p. 405). The only glycopeptide to arrive on the scene as a rival to vancomycin for human therapy is teicoplanin (originally called teichomycin), isolated in 1976 by Franco Parenti and his colleagues at Gruppo Lepetit in Italy from *Actinoplanes teichomyceticus*, an actinomycete obtained from soil collected in Nimodi, a village in Madhya Pradesh in Central India (71). Teicoplanin is easier to administer than vancomycin, which needs to be given by slow intravenous injection; it is also much more slowly eliminated from the body and these features have helped to increase its popularity. A semi-synthetic derivative of vancomycin, oritavancin is in clinical trial at the time of writing.

Lincosamides It was penicillins like methicillin and cloxacillin (see p. 123–4), which were able to draw on the reputation of benzylpenicillin for safety and efficacy, that came to dominate the market for drugs aimed at infections with resistant strains of staphylococci. Nonetheless, other compounds with antistaphylococcal activity were still an attractive proposition for pharmaceutical firms in the early 1960s. At Upjohn's research laboratories at Kalamazoo, Michigan, Donald Mason, Alma Dietz, and their colleagues, followed up their discovery of spectinomycin (see p. 235) and novobiocin (see p. 240) with a description in 1962 of lincomycin, a compound characterized by excellent activity against Gram-positive cocci (72). The antibiotic was a product of a soil micro-organism, *Streptomyces lincolnensis*, obtained from Lincoln, Nebraska. According to Wallace Herrell, who wrote a monograph on the substance, the discovery had been made and investigated many years before it was made public (73).

An attractive feature of lincomycin was its novel structure, which raised hopes, never to be realized, that it might be the forerunner of a new family of antibacterial agents. The molecule was amenable to chemical modification and from the start the Upjohn chemists sought semi-synthetic derivatives of lincomycin, but nothing of note emerged until 1966 when the simple expedient of replacing a hydroxyl group with a chlorine atom seemed to do the trick. The resultant compound, clindamycin, not only displayed a four-fold increase in activity, but also produced much better blood levels when given by mouth (74). Before long clindamycin had virtually replaced lincomycin as the preferred version of the antibiotic. A surprising added bonus was that clindamycin exhibited antimalarial as well as antibacterial activity, prompting a renewed search for compounds of this type (75). In the event only one other lincosamide proved to be commercially viable: pirlimycin, unveiled by Robert Birkenmeyer of Upjohn at the 20th ICAAC in New Orleans in 1980, a congener that was eventually put on sale as an antistaphylococcal agent for veterinary use in bovine mastitis.

Although it was the antistaphylococcal activity of lincomycin that had ensured its survival, activity against anaerobic Gram-negative bacilli was noted in 1965 (76) by the doyen of anaerobe studies, Sydney Finegold, Professor of Medicine and Microbiology at the University of California Los Angeles School of Medicine and founding president of the Anaerobe Society of the Americas. The discovery did not arouse much interest, since the activity was unremarkable and, in any case, awareness of the importance of anaerobes, especially the Gram-negative varieties, was only just beginning to become apparent. When clindamycin became available it was also marketed primarily as an antistaphylococcal agent, but its activity against Gram-negative anaerobes, notably *Bacteroides fragilis*—an important pathogen in post-operative intestinal and gynaecological infections—was very much better than that of lincomycin. Since *Bacteroides fragilis* is resistant to penicillins and cephalosporins, it came to be used widely in anaerobic infections.

Both lincomycin and clindamycin came through clinical trials with virtually unblemished safety records apart from transient diarrhoea, which accompanies the use of many antibacterial agents that affect the gut flora. It therefore came as an unwelcome surprise when the antibiotics were linked to deaths from a serious inflammatory condition of the large bowel, pseudomembranous colitis, which were reported with increasing frequency in the 1970s (77). Warning bells were sounded when a gastroenterologist, Jerome Ecker and his colleagues from Santa Barbara, California, presented a case report to the Annual Convention of the American College of Gastroenterology held in Houston, Texas in October 1969 (78). The 38-year-old wife of a physician had been given lincomycin for a pneumococcal sinusitis in February 1967; she developed diarrhoea and became critically ill with a classic pseudomembranous colitis. The disease was not new, but it was rarely seen, although a similar condition caused by overgrowth of staphylococci in the gut following antibiotic therapy had been described.* Many similar cases were reported in the following years and the disease became associated with treatment with lincosamides, although other agents including broad-spectrum β-lactam antibiotics were later incriminated.

The woman described in the original case report was extremely fortunate. She slowly recovered when given oral vancomycin, the recognized treatment at the time for staphylococcal enterocolitis. Vancomycin is now known to be one of the few useful drugs in pseudomembranous colitis, but the precipitating cause of the disease was not known at the time and there was no evidence of staphylococcal overgrowth to support the use of vancomycin in this case. It was some years later that animal experiments revealed that the disease is caused by toxins elaborated by a previously overlooked anaerobic Gram-positive bacillus, *Clostridium difficile*. Despite their anti-anaerobe activity, lincosamides are relatively ineffective against this organism and by suppressing the rest of the anaerobic flora of the gut allow it to flourish.

Antibiotic-associated diarrhoea caused by clostridial toxins does not always progress to a life-threatening colitis and lincosamides are by no means the only culprits. Moreover, the frequency with which the side effect occurs during therapy with lincosamides or other antibacterial agents in various population groups has long been disputed. Nevertheless, the lincosamides suffered more than other antibiotics from the reputation of causing severe diarrhoea. For this reason they failed to achieve the popularity that the manufacturers had hoped for. Despite the relative success of Upjohn's soil screening programme, the firm never managed to produce an antibiotic destined to become a market leader.

Streptogramins Regardless of their novel structure, the site of action of the lincosamides on ribosomes within the bacterial cells is very close—possibly even identical—to that of the macrolide antibiotics, and the same seems to be true of the streptogramins. One consequence of this is that a type of macrolide resistance caused by enzymic modification of the ribosomal binding site also renders the bacteria resistant to lincosamides and streptogramins; resistance is manifested only in the presence of a macrolide, since the other antibiotics do not induce production of the enzyme. These peculiarities, and activity biased towards staphylococci and streptococci, led Yves Chabbert and Jacques Baudens of the Institut Pasteur, Paris to propose that macrolides, lincosamides, and streptogramins should be considered as a homogeneous group (79). This association of the three families of antibiotics in a single group remains prevalent in the microbiological literature, though they are in fact very different.

The streptogramins have had a chequered history. The antibiotic that gave the group its generic name was described in 1953 by Jesse Charney and associates at Merck's Sharp and Dohme Division in Philadelphia (the companies had been merged in that year) as a product of *Streptomyces graminofaciens* isolated from soil in Texas (80). They noted that

* Staphylococcal enterocolitis was recognized as a complication of antibiotic therapy in patients undergoing surgery. Tetracyclines were most commonly incriminated and the staphylococci involved were usually tetracycline-resistant. Huge numbers of staphylococci were evident in faecal smears. The condition became mysteriously less common in the 1970s and is now rarely reported.

purified concentrates of culture filtrates of the organism exhibited activity against Gram-positive cocci and protected mice infected with β-haemolytic streptococci, but the most extraordinary aspect of the streptogramins was not appreciated at the time: the inhibitory potency arises from the co-operative action of two dissimilar antibiotic compounds* that alone have comparatively feeble antibacterial activity.

In the ensuing years Lilly, Parke Davis, Pfizer, and Squibb among others described similar antibiotics, but none seems to have been actively pursued. More enthusiasm for streptogramins was found in Europe and Japan; a few have been used for human therapy, though they have found their main market as growth promoters in animal husbandry. The first of these compounds was virginiamycin, which has occasionally been used in human staphylococcal infections, notably in Belgium, where it was discovered in 1955 in the laboratories of Recherche et Industrie Thérapeutiques, a vaccine manufacturing company in the village of Genval, near Rixensart south-east of Brussels; the company was acquired by Smith Kline in 1963 and is now part of GlaxoSmithKline. The antibiotic was discovered as a product of *Streptomyces virginiae*, an organism originally isolated in 1952 in a soil sample from Roanoke, Virginia and investigated by Abbott and Pfizer in the United States as the producer of an antimetabolite of the vitamin, biotin.

In 1956, a group led by Hiroshi Yonehara at the University of Tokyo described mikamycin, a streptogramin complex produced by *Streptomyces mitakaensis*. It was taken up by the Kanegafuchi Chemical Company in Japan and was briefly considered for human therapy and as a growth promoter for poultry (81). A very similar compound, osteogrycin, was investigated in the mid-1950s in Britain. Workers at Glaxo had obtained it from *Streptomyces osteogriseus* recovered from a soil sample from Jericho. Intravenous preparations were shown to be effective in staphylococcal septicaemia and endocarditis, but it was difficult to prepare and administer and was never marketed (82).

The most widely used streptogramin in human medicine, at least in France, where it was promoted under the splendidly jingoistic slogan 'Antibiotique 100 per cent Français' was pristinamycin, a compound discovered and developed by Jean Preud'homme and his colleagues in the laboratories of Rhône-Poulenc in Vitry-sur-Seine. The antibiotic complex, part of which is identical to the virginiamycin complex, was first isolated in 1958 from *Streptomyces pristinaespiralis*. Clinical use of oral pristinamycin started in France in 1962, predominantly for the treatment of staphylococcal infections (83). Little progress was made in introducing the drug into other countries, although it became available in Belgium, the Netherlands, and Germany. It was offered to May and Baker in Britain, a firm in which Rhône-Poulenc had acquired a majority shareholding as early as 1927.[†] Tentative clinical studies were started in 1963, but with the advent of semi-synthetic

---

* As with most other naturally occurring antibiotics, the two main active components of streptogramins are found in fermentation broth as a mixture of several closely related variants.

† The Poulenc brothers bought the controlling interest in May and Baker in 1927. Rhône–Poulenc was formed the following year by the merger of la Société chimique des usines du Rhône (founded in 1895) and the firm established by the Poulenc Frères in 1900. The composer Francis Poulenc (1899–1963) was the son of one of the brothers.

penicillins, development was halted. In 1970 another attempt was made to initiate clinical trials in Great Britain, but there was no enthusiasm for a drug seen to have little to recommend it and the trials were abandoned.

Making headway outside France obviously required a fresh approach. The opportunity came in the 1990s, when concerns over the spread in hospitals of strains of *Staphylococcus aureus* resistant to methicillin and other antistaphylococcal drugs reached a fever pitch. One of the drawbacks of pristinamycin is that it can be administered only by mouth, since preparation of a solution suitable for injection proved impracticable. The vagaries of intestinal absorption and the difficulty of oral therapy in critically ill patients who may be unable to swallow make an injectable form essential in serious staphylococcal infections. The answer was to create water-soluble derivatives of the two principal synergistic components of pristinamycin, to provide a preparation suitable for intravenous use. The two derivatives were called quinupristin and dalfopristin, though the commercial mixture is known by the less tongue-twisting name Synercid. It was marketed in Great Britain and the United States in 1999 and is one of the drugs that physicians turn to when older antistaphylococcal agents fail.

Fusidic acid The final antistaphylococcal agent to emerge in a highly productive period in the early 1960s came from what is probably the most unexpected source of any antibiotic: Japanese monkey dung. The find was made by scientists in the small Danish pharmaceutical company, Leo Pharma, in Ballerup, north-west of Copenhagen, a firm founded in 1908 by August Kongsted and Anton Antons in the basement of the pharmacy, Løveapoteket, which they had recently purchased in Copenhagen. The company became interested in antibiotics during the Second World War, when they started to manufacture penicillin. Later, in 1972, they produced the unusual penicillin derivative, mecillinam (see p. 126).

The discovery of fusidic acid in 1960 was a classic piece of serendipity. The research group were looking for fungal enzymes that would remove the side-chain from penicillin in order to provide the basic structure needed for the creation of semi-synthetic penicillins. As part of the investigation strains of fungi belonging to the *Fusarium* genus were purchased from the Dutch type culture collection, Centraalbureau voor Schimmelcultures, at Baarn, in the Netherlands. In the alphabetical list of the Baarn catalogue, *Fusarium* was followed by *Fusidium*, one species of which was *Fusidium coccineum*. When this species was bought—apparently in error or on a whim—and tested, it was found to be unsuitable as a source of the enzyme that the chemists had sought, but routine testing unexpectedly showed potent antistaphylococcal activity (84). *Fusidium coccineum* had originally been isolated in 1953 by the Japanese mycologist Keisuke Tubaki from the dung of a wild monkey caught in Settu, Japan. It was not at that time known to be an antibiotic producer. Ironically the fungus was later reclassified and has been described since 1971 in the Baarn collection as *Acremonium fusidioides*—far removed alphabetically from *Fusarium*.

The structure of fusidic acid is very similar to that of steroid compounds, but the stereochemistry of the molecule is different and it exhibits none of the pharmacological properties associated with steroids (85). The antibiotic is related to helvolic acid—a substance isolated by Howard Florey's team in Oxford in 1943 from the culture fluid of the fungus *Aspergillus fumigatus*—and to cephalosporin P_1, the component of Giuseppe Brotzu's *Cephalosporium* mould that was principally responsible for its activity against staphylococci (see p. 117); the activity of fusidic acid is, however, much greater than that of either compound.

Clinical trials were soon under way in Britain as well as continental Europe and fusidic acid was found to be a useful addition to the antistaphylococcal armoury. The manufacturers were unable to obtain a licence in the United States, probably because of fears over liver toxicity that materialized, especially after intravenous use, but the drug was marketed over the border in Canada.

Fusidic acid has an idiosyncratic spectrum of activity, which includes moderately good activity against *Mycobacterium tuberculosis* and some other mycobacteria, though there is little experience of its use in mycobacterial disease. Its place remains as an antistaphylococcal agent with a good safety record and excellent tissue permeability. Resistance develops readily in laboratory culture and, sometimes, in clinical use. For this reason it is usually administered together with an antistaphylococcal penicillin or other agent.

Spanish interlude

In 1954, at the height of the antibiotic discovery boom, a collaborative research programme was begun in Spain as the result of an agreement between Merck (by then merged with Sharp and Dohme) in the United States and Compañia Española de la Penicilina y do los Antibióticos (CEPA) in Madrid (86). The first discovery of any note from this venture was unveiled in October 1969 with the publication in *Science* of a joint paper from Merck and CEPA describing a new antibiotic, phosphonomycin (87), since shortened to fosfomycin. Sagrario Mochales and her colleagues at CEPA had isolated the antibiotic from a strain of *Streptomyces fradiae* found in a soil sample from Eastern Spain. Subsequent development took place in the Merck laboratories in Rahway, New Jersey, where an identical substance was found in two other soil isolates, *Streptomyces viridochromogenes* and *Streptomyces wedmorensis*. In contrast to the complex molecular configuration of most antibiotics, the structure of fosfomycin is appealingly straightforward, vying with cycloserine for simplicity (Fig. 6.4). Like cycloserine and chloramphenicol it is relatively easy to manufacture synthetically.

Fosfomycin bucked the trend of the string of new antibiotics distinguished by antistaphylococcal activity. In fact the overall antibacterial potency of fosfomycin is quite modest compared with many other compounds and Gram-positive cocci are among the least susceptible. The most noteworthy activity is against *Escherichia coli* and some other Gram-negative bacilli. Many factors affect the activity in laboratory tests and there has been much dispute about the most reliable way of conducting susceptibility tests of the drug. Resistance emerges quite readily in the test tube but seems to be surprisingly uncommon in countries in which it is used.

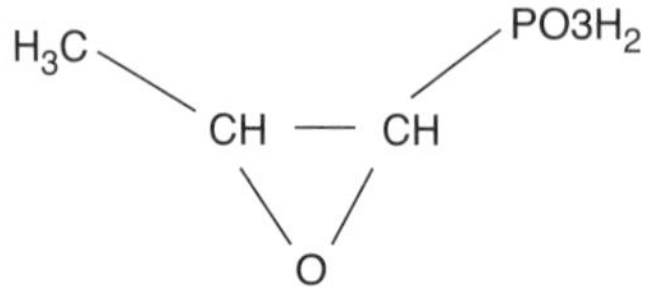

Fig. 6.4 Structure of fosfomycin.

Despite the energy Merck put into development of fosfomycin there was little enthusiasm in the United States or the United Kingdom for a compound with no obvious therapeutic place and it was not marketed in those countries. It went on sale in parts of Europe in the 1970s and reached Japan in 1980. Predictably, the greatest enthusiasm for the compound has been in Spain, where it is quite popular as a 'home-grown' antibiotic. Some further interest was revived during the 1980s when a small Italian pharmaceutical firm, Zambon, formulated fosfomycin in a chemical combination with the alkalizing agent tromethamine (trometamol). The salt is very soluble and is excreted into urine in high concentration making it particularly suitable for the treatment of uncomplicated urinary tract infection. The product was marketed in many countries, including the United States and Britain, as a single-dose treatment of cystitis—a common infection in young women. It was later discontinued in the United Kingdom, but is still available elsewhere.

The Merck-CEPA joint venture also provided the starting point for two important β-lactam antibiotics in the 1970s: cefoxitin (see p. 131) and imipenem (see p. 132–3). Both were developed from unusual β-lactam molecules found as natural products of streptomycetes isolated by the Spanish research group, though they played no part in turning them into commercial compounds. Merck took full control of the research centre in 1979, and the name was changed to Centro de Investigación Básica de España. In 1985, a mould that produced a new class of antifungal compound, the pneumocandins, was discovered there (see p. 361).

More antistaphylococcal agents

Mupirocin In the mid-1950s, Ernst Chain, by then working at the Istituto Superiore di Sanità in Rome (see p. 116), was being wooed by Imperial College in London. The Chair of Biochemistry at Imperial had been vacant since 1943 when the incumbent, Albert Chibnall, moved to Cambridge to succeed the famous biochemist and Nobel laureate, Frederick Gowland Hopkins. After the inevitable wrangling over Chain's exorbitant demands for laboratory and pilot plant facilities—finally resolved with the help of a grant from the philanthropist, Sir Isaac Wolfson—Chain was in due course appointed to the Chair of Biochemistry at Imperial College in 1961, though he did not actually take up his new position until 1964 (88).

Around 1970 Chain recruited to his new department a retired biochemist, Albert Fuller, who had a longstanding interest in antibiotics. Fuller had worked with Leonard Colebrook at Queen Charlotte's Hospital in the early days of sulphonamides and had helped to show that the activity of Gerhard Domagk's Prontosil was due to the breakdown product, sulphanilamide (see p. 74). Subsequently, he worked at the National Institute for Medical Research and isolated a number of substances with antibiotic activity. In 1955 he discovered an antibiotic produced by a strain of *Bacillus pumilis* found in a soil sample from East Africa provided by Dr Philip Spensley (later Director of the Tropical Products Institute), which attracted the attention of Edward Abraham at Oxford (89). It turned out to be identical, or very closely related, to a peptide antibiotic called micrococcin, which had been isolated from Oxford sewage by T. L. Su, a scholarship student from the National Medical College of Shanghai, around 1948 (90). The compound(s) were peptides related to bacitracin and were soon abandoned. Fuller continued his antibiotic studies at Imperial College in a characteristically desultory and leisurely fashion, much to the frustration of his notoriously impatient boss. He soon decided that retirement was preferable to life in Chain's hot-house and he departed, leaving behind his culture collection.

One of Albert Fuller's pet substances was an antibiotic produced by the bacterium *Pseudomonas fluorescens*, which he called pseudomonic acid (91). It was very active, notably against staphylococci and streptococci and was clearly worth following up. After Fuller left, further investigation of the substance was put into the hands of the biochemist Graham Mellows, who established during the 1970s that the structure and mode of action differed from those of other antibiotics then in use. Realizing that it had commercial potential, Chain passed the compound to Beecham Research Laboratories, where he was a consultant. The activity and safety of pseudomonic acid—now called mupirocin—were confirmed, but it was found that it was inactivated in serum and was thus unsuitable for systemic use. It was nevertheless marketed as a topical agent under the trade name Bactroban and has proved very useful, especially in the control of methicillin-resistant *Staphylococcus aureus* (MRSA; see p. 396–8)—for example in eradicating the bacteria from the noses of hospital patients and staff found to carry the organism.

Daptomycin In the mid-1980s, scientists at Eli Lilly recovered an antibiotic complex from *Streptomyces roseosporus* identified at that time only by the laboratory code A21978C. The substance was characterized by narrow-spectrum activity limited to Gram-positive cocci. The molecule turned out to be a cyclic peptide with a fatty acid tail and the structure was thus reminiscent of the polymyxins, though the spectrum of activity was clearly very different. Several derivatives were produced by chemical manipulation of the basic molecule and one, to which the name daptomycin was given, was judged to have the best safety profile in toxicity tests in animals (92).

Lilly obviously had high hopes for the new antibiotic, since a deluge of publications, mostly concerned with laboratory evaluation, appeared in chemotherapy journals between 1986 and 1990. However, in clinical trials, side effects—including neurotoxicity in some patients—were uncovered. Development stopped and it was assumed that nothing more would be heard of this interesting compound.

Renewed concerns over multiresistant staphylococci as the century drew to a close prompted a rethink. Daptomycin was licensed in 1997 to Cubist Pharmaceuticals, a company founded in 1992 to develop promising drugs, especially in the field of infection. After successful clinical trials in the United States, FDA approval was granted for the use of daptomycin in serious infections of skin and soft tissue in September 2003, clearing the way for its introduction on to the market.

Synthetic antibacterial agents

The golden age of antimicrobial agents coincided with a spectacular flourishing of the twin disciplines of microbial biochemistry and molecular biology. As information about metabolic pathways and transport mechanisms within the microbial cell accumulated exponentially, it was confidently predicted that 'designer' drugs aimed at essential cellular processes absent from mammalian cells—just as penicillin did—would inevitably follow. The optimism was misplaced. After more than 50 years, we still await a clinically useful antibacterial agent that has been designed to act through a premeditated attack on a unique and vulnerable microbial target. The search for natural products by random screening programmes has been much more rewarding in terms of the number of useful agents found. This should not be too surprising: in the sphere of biological protection, the micro-organisms have had a few million years start.

Several families of synthetic antibacterial drugs suitable for the systemic treatment of infection have nonetheless become available alongside naturally occurring antibiotics. In addition to the sulphonamides (Chapter 3) and an assortment of antimycobacterial compounds (Chapter 5) substances described chemically as nitrofurans, diaminopyrimidines, quinolones, and oxazolidinones have arrived on the scene by various routes. Few have provided rich commercial pickings with a single representative of each family accounting for nearly all the clinical use. The one exception is the large quinolone family; after a stuttering start, a profusion of interesting new quinolone derivatives appeared towards the end of the century triggering a bitter—and to those of us watching from the touchline, entertaining—struggle for market supremacy.

A major problem facing chemists trying to devise new synthetic agents was simply deciding where to begin. Attempts to produce safer derivatives of dyes and antiseptics earlier in the century had come to nothing, at least as far as substances active against bacteria are concerned, though there was some success with antiprotozoal agents (see Chapter 7). Nor could much be learned from natural products, since the structural features that led to the activity of most antibiotics were poorly understood. Moreover, starting from basic principles, no chemist, however ingenious, could hope to come up with a safe and effective chemical compound analogous to the complicated molecules that are a feature of most natural products. The sulphonamides showed what could be achieved, but other leads were hard to find. Chemical compounds like *para*-aminosalicylic acid and isoniazid, developed for their antimycobacterial action, turned out to be selective in their antibacterial range. As usual the vagaries of chance have played a considerable part in the discovery of such useful compounds as have materialized.

Nitrofurans

Furans are organic substances based on a simple 5-membered carbon ring linked by a single oxygen atom (Fig. 6.5). As early as 1832, Johann Wolfgang Döbereiner,* professor

---

* Döbereiner, son of a coachman from Bavaria and originally apprenticed to an apothecary, made several important contributions to chemistry. He is best remembered for the invention of the 'Döbereinersche Platinfeurzeug', an ingenious gas lighter in which hydrogen gas generated from zinc and sulphuric acid is ignited by being passed over activated platinum. See: Kauffman G. B., Johann Wolfgang Döbereiner's feuerzeug. http://www.nesacs.org/nucleus/0012Nuc/wolfgang_dobereiner.htm

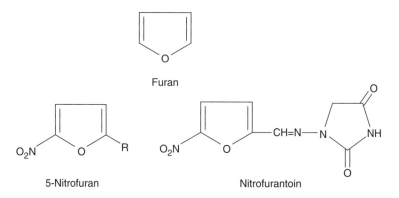

Furan

5-Nitrofuran   Nitrofurantoin

Fig. 6.5 Structures of furan, nitrofuran ('R' represents the variable side chain found in antimicrobially active derivatives), and nitrofurantoin.

of chemistry and technology at the University of Jena in Eastern Germany—and friend of the celebrated poet, Johann Wolfgang von Goethe—had fortuitously discovered a furan derivative called furfural during work on sugar distillation (93). Furfural, which has a variety of industrial uses, was later manufactured from the complex polysaccharides (pentosans) found in many vegetable products, notably grain husks (Latin furfur = bran). In 1922 the Quaker Oats Company in Cedar Rapids, Iowa started to make furfural from waste oat hulls and became the principal producer of the chemical. The following year the Irish–American Hugh McGuigan (born in Lisburn, County Down) head of the Department of Pharmacology at the University of Illinois reported that the substance exhibited antibacterial activity while being relatively non-toxic in experimental animals (94). Other furan derivatives were then investigated for antibacterial properties in the United States and Germany, but none of these attracted much interest.

Starting in 1939, the oddly named Norwich Pharmacal Company in Norwich, New York* revisited the antibacterial activity of furan compounds. By 1944 Matt Dodd and William Stillman of Norwich were able to report on the activity of 42 derivatives, 25 of which were 5-nitrofurans with the nitro (NO_2) group in the position shown in Fig. 6.5. All but one of these compounds showed enhanced antibacterial activity as compared to the non-nitrated analogue (95). Norwich was soon showing an interest in the therapeutic use of nitrofurans and had singled out one of Dodd's compounds, a derivative called Furacin (5-nitro-2-furaldehyde semicarbazone), as a likely candidate (96). Towards the end of the Second World War the American bacteriologist Marshall Snyder and his colleagues found Furacin to be effective in for the treatment of infected war wounds (97)

* Norwich Pharmacal was founded by Oscar G. Bell from a small pill making business that had been earlier started by a Baptist Minister, Lafayette Moore. Robert D. Eaton, a Norwich businessman was an early stockholder and his sons became presidents of the company. In 1945 a research offshoot, Eaton Laboratories, was started and the two merged in 1977 to form Norwich–Eaton. Procter and Gamble took over the firm in 1982.

and the compound was quickly put to use during the invasion of Normandy (93). It was later marketed as a topical antibacterial agent for skin infections. Known generically as nitrofurazone, it is still widely available, but is not on the market in the United Kingdom.

Several thousand nitrofuran derivatives were synthesized in subsequent years in the United States and Germany. A small number were subjected to brief clinical trial, but few survived for very long. The only one to have achieved an established place in the pharmacopoeias of most countries of the world is nitrofurantoin (Fig. 6.5), another product developed in the Eaton laboratories in the early 1950s. Nitrofurantoin is well absorbed when given by mouth, but it is unsuitable for the treatment of systemic infection because insufficient active drug reaches the tissues. It is excreted into the urine with a rapidity that matches the rate of elimination of penicillin and, although much is in a metabolized form, an adequate concentration of unaltered drug is achieved to deal with most common urinary pathogens. For these reasons nitrofurantoin was, from the start, promoted as a reliable oral agent for the treatment of urinary tract infection, especially in family practice. Resistance in bacteria within its spectrum is very uncommon. Its chief drawback is a tendency to cause nausea, an effect that can be mitigated by formulating the drug as macrocrystals, which are more slowly absorbed.

Although Matt Dodd had left Norwich for the Department of Bacteriology at Ohio State University in 1948, Eaton laboratories continued at the forefront of nitrofuran research and a further compound, furazolidone, was introduced in 1954, originally for veterinary use. Around 1959 use was extended to human medicine, mainly for the therapy of all kinds of infective diarrhoea, since effectiveness is claimed against most of the bacterial and protozoal causes. There has been much debate about the true value of furazolidone and it was withdrawn from the British market in the 1980s. The drug is now most often used in developing countries in which there is a high incidence of intestinal infections, but few readily available laboratory facilities to establish the cause. Even such use is questionable: furazolidone is certainly not the drug of choice for amoebiasis or giardiasis and many episodes of diarrhoea, especially among young children, are caused by viruses unaffected by nitrofuran derivatives.

Bacterial diarrhoea is a fertile ground for reliable 'cures' since most bouts last just a few days and recovery is usually imminent when the drug is taken. Except in severe bacillary dysentery and, possibly, cholera, antimicrobial drugs have only a minor part to play in bacterial diarrhoea. The pathological effects of acute diarrhoea are caused by massive loss of water and electrolytes, particularly the cation sodium, from the bloodstream; replacement of these ions is the most important intervention. Oral rehydration fluids, which act on the principle that loss of cations can be rapidly reversed by ingestion of salts in a glucose solution are promoted by the United Nations Children's Fund (UNICEF) and the World Health Organization (WHO) as routine therapy for diarrhoeal diseases caused by bacteria and viruses. As the writer of an editorial in the *Lancet* put it in 1978 with defensible hyperbole:

> The discovery that sodium transport and glucose transport are coupled in the small intestine, so that glucose accelerates absorption of solute and water, was potentially the most important medical advance this century (98).

The qualifier 'potentially' was necessary since at the time of writing it was calculated that the number of young children that were needlessly dying each year of diarrhoeal disease for want of oral rehydration therapy was a scandalous 5 million—around one every 6 seconds. The situation has improved somewhat since then, but a great deal still remains to be done (99).

Apart from nitrofurantoin, furazolidone, and nitrofurazone other attempts at the commercial exploitation of nitrofurans in medicine have met with little success. One compound, furaltadone was introduced in 1959, but hastily withdrawn soon afterwards—at least for human use—when neurotoxic side effects began to be reported. Nifuratel, a chemical modification of furazolidone, was described around 1968. It is available in some continental European countries for the treatment of urinary tract infection and as a vaginal pessary said to be effective against the protozoa, yeasts, and bacteria causing various forms of vaginitis. A derivative of nitrofurantoin, nifurtoinol, was marketed in Belgium and some other European countries in the 1990s, but has since been discontinued. One nitrofuran compound, nifurtimox, is exclusively used in Chagas' disease, South American trypanosomiasis (see p. 318).

Concerns have surfaced from time to time about the safety of nitrofurantoin and other nitrofurans. It has been known since the 1950s that many of them have mutagenic properties in microbial models of genotoxicity. However, nitrofurantoin and furazolidone have both been subjected to intensive scrutiny over decades of clinical use and no evidence of lasting harm has come to light.

Diaminopyrimidines

Amid the anonymity of most drug discovery in commercial research laboratories, two names stand out: those of Gertrude (Trudy) Elion and George Hitchings, whose work on drug discovery was to lead in 1988, to the award of the Nobel Prize in Physiology or Medicine jointly with the British pharmacologist James Black, pioneer of β-blockers.

Born in the coastal town of Hoquiam in Washington state on the West coast of United States, Hitchings trained as a chemist at Harvard. He was hired in 1942 by Burroughs Wellcome to develop a department of biochemistry at their American research laboratories, then situated in a converted rubber factory in Tuckahoe, New York.* Here he was able to indulge his passion for what was then the deeply unfashionable subject of nucleic acid chemistry. Elion, born in New York City of immigrant parents from Eastern Europe, joined him 2 years later. An extremely fruitful relationship developed between these two fertile minds that led to the discovery of many novel drugs.

The research programme originally initiated by Hitchings was chiefly concerned with finding analogues of purines and pyrimidines—the basic building blocks of nucleic acids—that might throw light on the process of nucleic acid synthesis. In 1945 an experimental system was devised with the help of an assistant with bacteriological experience, Elvira Falco, which made use of the bacterium *Lactobacillus casei*. It was known that in

* The Tuckahoe factory opened in 1928. In 1968, the laboratories moved to an extensive new site in North Carolina, which was named Research Triangle Park.

order to multiply this organism needed a then unknown growth factor—later identified as folic acid, one of the B-complex vitamins—or, alternatively, a mixture of thymidine (a pyrimidine) and a purine. They found that when chemically prepared analogues of purines and pyrimidines were introduced into the test system, growth of *Lactobacillus casei*, far from being stimulated, was actually prevented. Moreover, the inhibitory activity extended to pathogenic bacteria that did not require purines and pyrimidines for growth. When toxicity tests in animals showed the compounds to be relatively safe, they realized that the analogues might have therapeutic potential (100).

Among the inhibitory substances synthesized in 1947 by Elvira Falco was one with the chemical name, *para*-chlorophenoxy-2, 4-diaminopyrimidine. It was discovered that the addition of sufficient tetrahydrofolic acid (the active form of folic acid) could overcome inhibition by this analogue in *Streptococcus faecium* (now known as *Enterococcus faecium*) suggesting that the inhibitory activity was directed against an enzyme involved in tetrahydrofolate formation. The enzyme turned out to be dihydrofolate reductase, which, as the name suggests, converts inactive dihydrofolate to active tetrahydrofolate. Importantly, most bacteria cannot use preformed folic acid, but manufacture it themselves. Indeed, this is what makes them vulnerable to sulphonamides, which prevent the biosynthesis of folic acid, while at the same time avoiding mammalian toxicity since animals (including man) cannot synthesize folic acid and require the vitamin to be present in the diet. Plainly, Falco's compound was acting on the same metabolic pathway and might be presumed to have the same potential for safe use. Alas the presumption was wrong: although mammalian cells need preformed folic acid, they also need the enzyme dihydrofolate reductase, since, when tetrahydrofolate is used in the biosynthesis of the nucleic acid thymidine, it is oxidized back to the dihydrofolate form and needs to be constantly regenerated.

It soon became evident that diaminopyrimidines as a class were potent inhibitors of dihydrofolate reductase, but it became necessary to find compounds that were more selective in their enzyme preference. Happily, it transpired that different diaminopyrimidines displayed vastly divergent affinities for dihydrofolate reductases from various sources. This crucial fact allowed diaminopyrimidines to be successfully developed that were preferentially active against mammalian cells, bacteria, or protozoa. In seeking potential therapeutic compounds, Hitchings set his sights on developing anticancer, antibacterial, and antimalarial agents. The latter objective was prompted by a British member of the team, Peter Russell, a chemistry graduate from the University of Manchester,* who had noted a passing resemblance to ICI's Second World War discovery, proguanil (p. 296–7). As it turned out, it was an antimalarial agent, pyrimethamine, that gave the team one of their earliest successes (p. 301).

In collaboration with Cornelius P. Rhoades, director of the Sloan Kettering Cancer Research Institute in New York, many derivatives emanating from Hitching's laboratory

---

* Russell moved to Philadelphia in 1956 to become Director of Research at Wyeth Laboratories. See: Mackie, R., Roberts G. Biographical Database of the British Chemical Community, Open University. http://www.open.ac.uk/ou5/Arts/chemists/person.cfm?SearchID=10412

were tested for antitumour activity. Folic acid antagonists had been recognized as potential anticancer agents through the work at Lederle of Yellapragada SubbaRow, with whom Hitchings had worked at Harvard in the late 1920s in the laboratory of the biochemist Cyrus Fiske. SubbaRow's team at Lederle had synthesized folic acid in 1945. They went on to make a series of folic acid analogues, including aminopterin and methotrexate (amethopterin), which were used successfully in childhood leukaemia by Sidney Farber, an eminent paediatric pathologist at the Harvard Medical School. In the event, a breakthrough for the Burroughs Wellcome in anticancer compounds did not come with a pyrimidine, but with one of a group of purine analogues that Gertrude Elion had been investigating. In 1950, one of Elion's compounds, 6-mercaptopurine was found to be beneficial in inhibiting the multiplication of leukaemia cells in mice. Clinical trials at the Sloan Kettering Institute found that it was superior to methotrexate in inducing remissions in childhood leukaemia and in 1953 mercaptopurine was licensed for use in this condition (101).

A suitable antibacterial agent proved unexpectedly harder to find. Several candidate diaminopyrimidines were tentatively tested in human trials from 1953, but nausea proved to be a troublesome side effect with the doses administered. It was not until 1956 that a compound showing the requisite combination of antibacterial activity and freedom from side effects was synthesized. This substance was trimethoxybenzyl-diaminopyrimidine, soon concertinaed to provide the generic name, trimethoprim (87). The selectivity of the compound for the bacterial forms of dihydrofolate reductase was remarkable: the binding affinity for mammalian forms of the enzyme was found to be a hundred thousand times lower.

Silas Burroughs and Henry Wellcome had based the reputation of their company on meticulous attention to production standards and shrewd marketing techniques, but by the time trimethoprim was discovered the company that they had founded was much less aggressively commercial than other pharmaceutical firms. Wellcome was a philanthropist, whose philosophy was that money made from the relief of suffering should be reinvested for the same purpose. On his death in 1936 his will provided for the formation of the Wellcome Trust, a medical charity whose trustees were the sole shareholders of the commercial company, the Wellcome Foundation. Research workers such as George Hitchings enjoyed a company philosophy that allowed them to pursue their investigations at their own pace. This distinctive ethos may have contributed to the unhurried

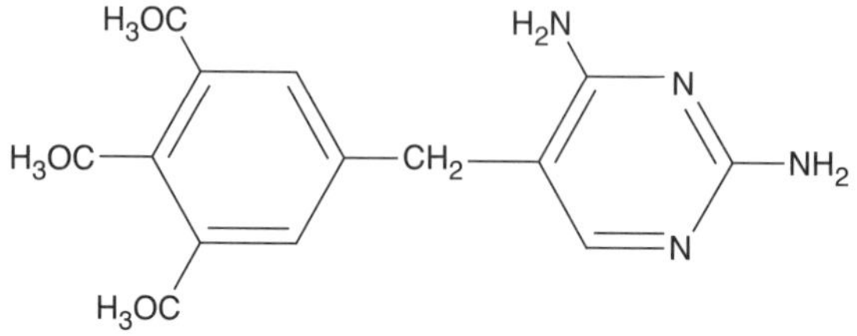

Fig. 6.6 Structure of trimethoprim.

commercial development of trimethoprim, for it was not launched on the market in Britain or the United States until well over a decade after its discovery.

A further delaying factor may have been the dilemma of how to formulate the drug. It was known as early as 1952, through the work of Don Eyles of the U.S. Public Health Service that diaminopyrimidines and sulphonamides interacted synergically against protozoa as a consequence of a sequential action on the metabolic pathway leading to the formation of folic acid (102). By 1968 Stan Bushby of the Wellcome Research Laboratories in Beckenham had demonstrated in laboratory tests that trimethoprim acts as a powerful potentiator of sulphonamides (103). The interaction was so striking that it was seen to be self-evidently advantageous to formulate the two drugs together—a tactic that was claimed to have the added benefit of reducing the likelihood of the development of resistance. Coincidentally, the period during which trimethoprim was being developed was also a time of intense debate about the wisdom of using fixed-dose combinations of antibacterial drugs. Several such combinations had appeared on the market on both sides of the Atlantic attracting criticisms of their irrationality and potential for increasing the likelihood of adverse reactions.

In the end, the degree of synergy observed between sulphonamides and trimethoprim *in vitro* was so prominent that the question of using trimethoprim alone seems hardly to have been considered. Various sulphonamides were tried as partners to trimethoprim in trials in the 1960s, but the sulpha compound that seemed to provide the best pharmacokinetic match for trimethoprim was sulphamethoxazole, a drug produced by the Japanese firm Shionogi, which had been licensed to Hoffmann-La-Roche in the United States. The combined product was licensed for use in 1969. Wellcome and Roche put together a joint marketing agreement, under the terms of which they would produce identical versions of the combination, but limit their promotional activities in rival territories. As a consequence the Roche product, Bactrim, became widely used in the United States and continental Europe; the Wellcome version, Septrim, being preferred in the United Kingdom. The rather cumbersome name co-trimoxazole was coined to designate the generic drug.

Polymyxins also interact synergically with trimethoprim and sulphonamides, probably by facilitating entry of those compounds into the bacterial cell. For a while a triple combination was contemplated and a few tentative trials were done. However, the inclusion of a polymyxin would have increased the potential for toxicity and the idea was wisely not pursued.

Co-trimoxazole was a great commercial success all over the world. It was enthusiastically used for a diverse range of bacterial infections from urinary tract and respiratory infections to enteric fever and brucellosis. But there was a sting in the tail. It transpired that the arguments adduced for combining trimethoprim with a sulphonamide were largely bogus; in most clinical situations the sulphonamide component was contributing little, if anything, to the overall antibacterial effect. More importantly, most of the side effects—including occasional fatalities—were attributed to the presence of the sulphonamide.

Doubts about the need for the inclusion of a sulphonamide began to surface in the early 1970s, when reports of the successful use of trimethoprim alone in urinary tract infection emerged from Finland and Britain. It was pointed out that, at the concentrations of trimethoprim achievable in urine on standard dosage, the sulphonamide component, which acts much more slowly than trimethoprim, had little opportunity to contribute to the overall effect. Similar doubts were expressed about the use of co-trimoxazole in respiratory infections, since trimethoprim and sulphonamides exhibit a differential capacity to penetrate into cells, so that the sulphonamide is effectively excluded from some sites accessible to trimethoprim. Again, clinical evidence suggested that trimethoprim alone might be just as effective as the mixture.

This debate prompted a re-evaluation of the use of co-trimoxazole, but the manufacturers were still reluctant to release trimethoprim alone. One reason was that it was claimed that the combination product was responsible for maintaining trimethoprim resistance at a low level. However, since sulphonamide resistance was already common when co-trimoxazole was introduced, trimethoprim was often the sole active component when the combination was used. Moreover, in trimethoprim-resistant bacteria, the resistance determinants for sulphonamide, and trimethoprim usually coexist on the same genetic element (plasmid), which can be transferred as a unit within sensitive bacterial populations.

In the end, good sense prevailed and trimethoprim alone became available in 1979. By this time co-trimoxazole was so well established that it continued to be widely preferred and, although serious side effects remained uncommon, many recipients of the drug suffered unnecessary toxic effects with a fatality rate calculated at around one per million prescriptions issued. Some of these reactions may have been attributable to the trimethoprim itself, but it was the sulphonamide component that came under greatest suspicion. Publicity given to the relative safety of co-trimoxazole and trimethoprim alone in the 1980s successfully reduced use of the combination product in general practice, but it was not until 1995 that the Committee on Safety of Medicines in the United Kingdom issued a recommendation to the effect that, although co-trimoxazole was useful in certain serious conditions (it is often used, for example, in AIDS sufferers who contract pneumonia caused by the fungus *Pneumocystis jirovecii*), it should be used in uncomplicated respiratory and urinary infections only if there are compelling reasons to prefer it to a single drug.

Despite early optimism that the antimicrobial activity of diaminopyrimidines might be further exploited (104), little headway was made in the development of analogues with novel properties. Various antibacterial diaminopyrimidines, including tetroxoprim (from Heumann Pharma, a small German firm in Nuremberg) and brodimoprim (from Roche), were introduced on to the market in some countries, but failed to make much impact. Trimethoprim itself has been partnered by other sulphonamides, including sulfadiazine (co-trimazine), sulphamoxole (co-trifamole) and sulphametrole (co-soltrim). None of these products, nor the combination of tetroxoprim with sulfadiazine (co-tetroxazine), has any discernable advantage over trimethoprim or co-trimoxazole.

Quinolones

Nalidixic acid, the first of an ever-expanding group of compounds that are related through a common structural feature that classifies them generically as quinolones (Fig. 6.7), was first described in 1962 by George Lesher and his colleagues in the medicinal chemistry

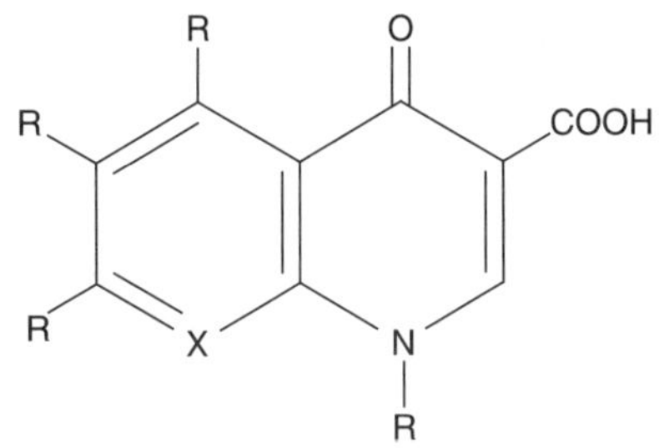

Fig. 6.7 General structure of quinolones. The various antibacterial compounds differ in chemical groupings indicated by 'R'. Some, including nalidixic acid, have a nitrogen atom at the position indicated by 'X' otherwise occupied by carbon and are properly called naphthyridines. Several other variants have also been described.

department of the Sterling–Winthrop Research Institute situated in Rensselaer across the Hudson River from Albany, New York State (105).

The Sterling Drug Company, founded in 1900 as the Neuralgyline Company* by William E. Weiss and his old friend Albert Diebold to peddle the latter's patent medicine, Neuralgine, missed out on the post-Second World War antibiotic revolution. The firm did, however, manufacture sulphonamides through a pre-war agreement with IG Farbenindustrie in Germany (see Chapter 7, p. 291) and had been one of the companies signed up by the War Production Board in the United States in 1944 to manufacture penicillin. Through the link with IG Farben, they also had a strong stake in antimalarial compounds (see p. 299). It was during experiments conducted in the late 1950s and early 1960s to investigate by-products of synthesis of the antimalarial agent chloroquine that Lesher and his colleagues stumbled on a compound that exhibited modest antibacterial activity against Gram-negative bacilli (106). The team went on to synthesize analogues of the substance and turned up several active derivatives, of which the one later given the name nalidixic acid seemed to possess the most desirable properties.

Sterling–Winthrop was reticent about revealing details of the discovery. The 1962 paper describing the antibacterial activity of nalidixic acid and related derivatives (105) tantalizingly states that a description of the original observation is 'to be published' by Sterling–Winthrop's chief scientist, the organic chemist Alexander Surrey, but no such article seems to have appeared. Details of the circumstances surrounding the discovery remained unclear until 1986 when George Lesher gave an account of the events at a symposium on quinolone agents in Chicago (107).

Surprisingly most of the early trials of nalidixic acid in urinary infection were carried out in Britain, where it was soon being marketed by the Bayer Products division of Sterling. It proved quite effective in uncomplicated cystitis, which is normally amenable to minimal treatment with antibacterial agents, but mutations to resistance occurred easily and treatment failures were common in more difficult infections. Occasional side

---

* In 1909, Weiss and Diebold bought the Sterling Remedy Company of Illinois. They changed the name of their company to Sterling Products Incorporated in 1917. The following year they created the Winthrop Chemical Company, later to become the Sterling–Winthrop Research Institute, to manufacture and sell prescription drugs. Sterling–Winthrop was acquired by Eastman Kodak in 1988 and was sold on to SmithKline Beecham (now GlaxoSmithKline) in 1994, but the 'over-the-counter' business, Sterling Health, went to Bayer.

effects began to be reported, but gave no great cause for concern and the drug achieved a useful, if undistinguished, place in the therapeutic armoury of general practitioners.

Nalidixic acid was no great shakes. It is extensively metabolized in the body to biologically inactive products and is ineffectual in systemic infection. Like nitrofurantoin (which for reasons that have never been satisfactorily explained abolishes the activity of nalidixic acid if the two drugs are tested together) its usefulness is virtually restricted to infections of the urinary tract caused by Gram-negative bacilli, though it has also found limited use in intestinal infections.

The unprepossessing properties of nalidixic acid did not prevent other firms from wanting to get in on the act. During the next 15 years hundreds of antibacterial quinolones were described (108) and several, including oxolinic acid (Warner–Lambert, 1968), cinoxacin (Lilly, 1973), piromidic acid (Dainippon, 1970), pipemidic acid (also Dainippon, 1972), and flumequine (Riker Laboratories, 1974) went on sale in various countries. None of these compounds offered much therapeutic benefit over nalidixic acid, though skilful promotion ensured healthy profits in selected markets.

By the mid-1970s, the antibacterial quinolones seemed played out: destined to be appended as a mere footnote in the history of antimicrobial agents. Around 1978, Lesher's group at Sterling–Winthrop developed a compound, rosoxacin (also called acrosoxacin), which attempted to break the mould by offering activity against sexually transmitted pathogens, notably the gonococcus, but it was less effective and more toxic than rival agents and made little progress. It was the indefatigable Japanese pharmaceutical industry that was to transform the fortunes of this family of compounds, when, in 1977, scientists at the Kyorin Pharmaceutical Company in Tokyo synthesized a compound that came to be called norfloxacin that exhibited much improved properties. The first English language description of the compound appeared in February 1980 in an article describing work on the antibacterial properties of norfloxacin carried out by Susuma Mitsuhashi's group in the Department of Microbiology in Gumma University School of Medicine (109).

What the Kyorin chemists had done was to combine the features of two of the earlier compounds: flumequine, in which addition of a fluorine atom at the C-6 carbon had the effect of improving the antibacterial activity against enteric Gram-negative bacilli like *Escherichia coli*; and pipemidic acid, in which addition of a piperazine group at C-7 had given the molecule modest activity against the difficult-to-treat opportunist pathogen *Pseudomonas aeruginosa*. When both features were linked in norfloxacin it was surprisingly found that the activity in both areas was boosted to levels previously unseen and Gram-positive organisms such as *Staphylococcus aureus* were brought within the spectrum (Table 6.1).

Kyorin was a small company, first established as a chemical company in 1931, but quickly expanding into pharmaceuticals before Japan entered the Second World War. Norfloxacin was its first major success and in 1980 the drug was licensed globally to Merck, one of the earliest American firms to take a serious interest in the Japanese pharmaceutical industry. Merck, whose own efforts to find a useful quinolone had been unsuccessful, were soon commissioning widespread laboratory evaluations of the new compound and clinical trials quickly followed. It became clear that, despite the improved

Table 6.1 Typical inhibitory concentrations (milligrams per litre) of nalidixic acid, flumequine pipemidic acid, and norfloxacin for three bacterial species.

Organism	Nalidixic acid	Flumequine	Pipemidic acid	Norfloxacin
Escherichia coli	4	1	4	0.5
Pseudomonas aeruginosa	Resistant	64	16	2
Staphylococcus aureus	Resistant	64	64	2

Resistant = not inhibited by a concentration of 64 mg/l.

activity, the chief role for norfloxacin was, like earlier quinolones, going to be in urinary tract infection. The drug was introduced in Japan in 1984, licensed in the United States in 1987 and reached the British market in 1989.

In the meantime, other firms took up the challenge to explore fluorinated, piperazine substituted quinolone derivatives. A multitude of similar compounds, some with barely distinguishable characteristics, appeared in rapid succession within a few years of one another: enoxacin (Dainippon, 1980; licensed to Parke, Davis); ofloxacin (Daiichi Seiyaku Pharmaceutical Company, 1982; licensed to Hoechst [Aventis] in Europe and to Ortho-McNeil [part of the Johnson and Johnson empire] in the United States); pefloxacin (Laboratoires Roger Bellon, Paris, 1981; licensed to Rhône–Poulenc); amifloxacin (Sterling–Winthrop, 1983); ciprofloxacin (Bayer, 1983); fleroxacin (Kyorin, 1983; licensed to Hoffmann-La Roche); and difloxacin (Abbott, 1984). In 1987, Daiichi in Japan had the bright idea of separating out the two optically active isomers of ofloxacin, selected the more active, and called it levofloxacin.

The reason for all this activity was that the manufacturers scented a greatly expanded market for drugs that were relatively cheap to synthesize. For the first time quinolones were described that offered sufficient activity and breadth of spectrum for them to break out of the urinary tract straitjacket into more generalized infections treated in hospitals as well as the community. Many could be formulated as more expensive injectable drugs to offer to institutional clientele for use against problem organisms such as *Pseudomonas aeruginosa*.

There followed a classic struggle for ascendancy in the marketplace, which kept micro-biologists and infectious disease experts entertained (in more than one sense of the word!) throughout the 1980s. Issues of intrinsic antibacterial activity, spectrum, safety, pharmacological behaviour, and clinical effectiveness of the rival compounds were pored over at endless industry-sponsored meetings and scientific symposia with the inevitable batteries of claim and counter-claim. It was ciprofloxacin, which proved to be the eventual winner, successfully backing up an undisputed edge in antibacterial potency with shrewd marketing, and aggressive promotional campaigns. Some of the competitors managed to maintain a worthwhile market share; others either fell by the wayside or sought to recoup their investment by promoting their product for the staple money-spinner, urinary tract infection. Several firms sought to widen their options by formulating their drug for particular markets with ophthalmic preparations or other specialized products.

One quinolone derivative, nadifloxacin, synthesized by chemists at the Otsuka Pharmaceutical Company in Tokyo in the 1980s, was specifically developed as a topical cream for use in acne. Nor was the veterinary market forgotten. Abbott's difloxacin resurfaced as a veterinary product to join enrofloxacin (Bayer) and, in due course, marbofloxacin (Pfizer), orbifloxacin (Schering–Plough), and another Abbott quinolone, sarafloxacin. Development of these animal health products was kept studiously independent of the drugs intended for human therapy. There has been considerable debate about the impact that their use has had on the prevalence of quinolone resistance.

Commercially successful though the fluoroquinolones (as they came to be called) were, there was still room for improvement. Despite strenuous efforts to claim the contrary, it rapidly became clear that they were clinically unreliable in serious streptococcal and staphylococcal infections. Consistent activity against the pneumococcus—the commonest cause of pneumonia acquired in the community—was essential if inroads were to be made into the lucrative market for the treatment of pulmonary infections. Improved potency against staphylococci was also highly desirable given the growing need for new agents to combat the threat of multiresistant strains. Poor activity against anaerobic bacteria was also seen by some as a deficiency, though there was a cogent argument in favour of compounds that did not interfere with the predominantly anaerobic flora of the gut.

Responding to these perceived needs, a rash of new quinolones were described. First from the starting blocks was a trifluorinated derivative, temafloxacin, developed in Abbott laboratories and first unveiled at the 26th ICAAC held in New Orleans in 1986. With high hopes of stealing a march on their competitors, temafloxacin was licensed and launched worldwide in 1992, only for the company to have to humiliatingly withdraw the product almost immediately when serious adverse reactions began to be reported.

Undeterred, other companies particularly those in the Far East continued to pursue the dream. During the early 1990s, a flood of candidate compounds were synthesized, among them: gatifloxacin (Kyorin Pharmaceutical Company, Tochigi, 1990); pazufloxacin (Toyama Chemical Company, Toyama, 1990; prulifloxacin (Nippon Shinyaku, Kyoto, 1991); sitafloxacin (Daiichi Pharmaceutical Company, Tokyo, 1991); grepafloxacin (Otsuka Pharmaceutical Company, Tokyo, 1992); trovafloxacin (Pfizer, 1992); gemifloxacin (LG Chemical Company, Tae Jon, Korea, 1995; olamufloxacin (Hokuriku Seikaku, Fukui, 1995); and moxifloxacin (Bayer, 1996). Most of these compounds were further developed in alliances with American or European Companies. In a replay of the events of the 1980s, a new rush for market dominance began and intensified as the first products were granted licences at the beginning of the new millennium.

From humble beginnings in the 1960s, quinolone antibacterial agents had, by the end of the twentieth century, come to occupy a significant place in the pharmacopoeia. It would be churlish to belittle this achievement, for these drugs certainly have an important role in the treatment of bacterial infections. Nonetheless, the extravagant publicity that has surrounded the fluoroquinolones has undoubtedly led to a great deal of overuse when cheaper, safer alternatives are ordinarily available. Although quinolones are generally free from serious adverse reactions, a wide variety of unwanted effects may occur. In addition to temafloxacin (see above), grepafloxacin was withdrawn because of suspected cardiotoxicity and trovafloxacin has a restricted licence because of its hepatotoxic potential. Increasing resistance has inevitably occurred, fuelled by excessive use in human and veterinary medicine, and threatens to negate much of the progress that has been made (110). Not for the first time in the history of antimicrobial chemotherapy, overenthusiastic acceptance by prescribers of valuable drugs has jeopardized their long-term prospects.

Oxazolidinones

When compounds categorized chemically as oxazolidinones were first described in 1987, they were hailed as a new class of synthetic agents (111). However, several earlier antimicrobial drugs, including the antibiotic cycloserine and the nitrofuran furazolidone, contain an oxazolidone grouping in their molecular structure. Nevertheless, the new compounds differ considerably in their structure, mode of action and spectrum of activity, so that their claim to be unique is certainly valid.

Renewed interest in antimicrobial properties of synthetic molecules of this type emerged at E.I. du Pont de Nemours and Company in Wilmington, Delaware, towards the end of the 1970s. The original intention was to find compounds suitable for the control of bacterial and fungal diseases, but in the late 1980s, several oxazolidinones were synthesized that offered the potential of useful activity against human pathogens such as staphylococci, streptococci, and certain anaerobic bacteria. Preliminary findings on two of these substances, known only by their laboratory codes, DuP 105 and DuP 721, were presented at the 27th ICAAC in New York in October 1987.

The brief flurry of interest that followed the report of the du Pont compounds soon subsided when animal tests indicated problems of serious toxicity. Development at du Pont was stopped, but the challenge to find safer derivatives was taken up by scientists at Pharmacia and Upjohn in Kalamazoo Michigan. After several false starts, two oxazolidinones emerged that offered attractive pharmacological properties and appeared safe in animal tests. Remarkably, the first of these compounds, subsequently known as eperezolid, displayed the two features that had transformed the prospects of quinolones (see p. 258), a piperazine ring and a fluorine atom. The other, later named linezolid, was a close analogue in which the piperazine ring had been modified (112).

By 1995, the Pharmacia scientists, in collaboration with colleagues from the Centers for Disease Control and Prevention in Atlanta, were ready to unveil their new drugs at the annual ICAAC meeting, held that year in September in San Francisco. This time there were no subsequent scares over safety and linezolid—chosen because of superior pharmacokinetic behaviour—was licensed for use in the United States in 2000 and in Europe the following year.

Although safety considerations have subsequently emerged, especially when the drug is used for an extended period, linezolid is a welcome addition to the antibiotic formulary. Its role is limited to that of a reserve drug for use in serious infections with staphylococci or other Gram-positive cocci, where the causative organism is resistant to more familiar and less expensive agents. These restricted indications highlight the dilemma facing pharmaceutical companies whose drug discovery policy demands adequate return for the investment.

The party's over?

By the end of the twentieth century, the flow of new compounds for the treatment of bacterial infection had slowed to a barely discernable trickle. Pharmaceutical firms could, of course, reflect on half a century of highly profitable trading during which the fortunes of some had been transformed by antibiotics—in Eli Lilly, for example, these drugs accounted for almost one third of total sales by 1975—but past success paradoxically reduced present incentives for investment in new compounds, which needed to be carefully tailored to fill a diminishing number of perceived gaps in the market. Mass screening programmes of soil samples had long been abandoned. Contrary to popular belief, they had seldom proved cost effective except for the lucky few. Some statistics, again from Lilly, are revealing. In the company's centenary volume published in 1976 (113) Ely Kahn cites the following figures for the screening programme for the period 1949–1959:

> Soil samples screened: 10,000
> Organisms isolated: 200,000
> Organisms showing some antibiotic activity: 25,000
> Organisms discarded: 24,700
> Antibiotics chemically isolated: 300
> New antibiotics discovered: 150
> New antibiotics that reached the clinical stage: 7
> New antibiotics that reached the market: 3

In fact, after the first flush of success of antibiotic discovery in the 1940s and 1950s, the industry has mostly relied on chemical reworking of older substances to keep the profits flowing. New derivatives of cephalosporins and quinolones have been the mainstay, but there have also been new tetracyclines, macrolides, glycopeptides, and streptogramins: mostly compounds that seek to exploit the fear of increasing resistance to older drugs. The only antibacterial drugs to have come forward in the last 30 years of the twentieth century with any claim to be truly novel are linezolid and daptomycin, narrow-spectrum compounds aimed at the market for antistaphylococcal agents.

Some new-found optimism has been provided by techniques of combinatorial chemistry that allow chemical screening on a scale formerly impossible. Similarly the ability to link biochemical and molecular know-how to advanced computer-generated molecular modelling procedures offers fresh hope of designing molecules that precisely disable susceptible targets within the bacterial cell. These approaches have yielded some success in the case of antiviral agents (see Chapter 8), but have so far had little impact on the development of new anti-infective drugs in other categories. Unfortunately, the best laid plans of laboratory scientists often come to grief in the real world in which bacteria—which have been in the game for eons—turn out to be adept at circumventing the new danger, or unexpected toxicities reveal themselves during development.

Part of the problem for the pharmaceutical houses in formulating policy on research into antibacterial agents is that we now have so many of them. Despite the threat of antimicrobial drug resistance (see Chapter 9), the market is awash with drugs to treat bacterial disease. The cost of developing a new antimicrobial compound and bringing it to market—often estimated at around $500 million—has caused even the richest pharmaceutical companies to hesitate, since the chances of recouping the investment is precarious. Understandably, they have chosen to divert resources previously directed at antibacterial agents into new antiviral and, to a lesser extent, antifungal compounds, where the needs are greater and the prospects of large profits for safe, effective compounds are somewhat more secure.

References

1. Florey HW, Chain E, Heatley NG, Jennings MA (1949). *Antibiotics: a survey of penicillin, streptomycin, and other antimicrobial substances from fungi, actinomycetes, bacteria, and plants.* Oxford University Press, Oxford.
2. McFadyen RE (1979). The FDA's regulation and control of antibiotics in the 1950s. The Henry Welch scandal, Félix Martí-Ibáñez, and Charles Pfizer & Co. *Bull Hist Med* 53, 159–69.
3. Johnson BA, Anker H, Meleney FL (1945). Bacitracin: a new antibiotic produced by a member of the *B. subtilis* group. *Science* **102**, 376–7.
4. Enochs BE (ed.). Columbia–Presbyterian Medical Center. *75 people, events, and contributions worth remembering: Bacitracin's beginnings* http://cpmcnet.columbia.edu/news/journal/75years.html
5. Hobby GL (1985). *Penicillin. Meeting the challenge* pp. 161–4. Yale University Press, New Haven.
6. Arriagada A, Savage MC, Abraham EP, Heatley N, Sharp AE (1949). Ayfivin: an antibiotic from *B. licheniformis*: production in potato–dextrose medium. *Br J Exp Pathol* **30**, 425–7.
7. Abraham EP (1953). *Biochemistry of some peptide and steroid antibiotics*, pp. 1–29. John Wiley, New York.
8. Meleney FL, Johnson BA (1956). Alimentary tract antisepsis with oral bacitracin and neomycin.In: Welch H, Marti-Ibañez F, eds. *Antibiotics annual 1956–57*, pp. 244–52. Medical Encyclopedia Inc, New York.
9. Maxted WR (1953). The use of bacitracin for identifying group. A haemolytic streptococci. *J Clin Pathol* **6**, 224–6.
10. Schwartz BS (1964). The polypeptides of the polymyxin group. In: Schnitzer RJ, Hawking F, eds. *Experimental chemotherapy, Volume III: Chemotherapy of bacterial infections part II*, pp. 217–70. Academic Press, New York.
11. Benedict RG, Langlykke AF (1947). Antibiotic activity of *Bacillus polymyxa*. *J Bacteriol* **54**, 24–5.
12. Stansly PG, Shepherd RG, White HJ (1947). Polymyxin: a new chemotherapeutic agent. *Bull Johns Hopkins Hosp* **81**, 43–54.
13. Stansly PG (1949). Historical aspects. *Ann N Y Acad Sci* **51**, 855–6. (contribution to a symposium on antibiotics derived from *Bacillus polymyxa* held in May 1948)
14. Ainsworth GC, Brown AM, Brownlee G (1947). 'Aerosporin', an antibiotic produced by *Bacillus aerosporus* Greer. *Nature* **160**, 263.
15. Brownlee G, Bushby SRM, Short EI (1952). The chemistry and pharmacology of the polymyxins. *Br J Pharmacol* **7**, 170–88.
16. Koyama Y, Kurosawa A, Tsuchiya A, Takakuta K (1950). A new antibiotic 'colistin' produced by spore-forming soil bacteria. (In Japanese) *J Antibiot* Series B3 457–8.
17. Wilkinson S (1949). Crystalline derivatives of the polymyxins and the identification of the fatty acid component. *Nature* **164**, 622.
18. Swift PN (1948). Treatment of pertussis with aeropsorin. *Lancet* **1**, 133–5.

19. Swift PN, Bushby SRM (1951). *Haemophilus influenzae* meningitis treated with polymyxin. *Lancet* **2**, 183–90.

20. Jackson DM, Lowbury EJL, Topley E (1951). *Pseudomonas pyocyanea* in burns. Its role as a pathogen, and the value of local polymyxin therapy. *Lancet* **2**, 137–47.

21. Dowling HF (1958–1959). The history of the broad-spectrum antibiotics. In: Welch H, Marti-Ibañez F, eds. *Antibiotics annual*, pp. 39–44. Medical Encyclopedia Inc, New York.

22. Ehrlich J, Bartz QR, Smith RM, Joslyn DA, Burkholder PR (1947). Chloromycetin, a new antibiotic from a soil actinomycete. *Science* **106**, 417.

23. Carter HE, Gottlieb D, Anderson HW (1948). Chloromycetin and streptothricin. *Science* **107**, 113.

24. Ehrlich J, Gottlieb D, Burkholder PR, Anderson LE, Pridham TG (1948). *Streptomyces venezuelae*, N. Sp., the source of chloromycetin. *J Bacteriol* **56**, 467–77.

25. Controulis J, Rebstock MC, Crooks HM (1949). Chloramphenicol (chloromycetin). V. Synthesis. *J Am Chem Soc* **71**, 2463–8.

26. Zinsser H (1935). *Rats, lice and history. Being a study in biography, which, after twelve preliminary chapters indispensable for the preparation of the lay reader, deals with the life history of typhus fever.* Routledge, London.

27. Smadel JE, Jackson EB (1947). Chloromycetin, an antibiotic with chemotherapeutic activity in experimental rickettsial and viral infections. *Science* **106**, 418–19.

28. Woodward TE (1990). Chloramphenicol, Kuala Lumpur, and the first therapeutic conquests of scrub typhus and typhoid fever. In: Moberg CL, Cohn ZA, eds. *Launching the antibiotic era*, pp. 43–55. Rockefeller University Press, New York.

29. Yunis AA (1989). Chloramphenicol toxicity: 25 years of research. *Am J Med* **87**, 44N–8N.

30. Wharton JC (1980). "Antibiotic abandon": the resurgence of therapeutic realism. In: Parascandola J, ed. *The history of antibiotics—a symposium*, pp. 125–36. American Institute of Pharmacy, Madison, Wisconsin.

31. Barber M, Garrod LP (1963). *Antibiotic and chemotherapy*, p. 124. Churchill Livingstone, Edinburgh.

32. Garrol LP (1959). Antibiotics and the common cold. *Lancet* **1**, 47.

33. Bassett EJ, Keith MS, Armelagos GJ, Martin DL, Villanueva AR (1980). Tetracycline-labeled human bone from ancient Sudanese Nubia (A.D. 350). *Science* **209**, 1532–4.

34. Cook M, Molto E, Anderson C (1989). Fluorochrome labelling in Roman period skeletons from Dakhleh Oasis, Egypt. *Am J Phys Anthropol* **80**, 137–43.

35. Hummert JR, Van Gerven DP (1982). Tetracycline-labeled human bone from a medieval population in Nubia's Batn El Hajar (55–1450 A.D.). *Hum Biol* **54**, 355–71.

36. Walker JC (1982). Pioneer leaders in plant pathology: Benjamin Minge Duggar. *Annu Rev Phytopathol* **20**, 33–9.

37. Bäumler E (1965). *In search of the magic bullet. Great adventures in modern drug research*, pp. 67–8. Thames and Hudson, London.

38. Duggar BM (1948). Aureomycin: a product of the continuing search for new antibiotics. *Ann N Y Acad Sci* **51**, 177–81.

39. Kane JH, Finlay AC, Sobin BA (1950). Antimicrobial agents from natural sources. *Ann N Y Acad Sci* **53**, 226–8.

40. Finlay AC, Hobby GL, P'an SY, *et al.* (1950). Terramycin, a new antibiotic. *Science* **111**, 85.

41. Various authors (1950). Terramycin. *Ann N Y Acad Sci* **53**, 221 et seq.

42. Blout E (2002). Robert Burns Woodward. *Biograph Memoirs Natl Acad Sci* **80**, 366–87. Available at: http://books.nap.edu/books/0309082811/html/367.html

43. Hochstein FA, Stephens CR, Conover LH, *et al.* (1953). The structure of Terramycin. *J Am Chem Soc* **75**, 5455–75.

44. Minieri PP, Firman MC, Mistretta AG, *et al.* (1953). A new broad spectrum antibiotic product of the tetracycline group.In: Welch H, Marti-Ibañez F, eds. *Antibiotics annual 1953–54*, pp. 81–7. Medical Encyclopedia Inc, New York.

45. James M. *Frances Kelsey. Government of Canada digital collections.* http://collections.ic.gc.ca/ heirloom_series/volume6/218–219.htm

46. Finland M (1974). Twenty-fifth anniversary of the discovery of aureomycin: the place of tetracyclines in antimicrobial therapy. *Clin Pharmacol Ther* **15**, 3–8.

47. Shyrock TJ (2000). Growth promotion and feed antibiotics. In: Prescott JF, Baggot JD, Walker RD, eds. *Antimicrobial therapy in veterinary medicine*, 3rd edn., pp. 735–43. Iowa State University Press, Ames.

48. Takeuchi T, Hikiji T, Nitta K, *et al.* (1957). Biological studies on kanamycin. *J Antibiot* **10**, 107–14.

49. Umezawa H, Okami Y, Hashimoto T, Suhara Y, Hamada M, Takeuchi T (1965). A new antibiotic, kasugamycin. *J Antibiot* **18**, 101–3.

50. Weinstein MJ, Luedemann GM, Oden EM, *et al.* (1963). Gentamicin, a new antibiotic complex from *Micromonospora*. *J Med Chem* **6**, 463–4.

51. Americo Woyciesjes. http://www.syracusehalloffame.com/pages/inductees/2003/ rico_woyciesjes.html

52. Weinstein MJ, Luedemann GM, Oden EM, Wagman GH (1964). Gentamicin, a new broad-spectrum antibiotic complex. In: Sylvester JC, ed. *Antimicrobial agents and chemotherapy–1963*, pp. 1–7. American Society for Microbiology, Ann Arbor, Michigan.

53. Jao RL, Jackson GG (1964). Clinical experience with gentamicin in Gram-negative infections. In: Sylvester JC, ed. *Antimicrobial agents and chemotherapy–1963*, pp. 148–52. American Society for Microbiology, Ann Arbor, Michigan.

54. Jackson GG (1969). Introduction. In: Finland M, guest ed. International symposium on gentamicin, a new aminoglycoside antibiotic. *J Infect Dis* **119**, 341–2.

55. Kawaguchi H (1976). Discovery, chemistry, and activity of amikacin. *J Infect Dis* **134** (November Suppl.), S242–S8.

56. Mason DJ, Dietz A, Smith RM (1961). Actinospectacin, a new antibiotic. I. Discovery and biological properties. *Antibiot Chemother* **11**, 118–22.

57. Oliver TJ, Goldstein A, Bower RR, Holper JC, Otto RH (1962). M-141, a new antibiotic. I Antimicrobial properties, identity with actinospectacin, and production by *Streptomyces flavopersicus*, sp. n. In: Finland M, Savage GM, eds. *Antimicrobial agents and chemotherapy–1961*, pp. 495–502. American Society for Microbiology, Detroit, Michigan.

58. Gardner AD, Chain E (1942). Proactinomycin: a "bacteriostatic" produced by a species of Proactinomyces. *Br J Exp Pathol* **23**, 123–7.

59. Mooney PR (1996). Forgotten parts; pirated diversity in the seas, soils and in ourselves. *Journal of the Dag Hammarskjöld Foundation. Development Dialogue, Special Issue.* Available at: http://www.dhf.uu.se/pdffiler/DD1996/DD1996_1-2_09.pdf

60. Bunch RL, McGuire JM (1953). *Erythromycin, its salts and method of preparation.* United States Patent Office. Available at: http://v3.espacenet.com/origdoc?DB=EPODOC&IDX=US2653899&F=0&QPN=US2653899.

61. Pratt WD (1988). *The Abbott Almanac: 100 years of commitment to quality health care.* Abbott Laboratories, Chicago.

62. Lepper MH, Moulton B, Dowling HF, Jackson GG, Kofman S (1953). Epidemiology of erythromycin-resistant staphylococci in a hospital population. In: Welch H, Marti-Ibañez F, eds. *Antibiotics annual 1953–54*, pp. 308–13. Medical Encyclopedia Inc, New York.

63. Pinnert-Sindico S (1954). Une nouvelle espèce de *Streptomyces* productrice d'antibiotiques: *Streptomyces ambofaciens* n. sp. caractères culturaux. *Annales de l'Institut Pasteur (Paris)* **87**, 702–7;

Pinnert-Sindico S, Ninet L, Preud'Homme J, Cosar C (1955). A new antibiotic—spiramycin. In: Welch H, Marti-Ibañez F, eds. *Antibiotics annual 1954–195*. Medical Encyclopedia Inc, New York.

64. Cosar C, Ninet L, Pinnert S, Preud'Homme J (1952). Trypanocide action of an antibiotic produced by a *Streptomyces*. *Comptes Rendu Hebdomadaire des séances de l'Academie de Sciences* **234**, 1498–9.

65. Ravina A, Pestel M, Eloy P, Duchesnay G, Albouy R, Rey M (1956). A new French antibiotic: spiramycin. In: Welch H, Marti-Ibañez F, eds. *Antibiotics annual 1955–1956*. Medical Encyclopedia Inc, New York; Kernbaum S (1982). Spiramycin. Therapeutic use in man. *Semaine des Hôpitaux* **58**, 289–97.

66. Pariza RJ (2006). From patent to prescription: paving the perilous path to profit. In: Chorghade MS, ed. *Drug discovery and development, Volume 1: drug discovery*, pp. 1–16. Wiley, Chichester.

67. Macey PE, Spooner DF (1964). Antibiotics with specific affinities. Part 2: novobiocin. In: Schnitzer RJ, Hawking F, eds. *Experimental chemotherapy*, Vol. III, pp. 291–327. Academic Press, New York.

68. McCormick MH, Stark WM, Pittenger GE, Pittenger RC, McGuire JM (1956). Vancomycin, a new antibiotic. I. Chemical and biologic properties. In: Welch H, Marti-Ibañez F, eds. *Antibiotics annual 1955–1956*, pp. 606–11. Medical Encyclopedia Inc, New York.

69. Philip JE, Schenck JR, Hargie MP (1957). Ristocetins A and B, two new antibiotics. Isolation and properties. In: Welch H, Marti-Ibañez F, eds. *Antibiotics annual 1956–57*, pp. 699–705. Medical Encyclopedia Inc, New York.

70. Cooper GL, Given DB (1986). *Vancomycin. A comprehensive review of 30 years clinical experience*. Park Row Publishers, Wiley, Philadelphia.

71. Coronelli C, Beretta G, Bardone MR, Parenti F. *Antibiotic substances*. United States Patent 4239751. Available at: http://www.freepatentsonline.com/4239751.html

72. Mason DJ, Dietz A, Deboer C (1963). Lincomycin, a new antibiotic. I. Discovery and biological properties. In: Sylvester JC, ed. *Antimicrobial agents and chemotherapy –1962*, pp. 554–9. American Society for Microbiology, Ann Arbor, Michigan.

73. Herrell WE (1969). *Lincomycin*, p. 13. Modern Scientific Publications, Inc, Chicago.

74. Magerlein BJ, Birkenmeyer RD, Kagan F (1967). Chemical modification of lincomycin. In: Hobby GL, ed. *Antimicrobial agents and chemotherapy–1966*, pp. 727–36. American Society for Microbiology, Ann Arbor, Michigan.

75. Magerlein BJ, Kagan F (1969). Lincomycin VIII. 4'-Alkyl-1'-demethyl-4'-depropylclindamycins, potent antibacterial and antimalarial agents. *J Med Chem* **12**, 780–4.

76. Finegold SM, Harada NE, Miller LG (1966). Lincomycin: activity against anaerobes and effect on normal human fecal flora. In: Hobby GL, ed. *Antimicrobial agents and chemotherapy–1965*, pp. 659–67. American Society for Microbiology, Ann Arbor, Michigan.

77. Editorial (1974). Lincomycin and clindamycin colitis. *BMJ* **4**, 65–6.

78. Ecker JA, Williams RG, McKittrick JE, Failing RM (1970). Pseudomembraneous enterocolitis—an unwelcome gastrointestinal complication of antibiotic therapy. *Am J Gastroenterol* **54**, 214–28.

79. Chabbert Y-A, Baudens J (1968). La pristinamycine et ses relations avec les macrolides et la lincomycine. *La Revue de Médecine* **9**, 625–8.

80. Charney J, Fisher WP, Curran C, Machlowitz RA, Tytell AA (1953). Streptogramin, a new antibiotic. In: Welch H, Marti-Ibañez F, eds. *Antibiotics annual 1953–54*, pp. 171–6. Medical Encyclopedia Inc, New York.

81. Tanaka N (1975). Mikamycin. In: Corcoran JW, Hahn FE, eds. *Antibiotics III. Mechanism of action of antimicrobial and antitumor agents*, pp. 487–97. Springer Verlag, Berlin.

82. Barber M, Garrod LP (1963). *Antibiotic and chemotherapy*, pp. 150–1. Livingstone, Edinburgh.

83. Various authors (1968). Traitment des staphylococcies par la pristinamycine. *La Revue de Médecine* **9**, 617–77.

84. Anonymous. *Fucidin. 1960–1970*. Leo Laboratories Ltd., Hayes, Middlesex. Undated.

85. Godtfredsen WO, Albretsen C, v. Daehne W, Tybring L, Vangedal S (1996). Transformations of fusidic acid and the relationship between structure and antibacterial activity.In: Hobby GL, ed.

Antimicrobial agents and chemotherapy-1965, pp. 132–7. American Society for Microbiology, Ann Arbor, Michigan.

86. Mochales S (1998). Ten years of CIBE symposia, 1989–1998. *Int Microbiol* **1**, 251–4. Also available at: http://www.im.microbios.org/04december98/03%20Mochales%20(F).pdf

87. Hendlin, D, Stapley EO, Jackson M, *et al*. (1969). Phosphonomycin, a new antibiotic produced by strains of *Streptomyces*. *Science* **166**, 122–3.

88. Abraham E (1983). Ernst Boris chain. *Biograph Memoirs Fellows R Soc* **29**, 43–91.

89. Fuller AT (1955). A new antibiotic of bacterial origin. *Nature* **175**, 722.

90. Su, TL (1948). Micrococcin, an antibacterial substance formed by a strain of *Micrococcus*. *Br J Exp Pathol* **29**, 473–81; Abraham EP (1957). *Biochemistry of some peptide and steroid antibiotics*. John Wiley, New York.

91. Fuller AT, Banks GT, Mellows G, Barrow, Woolford M, Chain EB (1971). Pseudomonic acid: an antibiotic from *Pseudomonas fluorescens*. *Nature* **234**, 416–17.

92. Debono M, Abbott BJ, Molloy RM, *et al*. (1988). Enzymic and chemical modifications of A21978C: the synthesis and evaluation of daptomycin (LY 146032). *J Antibiot* **41**, 1093–105.

93. Anonymous (1958). *The nitrofurans*, Vol. I. *Introduction to the nitrofurans*. Eaton Laboratories, Norwich, New York.

94. McGuigan H (1923). The action of furfural. *J Pharmacol Exp Ther* **21**, 65–75.

95. Dodd MC, Stillman WB (with the technical assistance of Roys M, Crosby C) (1944). The in vitro bacteristatic action of some simple furan derivatives. *J Pharmacol Exp Ther* **82**, 11–18.

96. Dodd MC (1946). The chemotherapeutic properties of 5-nitro-2-furaldehyde semicarbazone (furacin). *J Pharmacol Exp Ther* **84**, 311–23.

97. Snyder ML, Kiehn CL, Christopherson JW (1945). Effectiveness of a nitrofuran in the treatment of infected wounds. *Mil Surg* **97**, 380–4.

98. Editorial (1978). Water with sugar and salt. *Lancet* **2**, 300–01.

99. WHO/UNICEF joint statement (2004). *Clinical management of acute diarrhoea*. http://www.unicef.org/publications/Diarrhoea_FINAL.pdf

100. Hitchings GH (8 December 1988). *Selective inhibitors of dihydrofolate reductase*. Nobel lecture, Available at: http://www.nobel.se/medicine/laureates/1988/hitchings-lecture.html

101. Elion G (8 December 1988). *The purine path to chemotherapy*. Nobel lecture,. Available at: http://www.nobel.se/medicine/laureates/1988/elion-lecture.html

102. Eyles DE, Coleman N (1953). Synergistic effect of sulfadiazine and daraprim against experimental toxoplasmosis in the mouse. *Antibiot Chemother* **3**, 483–90.

103. Bushby SRM, Hitchings GH (1968). Trimethoprim, a sulphonamide potentiator. *Br J Pharmacol Chemother* **33**, 72–90.

104. Then RL, Bohni E, Anghern P, Plozza-Nottebrock H, Stoeckel K (1982). New analogs of trimethoprim. *Rev Infect Dis* **4**, 372–7.

105. Lesher GY, Froelich EJ, Gruett MD, Bailey JH, Brundage RP (1962). 1,8-naphthyridine derivatives. A new class of chemotherapeutic agents. *J Med Pharm Chem* **5**, 1063–5.

106. Rádl S (1996). From chloroquine to antineoplastic drugs? The story of antibacterial quinolones. *Archiv der Pharmazie. Pharm Med Chem* **329**, 115–19.

107. Wentland MP (1993). In memoriam: George Y. Lesher, Ph.D. In: Hooper DC, Wolfson JS, eds. *Quinolone antimicrobial agents*, 2nd edn., pp. 13–4. American Society for Microbiology, Washington, DC.

108. Albrecht R (1977). Development of antibacterial agents of the nalidixic acid type. *Prog Drug Res* **21**, 9–104.

109. Ito A, Hirai K, Inoue M, *et al*. (1980). In vitro antibacterial activity of AM-715, a new nalidixic acid analog. *Antimicrob Agents Chemother* **17**, 103–08.

110. Bakken JS (2004). The fluoroquinolones: how long will their utility last? *Scand J Infect Dis* **36**, 85–92.

111. Slee AM, Wuonola MA, McRipley RJ, *et al.* (1987). Oxazolidinones, a new class of synthetic antibacterial agents: in vitro and in vivo activities of DuP 105 and DuP 721. *Antimicrob Agents Chemother* **31**, 1791–7.

112. Zurenko GE, Yagi BH, Schaadt RD, *et al.* (1996). In vitro activities of U-100592 and U-100766, novel oxazolidinone antibacterial agents. *Antimicrob Agents Chemother* **40**, 839–45.

113. Kahn EJ (1976). *All in a century: the first hundred years of Eli Lilly and Company*. Eli Lilly, Indianapolis.

Chapter 7

Progress against parasites

Let us begin by imagining ourselves in an impoverished kala azar-stricken village. It is April and...

Robert S. Desowitz. *The Malaria Capers. Tales of Parasites and People Introduction*, p. 17. Norton, New York, 1993

The triumphant progress made in the treatment of bacterial infection in the quarter century that followed the appearance of the first sulphonamide in 1935 obscured the continuing inability of doctors to treat effectively other types of infection. In reality, by 1960—when there was (premature) talk in the air of an end to infectious diseases—relatively little had been achieved in improving the prospects for the many millions of people throughout the world suffering from parasitic, fungal, or viral disease. It is a melancholy truth that, until recently, serious parasitic diseases such as African sleeping sickness, kala-azar, and bilharzia, which afflict countless numbers of sufferers in developing countries, were— and sometimes still are—treated with arsenical and antimonial preparations of which Paracelsus would have approved.

Ironically, some parasitic diseases—protozoal infections like malaria and amoebic dysentery and intestinal worm infections—were among the few infective conditions for which reliable treatment pre-dated the antibiotic revolution by several centuries (see Chapter 2). Moreover, important advances in the treatment of certain parasitic infections in the twentieth century were made before effective antibacterial agents appeared on the scene.

Parasitic diseases are by no means confined to the tropics; nor, of course, are all tropical diseases associated with parasites. However, some of the most important parasites of human beings are restricted to warm countries because of the distribution of the obligatory arthropod or gastropod vectors; others are much more prevalent in warm climates and in conditions of poor hygiene. Consequently the discipline of parasitology, especially human parasitology, is almost synonymous with the study of tropical diseases.

As the European powers sought to exploit and expand their colonial empires in the late nineteenth century, tropical diseases took centre stage. In April 1899 the Liverpool School of Tropical Medicine opened its doors, kick-started by £350 provided by Alfred Lewis Jones, head of the Elder Dempster Shipping Line, who had business interests in the West African colonies (1). The opening occurred 6 months ahead (and to the great chagrin) of its rival, the London School, which was established in a branch hospital of the Seamen's Hospital Society in Albert Dock, East London in October 1899 after a protracted gestation (2). The German Institut für Schiff- und Tropenkrankheiten (Institute for Maritime and Tropical Diseases) in Hamburg was inaugurated the following year under the directorship of the naval physician, Bernhard Nocht. A School of Tropical Medicine was opened in Brussels in 1906, moving in 1931 to Antwerp to become the Prince Leopold Institute of Tropical Medicine. The Colonial Institute that was to become the Dutch Koninklijk Instituut voor de Tropen (Royal Tropical Institute) opened in 1910. With the Institut Pasteur also expanding into French possessions abroad, these developments greatly increased research into tropical diseases and stimulated efforts to find cures.

Academic groups such as those that formed around Ehrlich and Koch in Germany and French researchers at the Institut Pasteur in Paris, such as Ernest Fourneau, also took a close interest in tropical infections. Individuals in the field played their part as well, as exemplified by the efforts of Leonard Rogers in India to develop more efficient ways of tackling leprosy (see p. 192–3) and William Gorgas' fight against yellow fever and malaria during the construction of the Panama Canal. Strangely, America lagged somewhat behind in setting up formal structures for tropical disease research and training. Although the Rockefeller Institute for Medical Research (now the Rockefeller University) was established in 1901, diseases of the tropics were not at first among its main concerns. The Rockefeller Foundation, which was to play a major role in tropical research, was not created until 1913, although the ball had been set rolling in 1909 with finance for a Sanitary Commission for the Eradication of Hookworm Disease. In 1914 The Sanitary Commission became part of the International Health Commission (subsequently the International Health Division), with a wider remit. The Johns Hopkins School of Hygiene and Public Health, which became the principal centre for tropic research in North America, was not established (with Rockefeller money) until 1916.

At the time these developments were taking place the pharmaceutical industry was still at an embryonic stage. Few firms had any significant research base, and those that did took little interest in infectious diseases, let alone infections of the tropics, until sulphonamides came on the scene in the late 1930s. Notable exceptions were Burroughs Wellcome in England, inspired by Henry Wellcome's philanthropy and his love affair with tropical medicine, and the German dyestuff industry, most prominently and successfully the Bayer organization.

Henry Wellcome was extraordinarily committed to research and tropical medicine was his passion.* In addition to founding the Wellcome Physiological Research Laboratories (1894) with the famous physiologist Henry Dale in charge from 1906, and the Wellcome Chemical Research Laboratories (1896) with his friend Frederick Power at the helm (see p. 191), he also established: the Wellcome Tropical Research Laboratories in Khartoum

---

* Wellcome's interest in tropical medicine started early. In 1878, at the age of 25, he set out on an expedition to Ecuador in search of supplies of cinchona bark on behalf of his employer, the druggists McKesson and Robbins of New York (see James RR, reference 3, pp. 33–70 and 387–393).

(1902) with Andrew Balfour as director;* the Wellcome Bureau of Scientific Research (1913), dedicated to research in tropical medicine; and the Wellcome Entomological Field Laboratory in Esher, Surrey (1920) (3). Among Wellcome's other contributions to medicine in the tropics was the design of a medicine chest, the 'Congo chest', the first recipient of which was the journalist and explorer Henry Morton Stanley. These chests became essential equipment for future expeditions of all kinds.

But among pharmaceutical companies it was German expertise that made the most significant inroads into tackling the neglected therapeutic problems of tropical diseases, with the Bayer scientists making substantial progress in the years between the two World Wars. By the early twentieth century the German (and to a lesser extent the Swiss) dyestuffs and chemical industries had achieved a dominant position in world markets and were pioneering industrial research methods to develop new products (4). Diversification into new fields had gathered pace and pharmaceuticals were an area in which the inventive flair of their scientists, often in collaboration with academic institutions, was being exploited. The Bayer organization was among the most active of the dyestuff firms. From the start the company had attracted talented chemists and had encouraged research aimed at generating new dyes or other marketable compounds. In the wake of the success of phenacetin and aspirin (see p. 49), Bayer successfully increased its pharmaceutical portfolio with several products, including, from 1908, Antileprol for the treatment of leprosy (see p. 192). Spearheading the research effort was Carl Duisberg, the ambitious young chemist who had been recruited by Bayer in 1884, when he was just 23. Duisberg gathered round him an enthusiastic team, including Heinrich Hörlein, who joined the company in 1909 at the age of 27, was appointed head of scientific research the following year, and eventually became a director of IG Farben, the commercial partnership of which Bayer was a leading member (see p. 66). At the time of Hörlein's appointment to the firm Ehrlich's chemotherapy was very much in the air, and in 1910 a house in Elberfeld was adapted as a chemotherapy laboratory to exploit the new science (5).

Antiprotozoal agents

At the top of the list of diseases that were hindering the exploitation of overseas territories in the early twentieth-century heyday of European colonialism were two of Africa's most devastating protozoal infections: sleeping sickness (trypanosomiasis) and malaria. Indeed, these two diseases stimulated much of Paul Ehrlich's early researches in the field

---

* Balfour was instrumental in transforming the sanitary environment of Khartoum. It was he who suggested the idea of a floating laboratory on the Nile; Wellcome financed the venture, appointing, in 1907, the eminent protozoologist Charles Wenyon to take charge of scientific investigations. Balfour later (1923) became Director of the London School of Tropical Medicine and was knighted in 1930. As a young man he represented Scotland at Rugby and published several adventure novels. (See Gibson G The Edinburgh letter. *Canadian Medical Association Journal* 1931; 24: 576–578). Later in life he suffered from depression and was admitted to the Cassell Hospital, Kent for treatment. On 30 January 1931 his frozen body was found in the grounds after a fall from a window.

of chemotherapy (see p. 52f). Trypanosomiasis (and to a lesser extent its cousin, leishmaniasis) was particularly pressing, since the only drugs available for the treatment of this inevitably fatal condition were poisonous arsenical compounds; the most serious effects of malaria could, at least, be mitigated by the relatively safe quinine. Amoebic dysentery was the only other human protozoal infection that attracted much attention at that time, except in South America where an indigenous form of trypanosomiasis, quite different from the African variety, is prevalent. The importance of other protozoal diseases such as giardiasis, trichomoniasis, toxoplasmosis, and cryptosporidiosis, now known to be common and widespread infections—and by no means confined to tropical regions—were unrecognized in the early twentieth century.

African trypanosomiasis

African sleeping sickness is a cruel disease. It is insidious in its onset and inexorably fatal, killing sufferers after a protracted illness in which the victim becomes progressively disorientated, lethargic, and finally comatose. Infection is confined to tropical Africa, where two variants of *Trypanosoma brucei*, a flagellate protozoon that causes an economically important disease (nagana) in cattle, horses, and other ungulates, are transmitted to human beings by tsetse flies: *Trypanosoma brucei* subspecies *gambiense* is spread by a species of tsetse flies that inhabit forest areas of West and Central Africa alongside the Congo and other rivers; *Trypanosoma brucei* subspecies *rhodesiense* is transmitted by related flies found in the savannah regions of East Africa. The East African form of the disease tends to run a more rapid course than the West African type, which may take many months or even years to kill the victim.

Sleeping sickness and related trypanosomal infections in domestic animals presented a major threat to the development of European colonies in Africa. When a spreading epidemic that had followed the opening of trade routes occurred in Uganda and the Congo at the turn of the twentieth century, several expert commissions were sent by European powers with interests in Africa to investigate the disease. In June 1902 the Royal Society in England sponsored an ill-assorted group consisting of a Scot, George Carmichael Low, a medical adventurer, Cuthbert Christy, and a flamboyant young Italian, Aldo Castellani to travel to Entebbe in Uganda. Low and Christy were following up Manson's theory that the disease was caused by a filarial worm, while Castellani had a hunch that a streptococcus was responsible. Both theories proved wide of the mark. In 1903 the military doctor David Bruce* was dispatched to take over the investigation together with the bacteriologist David Nabarro and an Indian Medical Service doctor, a Scot, Edward Greig, who later did important work on the use of antimonials in kala-azar.

The British efforts to find the cause of sleeping sickness were widely publicized and caught the public imagination. The prevailing mood of England's middle classes, far

---

* Bruce, born in Melbourne, Australia to Scottish parents, but raised in Scotland, had earlier investigated an outbreak of nagana in cattle in Ubombo, northern Zululand (now KwaZulu-Natal). He established that it was caused by a trypanosome, now known as *Trypanosoma brucei* subspecies *brucei*. Even earlier, in Malta, he had found the bacterial cause of Malta fever, *Brucella melitensis*.

removed from the horrors of the disease, was nicely caught by their favourite magazine *Punch*:

Men of Science, you that dare,
Beard the microbe in his lair,
Tracking through the jungly thickness,
Afric's germ of Sleeping Sickness,
Hear, oh hear my Parting plea,
Send a microbe home to me!*

Bruce's team quickly confirmed that a trypanosome, found by Castellani in the cerebrospinal fluid of a victim, but thought at first to be an incidental finding, was the true cause. Both Bruce and Castellani had volatile temperaments and it is perhaps not surprising that a bitter dispute arose over who should take the credit (6).[†]

Bruce's team was also able to incriminate the tsetse fly in the transmission of sleeping sickness, so that attempts could at least be made to limit the disease by targeting the vector, but efforts to find an effective treatment remained stubbornly fruitless. Arsenic and the antimony-containing tartar emetic (potassium antimony tartrate) were the only compounds to have any effect and were too toxic for general use. Even when atoxyl was introduced as a purportedly safer way of administering arsenic (see p. 55–6 and below) it proved, despite its name, to cause blindness and other serious complications. After his setbacks with the performance of trypan red and other dyes, Ehrlich had pinned his hopes on improving on atoxyl, but the work led instead to the antispirochaetal compound Salvarsan (see p. 57f). The action of Salvarsan against the spirochaetes of syphilis brought Ehrlich fame, but the drug had disappointingly little effect against trypanosomes, which, at the time were thought to be related to spirochaetes, a belief that persisted for some years (7).

In the event scientists in Bayer's laboratories at Elberfeld made the first tentative steps towards an effective therapy for trypanosomiasis. The substance was given the splendidly nationalistic name 'Germanin', but has been known generically since the 1930s as suramin.

Suramin

In 1910, Bayer hired Wilhelm Röhl, a medical graduate of Heidelberg University who had worked as one of Ehrlich's assistants at the Georg-Speyer Haus in Frankfurt. The following year he was given the task of organizing the firm's chemotherapy laboratory, newly

---

* 'Lines by an insomniac' *Punch* 16 September 1903, p. 185. I am grateful to my daughter, Anna Crozier for unearthing this delightful snippet.

† The cause of sleeping sickness had, in fact, already been discovered in 1901 by Robert Michael Forde a colonial surgeon working in The Gambia. The parasitologist Joseph Everett Dutton was dispatched from the Liverpool School of Tropical Medicine to the Gambia in December 1901 to confirm the finding. Dutton called the parasite *Trypanosoma gambiense*. See Williams BI. African trypanosomes. In: *Illustrated history of tropical diseases* (Cox FEG ed.). The Wellcome Trust, London, 1996, pp. 178–191. Dutton died in 1905 from relapsing fever, while investigating the cause of the disease, aged just 29.

established in a small house in Elberfeld. Röhl had worked on atoxyl with Ehrlich and was familiar with the work on dyes and acridine derivatives, which he proceeded to extend in his new post.

In 1912 it was discovered that certain colourless derivatives of dyes retained their ability to bind to fibres and Röhl found that these substances remained active against spirochaetes. Realizing that this potentially removed one of the chief barriers to the use of dyes as antimicrobial substances—the fact that they caused pigmentation in the tissues of human beings and animals*—Röhl approached his colleague, Bernard Heymann, head of Bayer's main scientific laboratory asking him to provide colourless dye derivatives, to test in animal models of syphilis, trypanosomiasis, and malaria. Despite his initial scepticism, Heymann was persuaded and the chemists, Richard Kothe, Oskar Dressel, and Anton Ossenbeck duly started a programme of synthesis, basing their work on derivatives with urea linkages (a feature of the dye afridol violet which was known to have antitrypanosomal activity) that seemed to offer the best promise of success.

Although the work was interrupted by the First World War, when Röhl, a medical reservist, was drafted to serve on the eastern front and Ossenbeck was temporarily seconded to a factory manufacturing gas masks, Heymann's chemists continued their work and in 1916 synthesized a compound which the remaining personnel in Röhl's laboratory found to have excellent activity in a mouse model of nagana. The substance, originally called Detrilan,[†] became known as 'Bayer 205'. On his return to Elberfeld in 1918, Röhl confirmed the excellent antitrypanosomal activity and relative lack of toxicity of Bayer 205, a result reinforced independently in tests of animals infected with various trypanosomes by Drs Ludwig Haendel and Karl Wilhelm Jötten in Berlin and by Professor Martin Mayer and his colleagues at the Tropical Institute in Hamburg. The results encouraged Mayer to try the new drug in the therapy of sleeping sickness. Treatment of the first patient, a German who had returned home from West Africa with symptoms of the disease, was started in March 1920. The doctors had little idea of the correct dosage to use and this first trial was unsuccessful. When a cure was eventually claimed the following year, the honour of being the first successful case surprisingly went to a Welsh engineer, Christopher Gordon James, who had acquired sleeping sickness while hunting in the Serengheti in September 1920.

James had been unsuccessfully treated with various drugs including tartar emetic and atoxyl in East Africa and he returned to Britain, where he came under the care of Warrington Yorke at the Liverpool School of Tropical Medicine. Yorke was equally

---

* The problem did not inhibit the use of Prontosil in the 1930s, but the spectacular activity of that compound, which had a transient effect in imparting a pink colour to those receiving the drug, probably overrode such considerations.

† The chemists produced separate series for different organisms and they were named alphabetically. Compounds aimed at syphilis were thus called Asypin, Besypin, Cesypin etc; the antitrypanosome series were named Atrilan, Betrilan, Cetrilan, Detrilan etc. (see Dünschede, reference 5, p. 24).

unsuccessful in halting progress of the disease and, having read the German literature, wrote to Mayer in Hamburg asking for a sample of Bayer 205. Mayer refused, but offered to treat the patient if he were sent to Hamburg. Yorke was understandably hesitant:

> However, as notwithstanding the most rigorous treatment the patient's condition got steadily worse, I went critically through the above mentioned papers again and was so impressed by the results recorded, that I overcame my own scruples and those of the patient, with the result that he left for Hamburg on 5th July 1921 (8)

Treatment was started on 9 July under the care of Peter Mühlens and Walter Menk; by mid-August James was released from hospital, and in September he returned to Liverpool apparently cured:

> He appeared in excellent health, and stated that he never felt better in his life and plays two rounds of golf daily without the slightest distress...on 11th November he sailed for South Africa (8).

Gordon James was exceedingly lucky. He had been suffering from the more rapidly developing *rhodesiense* form of sleeping sickness for 10 months before treatment in Germany and suramin was later shown to be ineffective in advanced disease.

The fact that the first successfully treated case was British is all the more surprising since Germany had lost her possessions in Africa under the terms of the 1919 Treaty of Versailles and there was no love lost between the two countries. This was a period of great turmoil in Germany. Humiliated at Versailles, there was constant political instability and rampant hyperinflation. Between 1920 and 1923, money quickly lost its value, with prices sometimes doubling on a daily basis. Workers were paid with sacks of banknotes that rapidly became so worthless that they were used to feed the household stove. By 1923 the rate of exchange of the Reichsmark against the US Dollar was astonishingly in excess of 4 trillion (million million) to one. Industry was badly hit and Bayer was one of the firms to suffer severely: its assets in America, Great Britain, and France had been confiscated; the Rhineland was under Allied occupation; and the resources needed to conduct research were hard to come by. Moreover German firms had been excluded from the British and French markets after the war.

The loss of their African colonies created a headache for Bayer. Before Bayer 205 could be marketed, it was essential to test its efficacy for prophylaxis and treatment in the field and that meant tropical Africa, the only place in which human sleeping sickness occurred. Bayer's representative in England, Richard Hennings had to go cap in hand to Sir John Rose Bradford, an eminent physician at University College Hospital London, who acted as senior medical adviser to the Colonial Office, to obtain consent for trials to be undertaken in Rhodesia. Hennings had managed to get the support of David Bruce, who was a friend of Bradford and had suggested his name. In fact, through the influence of Bruce, Bradford already took a close interest in tropical medicine and, convinced by the claims made for the new drug, readily arranged the permission required for field trials to go ahead (9).

In October 1921 an expedition led by the tropical expert Friedrich Karl Kleine, who had earlier escorted Robert Koch on one of his scientific missions to Africa, set off once more for the Dark Continent. Accompanying him were Dr Walter Fischer, who had previous experience of trypanosomiasis with Kleine in the former German colony of the Cameroons, and Fräulein Hanna Ockelmann, who was later to become Kleine's wife. After a gruelling journey from Cape Town, where they landed in November 1921, they eventually set up a makeshift laboratory in the tsetse fly infested town of Ndombo in what is now Zambia, and started work in January 1922. While undertaking their investigations Kleine received a telegram from the governor general of the Belgian Congo offering facilities to carry out trials there, and in November 1922, the team set off once more on a 3-week cross-country trek to continue their researches in a new country. Towards the end of 1923, Kleine returned home to Germany, but Fischer moved on to the Spanish island of Fernando Po (Bioko) in the Gulf of Guinea, where 247 more patients were treated (9). The outcome of these three trials gave encouraging indications that Bayer 205 was indeed a valuable drug for the treatment of human trypanosomiasis, though the findings in cattle with nagana turned out to be disappointing. Bayer now had the information they needed to promote the drug and decided to go ahead with marketing it under the patriotic name 'Germanin'. The Oxford zoologist Julian Huxley wrote in the *Daily Herald* on New Year's Eve 1923:

> The discovery in Germany of a chemical substance—'Bayer 205'—which cures sleeping sickness is another and very important step forward in making the tropics inhabitable. This one single discovery is of such importance to all nations with tropical possessions that the criminal folly of bringing a great scientific nation like Germany to a pitch in which it is increasingly difficult for scientific research to be carried on at once becomes apparent. In the long run this discovery will probably be far more valuable financially to the Allies than the whole sum originally demanded for reparations (10).

The British press meanwhile howled that the key to Africa was now in German hands!

In fact there was much soul-searching within Bayer about how Bayer 205, which they realized could be of great benefit to mankind as well as being a potential money-spinner, should be protected for the national and company benefit. When the drug was eventually marketed in 1924, its formula was kept a closely guarded secret. Within the firm there was a satisfying feeling of poetic justice in finding a drug that would undoubtedly make a great deal of money from the countries that had taken possession of their colonies in East and West Africa. Later, when Hitler came to power, the argument was turned against them and the company (by now IG Farben) was castigated for concentrating its research effort—the antimalarials Plasmoquine and Atebrin were also by now on the market (see below)—on drugs of value to Germany's enemies (11).

Despite German attempts to keep details of the structure of the new product under wraps, a competing product emerged almost at once. In 1924, the same year in which Germanin was marketed, Ernest Fourneau of the Laboratoire de Chimie Thérapeutique at the Institut Pasteur in Paris, who had earlier worked on atoxyl (see p. 56), announced the synthesis of a colourless dye derivative with activity against trypanosomes that was given the laboratory designation Fourneau 309. Although the formula of Germanin was a trade secret, Fourneau had deduced from such information as was available in the patent literature the type of substance that it was likely to be and had set about synthesizing derivatives. He soon hit upon one that had the requisite activity and reasoned that since any modification to the structure reduced the potency, it must, in reality, be identical to that of Germanin. At first, the Germans contested this claim, but they were already excluded from the French market and soon came to an understanding with Fourneau. In 1925 a marketing agreement was reached between Bayer and the firm of Poulenc frères, with whom Fourneau had a long-standing relationship. Poulenc manufactured the French product, which was undeniably identical to Germanin, and put it on the market under the trade name Moranyl. Later, a British version, Antrypol, was marketed by ICI.

In the context of the 1920s, suramin was undoubtedly a major advance in the therapy of trypanosomiasis. Indeed, its value is attested by the fact that it is still used for the treatment of the early manifestations of the disease. In the remarkable tradition of drugs finding a place for unrelated conditions, it was later shown to be effective in onchocerciasis (see p. 332) and was briefly considered as a possible anti-HIV agent.

Arsenicals

Until suramin came along, the only drug of any real, if limited, value was atoxyl (Fig. 7.1). Following their successful use of the drug in mice, the Liverpool School of Tropical Medicine provided considerable quantities to doctors and missionaries for trials in West Africa (12) and it was soon being produced commercially. Although it was far from being a reliable cure, and one of its side effects was damage to the optic nerve with the risk of blindness, it speaks volumes for the parlous state of chemotherapeutic interventions at the time that it became quite widely used, often in combination with another toxic drug, tartar emetic. Addressing the Society of Tropical Medicine and Hygiene in London in 1907, the missionary doctor Albert Cook of the Church Missionary Society Hospital, which he had founded in Mengo, Uganda,* described atoxyl as 'by far the best drug that has yet been tried' though he fully recognized its limitations (13). Apart from unreliability and toxicity, one of the main problems with atoxyl was its expense—according to Cook, about £14 per pound. In response Burroughs Wellcome marketed a closely related formulation, Soamin (*para*-aminophenylarsonate)—synthesized in 1907 by Francis Pyman in collaboration with Marmaduke Barrowcliffe and Frederic Remfry (14)—at a fraction of the price. Prophylactic use of the drug was also tried, notably by the French military doctor, Eugène Jamot, who successfully controlled an outbreak of sleeping sickness in the French colony of Oubangui-Chari (now the Central African Republic) between 1917 and 1920[†] with a policy of 'atoxylation' carried out by mobile treatment teams (15). Atoxyl, despite its problems, still featured, though not as a first line treatment, in official War Office guidelines for the therapy of sleeping sickness

---

* Cook founded the hospital in 1897 with Katharine Timpson, a missionary nurse, as matron. They married in 1900; both received many honours and Albert Cook was knighted in 1932.

[†] Jamot led another celebrated expedition to control trypanosomiasis, this time to the French Cameroons between 1926 and 1932. It was captured in a fascinating film made on behalf of the Société Parisienne d'Expansion Chimique (Specia; now part of Aventis Pharma) in 1930. A video cassette version is held by The Wellcome Library for the History and Understanding of Medicine in London.

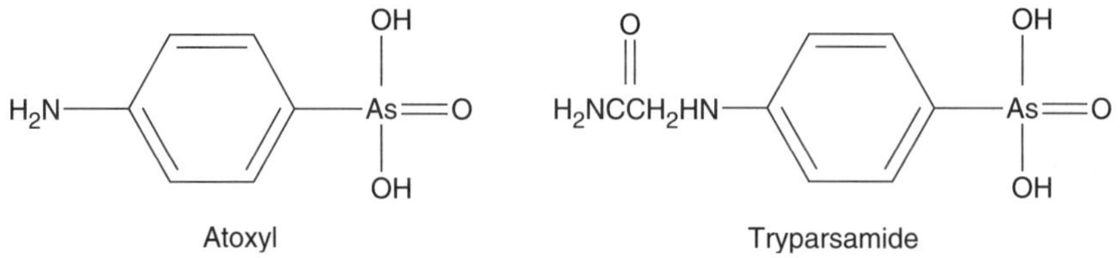

Fig. 7.1 The molecular structures of atoxyl and tryparsamide.

as late as 1941 (16). Even now it survives in veterinary use as sodium arsanilate for the treatment of swine dysentery as well as being used as a growth promoter (17).

Contemporaneously with the work at Elberfeld that was to lead to suramin, Ehrlich's dream of an arsenical compound with potent antitrypanosomal activity to replace atoxyl was being pursued at the Rockefeller Institute of Medical Research in New York. In 1912, Simon Flexner, the institute's director, had decided that the time was ripe to enter the new field of chemotherapy and set up a new division with Walter Jacobs in charge (see p. 64). Like many of his contemporaries, Jacobs had spent time abroad, studying for a PhD in Berlin from 1905 to 1907 under the famous chemist Emil Fischer. According to the American journalist Elmer Bendiner, the decision to investigate arsenicals was taken in 1914 as war broke out in Europe, because of the fear that American supplies of Salvarsan might be severely affected by British and French attempts to blockade German trade across the Atlantic (18). Synthesis of Salvarsan was soon accomplished, and the Rockefeller scientists set about trying to improve it. In a reversal of the direction that Ehrlich's researches had taken, it was an arsenical with striking activity against trypanosomes that was to be the chief outcome of this programme.

Jacobs' collaborators in the research investigation into arsenical compounds were the chemist Michael Heidelberger (who soon became a famous immunochemist), the pathologist, Wade Hampton Brown, and Louise Pearce, who was hired by Flexner in 1913 after completing a degree in physiology at Stanford University and medical training at the Johns Hopkins School. Jacobs and Heidelberger provided the chemical expertise, while Brown and Pearce carried out most of the biological testing, including extensive animal experiments. Over 230 different arsenical compounds were investigated, many of them glycine amides (containing the structure $NHCH_2CONH$) which simplified further chemical manipulation. Although these studies produced puzzling results in terms of relating structural changes to efficacy and toxicity, one of them, synthesized in 1915 and described chemically as the sodium salt of phenylglycine amide-p-arsonic acid, was found by Brown and Pearce to effect a rapid and permanent cure of various laboratory animals infected with trypanosomes at doses that did not cause serious toxicity (19). Unfortunately the drug was much less active against spirochaetes, but penetrated well into the cerebrospinal fluid raising hopes that it might also be of value in neurosyphilis. The results were published in the *Journal of Experimental Medicine* in 1919 (20), and the substance was patented with the name tryparsamide (Fig. 7.1).

Louise Pearce was, by all accounts, a determined and resourceful woman. She embraced physiology, medicine, and medical research at a time when these were almost exclusively the preserve of men, and she was by no means overshadowed. She was a champion of women's rights and in the 1930s she set up home with Dr S. Josephine Baker, who had been the first director of the New York Bureau of Child Hygiene (and had helped to track down the infamous 'typhoid Mary'; Mary Mallon), and the Australian writer and former suffragette, Ida Wylie. In later life Pearce became president of the Women's Medical College of Pennsylvania.

Pearce certainly was not one to shy away from a challenge. Once the potential of tryparsamide was realized and it became necessary to organize clinical trials in Africa, she volunteered to travel to the Belgium Congo (now the Democratic Republic of Congo; formerly Zaire) to carry out the first human trials. She left for Léopoldville (Kinshasa) in May 1920 spending about a year there treating patients in various stages of sleeping sickness at the Hôpital de la Reine and testing samples at the government laboratory. A meticulously detailed account of the findings was published on her return the following year (21). Three of the first four cases: men named as Eali, Bibaba, and Etumbu, showed some initial response, but died; the third of the first four to be treated, a woman called M'Boyo, survived. All were advanced cases that had previously been treated with atoxyl or other drugs. The overall results were, however, astonishing: 80 per cent of cases responded to the treatment, including many victims with advanced disease. The only major problem encountered was optic nerve toxicity, especially when high doses were given to those with late-stage disease. Pearce was fêted by the Belgium authorities; in 1953, by which time tryparsamide had saved many thousands of African lives, she went to Brussels to receive from the hands of King Baudouin the Ordre Royal du Lion (Royal Order of the Lion) and the King Leopold II prize on behalf of herself and her co-discoverers.

Before leaving the Congo, Pearce arranged that the director of the Léopoldville Laboratory, Frans Van den Branden and his colleague Lucien Van Hoof, should continue to follow-up the cases she had treated. It was also necessary to obtain independent confirmation of the findings. While in Léopoldville Pearce met the English medical missionary Clement Chesterman, who was on his way with his new wife Winifred to take up a position for the Baptist Missionary Society at Yakusu, near Stanleyville (now Kisangani), in the Upper Belgian Congo. Chesterman was greatly impressed with Pearce's capabilities and agreed to carry out a trial of tryparsamide at the Stapleton Memorial Hospital,* where he was to work. Supplies of tryparsamide were obtained through the Rockefeller from the firm of Powers–Weightman–Rosengarten† in Philadelphia, who manufactured the drug on licence.

....

* Founded by Walter Stapleton and continued by his assistant William Millman, who, after Stapleton's death in 1906 married his widow, Edith. For a fascinating account of her experiences See: http://myweb.tiscali.co.uk/janemarshallworld/MamaIntroCh1.htm

† An old established firm that manufactured quinine, opium, and mercurial compounds. The company merged with Merck in 1927.

From August 1921 Chesterman, with occasional help from his fellow missionary doctor, Frederick Gordon Spear—a radiologist who went on to become president of the British Institute of Radiology—used tryparsamide for the many advanced cases of sleeping sickness that came to the mission hospital. An admirably lucid account of the first 40 advanced cases of sleeping sickness treated with the drug—injected intravenously, and in some cases directly into the meninges, in boiled rainwater—was presented before the Royal Society of Tropical Medicine and Hygiene on 18 January 1923 while he was on leave (22). Chesterman recounts how many of the unfortunate men, women, and children who benefited from tryparsamide treatment had already received, with little success, not only atoxyl and tartar emetic, but also Soamin (from Burroughs Wellcome), Stibenyl (a German antimonial drug manufactured in England by Allen and Hanbury), and Bayer's Germanin; some were so emaciated that they had to be carried into the hospital for treatment. Chesterman returned to England the following year to deliver a progress report on 19 June 1924 (23), by which time 15 of 37 patients (40.5 per cent) who could be traced appeared cured: a success rate much better than any achieved up to that time and all the more remarkable as the correct dosage regimen was still a matter of conjecture. Seldom can a young missionary have received such encouraging results from a new treatment during his first tours of duty in the field.

Another arsenical entered the arena around this time. Ernest Fourneau and his colleagues (including the Tréfouëls, who were to be instrumental in elucidating the sulphonamides; see p. 70) described in 1921 a compound with activity against trypanosomes, which they called stovarsol. The name was a pun on Fourneau's name, which means 'stove' in English. Stovarsol was not a great success against sleeping sickness and became a drug searching for a disease, being subsequently used with little distinction for various parasitic and spirochaetal conditions from amoebiasis to yaws. Two similar compounds, orsanin and treparsol, emerged from the Fourneau laboratories a few years later, but suffered much the same fate.

Efforts to investigate arsenical derivatives for the treatment of trypanosomiasis and syphilis also continued in England in Warrington Yorke's laboratory at the Liverpool School of Tropical Medicine. From 1927 Yorke with his colleague Frederick Murgatroyd and, from 1930, Frank Hawking*—both of whom became distinguished tropical researchers in their own right—began testing potential candidate molecules with the help of small grants from the Medical Research Council's Chemotherapy Committee (24). The most promising arsenical derivative, given the name 'Neocryl' was one of those synthesized by Gilbert Morgan, director of the Department of Scientific and Industrial Research's Chemical Research Laboratory at Teddington, who provided many of the compounds for Yorke to test. Encouraging results, reported in 1936 (25), were obtained in 42 patients with syphilis in England and in 11 cases of sleeping sickness treated by the Liverpool school's staff in Nigeria. Neocryl was briefly marketed, but was never widely used.

* Father of the theoretical physicist, Stephen Hawking.

Improvement on tryparsamide had to await the fertile imagination of one of Chesterman's friends, the maverick Swiss chemist, Ernst Friedheim who described in 1949 a condensation product of melarsen oxide (a melamine derivative of arsenic which he had synthesized in 1941) and a substance known as British anti-lewisite. Friedheim called his new drug Mel B (short for melarsen–British anti-lewisite) long before a minor pop celebrity hijacked the name. Melamine is nowadays better known as a constituent of plastics and resins; British anti-lewisite (dimercaprol) was developed by the biochemist Rudolph Peters and his colleagues at Oxford during the Second World War to counteract the arsenical chemical warfare agent, lewisite, which it was feared might be used against Allied forces. Lewisite is named after the chemist, Winford Lee Lewis, who developed it as a blistering agent in 1918 while working for the United States Chemical Warfare Service research unit at the Catholic University of America in Washington DC. It had originally been discovered at the University in 1903 by a priest, Julius Nieuwland*, while working for his PhD.

Friedheim's investigation of arsenical compounds with reduced toxicity had been motivated by a tragic blunder by a military doctor in the Cameroons in 1932, when around 800 patients became blind after being given an overdose of tryparsamide. While working in the faculty of medicine in the University of Geneva, Friedheim converted the kitchen of his home in order to carry out research on antitrypanosomal compounds (26). His refreshingly idiosyncratic approach to science may be judged from a lecture that he gave at the Liverpool School of Tropical Medicine in October 1958 in which he describes some of the work that eventually led to Mel B. In selecting a suitable reagent for the synthesis of one arsenical compound he describes that it was chosen:

> for entirely unscientific reasons connected with a young lady who improved the shade of her auburn curls with a walnut rinse, i.e. 5-hydroxy-α-naphthoquinone (27).

No less appealing is his scientific philosophy, stated in the same lecture, which unwittingly reflects much of the history of antimicrobial chemotherapy:

> In my laboratory we are guided by a sentence from our English school grammar: "Have you seen the umbrella of my grandmother? Yes, but this parrot does not eat hard-boiled eggs." A hypothesis may point to granny's umbrella, but, while looking for it, try to keep your eyes wide open so as not to miss any useful eggs that may be hidden on the roadside.

Friedheim's search for less toxic arsenicals concentrated on melamine derivatives and in 1938 he described melarsen as a potential candidate. He travelled to Africa himself to test it, but sadly it turned out to be too toxic. A derivative, melarsen oxide, proved to be better in field trials, but Friedheim was still not satisfied. The idea of condensing melarsen oxide with the arsenical antidote, British anti-lewisite, in order to reduce its toxicity was a bold, if optimistic, step; but fortune favours the brave and this time Friedheim struck gold.

---

* Nieuwland, born in Belgium, but raised in Indiana, is more famous for his discovery of a synthetic rubber substitute, neoprene.

Friedheim's individualistic approach did not endear him to the chemical or medical establishments. Even after he moved in 1945 to the Rockefeller Institute in New York, where he had already spent 2 years in the early 1930s, he continued to plough a lonely furrow. When he first described Mel B in 1949, after another field trip to test the compound in collaboration with the sleeping sickness service of French West Africa (28), few took his discovery seriously. One who did was the British tropical specialist, Ian Apted (later assistant director of the Bureau of Hygiene and Tropical Medicine in London), who achieved remarkable results with the drug in the treatment of late-stage East African trypanosomiasis, against which tryparsamide had no useful effect (29). It subsequently became the standard treatment for advanced sleeping sickness. Mel B, now officially called melarsoprol, is very far from being an ideal treatment for sleeping sickness. Not only does it retain substantial toxicity—not helped by the fact that it is very insoluble and is administered dissolved in propylene glycol—but it is painful to inject and resistance of trypanosomes to arsenicals in general is quite common. Nevertheless, in the right hands it offers the prospect of cure for cases that are otherwise beyond help and remains the drug of choice for treating the *rhodesiense* form of trypanosomiasis.

Friedheim went on to produce a water-soluble melamine derivative, trimelarsen (Mel W), but it proved less effective and more toxic than Mel B. Another soluble version, cymelarsan, Mel Cy, is used exclusively against trypanosomiasis in animals, as is the related diminazene (Berenil).

Diamidines

The notion that diamidines—symmetrical organic molecules with a $HN=C–NH_2$ group at either end—might have activity against trypanosomes emerged in the 1920s when in-vitro culture of the parasites was being developed. It was found that glucose was essential to their survival and this led to the suggestion that drugs acting against glucose metabolism might starve the protozoa of an essential food. Working on this theory in the 1920s, Miklós Jancsó a pharmacologist at Szeged University in Hungary, showed that a compound then used in diabetes, Synthalin (decamethylene diguanidine) was effective in clearing trypanosomes from the bloodstream of infected mice. The idea was presently taken up by Warrington Yorke in Liverpool. Together with his colleague Emmanuel Lourie, who was to become director of the Department of Chemotherapy at the Liverpool School after Yorke's premature death in April 1943, it was shown that Synthalin was indeed active against trypanosomes, but the effect had nothing to do with interference with the supply of glucose (30). Clearly, Lady Luck had been at work once more.

Synthalin was too toxic for therapeutic use in man, but Yorke continued to pursue the idea. With the help of Harold King, head of organic chemistry at the National Institute of Medical Research in London and Arthur Ewins of May and Baker* (a firm that Yorke was

---

* Arthur Ewins had previously worked on arsenicals at the National Institute of Medical Research with Harold King and George Barger. The team had been brought together by Henry Dale to produce Salvarsan when supplies from Germany were cut off after 1914. Ewins moved to May & Baker in 1917 and was subsequently involved in the synthesis of sulphapyridine (see p. 75–6); Barger, a pioneering biochemist, was born in Manchester to a Dutch engineer and English mother and was brought up in Utrecht. In 1919 he became Professor of Medicinal Chemistry in Edinburgh, before moving to Chair of Chemistry in Glasgow in 1937.

courting as a financial sponsor for his research), related diamidines were found to be more active and less toxic. By the beginning of the Second World War, three potential therapeutic diamidines had been developed: stilbamidine, pentamidine, and propamidine. Stilbamidine was used for some years in antimony-resistant cases of the leishmanial disease, kala-azar (see p. 305) but was discontinued because of unacceptable toxicity; propamidine was developed for topical use, notably in eye drops and is still thought to be of value in *Acanthamoeba* keratitis, an amoebic infection that occasionally affects wearers of contact lenses. But it was pentamidine that was to be the most important of the three compounds.

Pentamidine was first used in sleeping sickness in the Gold Coast (present-day Ghana) in 1940 by George Saunders, an Irish medical officer based in Kintampo who was in charge of a local trypanosomiasis mass treatment campaign (31). The trial was conducted at the request of Warrington Yorke. Saunders had been in the Gold Coast since the late 1920s working with the entomologist Kenneth Morris on the epidemiology of sleeping sickness and control of the tsetse fly vector, and had earlier carried out a trial of Bayer's Germanin. Saunders treated 14 cases of sleeping sickness in the pentamidine trial, only 2 of which were early cases with no brain involvement. Although the drug brought about an improvement in the condition of nearly all the patients, with trypanosomes successfully eliminated from the bloodstream, most of the advanced cases still showed cerebral symptoms, indicating that a therapeutic concentration of pentamidine was probably not reaching the central nervous system. Side effects in this first trial were reported to be trivial (32).

Further testing by Lucien Van Hoof in Léopoldville and others confirmed the benefit of pentamidine against early infection with *Trypanosoma brucei gambiense*, but it turned out to be ineffective against the *rhodesiense* subspecies. Unsurprisingly, toxic side effects proved common, but were seldom life-threatening if the dosage was carefully controlled. Like suramin, it does not cross the blood-brain barrier and is only of benefit if used before the trypanosomes invade the central nervous system. It also shares another similarity with suramin: unsuspected activity against an unrelated pathogen. It was discovered to have useful activity against an unusual organism called *Pneumocystis carinii* (*jirovecii*), which can cause a serious pneumonia (see p. 361).

Eflornithine

Fresh hope for the thousands of sufferers from sleeping sickness in Africa emerged in the 1980s, in the shape of a new compound, eflornithine (difluoromethylornithine), which displayed unprecedented activity against the parasites and a safety profile which, while far from being unblemished, was considerably better than that of its predecessors. Sadly, the process of making eflornithine available for those who desperately needed it has been racked with uncertainties. Indeed, there are few better examples of the conflict between profitability and the humanitarian imperative—nor, some would say, of the impotence of the World Health Organization in fulfilling its mandate.

Eflornithine was originally developed in the late 1970s as an anticancer agent in the Merrell International Research Centre in Strasbourg, by a team of scientists led by Albert Sjoerdsma. In 1979 Sjoerdsma's research moved to the Merrell Dow laboratories in Cincinnati, Ohio and among those who moved with him was his senior scientist,

Peter McCann. For around 10 years, Cyrus Bacchi a biochemist working at the Haskins Laboratory in Pace University, New York, had pursued a research programme into potential antitrypanosomal agents centred on the notion that cancer cells and trypanosomes share some metabolic features and that antitumour compounds might offer a profitable avenue for study (33). At the time of the discovery of eflornithine Bacchi had recently turned his attention to polyamine metabolism in trypanosomes (34). These substances play an important role in living cells and eflornithine irreversibly inhibits an enzyme, ornithine decarboxylase, which is essential to their formation. Crucially, the trypanosomal enzyme is slightly different to the version found in mammalian cells, allowing the selective toxicity principle to operate. In collaboration with Peter McCann, Bacchi investigated whether eflornithine might inhibit polyamine metabolism in trypanosomes in the same way that it did in tumour cells. He gave the drug to mice infected with trypanosomes of the *Trypanosoma brucei* group by adding it to their drinking water, or by delivering the drug by a tube into the stomach, and found that doses that appeared to have no adverse effects eradicated the parasites from the bloodstream. These remarkable results were published in *Science* in 1980 (35) and the lengthy process of confirming the findings and establishing the safety and efficacy of eflornithine as a cure for sleeping sickness began.

According to Albert Sjoerdsma's daughter, Ann, who wrote a combative account of the trials and tribulations of eflornithine for *The Baltimore Sun* in 2000 (36), the first clinical use of the drug in Africa was arranged with little formal planning. A Belgian doctor from the Institute of Tropical Medicine in Antwerp, Simon Van Nieuwenhove, who was working in Southern Sudan for the Belgian–Sudanese Sleeping Sickness Control Project, had learned from a colleague, of Bacchi's work. While on leave in Europe Nieuwenhove arranged for an informal meeting with Paul Schechter, a clinical pharmacologist who was responsible for Merrell Dow's anticancer trials of eflornithine in Europe. At their meeting in Strasbourg Nieuwenhove put the case of need to Schechter, who agreed to provide supplies of the drug without further ado. Nieuwenhove returned to the Sudan with the eflornithine in his luggage and such information as was then known on how to administer it. Twenty patients, 18 of them with late-stage disease, but still conscious, were given eflornithine by mouth for up to 6 weeks. The oral route was chosen because of the difficulty of giving a course of injections under the rural conditions in which the trial was carried out. The results were unparalleled, with a marked response, few serious side effects and only one relapse during the period of observation. The first patient, identified only as 'K. A.', a 30-year-old woman who had previously been treated unsuccessfully with suramin and melarsoprol, started to receive eflornithine on 25 November 1982 and was still well nearly 2 years later (37).

Further trials, notably in the Côte d'Ivoire and the Congo (this time with eflornithine administered intravenously for the first 14 days) soon confirmed van Nieuwenhove's preliminary findings, although other studies disappointingly revealed that the *rhodesiense* form of the parasite was innately resistant. The effect in some late-stage cases, suffering from the commoner *gambiense* form of the disease, was so startling that eflornithine became dubbed 'the resurrection drug'. Unfortunately, several clouds appeared on this bright horizon: similar success was not being achieved in cancer trials in Europe and

America; a course of treatment of trypanosomiasis was far too expensive for poor countries with tiny health budgets; and production problems requiring expensive new plant emerged in the United States. What seemed to be the last ray of hope for the commercial viability of eflornithine—that it might be of value in pneumocystis pneumonia in AIDS patients—came to nothing.

In 1995, Hoechst Marion Roussel (since 1999 Aventis; now Sanofi–Aventis), who by then had acquired Merrell Dow, gave up the struggle and production of eflornithine ceased. The last supplies, enough for an estimated 5 years, were sold at cost to Médecins sans Frontières. Patent rights for manufacture of the trypanosomiasis formulations were transferred to the World Health Organization on the understanding that alternative sources of production would be found. Despite many attempts, no such source was forthcoming and in the Byzantine world of the World Health Organization, funding of trypanosomiasis projects was given little priority.

It seemed that eflornithine would be lost to medicine, but by an amazing stroke of luck, the drug was unexpectedly discovered in the nick of time to retard the growth of human hair. It needed little market research to confirm that facial hair was perceived as a problem by millions of women who would welcome a simple, straightforward solution. A new and lucrative application for the drug had been found. In August 2000 the United States Food and Drug Administration approved eflornithine cream as a topical agent to control the growth of facial hair. The preparation is now manufactured by Bristol Myers Squibb under a royalty agreement with Aventis and sold in association with the Gillette Company under the name Vaniqa.

Human vanity is a big market, whereas there are no dollars to be made from dying Africans. Nevertheless, victims of sleeping sickness were given fresh hope by the continued commercial production of eflornithine. The hopes received a boost in 2001, when Aventis concluded a 5-year agreement with the World Health Organization and Médecins sans Frontières committing them to support field programmes for trypanosomiasis control, including the provision of continuing supplies of eflornithine, together with melarsoprol and pentamidine. The company manufacturing Vaniqa, Bristol Myers Squibb, undertook to donate the first year's supply of the drug free of charge.

What the future holds is still uncertain. Sleeping sickness was almost eradicated in the 1960s, but war and associated population movements caused a resurgence of the disease, which still continues. Tsetse flies are not prolific breeders like the mosquitoes that transmit malaria and insect control measures combined with effective treatment to break the cycle of transmission could succeed if the political will exists in endemic areas and drug resistance does not intervene. It is a hope that millions of Africans would endorse.

Malaria

Ask any specialist in the field of tropical medicine to list their priorities for disease control and malaria would nearly always come top of the list. It was ever thus. Although strenuous efforts to eradicate the disease succeeded in Europe and other temperate regions of the world, it is still the most common cause of fever throughout the tropics and one of the commonest causes of death in young infants in Africa. The economic impact on productivity and development in endemic areas continues to be profound (38). Treatment alone is not the answer, but effective drugs remains crucial to the fight against malaria. Despite the availability of a sovereign remedy in the form of cinchona bark (quinine) since the seventeenth century (see p. 31f), new treatments are still urgently needed.

Alternatives to quinine have been actively sought since at least 1880 when the causative parasite was first recognized in the blood of a young soldier by Alphonse Laveran, a French army surgeon working in Algeria. Although quinine was plainly effective when correctly used, it was extremely bitter, was prone to unpleasant side effects and, most important of all, demand exceeded supply. Progress was at first slow; the chemical structure had not been completely elucidated and synthesis was out of the question. Attempts to find new antimalarial agents were restricted to the production of simple salts and esters of quinine and related alkaloids, or trying to exploit Ehrlich's observations of the selective susceptibility of malaria parasites to azo dyes (see p. 53). During the First World War difficulty in maintaining sufficient quinine for troops fighting in malarious areas of the Balkans and elsewhere were experienced by both the German and Allied armies. The bulk of supplies of quinine came from Dutch plantations in Java (see p. 39) and much of it was required for the protection of those working in the extensive European colonies (39).

Numerous remedies offering a speedy and effective cure of, or protection from malaria were being peddled in the 1920s, but none of them worked. Italy, where around a quarter of a million cases of malaria were reported each year with thousands of deaths (40), was a particularly rich marketplace for such nostrums. Two of the most popular were: 'Esanofele' pills (also formulated as a syrup 'Esanofelina' for children), a herbal concoction containing arsenious acid and quinine sold by the same firm that produced the quinine-containing aperitif 'Ferrochina Bisleri'; and 'Smalarina', an alarming mixture of mercury, antimony, and iodine devised by Professor Guido Cremonese of Rome, which was claimed to induce immunity to the disease.* Both attracted some attention outside Italy, but did not find much favour among tropical experts. Smalarina in particular was generally regarded as having absolutely no beneficial effect (41). Indeed, *Tropical Disease Bulletin*, a journal devoted to independent abstracts of papers on tropical diseases, took to annotating its index entry to Smalarina with the parenthetical comment '(useless)'.

Breakthrough at Bayer

Once again, it was left to a team of scientists in Bayer's research laboratories in Elberfeld to come up with a substance that offered the first glimmer of real hope for a synthetic drug that might help to combat the scourge of malaria: a compound marketed in 1927 under the name of Plasmochin (Plasmoquine in English), but known later in Britain as pamaquine. Over 40 years later, Fritz Schönhöfer, who had originally synthesized the

---

* Cremonese had other unorthodox views. He claimed in a book published in 1930 'I raggi della vita fotografati' to have photographed vital rays emanating from the human body indicating that life is an electromagnetic phenomenon.

compound, left a personal account of the events that led up to the discovery of Plasmochin, dictated just 4 days before he died in February 1965 (42).

Surprisingly, since Germany had been forced to cede its overseas territories in Africa, none of the enthusiasm for tropical diseases had been lost in the Bayer laboratories in the years following the First World War and malaria remained a priority target. In 1919 a medically qualified pharmacologist, Werner Schulemann, the urbane son of a business family from Saxony who later became an amateur expert on Tibetan art and culture, had been engaged by Heinrich Hörlein for the pharmaceutical research laboratories in Elberfeld. Between 1921 and 1923 an enthusiastic team of young chemists—Fritz Schönhöfer, August Wingler, and Fritz Mietzsch—was recruited to Schulemann's staff. Against the prevailing background of civil unrest and rampant inflation, scientific work had been continuing as best it could, but it was not until the German currency was reformed in November 1923 that a semblance of sanity was restored and facilities for research were gradually re-established.

In 1924 work to synthesize potential antimalarial compounds began in earnest. Studies with methylene blue had provided useful clues about the effect of various modifications on antimalarial activity and this information was now used for the synthesis of new quinine derivatives. Since quinine itself is too complex for routine synthesis (Mother Nature is a much more accomplished and adventurous chemist than mere mortals!) the basic quinoline nucleus, which was assumed to be the business end of the quinine molecule (Fig. 7.2), was chosen for investigation.

Schulemann assigned to Schönhöfer the task of creating quinolines, using substituents synthesized by his colleague August Wingler. The division of labour proved fortunate for Schönhöfer, because the processes needed to produce the intermediates made Wingler and his assistant ill. Acting mainly on what was known about quinoline chemistry, but also partly on their own chemical instincts of what might work, the team quickly homed in on 8-aminoquinolines and started to pass a stream of compounds to Wilhelm Röhl in the chemotherapy laboratory for biological testing.

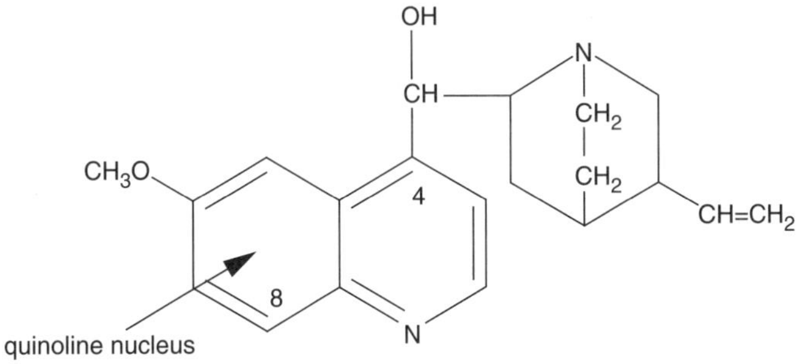

Fig. 7.2 The structure of quinine, showing the quinoline nucleus on which many synthetic antimalarial agents are based. Most are derivatives in which substituents are linked through an amino (NH_2) group introduced onto the carbon atom at position 4 (4-aminoquinolines) or the carbon at position 8 (8-aminoquinolines).

Röhl had cherished hopes of finding a cure for malaria ever since he joined Bayer before the Great War. In his annual research report for 1922 he reiterated his belief that a solution was possible and that with patience, he would succeed: 'Ich sehe darin eine der höchsten Aufgaben meines Lebens' ('I see it as one of the most important tasks of my life.') (43) A major stumbling block was the lack of a suitable animal model. In 1911 a Greek doctor, Phokion Kopanaris, at the Hamburg Tropical Institute had described the use of canaries infected with *Plasmodium praecox* (also called *Plasmodium relictum*) as a model for human malaria studies (44) and this seemed to provide a possible answer. Röhl's work was interrupted by the war and its aftermath, but in 1924 he adapted Kopanaris's technique* for his studies on malaria and satisfied himself of its relevance to the human disease. As pointed out by Ann Bishop who later maintained an aviary for the study of antimalarial agents at the Molteno Institute in Cambridge, hen canaries were used, since it was the cocks that were valued for their song and hens could be purchased cheaply (45).

Röhl found that Schönhöfer's 8-aminoquinolines (listed in the alphabetical series that Röhl used as A-prochin, Be-prochin, Ce-prochin, etc.), were several times more active than quinine and seemed to produce no serious side effects in his canary model. Most active of all was Be-prochin, which Schönhöfer had synthesized in December 1924. But bird malaria is one thing, human malaria another. In order to test the activity of the compounds in human beings, they were sent to Franz Sioli, the director of the psychiatric hospital in Düsseldorf, who carried out some preliminary toxicity tests and then used the compounds therapeutically in patients artificially infected with blood containing malaria parasites.

Infecting mental patients with malaria is not quite as unethical as it might seem at first sight. Treatment of neurosyphilis (then known as general paralysis of the insane) by inducing high fevers aimed at killing the spirochaetes, which were known to be temperature sensitive, was a standard procedure for many years. The technique had been popularized by the Austrian psychiatrist, Julius Wagner-Jauregg, who in 1917 introduced the practice of intravenous injections of blood containing malaria parasites of a species that causes a marked febrile response without killing the patient (46). The treatment was considered such an important advance that in 1927 Wagner-Jauregg was awarded the Nobel Prize in physiology or medicine. Fever therapy was largely rendered obsolete by penicillin, but survived in occasional use into the 1960s.

Wagner-Jauregg's method was widely used. It was introduced in Britain from about 1923 first at the Manor Hospital, Epsom, afterwards at the neighbouring Horton Mental Hospital where, in 1925, the Ministry of Health formally established the Horton Malaria Laboratory (later the Mott Clinic for Malaria Therapy and Malaria Reference Laboratory) with Colonel Sydney James as director (47). The laboratory provided blood and later infected mosquitoes for use in fever therapy at mental asylums around the country.

* According to the malariologist Leonard Bruce-Chwatt, Röhl adapted a method devised by the brothers Edmond and Etienne Sergent, Algerian-born French scientists working at the Institut Pasteur in Algiers (see Bruce-Chwatt, LJ. *Chemotherapy of Malaria* 2nd edn. WHO, Geneva, 1981, p.12). However, Dünschede (reference 43, pp. 62–63) who had access to the Bayer archives, states that Kopanaris was the source.

Around 10 per cent of all patients in mental hospitals in Britain were victims of tertiary syphilis when the malaria laboratory was set up, so there was a plentiful supply of patients.

The effectiveness of potential antimalarial compounds (including Plasmochin, a sample of which was obtained from Bayer in 1926) was tested at Horton Hospital in much the same way as Sioli had done in Germany, except that, after some disastrous early experiences with infected blood, malaria was induced through the bite of infected mosquitoes or by injecting sporozoites from the insect's salivary glands (48). The task of establishing a strain of malaria parasite that could be safely used,* and maintaining it in mosquitoes, was entrusted to James's assistant, Percy Shute. Shute, a baker by trade, had been invalided back to Britain in 1917 and served as a technician to Ronald Ross at the Manor Hospital. He was to become a world expert on malaria and deputy director of the Malaria Reference Laboratory, ably supported for 37 years by his assistant, Marjorie Maryon (49).

Franz Sioli had established by the summer of 1925 that Beprochin (Plasmochin) was more effective than quinine in restoring the normal temperature of patients once the treatment course for neurosyphilis was complete, although the drug was not entirely free from side effects. The effectiveness of Plasmochin in this trial is puzzling, since it later transpired that 8-aminoquinolines as a group have little curative effect on malaria parasites multiplying in the bloodstream, although they are quite effective in attacking the forms that invade the liver following the bite of an infected mosquito. Sioli followed the normal practice of inducing malaria by injecting blood from another patient with the disease, whereas in a natural infection sporozoites in the insect's salivary glands first invade liver cells and develop there before entering the bloodstream to multiply further and produce the characteristic fevers. By injecting patients with blood from other infected individuals, Sioli was bypassing the liver stage, which at that time had not been discovered.

Sioli's findings encouraged the view within Bayer (at that time concluding negotiations with five other German firms to form IG Farbenindustrie; see p. 66) that a synthetic antimalarial compound with great potential in the marketplace has been discovered. Unfortunately the method of synthesizing Plasmochin produced very low yields, but with the help of another Bayer chemist, Karl Schranz, Schönhöfer was soon able to increase the yield from 3 to 30 per cent. Plasmochin was patented in 1926 and the properties of the new drug were trumpeted in a special supplement of the *Archiv für Schiffs- und Tropenhygiene.*[†] When the drug was eventually listed in *The Extra Pharmacopoeia* in Britain in 1932, the editor William Martindale felt it necessary to add the petulant footnote 'England should have done it' (50)!

Peter Mühlens and his colleagues at the tropical institute in Hamburg carried out the first proper clinical trials of Plasmochin starting in 1925 (51). No doubt hoping to

---

* This was the so-called 'Madagascar' strain of *Plasmodium vivax* isolated from a lascar sailor who had been infected in Madagascar. The strain was established in mosquitoes and first transmitted to two female patients at Horton on 25 May 1925. (See reference 47).

† *Archiv für Schiffs- und Tropenhygiene* 1926; 30: beiheft 3.

re-establish their damaged reputation abroad by building on the success of Germanin in sleeping sickness with a breakthrough in malaria, Bayer moved quickly to arrange additional trials with America's United Fruit Company and with the British Empire's Indian Medical Service, for which Royal Army Medical Corps officer, John Sinton* and his colleagues were engaged in a comprehensive survey of malaria and its treatment.

The United Fruit Company was a natural choice for studies involving the United States. The firm dated back to a partnership formed in 1899 between Andrew Preston, founder of the Boston Fruit Company, his associate Lorenzo Dow Baker, a Cape Cod sailor trading in bananas, and Minor Keith an entrepreneur who, at great cost to human life (including those of his two brothers) built a railroad in Costa Rica and started a banana exporting business. The United Fruit Company rapidly expanded throughout what became disparagingly known as the 'banana republics' of the Caribbean and Latin America. The firm possessed great political power, which it was not slow to wield in its own commercial interest. It also brought much-needed jobs and economic development to the region and was regarded in the United States as a beacon of enlightened capitalism. Realizing that a healthy workforce was in his own business interests, Andrew Preston, the United Fruit Company president, built hospitals and championed research into prevalent tropical diseases. The Plasmochin study was carried out in 1925 by Wilhelm Cordes at the company's hospital in Cuba (named the Preston Hospital after Andrew Preston's death in 1924). Like Mühlens in Hamburg, Cordes found Plasmochin to be disappointing in the therapy of acute malaria (52) as did Sinton's 1927 trial, carried out with his colleague William Bird in India (53). The toxicity of Plasmochin also dampened any enthusiasm for the new drug.

Although these studies failed to confirm that Plasmochin was as effective as quinine in controlling malaria fevers, it was noted that the drug did have an effect, for reasons that were unclear at the time, in preventing relapse. Furthermore, microscopy revealed that it had the unexpected effect of eliminating the sexual forms of the parasite, which are responsible for continuing the life cycle in mosquitoes. Suggestions were made that Plasmochin might be suitable for the prevention of malaria, or be used in combination with quinine for the treatment of clinical attacks, but unacceptable toxicity militated against widespread acceptance of these ideas. Although Bayer put a combination product of Plasmochin and quinine sulphate on the market in 1930 with the trade name Chinoplasmin, it was not a great success. When the Malaria Commission of the League of Nations pronounced on the place of the drug in 1933, the sole purpose for which it was recommended was in eliminating the sexual forms (gametocytes) of the parasites in situations in which breaking the link of transmission to mosquitoes was the intention (54).

---

* Sinton, born in British Columbia, but raised in Ulster from where his parents came, was enthused to become a malariologist by the teachings of Ronald Ross at the Liverpool School of Tropical Medicine. He joined the Indian Medical Service as a soldier, but served in the civilian branch from 1921. He was award the Victoria Cross in 1916 for conspicuous bravery during the Mesopotamian campaign and has the distinction of being the only holder of that award also to be a Fellow of the Royal Society (see Porterfield JS. Sinton, John Alexander (1884–1956). *Oxford Dictionary of National Biography*, Oxford University Press, 2004 http://www.oxforddnb.com/view/article/61406).

By the end of the 1920s, changes were occurring in the chemotherapy team at Elberfeld. In March 1929, a few weeks before his 48th birthday, Wilhelm Röhl died from a staphylococcal septicaemia as a complication of a carbuncle that had developed on his neck. Meanwhile, in April 1928 August Wingler had moved to New York to promote Bayer's interests with the Winthrop Chemical Company, the prescription drug arm of the Sterling Drug Company (see p. 257). At the end of the First World War, when the assets of the American Bayer Company, were seized and put up for auction by the office of the Alien Property Custodian in the United States, the stock was bought by Sterling, who thereby acquired the rights to Bayer's best-seller, aspirin* However, Sterling had great difficulty in manufacturing the drug and had to go cap in hand to Bayer to seek help. As a price of the assistance, Bayer concluded a cartel agreement with the Winthrop Chemical Company, giving them renewed access to the American market for their drugs.

Wingler's departure had already been anticipated, by the recruitment to Schulemann's group in 1927 of Hans Mauss. Together with Fritz Mietzsch, he was set the task of synthesizing acridine derivatives as possible antimalarial compounds. These yellow dyes were already being widely used as topical antibacterial agents (see p. 63) and were the subject of much research at the time. Indeed, some of the compounds that Mauss and Mietzsch produced were passed on to Gerhard Domagk—also newly recruited in 1927—for testing for antibacterial activity. But it was their structural similarity to quinolones that suggested that they might offer a fruitful avenue of investigation in the antimalarial field. Applying the same chemistry that had been successful with Plasmochin, but attaching the substituent to an amino group on the carbon opposite to the nitrogen atom rather than to the adjacent ring, the chemists produced in 1930 a substance with the laboratory designation Erion, which was later marketed under the name Atebrin (Fig. 7.3). Biological testing for antimalarial activity was carried out by Walter Kikuth, who had been appointed to replace Wilhelm Röhl in October 1929. Kikuth was a doctor who had established a reputation as a researcher while working with Bernhard Nocht at the Hamburg Tropical Institute, and his appointment helped to cement ties with one of Europe's premier tropical institutes.

Kikuth, installed in a new purpose-built chemotherapy laboratory, rejected Röhl's canary model in favour of one in which reisfinken (Java sparrows) were infected with a blood protozoon of birds called *Halteridium* (now *Haemoproteus*), in which a sexual phase similar to that which occurs in human malaria parasites had been discovered in 1897 by a Canadian medical student, William MacCallum, a member of the first intake to the Johns Hopkins Medical School in Baltimore.[†] Kikuth reasoned that *Halteridium* infection of Java sparrows was more representative of human malaria than Röhl's canary

---

[*] During the takeover of Eastman-Kodak (which then owned Sterling-Winthrop), by SmithKline Beecham in 1994 (see footnote, p. 257), Bayer acquired the Sterling Health business and recovered the rights to the trade name 'Aspirin' which is still used in some countries.

[†] Ronald Ross, who discovered and demonstrated the transmission of malaria by mosquitoes in the same year acknowledged the contribution of MacCallum in his Nobel lecture in 1902.

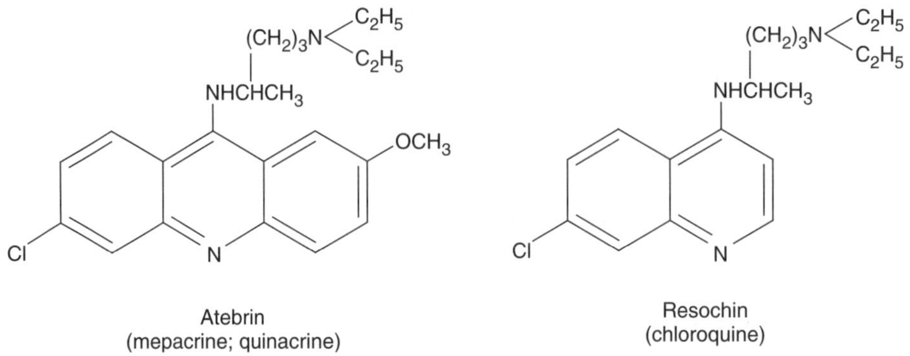

Fig. 7.3 The structures of Atebrin (later known as mepacrine or quinacrine) and Resochin (chloroquine).

model, since it could distinguish between the effect of quinine on parasites multiplying in the bloodstream and that of Plasmochin, which affected the sexual stages. The period of development in the liver, which Plasmochin also affects, was not recognized at that time, although Colonel James at Horton had proposed that the drug acted on some unspecified pre-erythrocytic phase of development initiated by the sporozoites injected by mosquitoes carrying malaria parasites. The involvement of the liver was not proven until experiments at the London School of Hygiene and Tropical Medicine by Henry Shortt and Percy Garnham put the matter beyond doubt in 1948 (55).

In Kikuth's reisfink model, Atebrin had a clear effect on developing parasites multiplying in the bloodstream that was better than that of quinine. Sioli again confirmed the effect in patients receiving malaria therapy for tertiary syphilis, but Kikuth was taking no chances and had already arranged for Franz Peter in the malaria research station in Gurbanesti, Romania and his former colleague Peter Mühlens in Hamburg to test the new compound in naturally acquired malaria. This time the drug was clearly shown to work. It also seemed to be relatively free from serious side effects. Once again independent studies were quickly initiated in Central America and British India. Lionel Napier, in collaboration with Birajmohan Das Gupta, tested Atebrin at the Calcutta School of Tropical Medicine in 1932 with good results (56). In the same year Richard Green, a Liverpool-trained Australian research officer working at the Institute for Medical Research in Kuala Lumpur, treated 50 patients with the new drug and found it to be at least as good as quinine (57). These studies encouraged the use of Atebrin in the control of a particularly severe malaria epidemic which occurred in Ceylon—the original Serendip—in 1934–35 and this provided further convincing evidence of its value (58).

There was no doubt about the effectiveness of Atebrin in the treatment of malaria, though there were reservations as to its safety, especially when used for prolonged periods as a prophylactic. Its main drawback was that it imparted a yellow colour to the skin and eyes, an effect that fuelled suspicion that it might cause liver damage leading to jaundice. Schulemann's team embarked on a project to produce a derivative of Atebrin that retained its activity, but lacked its shortcomings. In April 1928 the antimalarial research group had been strengthened by the addition of Hans Andersag, who had studied under Hans Fischer at Munich's Technische Hochschule (Technical University). Together with another of Fischer's former students, Stefan Breitner, who had just joined the project, a compound was synthesized in 1934 that seemed to have the right credentials. The molecule was identical to that of Atebrin, except that a methoxy-substituted benzene ring had been removed (Fig. 7.3). The new compound, which was given the name Resochin, was very similar in structure to Plasmochin, but crucially, the side chain was attached to carbon atom number 4 of the quinolone ring, making it a 4-aminoquinoline (see Fig. 7.2). This apparently simple change altered the activity, which was now directed against the parasites in the bloodstream that were responsible for acute malaria. Resochin was passed to Sioli for testing in patients undergoing malaria therapy, but he found it to be somewhat more toxic than Atebrin. In 1936, a methylated version of Resochin, called Sontochin, was also found to exhibit excellent activity. This time Sioli gave the drug the all clear.

With uncharacteristic tardiness, patent applications on Resochin and Sontochin were not submitted until 1937, and not granted until 1939. The first clinical trials in naturally acquired malaria by Walter Menk and Werner Mohr at the Hamburg Tropical Institute were started only towards the end of 1938 (59). Thus, at the start of the Second World War, evaluation of the two compounds was still far from complete.

The spoils of war

The interwar years. The British and American responses to the developments in continental Europe between the wars were lacklustre. German success in developing drugs useful in the treatment of tropical diseases like sleeping sickness and malaria had dented British pride in the 1920s. In 1927 the Medical Research Council in partnership with the Department of Scientific and Industrial Research set up a Chemotherapy Committee under the chairmanship of Henry Dale. The intention was to coordinate academic and commercial research into drugs for diseases that were hindering the exploitation of Britain's imperial territories. Facilities for the biological testing of potential antimalarial compounds were established at the Molteno Institute of Parasitology in Cambridge, which was already active in protozoal research under its Director George Nuttall, and the Department of Protozoology at the London School of Hygiene and Tropical Medicine in its splendid new building in Keppel Street, completed in 1929. Warrington Yorke was a founder member of the Committee and took the opportunity to seek funds for his own research in Liverpool. From 1934, studentships were also provided, funded by ICI, for studies in the laboratories of Robert Robinson in Oxford and William Kermack in Edinburgh.*

It was all in vain. Nothing of any value came of the venture, which, judging from the Chemotherapy Committee minutes held in the National Institute for Medical Research

---

* Kermack was blinded in a laboratory accident in 1924 and nearly gave up research. The funding for antimalarial research by ICI continued until the end of the Second World War. I am grateful to William C Hutchison for this information. He was a PhD student working under Kermack in Edinburgh from autumn 1943 and a beneficiary of one of ICI's grants.

archives, was characterized by distrust of commercial motives, concerns about academic freedom and squabbles over patent rights should anything useful emerge. By 1935, as the minutes reveal, chemotherapeutic research was 'quite inadequate, and not in proportion to the obligations of the country as a great Colonial power' (39).

In America the developments in Germany seem to have been viewed with detachment. Although Jacobs and Heidelberger at Rockefeller were pursuing a programme of research into potential chemotherapeutic agents, the studies focused mainly on cinchona alkaloids with the aim of finding an antibacterial agent of the optochin type (see p. 64). The Rockefeller team also investigated arsenicals and were successful in the invention of tryparsamide (see p. 278), but there seems to have been little interest in malaria. If any other research into antiprotozoal drugs was being pursued in the United States in the 1920s and 1930s, it appears to have been no more productive than the British efforts.

All this was to change with the outbreak of war in Europe in 1939.

Atebrin for the Allied war effort. Mindful of the shortages of quinine during the First World War, and aware that supplies of Atebrin and Plasmoquine would be cut-off if the country went to war with Germany, British drug companies, including Burroughs Wellcome, May and Baker, Boots, and ICI were being encouraged as early as 1937 to provide independent supplies of these and other essential products. Production of the anti-malarial compounds was not an easy task since the details of the methods of synthesis had been left vague in the patent literature. Fortunately, suitable manufacturing processes were quickly worked out on both sides of the Atlantic. In Britain it was scientists at ICI that came up with the goods and production started in 1939 at their new laboratories at Blackley, North Manchester.

ICI's Blackley site had belonged at the turn of the nineteenth century to the exotically named Angel Raphael Louis Delaunay, a French dye manufacturer whose most successful product was turkey red. The factory was bought in the mid-1860s by an ambitious young German chemist, Ivan Levenstein, who greatly expanded Delaunay's operations. A few years after Levenstein's death the firm merged with British Dyes Ltd of Huddersfield, to form the British Dyestuffs Corporation. In 1926, three other firms, Nobel Industries, Brunner, Mond* of Winnington, Cheshire, and its affiliate United Alkali, joined forces to form the Dyestuffs Division of Imperial Chemical Industries. By 1936 ICI was taking an increasing interest in pharmaceuticals, and new laboratories were built at Blackley and brought into use in 1938 (60).

---

* Formed in 1873 by John Brunner and the German chemist Ludwig Mond. It was originally a producer of soda ash and returned to its roots as an independent company in 1991. In 1950 ICI bought Alderley Park in Cheshire, which formerly belonged to Brunner, Mond, and in 1957 moved their research to this larger and more congenial location. ICI pharmaceuticals, which was established during the Second World War (see footnote p. 196), demerged from the main business in 1993 with the formation of a wholly owned subsidiary, Zeneca (since 1999 AstraZeneca)

In the first year of the manufacture of Atebrin at Blackley, 22 lb (about 10 kg) were produced; this grew to 12,500 lb (5675 kg; enough for 50 million tablets) by 1942, and to more than 100,000 lb (45,400 kg) by 1943. Plasmoquine (pamaquine) was also manufactured at Blackley, achieving production sufficient for 32 million tablets by 1942 (61). Similar success followed in the United States after American chemists worked out a method of synthesizing the drug in 1941. By the time antimalarials were needed for the Far East campaign, adequate supplies were available. However, there was a dearth of information on the way the drug was handled by the body and optimal regimens for prophylaxis had not been established. Consequently, in the first 2 years of the war in the Far East cinchona alkaloids, which were in short supply after the fall of Java, were still used. Because of the limited availability of quinine, totaquine (a mixture of the active alkaloids of cinchona bark) was often used and supplies were reserved mainly for treatment rather than prophylaxis.

The effectiveness of Atebrin (from 1941 called mepacrine in Britain; known as quinacrine in the United States and marketed as Atabrine in that country) in the prevention of malaria was established in classic studies carried out in tests on volunteer soldiers in Cairns, Northern Queensland, Australia by a team led by Neil Hamilton Fairley (62). The investigation did not get off to an auspicious start. In late 1942, Fairley, then director of medicine for the Australian Army, travelled to England with Adrian Albert, a lecturer in organic chemistry from the University of Sydney who had been given a Commonwealth Research Scholarship to fund work on drugs essential to the war effort. Their task was to make representations in Britain over the urgent need for antimalarials in the Far East. The advice they got was that certain sulphonamides might be of use and on their return to Australia valuable time was wasted showing that these compounds had no worthwhile activity in the prevention or treatment of malaria. It was not until September 1943 that experiments with Atebrin began. By early 1944, the drug was shown to be highly effective in suppressing infection with the two types of malaria most prevalent in the Far East, *Plasmodium falciparum* and *Plasmodium vivax*. In order to test whether the results were likely to be valid under the stressful conditions of battle, Fairley came up with a tough and imaginative ordeal for the soldier volunteers. The regimen has been vividly described by the renowned virologist Frank Fenner, who served with the Australian Army Medical Corps in New Guinea, and the medical entomologist and historian of the Australian war effort against malaria, Tony Sweeney:

> Subjects on 100 mg of atebrin a day were infected using large numbers of mosquitoes and then subject to severe exercises—chopping wood all day for five days in tropical heat, swimming upstream until they sank with fatigue, being marched over hills at as fast a pace as possible by a specially trained sergeant-major—"without even the chance for a nice lie-down in hospital"—but they did not get clinical malaria. Then to simulate conditions of aircrew operating in unpressurised aircraft at high altitudes; dressed only in boots and trousers, they were packed into a refrigerated room at –9°C for an hour, or put into a decompression chamber for two hours each day at the equivalents of 15,000 and then 18,000 feet. Although "somewhat battered" from these experiences, not one of them suffered from malaria (63).

Elsewhere, pharmacological studies on Atebrin were underway in the United States, masterminded by James Shannon at the Goldwater Memorial Hospital, New York; at an American unit in Brisbane, Australia; and at the Army Malaria Research Unit in Oxford, where student volunteers were recruited. Neil Hamilton Fairley presented the results of the experiments at Cairns at a conference in Atherton, Queensland in June 1944, and in September that year instructions were issued under the authority of General Thomas Blamey, commander-in-chief of the Allied Land Forces in the south-west Pacific area, that troops in malarious areas should take a tablet of Atebrin daily as a matter of military discipline. Disciplinary action was taken against officers who did not adequately enforce the order. Administration of the daily tablet was closely supervised leading to some resentment in the ranks (64). The inevitable yellowing of the skin and eyes also caused some disquiet, and some soldiers were startled to discover that their urine fluoresced in the moonlight.

It was all worthwhile. Serious side effects appear to have been minimal and the incidence of malaria among Australian troops in the south-west Pacific fell from ~750 per 1000 men per year in 1943 to ~25 per 1000 per year by early 1945. American forces benefited by similar falls in incidence (65). In the words of Leonard Bruce-Chwatt 'There is no exaggeration in saying that this probably changed the course of modern history' (66).

Paludrine: a new antimalarial. Back in England, scientists at ICI were turning their attention to finding new antimalarial drugs. In 1941, British pharmaceutical firms had agreed to pool their expertise for the duration of the war in a consortium called the Therapeutic Research Corporation, but ICI did not join the corporation until Imperial Chemicals (Pharmaceuticals) was formed during 1942. The Therapeutic Research Corporation was chiefly concerned with penicillin, sulphonamides, and potential antituberculosis compounds (67), and declined to become involved in antimalarials. Encouraged by Warrington Yorke before his untimely death in 1943, and by Robert Robinson, who had long been a senior consultant to the firm, ICI took up the challenge by offering to use its testing facilities at Blackley for the evaluation of potential antimalarial drugs. The intention was to include substances provided by the National Institute for Medical Research and any commercial source that cared to submit samples, but drug companies were wary of the scheme and in the event most test compounds originated in ICI's own laboratories. From late 1943, two chemists in the Blackley laboratories, Frank Rose and Francis Curd, supplied their colleague Garnet Davey, a Cambridge trained parasitologist who had joined ICI in 1942, with material for biological testing. Preliminary testing was against *Plasmodium gallinaceum* infection in chickens, which had by now become the favoured model.

The starting point for the investigation was the feeble antimalarial activity of certain sulphonamide derivatives, such as sulphadimidine, that featured a pyrimidine group. Extensive manipulation of the molecule eventually yielded two pyrimidine-containing compounds, designated M2666 and M3349, which exhibited reasonably good activity in birds. Preliminary trials carried out at the Liverpool School of Tropical Medicine showed compound 3349 to have promise in the treatment of acute malaria, but did not prevent subsequent relapse.

By the summer of 1944, the ICI scientists had started to synthesize a series of compounds in which the pyrimidine ring had been opened to create a linear rather than a cyclic molecule. One of these substances (technically called biguanides) designated M4430, showed striking activity in chicken malaria; moreover, it prevented the birds from developing the infection suggesting that it might be of value as a prophylactic drug—a major aim of the antimalarial programme. Clinical trials of M4430 in Liverpool were encouraging, but in November 1944 a closely related biguanide, M4888, had been synthesized and Garnet Davey was able to report in February 1945 on its superior activity in chickens. With commendable speed, M4888, now called Paludrine (generic name proguanil; chlorguanide in the United States) was being tested as a chemoprophylactic agent in Fairley's unit in Cairns by April 1945, while Alfred Adams and Brian Maegraith undertook clinical studies at the Liverpool School. It soon became clear that Paludrine possessed the valuable property, unique among antimalarial drugs at that time, of safely and effectively preventing the development of malaria following the bite of infected mosquitoes.

Paludrine was hailed as another triumph for chemical expertise, but Lady Luck, as always mischievously seeking to undermine human pride, had again been at work. When the ICI scientists described their painstakingly logical approach to the discovery of Paludrine in a special issue of *Annals of Tropical Medicine and Parasitology* nominated as *The Warrington Yorke Memorial Number* in 1945, they explained how they had sought a stepwise simplification of the structures of compounds M2666 and M3349 to determine at which point antiparasitic activity disappeared. They came to the conclusion that the cyclic pyrimidine structure was unnecessary and proposed that it should be modified. 'If the function of the pyrimidine ring was solely to provide two tertiary nitrogen atoms suitably orientated...it might be considered inessential and cyclic systems could be dispensed with' (68). What they had not reckoned with was that the open-ring biguanides that had apparently proven the soundness of their approach actually exhibited very limited antimalarial activity. In 1947 Frank Hawking at the National Institute for Medical Research presented evidence leading him to the conclusion that 'probably paludrine does not in itself possess antimalarial activity, but that it is converted by the body into something which is active' (69). The truth was later confirmed by the ICI scientists (70): the straight chain biguanide structure of Paludrine, once absorbed into the bloodstream, was enzymically turned back into a cyclic derivative, cycloguanil, which was responsible for most of the antimalarial activity.

The ICI team at Blackley went on to produce another drug that was to prove useful in the tropics. In 1948, shortly before Francis Curd died in a railway accident in November that year, they synthesized a quinoline derivative, later given the name Antrycide, which was active against trypanosomes (71). It turned out to be too toxic for human use, but was a useful addition to the veterinary pharmacopoeia.

The saga of chloroquine. Before the German army unceremoniously occupied Tunisia in November 1942 to try to stem the Anglo-American advance in North Africa, the country was under French control as part of its overseas Empire. The French drug firm, Specia, which had a licensing agreement with IG Farben covering French territories, were undertaking a trial of Bayer's Sontochin. The trial was led by Philippe-Jean Decourt, a tropical diseases expert based at the Hôpital Ernest Conseil in Tunis, who had considerable experience of malaria in North Africa and acted as a medical consultant for Specia. When he returned to France in September 1942, Decourt handed over the trial to Jean Schneider, another French doctor who had recently joined him at the hospital.

On 7 May 1943, the British First Army entered Tunis. Within a week all the German and Italian forces in Tunisia had surrendered to the American and British commanders, marking the end of the North African campaign. Schneider, who had been obtaining impressive results with Sontochin, offered to disclose his findings to the Allies and on 25 May 1943 he was flown in an American plane to Algiers, where he handed over 5000 tablets of Sontochin and all his clinical data to Colonel Loren D. Moore, commander of the local malaria control detachment of the US army. The unexpected prize was sent to the US army surgeon general in Washington on 8 July 1943 and passed on to William Mansfield Clark, chairman of the Division of Chemistry and Chemical Technology of the National Research Council.

By the time Sontochin reached the United States, research on new antimalarial agents was finally in full swing. In 1939, the chemist Lyndon Small—better known for his work on drug addition—had started a project aimed at the synthesis of new antimalarial drugs at the National Institute of Health. When America entered the war in late 1941 the American effort was stepped up through a programme organized by the Committee on Medical Research of the Office of Scientific Research and Development. An unprecedented scientific undertaking involving cooperation between government agencies, universities, and commercial organizations, including all the big drug firms, set about synthesizing and screening over 14,000 compounds for antimalarial activity. A record of this prodigious effort, which was coordinated by Frederick Wiselogle in the Department of Chemistry at Johns Hopkins University, is preserved in two large volumes published when the war had ended (72). Throughout the programme, Fairley's group in Australia and the Medical Research Council in Britain were kept fully briefed on progress and received in return reports of developments in each country. When Henry Dale who, as chairman of the Scientific Advisory Committee to the War Cabinet, was trying to set up a similar co-operative venture among British drug firms in early 1943, he sought details of the operation of the American survey from Mansfield Clark. The British scheme had been beset with arguments over patent rights, whereas it was clear from Mansfield Clark's reply that the Americans had adopted a much more pragmatic view. In a letter dated 17 April 1943 to Edward Mellanby, secretary of the Medical Research Council, Dale snootily observed:

> The Americans are always more casual about matters of that kind than we are. I suppose that they take the view that the matter of paramount importance is to get better antimalarials, and that, if somebody is incidentally helped to make a fortune out of it, with the help of public expenditure, that does not matter. I think such an attitude would not be in violent disharmony with American standards of public life in general.*

---

* The letter is among the Henry Hallett Dale papers held in the Royal Society library.

Among the compounds submitted to the American co-operative survey team was one synthesized by chemists at the Winthrop laboratories and given the Survey Number SN-183; no special attention had been paid to this substance at the time, though it had been submitted to the Rockefeller Institute in 1941 for testing against *Plasmodium cathemerium* in canaries and found to be active. When Walter Jacobs' group at the Rockefeller Institute elucidated the structure of Sontochin, it was realized that it was the same as that of SN-183. Plainly an opportunity had been missed. To make matters worse, it transpired that Winthrop already held information on Sontochin and various related compounds, all 4-aminoquinolines, which they had received as early as 1939 from Bayer under the terms of their mutual agreement (see p. 291), and patented in the United States in 1941. None of the other 4-aminoquinolines had been synthesized in the United States and Winthrop was now requested to investigate these compounds further. Sufficient quantities were quickly produced for screening tests and by March 1944 it emerged that Sontochin (now renumbered SN-6911) and a molecule given the number SN-7618 displayed excellent antimalarial activity in neurosyphilis patients receiving malaria therapy.

Without further delay, these compounds were sent to Hamilton Fairley's team in Australia and trials were carried out in soldier volunteers at Cairns between July and October 1944 (73). By the autumn of 1944, when Fairley flew to Washington to discuss antimalarials with James Shannon and Kennerly Marshall,* it was clear that SN-7618 stood out in terms of its favourable activity and lack of toxicity. SN-7618 was given the non-proprietary name chloroquine in November 1945 and Harry Most and his colleagues published the first successful clinical trial results in naturally acquired malaria caused by *Plasmodium vivax* in July 1946 (74). Resochin had been rediscovered.

The strange story of chloroquine, from which many of the above facts have been gleaned, was vividly described by the eminent malariologist Robert Coatney in his presidential address to the American Society of Tropical Medicine in Atlanta in November 1961 (75). It is a remarkable tale, which well illustrates the uncertain course that drug discovery and development sometimes takes. Chloroquine, which under the name Resochin had been rejected by its inventors became the drug of choice for the prevention and treatment of malaria before widespread resistance intervened in the 1960s. In 1945, when Allied forces occupied Germany, Walter Kikuth handed over information on Resochin and Sontochin to American and British intelligence teams, but the data—and Kikuth himself—strongly favoured Sontochin. But for the fortunate events that had earlier taken place in America, chloroquine could so easily have been overlooked.

---

* Kennerly Marshall, Professor of Pharmacology and Therapeutics at Johns Hopkins Medical School, was much involved with the antimalarial survey. He had already contributed to the war effort through his role in the development of sulfaguanidine (see p. 75).

Late harvest

The American co-operative survey of antimalarial drugs turned up a number of new leads that were to bear fruit in useful compounds. A derivative of chloroquine developed at Parke, Davis, amodiaquine, was marketed soon after the end of the war and was widely used until it was found to be occasionally responsible for a fatal agranulocytosis in persons who had taken the drug prophylactically. Other 4-aminoquinolines closely related to amodiaquine appeared elsewhere, but made little impact: cycloquine (Halochin) was developed in the former Soviet Union; amopyroquine (Propoquine) was manufactured in France and mainly used in Francophone countries.

Primaquine. The search for safer and more effective 8-aminoquinolines to replace pamaquine (Plasmochin) had also continued. Even before the war Fourneau in France had synthesized a variant molecule, Rhodoquine (Fourneau 710) that was used chiefly in French territories as a substitute for pamaquine (Plasmochin), and Schönhöfer himself had developed a derivative of Plasmochin, which was briefly marketed in 1938 as Certuna (originally called Cilional).* In the former USSR a home-grown version, quinocide, was often used, but it proved to be even more toxic than pamaquine. The American wartime survey yielded one promising lead, pentaquine, and the Malaria Study Section of the National Institutes of Health, which succeeded it for a time after the war, generated dozens of other molecules of the 8-aminoquinoline type synthesized by a team at Columbia University led by the organic chemist Robert C Elderfield (76). The best of these compounds turned out to be primaquine, synthesized in 1945 by Elderfield's group. Elderfield, who had started his career with Walter Jacobs at the Rockefeller Institute, served as a regional director of the Panel on Synthesis during the wartime antimalarial survey. The molecules that he produced were sent for animal testing to Leon H Schmidt of the Christ Hospital Institute, Cincinnati, Ohio, who used primates as a model in order to more closely mimic human malaria.

The proving of primaquine was carried out to the background of the Korean War in 1950–53 (77). Malaria was common in the Korean campaign and although chloroquine was very effective in preventing infection and in treating acute attacks, troops often experienced relapses on their return to the United States. Shortt and Garnham in England had by now established the existence of the cycle of development of malaria parasites in the liver (see p. 292) and it was these parasites, unaffected by chloroquine, mepacrine, or quinine, but susceptible to 8-aminoquinolines like primaquine, that were responsible for recrudescence of fevers up to 2 years after the initial exposure. It was at first thought that there was an ongoing recycling of parasites within liver cells during this latent period, but it was later shown that some parasites entered a dormant (so-called 'hypnozoite') phase in the liver. These hypnozoites are absent in malaria caused by *Plasmodium falciparum*, but regularly occur with the species prevalent in Korea, *Plasmodium vivax*.

---

* Another Plasmochin analogue called Uprochin (also known as Antiplasmin), was also developed by Bayer around the same time. See Dünschede, reference 5, p. 80.

Preparatory trials of primaquine were carried out in prisoner 'volunteers', chiefly at Stateville Penitentiary, just North of Joliet, Illinois, under the direction of Alf S. Alving, Professor of Medicine at the University of Chicago (78), and at the Federal Penitentiary in Atlanta, Georgia under the guidance of Robert Coatney of the United States Public Health Service. Malaria research units had been established at both prisons as early as 1944 and trials of primaquine were underway at Stateville by 1948. Although such experimentation on human guinea pigs is now rightly condemned as an affront to human dignity, it was widely condoned at the time. Even after revelations about human experimentation at the Nuremberg war trials, American practices were defended on the grounds that the prisoners had given their consent. It was not until 1976 that the practice was finally outlawed in the United States (79).

Pyrimethamine. Meanwhile, at the Wellcome laboratories in Tuckahoe, New York, George Hitchings and his colleagues were investigating diaminopyrimidines—analogues of the crucial enzyme, dihydrofolate reductase—for antibacterial, antimalarial, and anticancer activity (see p. 253). The decision to include antimalarial properties into the study programme was done at the suggestion of a British member of the team, Peter Russell, who in 1947 had spotted the similarity of ICI's proguanil (Paludrine) to the diaminopyrimidines (80). The structural analogy between proguanil and the diaminopyrimidines was noticed before the discovery was made that proguanil is converted in the body to a heterocyclic compound resembling a diaminopyrimidine, and was a particularly astute observation.

From 1948, the Wellcome scientists synthesized hundreds of diaminopyrimidines The antimalarial activity of more than 150 of them was described in a paper published in 1951 (81). Screening tests, in chicks infected with *Plasmodium gallinaceum* and mice infected with *Plasmodium berghei*, were carried out by Len Goodwin and Ian Rollo in the Wellcome laboratories in London. Selected compounds were also tested on monkeys infected with *Plasmodium cynomolgi*, which is closely related to the human parasite, *Plasmodium vivax*. The most potent substance found in this extensive study was one with the laboratory number 50–63—pyrimethamine—later marketed as Daraprim. Goodwin was soon testing the ability of Daraprim to protect against malaria in volunteers, and looked no further than himself for the first candidate:

> From January to June, 1951, I was working in Africa, and therefore had the opportunity of making personal trials with daraprim. The aims of the trial were (a) to take the drug at a higher dose level higher than was necessary for the suppression of malaria and watch carefully for any toxic effects, and (b) to ensure that I came into contact with infected mosquitoes (82).

Just to make sure (it was the dry season in Kenya and although he took every opportunity to be bitten he could not be absolutely certain that he had been naturally exposed) Goodwin arranged to be infected with *Plasmodium falciparum* sporozoites from infected mosquitoes obtained from the ICI research station conveniently but mystifyingly situated in Nairobi gaol. Goodwin continued to take Daraprim on his return to London until February 1952. Blood tests at University College Hospital carried out by the eminent haematologist Monty Maizels indicated that he had suffered no ill effects and he even submitted himself to a sternal puncture to confirm that there were no abnormalities of the bone marrow. A group of 13 other volunteers in England were then given the drug twice a week for 3 months and similarly experienced no serious side effects.

While Len Goodwin was embarking on his one-man trial, Munro Archibald of the Nigerian Medical Department's malaria service was testing Daraprim in 5–10-year-old children from schools in and around Lagos (83). Between August and November 1951, Ian McGregor and Dean Smith at the Medical Research Council's Field Research Station at Fajara in the Gambia undertook a similar trial in infants, children, and adults (84). Both studies gave the drug a clean bill of health and Daraprim was soon being extensively used for the treatment and prophylaxis of malaria.

In the belief that sulphonamides would interact synergically with Daraprim—a belief supported by experiments by Ian Rollo in chick malaria (85) and later by trials in human malaria in the Gambia (86)—combination products with the long-acting sulphonamide, sulfadoxine (Fansidar; launched in 1971 by Hoffmann-La Roche, the company that had developed sulfadoxine), and dapsone (Maloprim) were later introduced, but occasional serious side effects have limited the use of these formulations, especially for antimalarial prophylaxis. From the mid 1950s, the combination of pyrimethamine with sulphonamides (usually sulphadiazine) was introduced for the treatment of another protozoal disease, toxoplasmosis, following on work started in 1952 by the malariologist Don Eyles and his colleagues in the United States Public Health service Laboratory of Tropical Diseases at Memphis Tennessee (87).

Mefloquine and halofantrine. When America became embroiled in Vietnam, malaria was once more a major problem. From March 1965 when the first American combat troops arrived in the country, until they left almost exactly 8 years later, well over a million sick days were lost to malaria among the army and naval forces, with 124 deaths attributable to the disease, despite the availability of chloroquine and other drugs (88). In Vietnam, unlike Korea where *Plasmodium vivax* was the prevalent type, the much more lethal *Plasmodium falciparum* was common. Moreover, in Vietnam there was another problem: multidrug resistant strains of the parasites began to turn up (see p. 400–1), threatening the effectiveness of the chloroquine prophylaxis policy.

With impeccable timing, the United States Army Medical Research and Development Command commenced a programme aimed at discovering new antimalarial agents in 1963. The task was given to the Walter Reed Army Institute of Medical Research in Washington DC, which embarked on a project that dwarfed even the wartime survey in its extent. As might be expected, research activity and the necessary government funding to underpin it reached a peak during the Vietnam War, but it was not until the conflict ended in 1973 that a suitable candidate, mefloquine, emerged. Mefloquine belongs to a group of compounds known as the quinoline methanols. Analogous structures had been investigated after the end of the Second World War. They were found to exhibit high antimalarial activity, but were rejected after phototoxic side effects were found in experiments in prisoner volunteers at Stateville Penitentiary. By 1975, tests, again conducted at Stateville, indicated that mefloquine was safe and effective in the treatment of malaria (89). Worryingly, some of the inmates were infected with multiresistant strains of *Plasmodium falciparum* in this study, but fortunately, the experimental treatment was successful. After its discovery by the Walter Reed scientists, mefloquine was jointly developed by Michel Fernex's group at Hofmann-La Roche in Basel and the World Health Organization's Special Programme for Research and Training in Tropical Diseases—a collaborative initiative between the United Nations Children's Fund, the United Nations Development Programme, the World Bank, and the World Health Organization which had been established in 1975 to facilitate research in neglected tropical diseases.* Roche launched the drug alone under the trade name Lariam, and in a formulation with Fansidar (Fansimef) in 1985. It immediately attracted controversy because of the occurrence of neuropsychiatric side effects, ranging from mild sleep disorders to hallucinations and paranoia, in some people taking the drug as an antimalarial prophylactic.

Hard on the heels of mefloquine came halofantrine, another Walter Reed product developed by Craig Canfield and his colleagues and initially tested on United States Army personnel alarmingly—as in the mefloquine trial in Stateville—infected with multiresistant *Plasmodium falciparum* (90). The drug was later marketed as Halfan by SmithKline Beecham (now Glaxo SmithKline). Its progress has been as problematic as that of mefloquine: it suffers from the disadvantage of variable absorption when taken by mouth and has been associated with occasional, but serious problems of cardiotoxicity.

Antibacterial agents. Soon after the tetracyclines were established in therapeutic practice it was discovered that these antibiotics exerted some effect on malarial parasites, but it was not until the 1970s with the rise of chloroquine-resistant *Plasmodium falciparum* that the possibility of using tetracyclines was taken seriously. Barney Magerlein and Fred Kagan reported from Upjohn in the late 1960s that clindamycin and related lincosamide derivatives also exerted useful antimalarial activity (91), an effect that Leon Schmidt in Cincinnati confirmed in experiments with monkeys (92). These compounds still have a place in malaria, especially for prophylaxis in areas of the world where resistance to other antimalarial agents is prevalent.

Artemisinin. Despite the monumental exertions of the Walter Reed chemists, the most promising antimalarial agent to emerge in the final decades of the twentieth century came from Mother Nature: a common weed, qinghao, used in Chinese traditional medicine. Known in the west as sweet wormwood—*Artemisia annua*—it was later found growing under the noses of the Washington scientists on the banks of the Potomac River.

Chinese scientists started a systematic examination of the antimalarial properties of indigenous herbal compounds in 1967, reputedly at the request of Ho Chi Minh, whose supporters suffered from drug resistant malaria just as American troops did during the Vietnam War. There is a recipe recommending infusions of qinghao to relieve the pain of haemorrhoids dating back to the early Han dynasty period in the second century BC and use of the

---

* The six diseases targeted by this ambitious scheme were malaria, leishmaniasis, trypanosomiasis, filariasis, schistosomiasis, and leprosy.

herb to combat fevers recognizable as malaria is described in Chinese medical texts from the late seventeenth century. However, it is unlikely that these decoctions had a true antimalarial effect, since aqueous solutions examined in modern studies are devoid of activity. It was only when organic solvent extracts of the leaves were fractionated and crystallized by Chinese chemists in 1971 that an active substance was isolated. It was given the name qinghaosu (literally, the active ingredient of qinghao) and later called artemisinin (93).

Artemisinin is a terpene (more precisely, a sesquiterpene), volatile oils with a hydrocarbon structure that are often aromatic. Such substances are common in nature and are widely used as fragrances and flavouring agents, but none had previously been found to display any activity against malaria parasites. Yields of artemisinin from plants grown in different locations vary enormously depending on the soil conditions; samples gathered in Washington DC for studies at the Walter Reed Institute in 1983 produced very small amounts of the active principle and the best yields have been found in plants harvested in China and other parts of the Far East.

With exemplary efficiency, dedicated research groups were set up to study the structure and properties of the new discovery. A major problem was the production of suitable formulations of the active principle, which is essentially insoluble in water and unstable in some organic solvents. Oily suspensions suitable for administration by injection, in tablet form or as suppositories were produced. Human trials were organized through a Qinghaosu Antimalarial Coordinating Research Group. By 1979, the ability of artemisinin to cure malaria, including chloroquine resistant malaria and advanced cerebral malaria, had been unequivocally established in China after studies in over 2000 patients. Not only was the drug found to be safe and outstandingly effective, but it also appeared to act more rapidly than previously known antimalarial agents. Development of artemisinin continued in China and a metabolite with improved potency, dihydroartemisinin, was used as the basis for the marketed formulations, artemether (for oral use) and artesunate (for injection) (94).

In view of the inexorable spread of chloroquine and antifolate resistant strains of *Plasmodium falciparum*, it might have been expected that the development and use of artemisinin derivatives outside China would have been fast-tracked, but, in fact, acceptance of the drug was painfully slow. Although the Walter Reed Institute started to investigate the compound in the mid-1980s, interest elsewhere was sporadic. Cost, concerns about toxicity based on high-dose tests in laboratory animals, and the reluctance of pharmaceutical firms to invest resources in drugs for the tropical market all conspired to delay general acceptance of artemisinin as a valuable addition to the fight against malaria. Few clinical studies were done outside China until 1992, when the Oxford malariologist Nick White, based in Thailand at Mahidol University, Bangkok began to champion its use in south-east Asia. It was at first spurned by the major aid agencies and it is only in recent years that formulations of the drug have become generally available in Africa and other countries where it was desperately needed. Although naturally-occurring resistance has so far not been described, fears that it may emerge have led to recommendations that artemisinin derivatives should be used in combination with mefloquine, doxycycline (the tetracycline derivative usually favoured in malaria), lumefantrine (benflumetol; another Chinese antimalarial compound originally synthesized by the Academy of Military Medical Sciences in Beijing in the mid-1990s), or piperaquine (synthesized independently by Rhône-Poulenc in France and in China at the Shanghai Pharmaceutical Research Institute in the 1960s, but developed and manufactured in China).

Pyronaridine and atovaquone. Among other antimalarials to emerge in the latter part of the twentieth century, most interest surrounds two compounds, pyronaridine and atovaquone. The former, yet another Chinese discovery, first synthesized in 1979, is very active, but resistance develops readily. Atovaquone belongs to a group known as the hydroxynaphthoquinones that have broad antiprotozoal activity. It is structurally related to the natural product, lapachol, derived from the wood of various species of tree, and was developed in the early 1980s by Win Gutteridge and his colleagues at the Wellcome Research Laboratories at Beckenham, Kent. Original trials in malaria in the early 1990s were disappointing, but it has been given a new lease of life as a combination product with proguanil and is now marketed by Glaxo SmithKline as Malarone.

Leishmaniasis

The term 'leishmaniasis' embraces a constellation of diseases cause by closely related protozoon parasites transmitted to human beings and other animals by sandflies belonging to the genus *Phlebotomus* (in India, the middle East, Africa, and Southern Europe) or *Lutzomyia* (in South America). Manifestations of the disease range from single boil-like lesions on exposed areas of the body (often the face), which resolve spontaneously leaving a characteristic scar, to a serious systemic disease, visceral leishmaniasis— often called kala-azar (Assamese = black disease; so-called because of associated skin changes)—with a high mortality. Treatment has always been problematical. Until recently management depended almost entirely on compounds familiar to Paracelsus and his followers: antimonials.

Antimony compounds

When early twentieth-century physicians in the tropics were faced with infections, the pathology of which they understood little, and approaches to management even less, it was natural that they should turn to time honoured remedies in which they had a touching if groundless faith. Hence the long love affair with arsenicals. Hence, too, the use of another favourite Victorian metallic remedy, tartar emetic. When it turned out to be modestly efficacious, as it did in leishmaniasis and the worm infection bilharzia (see p. 327), they must surely have felt vindicated, though there was little rational basis for application of the remedy in either disease.

Although the use of antimony in medicine was always controversial owing to its evident toxicity, the tartrated salt of antimony and potash (potassium antimony tartrate)—tartar emetic—has had a better press. Its supposed value first came to prominence in Italy in the early seventeenth century, probably based on wonderful cures obtained by *pulvis Warwicensis*, a recipe of scammony (a gum-resin obtained from the roots of *Convolvulus scammonia*, used as a purgative), antimony sulphide, and tartar, concocted around 1614 by Sir Robert Dudley, Earl of Warwick,* during his exile in Florence (95). The heyday of tartar emetic was the nineteenth century, when it was enthusiastically promoted by many of the most influential physicians of the day, including René Laennec, inventor of the stethoscope (96). The celebrated Victorian physician, Thomas Watson, in his lectures delivered at King's College, London, praised the use of tartar emetic in pneumonia, recommending that the unfortunate patient, exhausted by repeated blood-letting that had sapped the strength required to cough up the suffocating pulmonary secretions, be switched to an equally taxing regimen of tartar emetic and mercury (97).

At the turn of the twentieth century, when the various manifestations of leishmaniasis and their interrelatedness were just beginning to be recognized, even such an eminent tropical expert as Patrick Manson had nothing worthwhile to suggest by way of treatment. The beneficial effect of tartar emetic was first detected by the young Brazilian physician Gaspar Vianna, who used the drug to treat mucocutaneous leishmaniasis, a form of the disease prevalent in South America in which the nose and mouth are attacked with disfiguring consequences. In April 1912, Vianna could report to a meeting of the Sociedade Brasileira de Dermatologia held in Bello Horizonte that injections of tartar emetic—chosen because of reports that it had been successfully used in trypanosomiasis—produced much better results than Salvarsan in mucocutaneous leishmaniasis (98). By June 1914, Vianna was dead, a victim of tuberculosis, probably contracted while carrying out autopsies. He was also the first person to describe *Leishmania braziliensis* as a separate species; this and other New World species are often given the Genus name *Viannia* in his honour.

Vianna's results soon came to the attention of Giovanni Di Cristina, director of the paediatric clinic in Palermo, Sicily. Aware of the connection between cutaneous and systemic manifestations of the disease, Di Cristina decided to test tartar emetic in infants and young children suffering from visceral leishmaniasis, which was prevalent at that time in Sicily and Southern Italy and was virtually a death sentence. Together with his colleague Giuseppe Caronia he treated 10 cases; two died before the therapy could have any effect, but seven of the remaining eight responded to the treatment. Caronia remained in Palermo to test other antimonials (see below), but eventually left to take up a post in Rome in 1922. His political views set him at odds with the newly elected fascist government and in 1928 he was forced to move to Naples. He returned to Rome in 1944 and was able to use his position to help Jews and political dissidents by falsifying their health records. After the war he briefly served as a politician and was for a time president of the Società Italiana di Pediatria.

---

* The son, probably illegitimate, of Robert Dudley, the favourite of Queen Elizabeth.

The results of Di Cristina and Caronia's study with tartar emetic were published in Italian (99) in February 1915. A translation of the paper appeared in the *Journal of Tropical Medicine and Hygiene* in May 1915 (100) where it was spotted by Leonard Rogers, doyen of the Indian Medical Service. By July, Rogers, never slow to blow his own trumpet, had dashed off a letter to the *British Medical Journal*:

> ...to place on record that I had previously commenced similar treatment of the India form of kala-azar with most promising results. As a matter of fact, I had arranged to try this plan of treatment as far back as October last (1914), quite independently of any other worker, and even before I was aware of the success of Gaspar Vianna in the case of cutaneous leishmaniasis in Brazil, basing my hopes that it would very possibly prove to be a cure for kala-azar on the success of antimony treatment in some cases of the closely-allied sleeping sickness...I may therefore claim to have originated the intravenous use of tartar emetic in kala-azar quite independently of any other worker (101)

Tartar emetic is, of course, highly toxic and survival from the 2-month course of treatment needed in kala-azar was by no means assured. As with arsenicals for sleeping sickness and syphilis, the search for safer substitutes soon got under way. In 1912, Paul Uhlenhuth, who had just moved from the Department of Bacteriology of the German Reichsgesundheitsamt (Imperial Public Health Office) to become Professor of Hygiene in Strasbourg, concluded an agreement on behalf of the Reichsgesundheitsamt to investigate antimonial compounds in collaboration with the firm of von Heyden in Dresden. Uhlenhuth, who had worked with Robert Koch in Berlin, had considerable experience of tropical diseases and had investigated the use of atoxyl with Koch in German East Africa; in 1914 he was joined on the antimony project in Strasbourg by a former colleague, the splendidly named Philalethes Kuhn.* But it was in Dresden that the first breakthrough came. By 1920 Hans Schmidt, a chemist working for the von Heyden company, had devised a method for the synthesis of an antimonial compound, *para*-aminophenylstibonic acid, in which the antimony linkage was pentavalent rather than trivalent as in tartar emetic. This molecule formed the basis for the preparation of a range of derivatives that were to prove more effective in leishmaniasis than tartar emetic; an important advantage was that, although they retained much of the considerable toxic potential, these compounds lacked the unpleasant nauseous side effect. The first of Schmidt's antimonials to show promise in medicine was Stibenyl, which was submitted to Giuseppe Caronia in Palermo for preliminary testing and was given a more extensive trial in Calcutta in 1923, by Leonard Rogers' colleague, Lionel Napier. A similar substance, Stibosan, quickly followed. Stibenyl and Stibosan were synthesized while Schmidt was still with von Heyden, but Bayer, noting Schmidt's success in an area that they regarded as their preserve, persuaded von Heyden to let Schmidt join the firm in November 1926.

---

* Kuhn, had been a military doctor with the German colonial service in East Africa and Cameroon. He was a member of the German Society for Racial Hygiene and became an avid supporter of Hitler's policies. See Meusch, M. Die Medizinische Fakultät Gießen im Nationalsozialismus (1933–45), http://www.med.uni-giessen.de/infoweb/allgemein/ns_geschichte.html

As part of the deal, Bayer acquired the von Heyden antimonial compounds for their product range. Stibenyl was later manufactured in England by Allen and Hanburys.*

Hans Schmidt's move to Elberfeld provided him with improved research facilities and collaboration with an experienced pharmacologist, Fritz Eichholtz—later director of the Pharmacological Institute of the University of Heidelberg. He also acquired the reliable animal testing services of Wilhelm Röhl and (after Röhl's death in 1929) Walter Kikuth. At first Röhl had to make do with mice infected with trypanosomes as an experimental model of the effectiveness of antimonial preparations. Their value in leishmaniasis could only be tested in human beings. By August 1926, however, Röhl had learned that the hamster was susceptible to leishmanias and he immediately began to acquire Chinese hamsters and, later, the more readily available European species in order to establish a model that could be reliably used to test potential therapeutic drugs (102). It was the last important work that he undertook before his untimely death at the beginning of March 1929.

An Irish doctor, Jocelyn Smyly and his colleague Charles Young had introduced the Chinese hamster as a research animal for the study of visceral leishmaniasis at the Peking Union Medical College in 1924 (103). The animals were introduced to Europe by the Sheffield-born zoologist Edward Hindle, who used them during a Royal Society expedition to investigate the problem of visceral leishmaniasis in Northern China between 1925 and 1927. Chinese hamsters proved difficult to breed in captivity, but following Smyly and Young's lead, Martin Mayer, head of bacteriology at Bernhard Nocht's tropical institute in Hamburg, had succeeded in infecting European hamsters with leishmania parasites by 1927 (104). Presumably he used animals caught in the wild, since it is claimed that the first breeding colony of golden (European) hamsters was not established until 1930 (105). This was achieved in Jerusalem by the eminent parasitologist, Saul Adler with animals captured by his colleague, the zoologist Israel Aharoni from a site in Aleppo, Syria. Adler was born in Russia but his family had settled in Leeds when he was a small boy. After studying medicine at the University of Leeds, he served with the Royal Army Medical Corps before being recruited in 1924 by Chaim Weizman to head the new Microbiological Institute in Jerusalem.

Hans Schmidt's researches in Elberfeld with Eichholtz and Röhl led to an improved derivative of Stibosan, Neostibosan, which was added to the product range in 1928. These compounds represented a useful advance, but they had already been upstaged in India, by urea stibamine, a compound of urea and *para*-aminophenylstibonic acid developed at the Campbell Medical School in Calcutta by an Indian chemist, Upendranath Brahmachari. Brahmachari first produced urea stibamine in his ill-equipped laboratory in 1920, but he did not patent it. It was successfully used in Calcutta and extensively tested in 1923 in Assam, where the risk of kala-azar often reached epidemic proportions. By 1928, it was being used for mass therapy and remained the treatment of choice for

* A firm founded by William Allen and his nephew Cornelius Hanbury in Bethnal Green, London. It merged with Glaxo in 1958.

leishmaniasis for many years. Meanwhile in 1925 clinical trials of another antimonial compound, Neostam (stibamine glucoside), prepared in England by William Herbert Gray of the Wellcome Chemical Research Laboratories in London, were under way.

All the pentavalent antimonials, though effective—mortality in kala-azar was reduced from over 90 per cent to around 5 per cent—were unstable in aqueous solution. To overcome this impediment Schmidt's group developed Solustibosan, in which a pentavalent antimony preparation is complexed with sugar. Trials started in 1935 indicated that it was not only easier to administer but was also less toxic and in 1937 Bayer marketed Solustibosan as a stable solution ready for use for intravenous administration. With war looming William Solomon of Wellcome was given the task of finding a substance to rival Solustibosan. Len Goodwin carried out the biological testing of candidate molecules in hamsters—and later on himself—and by 1946 sodium antimony gluconate (sold as Pentostam), a substance very closely related to Solustibosan, was ready for clinical trial by the Scotsman, Robert Kirk and his colleagues in the Sudan (106). Not to be outdone, Specia in France went on to produce their own version, meglumine antimonate (Glucantime), which was under clinical investigation in Italy by 1948.

Alternatives to antimonials

Pentostam and Glucantime became the mainstay of therapy for leishmaniasis, with the latter being used mainly in Latin countries and the former in India and elsewhere. Inevitably, treatment failure associated with resistance began to arise with increasing frequency. It had become a major problem in parts of India by the 1990s. Pentamidine has been used with some success in such cases, but serious side effects are common and safer options were also sought. Studies by Tancredo Furtado of the National Institute for Rural Endemic Diseases in Belo Horizonte in Brazil had shown as early as 1959 that the antifungal antibiotic, amphotericin B (see p. 352–3) was effective against South American forms of leishmaniasis (107). Furtado had attempted to avoid the considerable toxicity of amphotericin by administering it by mouth, but, not surprisingly, this was unsuccessful. The availability of safer formulations of the drug that appeared in the 1990s made it a viable, if expensive, proposition. Various other alternatives were tried, including antifungal azoles (see p. 358–60) and the gout remedy, allopurinol, which was trialled in Kenya and India in the early 1980s following work by a group headed by Wallace Peters at the London School of Hygiene and Tropical Medicine (108). But more success was obtained with a resurrected antibacterial antibiotic, paromomycin (see p. 234).

Following up a report from Russian physicians, working in the Southern states of the former USSR, of the effectiveness of paromomycin in cutaneous leishmaniasis in 1968, Ralph Neal at the Wellcome Laboratories of Tropical Medicine in Beckenham, Kent, included the drug in a survey of the activity of aminoglycosides in experimental animals (109). However it was not until 1984, when Joseph El-On and his colleagues in the Hebrew University–Hadassah Medical School in Jerusalem, popularized use of an ointment containing paromomycin and methylbenzethonium chloride (which also exhibits antileishmanial activity) that a serious interest began to be taken in the antibiotic (110). Teva Pharmaceutical Industries in Israel marketed el-On's formulation as Leshcutan. Unfortunately, it proved too irritating for general use and paromomycin alone was ineffective, but Tony Bryceson and his colleagues at the Hospital for Tropical Diseases in London and the London School of Hygiene and Tropical Medicine developed alternative formulations that appeared to be less toxic (111). There have also been trials in India and Africa of injectable formulations of paromomycin (used alone or in combination with antimonials) for the treatment of the systemic form of leishmaniasis, kala-azar. However, the potential for toxicity is not in its favour and since paromomycin is no longer readily available, prospects for its further development rest with not-for-profit organizations such as the Drugs for Neglected Diseases Initiative or the Institute for One World Health (112). Other drugs, most notably sitamaquine, an 8-aminoquinoline discovered through the Walter Reed Army Institute's antimalarial programme, have been investigated, but have made little progress.

The latest hope for safe, reliable treatment of kala-azar rests with a group of drugs known as alkylphosphocholines, which were originally investigated as cytotoxic agents for the treatment of cancer. One of these drugs, miltefosine, already shows great promise. William Pendergast and J. H. Chan first synthesized the compound at Burroughs Wellcome's Research Triangle Park in the 1980s as part of an anticancer research programme. Sensing that such molecules might have some potential as antileishmanial agents, Simon Croft (who had just moved from Wellcome's Beckenham Laboratories to the London School of Tropical Medicine and Hygiene), persuaded his colleague Ralph Neal to test them in a mouse model of leishmaniasis. The experiments showed that miltefosine and related compounds had a pronounced affect against leishmania when injected subcutaneously, though, disappointingly, they were not free of toxicity (113). Miltefosine was later shown to be almost completely absorbed when given by mouth—an important feature in keeping the cost low—and a clinical trial in the Muzaffarpur district of Bihar by Shyam Sundar and his colleagues at the Indian Kala-Azar Research Centre, showed the drug to be remarkably effective when administered by this route (114). Miltefosine was developed commercially by the German firm of Zentaris* with the help of the World Health Organization's Tropical Disease Research Programme. It is already licensed in India, where it is badly needed and has given rise to new optimism in the control of this age-old scourge. Residual toxicity and the potential emergence of resistance have tempered the confidence somewhat and time will tell whether it will be truly justified.

Amoebiasis

Amoebic dysentery is one of the few infections that responded to treatment available before the start of the twentieth century; namely ipecacuanha root and its active ingredient, emetine (see p. 40). As described in Chapter 2, Leonard Rogers in Calcutta first championed the use of emetine injections in both amoebic dysentery and amoebic liver abscess in 1912. By the end of the First World War it was established as the drug of choice in these conditions. The treatment is generally effective in expert hands, but requires a

---

* A subsidiary of the Canadian firm, Æterna Zentaris Inc.

prolonged stay in hospital for the patient. In any case, the frequency of side effects—some life-threatening—when emetine is given by injection and the profound nausea of oral formulations such as emetine bismuth iodide, ensured that the search for alternatives was not long delayed.

Arsenicals, including Fourneau's stovarsol (see p. 280) were tried with modest success sometimes in combination with emetine. Another arsenical, a derivative of atoxyl that had been investigated in Paul Ehrlich's laboratory, but rejected for lack of activity against trypanosomes and spirochaetes, was resurrected in 1930 under the name carbasone by the pharmacologist Chauncey Leake at the University of California School of Medicine, San Francisco. Neither stovarsol nor carbasone produced benefits worth the toxic risk and though there were vogues for their use in France and America, respectively, they were soon discredited.

Chauncey Leake, a polymath who was a notable historian of science, medical ethicist, and minor poet, was also instrumental in the development of iodochlorhydroxyquin (clioquinol) as an anti-amoebic agent. Like carbasone, it was clinically unimpressive, but it remained popular for many years under the name EnteroVioform for the treatment of traveller's diarrhoea. Its reputation suffered when it was associated with neurotoxic effects, sometimes leading to paralysis and blindness, in Japanese subjects taking the drug in the late 1950s and 1960s. It is still on the market in some countries as a topical treatment for certain skin conditions (a use which precedes the demonstration of its activity against amoebae) but is now banned as an antidiarrhoeal drug. A similar substance, diodoquine (iodoquinol), was introduced in 1935 by the distinguished American parasitologist Charles Craig and Joseph D'Antoni of Tulane University. It has not suffered the same fate as clioquinol, although it has been implicated in similar side effects. It is still available as an oral treatment for the eradication of amoebic cysts from the intestinal tract, but is no longer recommended.

The value of iodinated quinolines in amoebic dysentery was not an American discovery. Peter Mühlens and Walter Menk at the Hamburg Tropical Institute had pioneered the use of such a compound, known as Yatren (chionofon) as early as 1921. These compounds were commonly used in combination with emetine, which relieved the acute symptoms, but often allowed relapse of infection when used alone owing to persistence of the more resistant cyst form of the parasite in the intestinal tract. Eradication of cysts from patients recovering from acute amoebiasis is important, since even if a relapse of disease does not occur, continued carriage and excretion of virulent strains of the protozoa present a hazard to the community in the absence of good hygienic facilities. Quinolines, like the arsenicals, stovarsol, and carbasone, have more activity against cysts than emetine does and their chief role in combination with emetine was to eradicate amoebic cysts. Rivanol, an antibacterial acridine derivative introduced by Julius Morgenroth in the 1920s (see p. 62) was also sometimes used in this way. In the 1960s these compounds were replaced by a safer, more effective agent for the eradication of amoebic cysts, diloxanide furoate, developed by the Boots Company in Nottingham, and marketed by them after successful trials in Burma (115).

It was presumably the reputation of iodinated quinolines such as clioquinol and diodoquin that prompted investigations of antimalarial quinolines in amoebiasis. As sometimes happens, such speculative trials brought rewards, when numerous reports in the early 1950s indicated that chloroquine and amodiaquine were effective in amoebic liver abscess. Exploration of other antimicrobial agents was less successful. When antibacterial antibiotics became available after the Second World War, attempts were naturally made to evaluate their activity against protozoa, and *Entamoeba histolytica* the cause of amoebic dysentery and hepatic amoebiasis was no exception. Little came of these optimistic forays, although there was some short-lived excitement over results obtained with the first tetracyclines, especially Aureomycin (116). In 1951, Max McCowen and his colleagues at Lilly Research, Indianapolis described the antiamoebic activity of an antibiotic called fumagillin that workers at Upjohn had found in *Aspergillus fumigatus* (117). This too came to nothing, though the compound survived as a useful agent for the control of *Nosema apis* infections in bees and later resurfaced in human medicine for the treatment of the rare protozoan infection, microsporidiosis (118). A little more success was achieved with paromomycin when it became available around 1960. Indeed, use in amoebiasis was one of the reasons for continuing interest in this otherwise unremarkable antibiotic (see p. 234). But the biggest advance in the treatment of hepatic and intestinal amoebiasis came from another quarter with the discovery in the late 1950s of metronidazole, a remarkable drug originally developed for the treatment of an unrelated protozoan disease, trichomoniasis.

Metronidazole

In 1953, a few years before the discovery of kanamycin (see p. 230), Hamao Umezawa, and his colleagues in Tokyo isolated a new antibiotic from a species of *Streptomyces*, which they called azomycin. The compound had a very simple structure, which showed it to belong to a class of chemicals called nitroimidazoles. The nitro group was on the number 2 carbon, making it a 2-nitroimidazole (Fig. 7.4).

Azomycin aroused little interest and soon disappeared without trace, but its legacy has been astonishing. It became the precursor of a family of synthetic compounds, of which metronidazole is the best known, which established themselves as the drugs of choice in human and veterinary medicine for the therapy of a range of diseases caused by protozoa and anaerobic bacteria. Nitroimidazoles also aroused considerable interest as

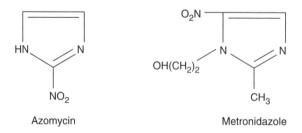

Fig. 7.4 Structures of azomycin (a 2-nitroimidazole) and metronidazole (a 5-nitroimidazole).

radiosensitizers, drugs that potentiate the activity of radiotherapy in cancer. In addition, azoles more remotely related to azomycin and metronidazole have emerged as front-line drugs in the treatment of fungal diseases (see p. 358–60) and worm infections (see p. 325–6), though their antecedents are different.

The metamorphosis of azomycin into an innovative antimicrobial agent occurred not in Japan, but in France. Investigators at Rhône-Poulenc rediscovered the antibiotic during examination of *Streptomyces* species from soil samples obtained from the island of Réunion in 1955 (119). One of the features of azomycin was that it possessed activity against trichomonads, flagellate protozoa responsible for abortion and infertility in cattle (*Trichomonas fetus*) as well as an ordinarily mild, but troublesome vaginal discharge in women and urethritis in their male sexual partners (*Trichomonas vaginalis*). Although azomycin has a simple structure, it proved difficult to synthesize, but compounds with the nitro group attached to the number 5 carbon were more amenable and in 1957 one of these, subsequently called metronidazole (Fig. 7.4), was found by Charles Cosar and Louis Julou at Rhône-Poulenc to display impressive activity and low toxicity in laboratory animals infected with *Trichomonas vaginalis*.

Cosar and Julou's laboratory studies were reported at a session of the Société Française de Microbiologie on 4 December 1958 (120). On 16 October 1959 the French venereologist Pierre Durel of the Hôpital Saint Lazare in Paris read a paper before the General Assembly of the International Union against Venereal Diseases in London giving preliminary details of the clinical efficacy of the drug in trichomonal vaginitis (121). The results were soon confirmed in venereology clinics throughout Great Britain and in Canada at the Hôpital Notre Dame in Montreal.

Whether such a drug would be commercially viable was by no means certain. In fact there is a persistent suggestion in the folklore of British microbiology that the French company considered the drug to be commercially uneconomic and were more than willing to hand it over to the British firm of May and Baker (which was part owned by Rhône-Poulenc; see footnote p. 75). Fifty years on it is difficult to establish the accuracy of this tale, but metronidazole was subsequently marketed by May and Baker under the name 'Flagyl' and the drug was most enthusiastically taken up in Britain. If the story is true an antimicrobial agent of remarkable range could easily have been lost to medicine.

Prompted by reports of the successful use of metronidazole in trichomonal infection, Jean Schneider at the Hôpital Beaujon in Clichy la-Garenne, north-west of Paris hit on the idea of trying the new compound in giardiasis, a diarrhoeal infection caused by a distantly related flagellate protozoon for which contemporary treatment, even with mepacrine (see below) was not entirely reliable. Schneider had pioneered the use of Sontochin for malaria in North Africa (see p. 298) and had investigated treatment of giardiasis with various antimalarials besides mepacrine with little success. It was in May 1960 that he started to use metronidazole with little idea of the correct dose. The initial results were not very promising: the first patient, a 59-year-old Algerian woman, failed to respond in the 2 weeks before she left France to return to Algeria; the second quickly relapsed after two apparently successful courses of treatment. It was then realized that the patient was probably reacquiring the parasite from his daughter who was also infected. Encouraged by this discovery, Schneider went on to treat another 25 patients with few serious side effects and almost uniform success (122).

Many of Schneider's patients had contracted giardiasis in tropical countries and several of them also suffered from amoebic dysentery. Such patients were given conventional treatment for amoebiasis before metronidazole was administered for the infection with *Giardia*, but Schneider had missed a trick. By 1966, a team led by the South African parasitologist, Ronnie Elsdon-Dew, Director of the Amoebiasis Research Unit in Durban, was reporting the success of metronidazole in intestinal and hepatic amoebiasis (123). Confirmation swiftly followed and in the following years metronidazole became the drug of first choice for treating all serious infections with *Entamoeba histolytica*. For the first time, a simple, safe, and effective oral therapy to replace emetine was available. It was a major breakthrough in the management of this globally important infection.

Meanwhile, more good news had come out of the blue in 1962: a woman being treated with metronidazole for trichomonal vaginitis remarked to her dentist at King's College Hospital Dental School, London, that she had not only responded well to the treatment, but her acute gum infection had inexplicably cleared up as well. The young dentist, David Shinn, intrigued by this apparent coincidence, was emboldened to give metronidazole to six other patients suffering from severe ulcerative gingivitis with startlingly rapid results (124). The finding was puzzling. Although protozoa—*Entamoeba gingivalis* and *Trichomonas tenax*—are found in the gums, they were generally regarded as harmless commensals and the expert consensus was that acute ulcerative gingivitis was probably an exclusively bacterial disease. To add to the mystery, nitroimidazoles had been regularly tested for antibacterial activity with uniformly negative results.

Ulcerative gingivitis is often called Vincent's gingivitis, after the French military physician Jean Hyacinthe Vincent, who first described the association of spirochaetes and fusiform (spindle-shaped) bacteria in serious infections in the mouth and throat in 1896. These bacteria grow in the absence of oxygen and flourish in the anaerobic conditions that exist in the gum pockets. Further testing of metronidazole revealed that the drug had unprecedented and previously unsuspected activity against virtually all anaerobic bacteria, but was completely inactive against those that require oxygen for growth.

It transpired that the feature that linked *Trichomonas vaginalis, Giardia lamblia, Entamoeba histolytica,* and anaerobic bacteria was anaerobic metabolism. Metronidazole acts when it is reduced under anaerobic conditions to a highly reactive intermediate form that causes damage to the DNA of the organisms. Because of its action against DNA the drug was viewed with understandable suspicion in some quarters—it remained unavailable for many years in the United States—but extensive monitoring has failed to reveal any link with the development of tumours in human beings.

The introduction of metronidazole for the treatment of anaerobic infections did not immediately follow David Shinn's successful but small-scale trial. The principal indication for the drug remained trichomonal vaginitis in which it gained a growing reputation for reliability. Most anaerobic bacteria, including those that cause Vincent's gingivitis, are very susceptible to penicillin, which had an impeccable safety record apart from its propensity to cause allergic reactions. It was only when an anaerobe called *Bacteroides fragilis*, which is relatively resistant to penicillin, rose to prominence in the 1970s as an organism implicated chiefly in infections following intestinal and gynaecological surgery, that the value of metronidazole as an anti-anaerobe agent became widely appreciated.

Metronidazole was first marketed in France and the United Kingdom in 1960. Numerous nitroimidazole derivatives were synthesized in subsequent years. Apart from metronidazole, the most widely used is tinidazole, developed in the United States by Arthur English and his colleagues in the Pfizer medical research laboratories in Groton, Connecticut in 1969. Various related compounds, most of which have properties virtually indistinguishable from metronidazole or tinidazole have been marketed round the world for human or veterinary use.

Giardiasis

In the seventeenth century Antonie van Leeuwenhoek observed motile flagellate organisms in faecal material that are recognizable from his contemporary drawings as *Giardia lamblia*.* The Czech pathologist Vilém Lambl described in 1859 the same organism (and, a year later, its cysts), which he had found in the faeces of children suffering from mild diarrhoea. The presence of the protozoon was at first regarded as an incidental curiosity and its role as an intestinal pathogen was not taken seriously until the time of the First World War (125). It is now known to be a very common cause of chronic diarrhoea, especially in countries in which faecal contamination of water supplies occurs through inadequate treatment of the water or of the supply infrastructure. In the 1970s, the chance of acquiring giardiasis from the public water supply in Leningrad (now St Petersburg) was so reliable that several epidemiological studies were carried out on students crossing from Helsinki for visits.

Even when *Giardia* was recognized as a pathogen, treatment with the usual array of drugs used in other intestinal infections—anthelminthics, emetine derivatives, internal disinfectants, and arsenicals—was of little avail. All this was to change as Second World War approached, when scientists searching for a cure for giardiasis turned their attention to the antimalarial drug, mepacrine.

Mepacrine: death and resurrection

After the war mepacrine (quinacrine; Atebrin) became a casualty of the success of chloroquine, which was safer, more effective, and free of the pigmentation that was a major drawback of the acridine dye. By 1947, George Findlay of the Wellcome Bureau of Scientific Research† in reviewing the toxicity of mepacrine, so successfully used for the prevention of malaria in the Second World War, could write that the drug was 'now largely of historical

---

* Several names are used interchangeably for this parasite; some prefer *Giardia duodenalis*, others *Giardia intestinalis*.

† 1947 was also the year Findlay left the Bureau to become editor of the British Medical Association's abstracting journals.

interest—except for claims for compensation or pension' (126). But it was too soon to write off this remarkable compound.

At a meeting of the Société de Biologie in Paris on 10 April 1937, Lucien Brumpt, reported that, while working in the laboratory of his father, the eminent French parasitologist, Emile Brumpt, he had found that mepacrine (manufactured in France under the name quinacrine) cured mice of infection with *Giardia muris* (127). Later the same year Bruno Galli-Valerio Professor of Veterinary Medicine at the University of Lausanne, revealed in an article in the *Schweizerische Medizinische Wochenschrift* that the Bayer product, Atebrin, had been successfully used in two children by his student Edgar Heim as early as 1935 and that the French version, quinacrine, had subsequently proved curative in 53 of 54 cases of human giardiasis treated by a Doctor Martin in the spa town of Châtel-Guyon (128). In 1940, Bayer marketed another acridine derivative, Acranil, for the treatment of giardiasis, but it made little impact. After the Second World War mepacrine became the drug of choice for the therapy of giardiasis, but was gradually ousted in the 1960s by metronidazole, which proved to be superior in safety and efficacy.

The frequency with which drugs developed for one purpose are subsequently discovered, usually fortuitously, to have unanticipated beneficial effects in completely unrelated conditions is truly astonishing. There are dozens of such examples in the pharmacopoeia and the history of drugs used in parasitic diseases is littered with clear instances of this variant of the serendipity principle at work. None is more extraordinary in its variety than mepacrine, which, within a few years of its launch for the treatment of malaria, was not only successfully employed in giardiasis, but was also found to be remarkably effective in a quite different parasitic disease: tapeworm infection (see p. 322–3). Outside the realm of infection mepacrine has been used since the 1950s in the autoimmune diseases, systemic lupus erythematosus, and rheumatoid arthritis. Quinine had been used speculatively in rheumatic diseases since at least the nineteenth century and when other antimalarials, including chloroquine, hydroxychloroquine, and mepacrine, became available they were found to suppress the symptoms in some cases. The value of mepacrine in lupus was discovered by chance by Francis Page, a Medical Registrar at the Middlesex Hospital in London. Faced with a patient who had received various treatments, including quinine without success, Page decided to give mepacrine a try with, according to the patient—a highly articulate solicitor—astonishing results (129).

In the 1970s this rather undistinguished acridine dye was once more resurrected by the Chilean gynaecologist, Jaime Zipper at the Sótero el Rio Hospital, Santiago, who controversially introduced the use of quinacrine pellets inserted into the uterus as a method of female sterilization (130). Zipper had been alarmed at the number of women presenting with life-threatening septic abortions in a country where contraception was proscribed and mepacrine was found to cause tissue fibrosis specific to the fallopian tubes. Most recently and most remarkably, quinacrine had been proposed by the Nobel laureate Stanley Prusiner and his colleagues at the University of California, San Francisco as a possible candidate for the treatment of prion diseases such as Creutzfeldt–Jakob disease (131).

South American trypanosomiasis

Trypanosomes that are quite different from those found in Africa cause a serious infection called Chagas' disease in South America. The disease is named after Carlos Chagas the brilliant Brazilian doctor who between 1907 and 1912 not only described the presence of the flagellate protozoa in human blood, but identified the insect vector and showed that armadillos act as reservoirs of infection in the wild (132). Most of this work was done in Lassance, a small settlement in the state of Minas Gerais in the interior of Brazil, where Chagas had been sent to study malaria by Oswaldo Cruz, a Paris-trained medical microbiologist who is justifiably fêted as the founder of Brazilian public health medicine. Chagas named the trypanosome *Trypanosoma cruzi* in his honour.

Chagas' disease is transmitted by bugs roughly the size of cockroaches that commonly inhabit the homes of poor people living in rural areas. The insects feed around the mouths of sleeping individuals and are known as 'kissing bugs' (see p. 15). Unlike African trypanosomes, the parasites do not multiply in the bloodstream; they invade muscle, including heart muscle, lose their flagella and multiply in a form closely resembling that of their cousins, the leishmania. They are responsible for various types of pathology, among the most serious being progressive heart failure. Infection is often eventually fatal, but the first patient described by Carlos Chagas in 1909, a 2-year-old child named Berenice, lived until 1981. Shortly before her death of heart failure—apparently unrelated to her infection—trypanosomes could still be isolated from her bloodstream (133).

Evidence of Chagas' disease has been found in Peruvian mummies predating the Spanish conquest and the disease has probably existed there for several thousand years (134). Despite its antiquity and the continued importance of the disease in countries of Central and South America, the treatment cupboard is almost bare. Numerous compounds, including all the usual suspects—arsenicals, antimonials, antimalarials etc., etc.—were tried during the first half of the twentieth century, but all to no benefit. When antibiotics came along there was a brief flirtation with tetracyclines, but these, too, proved singularly ineffective.

Some transient interest was shown in a complex organic molecule, Bayer 7602—distantly related to the early quinolines—which had been synthesized at Elberfeld and came to light when Allied intelligence officers visited the IG Farben sites after the Second World War (135). Clinical trials of Bayer 7602 were carried out in Argentina from 1937, notably by Salvador Mazza, a medical bacteriologist who took a special interest in Chagas' disease. It was found to have a symptomatic effect, but was not curative. After the war the drug was developed by ICI in England under the name Cruzon, but it was soon abandoned. A phenanthridine compound, Carbidium, synthesized by Leslie Walls at the Wellcome Chemical Research Laboratories in London, suffered a similar fate after a clinical trial in Brazil.

The first glimmer of hope came in the 1950s when an American of Armenian ancestry, Ardzroony Packchanian at the University of Texas Medical Branch, Galveston, showed that certain nitrofurans, notably the Eaton Laboratories product, nitrofurazone (see p. 251), exhibited activity against the trypanosomes of Chagas' disease. Nitrofurazone proved too toxic in preliminary human trials (including some trials in African trypanosomiasis), but following up this lead, Rudolf Gönnert and his colleagues Marianne Bock and Axel Haberkorn in Bayer's Institute of Parasitology and Veterinary Medicine developed a nitrofuran derivative in 1969, which they called nifurtimox (136). Early trials of nifurtimox were encouraging and hopes were raised that a reliable therapy for Chagas' disease had at last been found.

Around the same time, scientists at Hofmann–La Roche in Nutley, New Jersey led by Emanuel Grunberg were turning their attention to nitroimidazoles as potential chemotherapeutic agents, no doubt stimulated by the success of metronidazole. In collaboration with the Brazilian trypanosomiasis expert Zigman Brener activity against *Trypanosoma cruzi* was included in the screening programme (137). Further investigation of these compounds by Roche scientists in Basel yielded a 2-nitroimidazole, which appeared active against trypanosomes. It was given the name benznidazole and marketed in 1978 as Radanil or Rochagan.

Neither nifurtimox nor benznidazole proved to be the answer to Chagas' disease. Both have toxicity problems and much of the useful antitrypanosomal effect is restricted to the early stages of infection, when symptoms are not always apparent. The best hope for control of the disease still lies in control of the insect vectors and the provision of better housing and education for the populations at risk.

Anthelminthic agents

It might seem odd to include worms, all of which can be seen without the aid of a lens and some of which (certain tapeworms) can attain a length of several metres, in a book dealing with antimicrobial agents. But it would be perverse to ignore these agents of infection. The sheer number of persons harbouring helminths and suffering their ill effects (see p. 17) demands that they be given consideration. Moreover, the quest for drugs capable of casting out worms from the body is as least as old as the search for other remedies. At first the focus was on intestinal worms, but once it was realized that worms were responsible for serious systemic diseases such as schistosomiasis (bilharzia), filariasis (elephantiasis and river blindness), and hydatid disease, these infections began to move centre stage.

Not surprisingly, natural products that had the effect of expelling intestinal worms easily visible to the naked eye were recognized from the earliest times. By the turn of the twentieth century several effective products, including santonin and oil of chenopodium (for ascaris and threadworms) and extract of male fern (for tapeworms) were in regular use in human beings and domestic animals (see p. 29–31) and survived beyond the introduction of more modern treatments for other microbial diseases.

Intestinal worms

Ascaris and threadworm

Various synthetic drugs, including hexylresorcinol and carbon tetrachloride threatened to oust traditional remedies from their perch as specifics for ascaris and the common threadworm of children during the mid-twentieth century. For threadworm, formulations of gentian violet given by mouth also became popular. Hexylresorcinol had a brief vogue in the 1920s as a urinary antiseptic and was found to have anthelminthic properties around 1935. For threadworm infection administration of hexylresorcinol by enema—which seems almost tantamount to child abuse—was popular for a time, especially in America (138). The source of hexylresorcinol for the original investigation carried out by the pharmacologist Paul Lamson and his colleagues at Vanderbilt University at the behest of the Rockefeller Foundation, was the firm of Sharp and Dohme, which marketed it as a mouthwash called 'S.T. 37' (139). The antiseptic properties of hexylresorcinol are still exploited today in some throat lozenges.

The American veterinary parasitologist Maurice Hall introduced carbon tetrachloride as an anthelminthic around 1921. Hall had noticed that animals anaesthetized with chloroform often passed worms in their faeces and went on to experiment with the related carbon tetrachloride (140). After safety tests on animals (and Hall himself), the chemical was tried with some success in human medicine, especially in hookworm infection (see below). All these compounds were upstaged in the 1950s by a much safer drug, piperazine.

Piperazine has a remarkable history, much of which was recounted by Len Goodwin in his presidential address to the Royal Society of Tropical Medicine and Hygiene in October 1979 (141). In 1890, Ernst Schering's pharmaceutical company in Berlin marketed piperazine as the first product of its new chemical research laboratory, headed by Albrecht Schmidt,* a pupil of Robert Wilhelm Bunsen of Bunsen burner fame. Schering advertised the product as a rejuvenating tonic, but in 1892, after a fierce patent battle, Bayer started to offer the same drug as a remedy for gout—albeit one that proved to have dubious efficacy. The activity against ascaris was first revealed in a thesis by C Fayard published in Paris in 1949 (142), but according to Goodwin, Fayard got the idea from a pharmacist in Rouen, called M Boismare, who was selling a preparation called 'Lumbrical' after learning that customers taking piperazine for gout had reported passing roundworms. Other workers, who had published their findings in French journals, had followed up Fayard's observations and the helminthologist Owen Standen at the Wellcome Laboratories of Tropical Medicine in London picked up these results through a close scrutiny of the literature on compounds alleged to act against intestinal worms. Standen was looking for a substance to replace diphenan, a toxic drug of poor efficacy originally synthesized by Werner Schulemann in Bayer's Elberfeld Laboratory in 1921 (marketed as Butolan) and promoted by Wellcome in Britain and America for threadworm infection. Standen tested hundreds of potential compounds and to everyone's surprise piperazine emerged as much the most active. A clinical trial by Richard White, a House Physician at Guy's hospital, in 1953 confirmed the efficacy of piperazine in eliminating threadworms (and a couple of cases of ascaris, which is much less common in the United Kingdom). In 1954 Goodwin and Standen took a supply of piperazine citrate with them to East Africa to test the effect on roundworm infections during an expedition the prime purpose of

* In 1898 Schmidt moved on to become head of research at Meister Lucius & Brüning at Hoechst, Frankfurt am Main.

which was to undertake work on schistosomiasis. Piperazine citrate was subsequently marketed by Burroughs Wellcome as Antepar. Various other salts followed, notably piperazine adipate (Entacyl) which was being developed at the same time as Antepar at British Drug Houses*

None of the mentioned anthelminthic agents, including piperazine, had much effect on whipworm (*Trichuris trichiura*), a very common, but generally benign inhabitant of the human large intestine. The first inroads into treatment were made by dithiazanine (Telmid), developed by Eli Lilly and introduced in 1957 by Clyde Swartzwelder and his colleagues at Louisiana State University, New Orleans (143). Dithiazanine is a green dye, which imparts a macabre colour to the faeces of patients treated with the drug, but it is fairly effective in removing whipworms. It also has some effect on *Strongyloides stercoralis*, a worm known for its long persistence in the human gut—strongyloides larvae were still being found in some prisoners of war who had acquired the infection in the Far East over 30 years earlier during Second World War (144). Persistence of infection first came to light when ex-prisoners of war received systemic corticosteroid treatment for other diseases; the resulting immunosuppression sometimes allows a potentially fatal dissemination of the larvae outside the intestinal tract, a condition known as 'hyperinfection'. Publicity among ex-prisoners of war groups encouraged them to be examined for persistence of the worm and numerous other cases were discovered and treated during the 1980s.

Hookworm

By the end of the nineteenth century it was clear that at least one type of intestinal worm—hookworm—was worth taking much more seriously than the others. Avicenna (Ibn Sina) had recognized worms inhabiting the small intestine (assumed from their location to be hookworms) around the first millennium, but no one had taken much notice of them. In 1838 Angelo Dubini an Italian doctor who has just joined the staff of the Ospedale Maggiore in Milan after qualifying in medicine at the University of Pavia, found the helminths in the body of a young peasant woman. After further study of other cases he published his findings and named the worm *Ancylostoma* (originally *Agchylostoma*) *duodenale*. Dubini had noticed that hookworm infection is sometimes accompanied by intestinal bleeding and the German pathologist and pioneering psychiatrist, Wilhelm Griesinger was among those who realized that serious, even fatal, anaemia can follow from bleeding lesions directly attributable to the worms. While investigating intestinal worm infections of labourers—many of who were Italian— building the St Gotthard railway tunnel (built 1872–80), Edoardo Perroncito, Professor of Parasitology in Turin, found that heavy hookworm infections were particularly common (145). Together with Luigi Pagliani and Camillo Bozzolo he recognized that a massive infection with *Ancylostoma duodenale* was contributing to the severe anaemia afflicting the workers.

---

* British Drug Houses, was established in 1908 as a drugs wholesaler and manufacturer. It was absorbed by Glaxo in 1968.

Although it was not realized at the time, hookworm infection is usually acquired by walking barefoot in soil contaminated with human faeces containing the eggs. Larvae are able to penetrate unbroken skin and migrate through the bloodstream to the lungs from where they climb up the trachea, are swallowed and grow to maturity attached to the lining of the small intestine. The adult worms ingest blood and also leave behind bleeding lesions when they move from place to place; the effect of heavy infections is to cause life-threatening iron-deficiency anaemia. Providing buckets for workers wishing to defecate proved effective in curbing hookworm disease, but treatment for established infection was also plainly necessary. It was Camillo Bozzolo who discovered that thymol, previously employed only as a topical antiseptic, was effective in expelling hookworms in 1879 during the St Gotthard tunnel incident.

Caspar Neumann, who served as apothecary to the court of the Prussian King Friedrich Wilhelm I in Berlin and helped to establish chemistry as an academic subject, originally obtained thymol as a crystalline extract from the garden herb *Thymus vulgaris*. Neumann described the extract in 1719 as camphor of thyme and it was not until 1853 that it was given its present name thymol by the French chemist A Lallemand.

Thymol was not much used in medicine until Bozzolo described its action against hookworm, but it played an important part in two important episodes in the history of tropical medicine in the United States. In turn of the twentieth century America hookworm anaemia was common among the poor of the southern states, where it was partly responsible for the prevailing stereotype of 'poor white trash'—a lazy, lethargic, and supposedly genetically predisposed underclass. The role of hookworm disease in this myth was exposed by the work of two men: Charles Stiles, a parasitologist who had studied in Leipzig under Rudolf Leuckart; and one of his students at the Army Medical School, Bailey Ashford, who went to Puerto Rico after the American invasion in 1898 and was put in charge of hospital facilities in the Southern city of Ponce.

Stiles discovered that the American species of hookworm, which he called *Uncinaria* (later *Necator*) *americanus*, differed from the so-called 'old world' variety, though it was probably imported with slaves from Africa, where it is common. In 1899 Ashford deduced that endemic hookworm infection was responsible for the anaemia afflicting the peasant population of Puerto Rico, lately colonized by the American government. The clinching observation was that treatment to remove the hookworms relieved the anaemia, whereas dietary efforts singularly failed. Ashford had most success in the use of thymol to expel the worms, but also used filix-mas, which was popular in Europe for the treatment of hookworm, until it became clear that it was ineffective. β-Naphthol, which was introduced with success in India in 1902 by Charles Bentley, was also favoured for a while, but was found to be inferior to thymol. Ashford subsequently wrote, together with, Pedro Gutierrez Igaravidez, Director of the Tropical and Transmissible Diseases Service of Puerto Rico, an exhaustive and combative account of the history of hookworm infection in Puerto Rico, its effect on the population and the fight to control the disease (146).

Meanwhile, back in America, Stiles was pursuing a campaign to tackle the scourge of hookworm infection in America. In 1909 he persuaded Rockefeller to fund the 'Rockefeller Sanitary Commission for Eradication of Hookworm Disease' (see p. 270).

It was one of Rockefeller's first major excursions into medical philanthropy and anticipated the creation of the Rockefeller Foundation in 1913. Once again thymol was the drug used as the chief weapon for treatment in spite of its known harmful effects. Later oil of chenopodium was substituted for a time. In 1921 the veterinary parasitologist Maurice Hall introduced carbon tetrachloride. It was more effective than thymol, but it was just as harmful to the liver and both had to be used with purgatives to ensure that they did not remain long in the digestive tract. In 1925, Maurice Hall reported that tetrachlorethylene was as effective as carbon tetrachloride and much safer. After further testing it was marketed in 1929 and became the drug of choice for the treatment of hookworm for many years.

It was at the Wellcome Research Laboratories in Beckenham, Kent that a challenger to the supremacy of tetrachlorethylene emerged. The chemist Fred Copp was working on quaternary ammonium salts and on the hunch that some of these substances might have selective activity against helminths, he submitted suitable candidate molecules to his colleague Owen Standen for testing at the Wellcome Laboratory of Tropical Medicine in Euston Road. As luck would have it, the first of the compounds to be submitted, bephenium, displayed activity against a variety of roundworms, including *Ancylostoma caninum* in dogs, which was far superior to that of any of the numerous others that he subsequently synthesized. Bephenium was briefly tested in patients in a London hospital before Goodwin and Standen again set off on their travels, this time to Sri Lanka. With the help of the Singhalese doctor, Gladys Jayewardene—who was assassinated in 1989 for defying a boycott of Indian goods by allowing the import of medicines—the effectiveness of bephenium against hookworms was established in 1958 and the drug was marketed as 'Alcopar' the following year (147).

Tapeworms

It was known in antiquity that extract of male fern (*Dryopteris filix-mas*) could expel tapeworms (see p. 31). Although other plant extracts had sometimes been tried and a vogue for using carbon tetrachloride emerged in the 1930s, nothing better was found to replace male fern. Extract of male fern is a thick, dark green, smelly liquid, and quite nauseating. It is so unpalatable that it was often given through a duodenal tube, but so effective is the drug that it remained in regular use in until the 1960s, when it was replaced first by the remarkable acridine dye, mepacrine, and then by a novel organic molecule, niclosamide.

The Australian historian of medical helminthology, David Grove unearthed a reference from 1939 (148) establishing the priority of the Chilean parasitologist, Amador Neghme for the discovery that the antimalarial acridine dye, mepacrine (Bayer's Atebrin sold in America as Atabrine) was effective in tapeworm infections. The observation was probably made during a malaria control campaign in which Neghme, who went on to become Professor of Parasitology at the University of Chile in Santiago* and a champion of medical education, was an active participant.

---

* The library of the Medical School in Santiago is named in Neghme's honour.

The ability of mepacrine to act against tapeworms was also recognized in 1940 by James T Culbertson at the College of Physicians and Surgeons, Columbia University, New York, who apparently had no knowledge of Neghme's work. Noting the unexpected effectiveness of mepacrine in giardiasis (see p. 316), and working on the flimsy hypothesis that, in infected mice, the dwarf tapeworm *Hymenolepis fraterna* is located in the same part of the intestinal tract as *Giardia muris*, Culbertson examined the action of mepacrine in mice harbouring the tapeworm (149). Surprisingly, it worked and Culbertson suggested that a trial in human tapeworm infections was strongly indicated. Several small studies in Latin America and by the parasitologist Paul Beaver in New Orleans at the end of the Second World War confirmed the effectiveness of mepacrine in *Taenia* infections, but the value of the drug was not generally appreciated until 10 years after Neghme's and Culbertson's discovery. The publication that triggered wider interest was a report in 1951 by Mark Hoekenga, working for the United Fruit Company at La Lima Hospital on the North coast of Honduras, of the successful use of Atabrine in 40 Honduran children and adults infected with *Taenia saginata* or the human dwarf tapeworm, *Hymenolepis nana* (150). Even then mepacrine was accepted only slowly. In the mid-1960s reports began to appear that the aminoglycoside antibiotic paromomycin—that classic example of a drug in search of a purpose (see p. 234–5)—was effective in taeniasis and there was a short fashion for its use against various tapeworms. By this time, a more attractive compound, niclosamide, had appeared on the scene.

Ernst Schraufstätter and Rudolf Gönnert synthesized niclosamide in the Bayer chemotherapy research laboratories in 1953. It was originally developed as an agent designed to kill the snails that act as the intermediate host of schistosomiasis and was marketed for this purpose in 1959 as Bayluscid. The following year the Bayer scientists were able to report that it also exhibited activity against tapeworms (151). Various small trials around the world revealed that it was safe and effective against human tapeworms and it was relaunched as Yomesan in 1962. Niclosamide was found to be so reliable that it became the favoured drug for the eradication of tapeworms, although a question mark remained over its use against the pork tapeworm, *Taenia solium*, because it causes disintegration of the worm, potentially releasing numerous eggs within the intestinal tract. Unlike the eggs of the beef tapeworm, those of *Taenia solium* can develop to the larval stage in man, sometimes migrating to the brain where they can give rise to a form of epilepsy—a condition known as cysticercosis. This danger was never substantiated and niclosamide remained in widespread use until an antischistosomal drug, praziquantel (see below), largely replaced it after it became available in the late 1970s.

Broad-spectrum anthelminthic agents

Intestinal helminths display a wide variety of forms and it was generally thought that broad-spectrum activity that was a feature of many antibacterial agents was not likely to be feasible for worms. Surprisingly, this turned out to be untrue. The first anthelminthic drugs that might legitimately be considered to be broad spectrum emerged in the 1960s. They include pyrantel and levamisole, but it was a series of compounds known as benzimidazoles that provided the real breakthrough in the treatment of worm infections in human beings and animals.

Pyrantel belongs to a group of chemicals called tetrahydropyrimidines. Various congeners were synthesized and developed in the mid-1960s in a research programme carried out at Pfizer's Central Research Laboratories in Sandwich, Kent in collaboration with the company's Chemotherapy Research Department in Groton, Connecticut (152). The nominated co-inventors of pyrantel were WC Austin, James McFarland and Lloyd Conover (who also produced the first semisynthetic tetracycline; see p. 227). Pyrantel is most active against hookworms, but also has useful effect on other worms, including the human parasites, *Ascaris lumbricoides* and *Enterobius vermicularis*. The original product, pyrantel tartrate, was restricted to veterinary use, but after a successful trial by Pfizer company's doctors against hookworm infection in East Africa in 1971 (153), the closely related pyrantel pamoate (which is less soluble and safer since it remains in the intestinal tract when given orally) was also made available for human therapy. A derivative, oxantel, was later to prove useful in whipworm infection.

Another anthelminthic agent with a claim to broad-spectrum activity, at least in its veterinary applications, is levamisole. It belongs to a group of heterocyclic molecules synthesized in the 1960s at Janssen Pharmaceutica, the company developed from 1953 by Paul Janssen from his father's pharmaceutical import business in the Flemish town of Turnhout. Paul Janssen joined the family firm in 1953 after qualifying in medicine and studying chemistry and pharmacology in several countries. He built up a team of innovative researchers and succeeded in discovering a number of important antimicrobial agents, notably the antifungal azoles (see p. 358).* After numerous fruitless attempts to find a molecule that would offer inroads into the lucrative veterinary anthelminthic market, a compound that seemed to fit the bill, tetramisole, was discovered in 1966. The discovery was a classic example of scientific serendipity in that an unexpected finding bore fruit when puzzled scientists sought an explanation of aberrant results. The American Parasitologist, William Campbell, has described the chain of events (154). Unlike most parasitological researchers, the Janssen team used chickens rather than small mammals for primary screening of potential anthelminthic compounds. One substance that seemed to work in chickens, thiazothienol, was mystifyingly found to be inactive when tested in rats and mice. However, a chemical harvested from the faeces of the chickens, identified as a metabolite of thiazothienol, did successfully eliminate helminths from infected rodents. It was a further modified variant of this active molecule that was eventually put on the veterinary market as tetramisole. As Campbell points out, it was the chickens, not the chemists, who synthesized the active compound.

Tetramisole is a mixture of different isomeric forms of the molecule and the L-isomer, levamisole, was later found to found to be responsible for most of the activity. Since it

---

* Janssen's company agreed a merger with Johnson & Johnson in 1961, but negotiated terms that allowed it to operate independently within the group. It now trades as Janssen–Cilag having joined forces with Cilag Chemie, a Swiss firm that became part of the Johnson & Johnson group in 1959.

could be given in a lower dose, it was safer to use and by 1969 was in trial in human infection with ascaris (155). Levamisole subsequently proved useful in hookworm infection, though it has little activity against threadworm or whipworm. In the mid-1970s the drug aroused considerable interest when it was found to have immunostimulant and anti-cancer effects, but as with many such compounds, these claims were soon found to be overoptimistic.

Benzimidazoles

Benzimidazoles revolutionized the treatment of intestinal worm infections in human beings and animals. They were originally investigated as anthelminthic agents in the Animal Health Division of Merck in America.

Wayne Woolley, a Canadian biochemist at the Rockefeller Institute, had floated the notion that benzimidazoles might exhibit antimicrobial activity as early as 1944 (156). Commercial interest was kindled in the 1950s when Karl Folkers, Merck's distinguished chemist who had purified the anti-pernicious anaemia factor vitamin B_{12} in the 1940s, recognized benzimidazoles as degradation products of the vitamin. Folkers, together with his colleague Clifford H Shunk, collaborated with Igor Tamm, a virologist at the Rockefeller Institute, in investigating benzimidazole derivatives as potential anti-influenza compounds, but without success. In the late 1950s, Shunk and Folkers (by now executive director of fundamental research) passed on 2-phenylbenzimidazole to Ashton Cuckler and Bill Campbell working on the anthelminthic programme in Merck's Animal Health Division. It was only after this circuitous journey that a benzimidazole was found to exhibit broad-spectrum anthelminthic activity in sheep, encouraging further investigation of this group of compounds.

Thiabendazole, the first benzimidazole to find its way onto the market, was synthesized by the chemist Horace D Brown and his colleagues at Merck and described in the literature in 1961 (157). It was marketed the following year for use in sheep and cattle. In 1964 it became available for the treatment of human infections after successful trials in the treatment of strongyloidiasis in Brazil. Thiabendazole is active against most of the common intestinal nematodes. It is also effective against the larvae of certain animal parasites that may give rise to such human problems as cutaneous larva migrans, in which the larvae of hookworms of the dog, *Ancylostoma caninum*, invade the skin causing an intense itching; and visceral larva migrans in which larvae of the dog ascarid, *Toxocara canis*, invade tissues, sometimes reaching the retina to cause problems with vision or even blindness.

Once the effectiveness of thiabendazole had been established other firms began to take a close interest in the potential of these compounds. Dozens of benzimidazoles were produced, and by 1990 at least 10 of these broad-spectrum anthelminthic drugs were available on the lucrative veterinary market. In terms of human helminth infection two of the new compounds proved particularly important: mebendazole, a product of research at Paul Janssen's organization in Belgium in the late 1960s; and albendazole developed by Smith, Kline and French (now GlaxoSmithKline) in the 1970s and marketed for human use in 1982.

The chief disadvantage of thiabendazole is that it is extremely unpleasant to take, causing nausea and sometime more serious side effects. For infections with most intestinal worms, apart from *Strongyloides stercoralis*, a difficult to treat infection for which thiabendazole still remains the drug of choice, it was superseded first by mebendazole and then by albendazole, which is the most active member of the group, though significantly more expensive.

The broad-spectrum activity of benzimidazoles is not confined to helminths. Soon after it was described, thiabendazole was shown to inhibit the growth of fungi of various kinds and it is still widely used in crop protection. Traces can frequently be found on supermarket fruit. In 1968 the DuPont Company in the United States reported the antifungal activity of a related benzimidazole, benomyl; it was marketed the following year in the United States and in 1971 reached the United Kingdom. Benomyl was widely used as a fungicide in domestic gardens as well as in agriculture. Its toxicity is low, but during the 1990s evidence emerged that implicated the substance in serious damage to the eyes in the foetuses of pregnant women who had been exposed to high concentrations. Benomyl was subsequently withdrawn from sale, though its breakdown product, carbendazim, is presently still used in crop protection. There is no evidence of similar problems with other benzimidazoles, but these compounds are known to be teratogenic and use in human medicine is contra-indicated during pregnancy.

Further investigation of the medical uses of benzimidazoles revealed activity in such diverse diseases as cerebral cysticercosis, a rare condition in which tapeworm larvae invade the brain, and hydatid disease, in which human beings act as intermediate host of the canine tapeworms, *Echinococcus granulosus* or *Echinococcus multilocularis*. The chief problem with chemotherapy of these conditions is the failure to achieve adequate concentrations of active agents at the site of infection. Albendazole (or its metabolic product albendazole sulphoxide) seems best able to do this and encouraging results have been obtained with this drug, alone or in combination with praziquantel (see below), which also has some effect in these conditions (158). An important additional use of albendazole that emerged is in the treatment of filariasis. The drug now features together with ivermectin or diethylcarbamazine in schemes to control lymphatic filariasis in the tropics (see p. 335). Most surprisingly, workers in China (including Jean-François Rossignol, who later discovered nitazoxanide; see p. 336) reported in 1986 that albendazole was also effective in the giardiasis, a disease caused by flagellate protozoa (159).

Schistosomiasis

As Professor Rosalie David and her team have convincingly demonstrated by their pioneering work on the use of non-invasive techniques to examine Egyptian mummies at the KNH Centre for Biomedical Egyptology at the University of Manchester, schistosomiasis (bilharzia) has been a problem in Egypt for at least 5000 years. The disease has always been particularly associated with the Nile delta, but it is also prevalent in many other parts of the continent, including the lakes of East Africa, as well as in parts of the

Middle East. The main species affecting human beings in these areas are *Schistosoma mansoni* (found in the mesenteric veins of the gut) and *Schistosoma haematobium* (which affects the urinary bladder). Schistosomes were exported with the slave trade to the New World and *Schistosoma mansoni* was able to establish itself and flourish in the West Indies and parts of South America. An oriental variety, *Schistosoma japonicum*, is endemic in Japan and parts of China, where paddy field workers are especially at risk, and a related species called *Schistosoma mekongi* is found, as the name suggests, along the valley of the Mekong River. Schistosomes—known as the blood fluke because the adult worms live in the bloodstream—are responsible for a great deal of morbidity and mortality principally caused not by the presence of the worms themselves, but by the long-term deposition of their eggs.

Before the twentieth century, effective treatment for bilharzia was non-existent. Patrick Manson summed it up thus:

> Our knowledge of the situations occupied by the parasite indicates the futility of attempting a rad-
> ical cure by means of poisonous substances, whether introduced by the bladder, by the rectum, or
> by the stomach. As yet we know of no direct, or other, means by which the bilharzia can be
> destroyed...Our efforts must, therefore, be confined to palliating the effects of the presence of the
> parasite (160).

Tartar emetic

Not everyone was put off by Manson's negative talk. Emetine was tried with some apparent success in China as early as 1913 and in Egypt soon afterwards (161). In 1917, John
Brian Christopherson, Director of the Civil Hospitals of Khartoum and Omdurman,
having confirmed the efficacy of tartar emetic in leishmaniasis in the Sudan, irrationally
hit on the idea of trying the same drug in bilharzia. Amazingly it seemed to work (162).
By 1921, colleagues in the Church Missionary Society's hospital in Cairo were able to
report on the largely successful application of Christopherson's treatment regimen in
1000 cases, albeit with '10 deaths which could in anyway be attributed to the treatment or
to the disease itself' (163).

In fact, Christopherson did not have priority for the discovery of the efficacy of tartar
emetic in schistosomiasis, as another claimant, James McDonagh was quick to write to
The Lancet to point out. McDonagh, a surgeon to the London Lock Hospital*—and the
first practitioner in the country to adopt Ehrlich's Salvarsan—had, in a book on venereal
diseases published in 1915, slipped in the following short passage:

> Although not a venereal disease, I should like to mention here that I have had great success in
> treating cases of bilharzia with intravenous injections of antimony (164).

---

* Lock hospitals catered for patients with venereal diseases. They were originally setup for patients with
leprosy, but turned to venereal diseases in the eighteenth century. In McDonagh's time, the London
Lock Hospital had two departments: one for women in Harrow Road, close to the Paddington work-
house, the other for men and out-patients in Dean street, Soho.

Despite the toxicity of tartar emetic and the difficulty of delivering the repeated intra-venous injections that were required, it became standard treatment for schistosomiasis between the two World Wars and beyond. Plainly, this situation was unsatisfactory and prevention was energetically pursued as an alternative.

Bilharzia is transmitted by contact with water inhabited by certain types of snails that provide an essential host in which the infective forms—called cercariae—develop. In the absence of satisfactory therapeutic drugs much largely fruitless effort went into elaborate strategies to try to persuade local populations to adopt more hygienic practices and to eradicate the snail intermediate hosts, thus breaking the cycle of transmission. One such scheme funded by the Rockefeller's International Health Division took place in Egypt, where the former Chinese medical missionary, Claude Barlow and M Abdel Aziz conducted a vigorous campaign at the aptly named Bilharzia Snail Eradication Section (165). The scale of the problem, the difficulty of imposing the hygiene message and the ingenuity of the molluscs all conspired to thwart the good intentions of this scheme. In the event, matters got worse as irrigation and major dam projects extended the habitat of the snails.

Attempts to improve on tartar emetic were pursued by Hans Schmidt and his colleagues in Elberfeld as part of their research into agents suitable for the treatment of leishmaniasis (see p. 307–9). In 1927 or 1928 Schmidt's team (now including the newly recruited Gerhard Domagk) synthesized a trivalent antimony compound, which they called sti-bophen. As well as submitting it for clinical trial in leishmaniasis, they had the foresight to offer the compound to Mohamed Khalil, Professor of Parasitology in the University of Cairo and a former pupil of the famous helminthologist, Robert Leiper[*] at the London School. Stibophen was less toxic than tartar emetic and Khalil, who was acquiring a grow-ing reputation in Egypt as an expert in schistosomiasis,[†] enthusiastically endorsed the new drug (166). Bayer launched it in 1929 as Fouadin, a name chosen to honour King Fuad the first king of modern Egypt. Sadly, Fouadin failed to live up to Khalil's optimistic assess-ment of its royal potential. Although it continued to be used to modest effect for many years it never supplanted tartar emetic as the favoured drug among tropical physicians. Much the same fate befell three antimonials that emerged in the 1950s: Triostam, a triva-lent version of sodium antimony gluconate (see p. 309), investigated by Owen Standen's group at the Wellcome Laboratories of Tropical Medicine; antimony dimercapto succi-nate, synthesized by Ernst Friedheim and marketed by Roche as Astiban; and antimony lithium thiomalate, a Rhône–Poulenc compound marketed as Anthiomaline.

New approaches to bilharzia treatment

The first real alternative to antimonial compounds, lucanthone (Miracil D), came from work carried out by Walter Kikuth, Rudolf Gönnert, and Hans Mauss in the Bayer

---

[*] Leiper had himself studied in Cairo in 1907 under the equally famous German helminthologist, Arthur Looss.

[†] Khalil was a strong advocate of the use of copper sulphate in the eradication of snails. Claude Barlow scornfully criticized his methods and the two men became bitter enemies. See Farley, reference 165.

Laboratories. By 1936, Kikuth had managed to establish not only a suitable snail colony, but also a model of schistosomiasis in monkeys, and a rather cheaper one in mice, which were exclusively used when monkeys became unavailable after the outbreak of war. Experiments were started on a series of chemically modified xanthones—naturally occurring chemicals that form the basis for many dyestuffs—prepared by Hans Mauss. Xanthones have a tricyclic structure reminiscent of acridines and Mauss used substitutions that had been successful in the development of Atebrin (mepacrine). The first of these compounds to exhibit antischistosomal activity was synthesized in 1938 and given the name Miracil A. Closely similar variants, Miracil B and Miracil C were also active, but it was the fourth molecule in this series, Miracil D, in which a sulphur atom had been introduced to form a thioxanthone, which generated most interest.

Miracil D was synthesized by Hans Mauss in December 1939 and developed during the Second World War. It was one of the compounds revealed during Allied interrogation of Bayer scientists at the end of the war. According to John Farley, who researched British Colonial Office documents of the period, Kikuth had exaggerated the value of the compound by suppressing information about its harmful effects in order to protect his staff from military service (167). Whatever the truth of the matter, the German workers continued to claim that the compound was well tolerated in animal experiments when their work was eventually published in 1946 (168).

The great advantage of lucanthone, as the German scientists realized, was that it could be given by mouth and was effective in a short course of therapy. These attractive features compared with the currently available alternatives led to marketing of the drug as Miracil D by Bayer after extensive testing in Africa, notably by Dyson Blair in Southern Rhodesia (now Zimbabwe).* Ironically, it proved more effective against urinary schistosomiasis than against the intestinal form that had been the subject of the original animal tests. An alternative route to the synthesis of lucanthone was developed in the Wellcome Laboratories in London and marketed as Nilodin by Burroughs Wellcome. The helminthologist John Watson, who was involved in this work, helped to organize early clinical trials in Cairo in 1948; fascinated by the Arab world, he converted to Islam, changed his name to Mohammed Ali Watson and became a professor in the University of Baghdad (169).

Notwithstanding its obvious attractions, lucanthone soon fell out of favour, partly because it proved unreliable, but also because of the frequency of side effects, which were sometimes severe. In the 1960s Reimer Strufe at Bayer in Germany and a group led by Sydney Archer at the Winthrop Research Laboratories in America discovered that a metabolite of lucanthone was responsible for the antischistosomal activity. The active substance, hycanthone was somewhat less toxic and was marketed by Sterling Winthrop as Etrenol. By this time alternatives were beginning to appear and both compounds were largely abandoned for human use. First on the scene were niridazole, metrifonate, and oxamniquine.

* Dyson Milroy Blair founded the Bilharzia Research Laboratory in 1939. It was renamed the Blair Research Laboratory after he died in 1978 and in now incorporated in the Blair Research Institute in Harare.

Niridazole emerged from a programme of research into nitrothiazole derivatives related to the nitroimidazoles (see p. 312) carried out by Paul Schmidt and his colleagues in the Ciba Research Laboratories in Basel (170). It turned out to be something of a 9-day wonder. It soon revealed an array of unpleasant side effects and proved to be unreliable in intestinal schistosomiasis. Use of niridazole was consequently abandoned after a few years, though it survived for a while as a drug reputed on slender grounds to be useful in infection with the guinea worm, *Dracunculus medinensis*.

Metrifonate, known in the United States as trichlorfon, is an organophosphate, originally introduced in the 1950s as an agricultural insecticide. Its activity against schistosomes was investigated in the early 1970s and it became immediately popular. Although its activity is restricted to *Schistosoma haematobium*, it is well tolerated in the doses used therapeutically and has the undoubted attraction of being cheap.

In contrast to metrifonate and niridazole, oxamniquine is much more effective against *Schistosoma mansoni* than against other schistosomes. It was developed in the Pfizer Central Research Laboratories in Sandwich, Kent and first described in 1973 at the most active of a group of compounds that had been that had been the subject of a research programme started in the late 1960s (171). After clinical trials in South America, and Africa it was widely used in a large schistosomiasis control programme in Brazil, a role for which it is well suited, since it is well tolerated and effective when administered as a single dose. However, its lack of broad antischistosomal activity limited its popularity, particularly after a more active and reliable agent, praziquantel, came on the scene in the late 1970s.

Praziquantel

Praziquantel emerged through a programme of research started by scientists at the firm of E Merck in Darmstadt and in an unusual example of inter-company collaboration, brought to fruition at Bayer's chemotherapy institute. In the early 1970s the Merck scientists were looking for effective tranquillizers and had found that substances with a structure described chemically as pyrazinoisoquinolines provided promising leads. The compounds turned out to have no advantages over existing tranquillizing drugs and under an agreement with Bayer they were passed over to Rudolf Gönnert at Elberfeld for testing for possible veterinary use (172). Gönnert's team discovered in 1975 that one of these compounds, given the name Embay 8440 in acknowledgement of the joint involvement of E Merck and Bayer, rapidly inactivated tapeworms in experimental animals. The drug was subsequently introduced on the veterinary market as Droncit for use in tapeworm infections of cats and dogs. Further investigation by the Bayer scientists soon revealed that the drug was also active in mice experimentally infected with the human blood fluke, *Schistosoma mansoni*.

Collaboration with Merck continued and in January 1977, the Merck inventors of Embay 8400 were able to submit a paper to the Swiss journal *Experientia* claiming excellent activity not only against tapeworms, but also all schistosomes pathogenic to man (173). The evidence for this last claim was revealed in March 1977 at a meeting of the Deutschsprachige Tropenmedizinischer Gessellschaften (German-speaking tropical medicine societies) in Lindau, Lake Constance, where the English schistosomiasis expert, Gerry Webbe, Professor of Parasitology at the London School of Hygiene and Tropical Medicine, presented results indicating the broad-spectrum antischistosomal activity of the new compound.

Fortuitously, Gerry Webbe had briefly worked in Bayer's clinical trials department before joining the London School in 1967 and had retained contact with his former colleagues. In collaboration with George Nelson, Professor of Medical Helminthology, Webbe had successfully established at Winches Farm, the London School's field station near St Albans,* animal models of all three species responsible for most human schistosomiasis: *Schistosoma haematobium* in baboons; *Schistosoma mansoni* in monkeys and baboons; and *Schistosoma japonicum* in cats. Webbe and Nelson, together with other colleagues at Winches Farm, showed that praziquantel was very effective against each of these species when administered orally.

According to Nelson, Bayer was interested in the drug only as a veterinary product and needed convincing of its potential in the human field (174). Fortunately, good sense prevailed and field trials in human schistosomiasis were subsequently conducted under the auspices of the World Health Organization. By 1979 it was clear that praziquantel represented an important breakthrough in the treatment and control of all types of human schistosomiasis. Crucially the drug was effective after administration of a single oral dose making it an important tool, together with molluscicides, in attempts to eradicate bilharzia from endemic areas. As a bonus, the drug proved very effective against human tapeworms and most trematodes other than schistosomiasis, including the Chinese liver fluke, *Clonorchis sinensis*, which is widespread in parts of the Far East. The only disappointment was that praziquantel proved ineffective against the sheep liver fluke, *Fasciola hepatica*, which occasionally causes human infections in many sheep-rearing areas of the world, including Britain. Treatment of this infection remains problematic. Bithionol, a toxic phenolic compound, or triclabendazole, a veterinary imidazole derivative, seem to be the only compounds with much activity.

Filarial worms

Various types of filarial worms commonly infect human beings in the tropics and subtropics. Several of them cause remarkably few problems, although the blood of those harbouring the worms may contain numerous larvae—microfilariae. Some species, however, are involved in serious disease: none more so than *Onchocerca volvulus* and *Wuchereria bancrofti*. *Onchocerca volvulus* is a common cause of blindness—so-called river blindness—a scourge in parts of tropical Africa, where, in some localities the entire population is affected; *Wuchereria bancrofti* (and, in south-east Asia, the related *Brugia malayi)* is responsible for lymphatic filariasis, which sometimes leads to the horrifically deforming condition elephantiasis in many countries throughout the tropical belt (see p. 17).

---

* The London School of Hygiene and Tropical Medicine acquired Winches Farm as an animal parasitology research unit in 1953; Gerry Webbe was appointed Scientific Director there in 1967. The unit closed in 1992.

Although Leonard Rogers had experimented with tartar emetic in the therapy of lymphatic filariasis in India in 1920 and other antimonials were also tried, nothing of any consequence could be done to treat any of the filarial infections until after the Second World War. Attempts to control the diseases were largely restricted to the use of insecticides against the insect vectors and, in the case of elephantiasis, surgery to alleviate the worst effects of the condition. Insect control campaigns were successful in reducing the incidence of new infections in some places, but it was the arrival of effective drugs that gradually altered the prospects for the unfortunate victims of filariasis.

The first ray of hope for those suffering from river blindness came in 1945, ironically with a drug that had been available for 20 years: the antitrypanosomal compound, suramin (see p. 274–7). The discovery was made in what was then the Belgian Congo under circumstances that illustrate the extraordinary and questionable lengths to which colonial doctors would go in pursuit of cures for tropical diseases. According to his own account (175), the Belgian physician, Lucien Van Hoof had been pursuing the laudable aim of finding an effective medication for onchocerciasis since 1931; he had tried without success various arsenical and antimonial compounds as well as acridine dyes such as Atebrin. In 1944 the systematic search for a cure was resumed with the hapless sufferers being subjected to injections of anthelminthics such as oil of chenopodium, pyrethrins, oil of eucalyptus and thymol. Many of the older antiprotozoal drugs were also tried again, and one, a proprietary preparation called Tryparosan—a derivative of the dye parafuchsin—was found to have a clear, but transient effect. Van Hoof was encouraged to take a fresh look at other antitrypanosomal agents, and the merit of this approach received an immediate boost from an unexpected source: two 'volunteers' who had taken part in an experiment in 1942 to study the transmission of onchocerciasis by blackflies (*Simulium damnosum*) had also foolishly agreed to be infected with trypanosomes in order to examine the prophylactic efficacy of the new drug pentamidine (see p. 283). Prophylaxis evidently failed, since the volunteers developed trypanosomiasis and received ICI's version of suramin, Antrypol, to control the infection. In 1945, 2 years after the treatment, when the volunteers were recalled for a follow-up examination, it was discovered that they had also been cured of their onchocerciasis. A formal trial of Antrypol or Belganyl (a Belgian variety of suramin) in onchocerciasis was started in July 1945. The drug successfully cured the infection, but the dosage that had been safely used in sleeping sickness (2 g twice weekly) produced severe reactions caused by substances released from the dying worms. Fortunately, a reduced dose of 1 g per week proved to be still effective. The findings of Van Hoof's study were confirmed in a study of 13 children with mild ocular onchocerciasis conducted in the Gold Coast by the British ophthalmologist (and, in later life, Anglican priest) John Sarkies (176). Suramin is still the only drug that is able to kill the adult worms rather than the larval forms (microfilariae), but it is seldom used because of its toxicity.

Diethylcarbamazine

Van Hoof's results were published in 1947, and in the same year Yellapragada SubbaRow's group at Lederle Laboratories published a series of papers detailing their work on potential antifilarial compounds. Many American troops had returned from the Pacific war zone with filarial infections and in 1944 SubbaRow, an Indian with first hand experience of filariasis, recruited Redginal Hewitt—formerly an expert on bird malaria from Alabama—to take up the challenge of finding a drug to treat this condition. Hewitt's preferred model was naturally acquired infection with the filarial worm *Litomosoides carinii* in cotton rats. In April 1945 a piperazine compound originally investigated as a possible painkiller, but discarded for that purpose, was found to display antifilarial activity in the animal model. Numerous piperazine derivatives were subsequently synthesized and tested. The most active turned out to be one given the laboratory code 84-L synthesized by the organic chemist, Sam Kushner; it was subsequently called diethylcarbamazine, quickly given the trade name Hetrazan, and now known universally as DEC. Hewitt had found that DEC had a profound effect on infection in cotton rats and dogs without causing any serious toxicity (177). Subsequent testing by Hewitt and others in human lymphatic filariasis in Puerto Rico and the Philippines, and in onchocerciasis in Mexico, confirmed the value of DEC—though not the lack of toxicity: it sometimes leads to severe reactions to the dying microfilariae.

DEC became the mainstay of treatment for filarial infections throughout the world. In truth, apart from the very toxic suramin, there was little else on offer. Around 1959, the irrepressible Ernst Friedheim synthesized a derivative of his antitrypanosomal drug Mel B (see p. 281) for which he had high hopes. He called the new drug Mel W and it was originally intended as an improved form of Mel B. Sadly, it proved equally harmful and he tried his luck instead with filariasis. Although Mel W appeared to have some effect it was no match for DEC and was soon dropped. A further derivative, Mel D, fared no better. It was not until the 1980s, when a remarkable antibiotic called ivermectin was introduced, that prospects for the millions of sufferers from filariasis around the globe began to improve.

Ivermectin

The avermectins are a group of naturally occurring antibiotics produced by a strain of *Streptomyces avermitilis* grown from a soil sample collected near Kawana Golf Club in Shizuoka Prefecture, Japan around 1975 (178). Satoshi Ōmura and his colleagues at the Kitasato Institute in Tokyo isolated the producer organism. Ōmura had met Boyd Woodruff (who had strong connections with Japan) and other representatives of the Merck, Sharp, and Dohme Company while working in the United States from 1971–1973. Together they had negotiated a collaborative research deal under the terms of which novel antibiotics discovered in the Kitasato Institute should be sent to Merck in America for testing as potential anthelminthic agents. When the new streptomycete was discovered it was therefore passed on to Merck's Laboratories in Rahway, New Jersey, where Bill Campbell headed an anthelminthic research programme in the company's Animal Health Division. Tests in mice rapidly revealed the potency of avermectins against nematode worms and field trials confirmed that the activity extended to a wide range of nematode parasites that are troublesome in animals.

The most potent component of the mixture of closely related antibiotics produced by *Streptomyces avermitilis* was found to be avermectin B_1 (abamectin), which was soon marketed for veterinary use. By 1977 Campbell's group had found that a derivative in which two hydrogen atoms had been introduced at an appropriate point in the intricate heterocyclic structure of avermectin B$_1$ was at least as active and was less toxic. This compound, ivermectin, was also launched onto the veterinary market in 1981. Meanwhile, the avermectins had also been found to exhibit the remarkable property of killing many insects and other arthropods, such as ticks and mites. This surprising discovery was made when ivermectin was administered to a mite-infected rabbit in Merck's animal colony. Confirmation came during the investigation of the efficacy of ivermectin in the treatment of a form of onchocerciasis in horses: one of the horses was suffering from an unsuspected bot fly infection of the stomach and both the diagnosis and cure were indicated by the appearance of bot fly larvae in the horse's faeces (154). Ivermectin, as a safe drug that was not only able to control worms, but arthropod parasites such as bot flies, warble flies, mange mites, and ticks as well, was a runaway success. Within a decade it was among the world's bestselling animal health care products.

The work of Campbell's group on equine onchocerciasis pointed the way to the possible use of ivermectin in human infection. The first tentative step was to test the effectiveness of the new drug in other types of onchocerciasis in cattle. With the help of the Special Programme for Research and Training in Tropical Diseases a field trial of bovine onchocerciasis was organized in Australia. By the end of 1978 Campbell, who was a member of the Filariasis Scientific Committee of the World Health Organization tropical disease research programme, had assembled enough evidence to convince the Merck management that the company should put resources into investigating the use of ivermectin in human onchocerciasis (179). With the support of the World Health Organization, a preliminary dose-finding study was started in February 1981 in Senegal, West Africa, by a team led by one of Merck's doctors, the Bangladeshi, Mohammed Aziz. It showed that ivermectin, if given in sufficient dosage, was, as hoped, able to reduce the numbers of microfilariae found in skin (180). Further work by Aziz and others during the next few years established the unprecedented efficacy of ivermectin in curing, if not the blindness—which was irreversible—at least the intense itching and skin changes caused by the larval forms. As an incidental windfall, the drug also relieved sufferers of many of their intestinal roundworms.

Ivermectin is not a cure for onchocerciasis, since the adult worms may survive. Repeat treatment is needed in endemic areas and a scheme was devised whereby patients are given the drug at 6-monthly or yearly intervals. But first a major barrier had to be overcome. Ivermectin is expensive and the cost of treatment was far beyond the resources of the countries where it was most needed. In 1987 Roy Vagelos a former National Institute of Health medical biochemist who had risen to become chief executive officer of Merck, announced that the company had reached an agreement with the World Health Organization to donate ivermectin free for use in human onchocerciasis control programmes (181). The distinguished British filariasis expert Brian Duke, who had suggested to a reporter in a magazine interview that Merck ought to provide ivermectin free for human use, reputedly sowed the seed of this philanthropic gesture (182). The scenario is entirely plausible: Duke's voice was an influential one. He had worked tirelessly on filariasis in Africa since joining the Colonial Medical Service in 1953 and subsequently became head of the World Health Organization filariasis unit and medical director of the Carter Center's* River Blindness Foundation.

The 'Mectizan Donation Program' as it came to be known (Mectizan is Merck's trade name for ivermectin) went ahead from 1988. It was a pioneering initiative in corporate philanthropy made possible by the happy conjunction of three circumstances: a drug that was reaping enormous profits in the veterinary market, but had little prospect of sales in human medicine; a company ethos dating back to George Merck, son of the American company's founder,[†] that encouraged bold gestures; and favourable United States tax laws for charitable donations. It served as the model for other commercial schemes to make unaffordable drugs available in poor countries.

Early indications were that ivermectin was not reliably active against filarial worms other than *Onchocerca volvulus* and it took some further time for its wider role in the therapy of filarial diseases to become clear. From 1987 reports began to appear of the effectiveness of the drug in lymphatic filariasis caused by *Wuchereria bancrofti* and numerous studies confirmed the finding in the ensuing decade (183). In the meantime a benzimidazole derivative, albendazole (see p. 325–6), was also found to be effective in bancroftian filariasis. Thus, three effective drugs, DEC, ivermectin, and albendazole became available for the treatment of this long-neglected condition. None seemed superior to the others and a number of studies indicated that combination therapy might be best of all. The World Health Organization opted to promote the use of a permutation of any two of the three drugs in control programmes for lymphatic filariasis. In 1998 Merck extended the Mectizan Donation Program to include lymphatic filariasis in Africa and in the same year SmithKline Beecham (now GlaxoSmithKline) added their weight by agreeing to donate albendazole.

Ivermectin has certainly transformed the prospects for the millions of sufferers from filariasis in tropical regions. Its value in human infections in the rest of the world has been on a lesser scale, but the activity of this remarkable compound against arthropods offers one valuable benefit. The skin infection, scabies, caused by the mite *Sarcoptes scabei*, which burrows into the skin causing intense itching, is far from eradicated in Britain and other developed countries. Ivermectin is effective in this condition and is often used when topical treatment fails.

Perhaps the most astonishing development in the treatment of filariasis in recent years has been the discovery that targeting *Wolbachia*, a rickettsia-like bacterium that exists in an endosymbiotic relationship with filarial worms, prevents the adult worms from producing microfilariae. In 1999 Achim Hoerauf and co-workers at the Bernhard Nocht

---

* Founded in 1982 by former American President Jimmy Carter and his wife Rosalynn in partnership with Emory University in Atlanta, Georgia.

† The American firm under Georg Merck senior became independent of the parent company in Darmstadt (which still trades as E. Merck) after the First World War (See footnote, p. 131).

Institute for Tropical Medicine in Hamburg, together with colleagues in Edinburgh and Berlin, showed that eliminating these bacteria with tetracyclines, causes a marked reduction in the number of microfilariae circulating in the bloodstream of rodents harbouring *Litomosoides sigmodontis*. The scientists had not been seeking a cure, but were trying to find evidence of whether the bacteria existed in a mutually beneficial relationship with the worms, or were present in some pathogenic role. But they were not slow to realize that their finding had practical therapeutic implications (184). By Spring 2000, they were able to report preliminary results showing that 6 weeks daily therapy with doxycycline significantly reduced microfilariae in volunteer onchocerciasis patients in Ghana (185).

Shortcomings and challenges

Protozoal infections

As the twentieth century drew to a close, doctors dealing with parasitic diseases could look back on 100 years of considerable progress. Effective drugs are now available to treat most protozoal infections, but many problems remain. Therapy for several diseases, notably African trypanosomiasis and leishmaniasis, still relies largely on drugs that carry considerable risks of toxicity and is far from satisfactory. Suitable agents with which to treat South American trypanosomiasis remain elusive.

Even where safe and effective treatment is available for protozoal infections therapeutic options remain precarious. Many fewer alternatives are available than is the case for most bacterial infections. Treatment of malaria—still, with tuberculosis and AIDS, among the world's top three killers—is constantly threatened by the development and spread of resistance to available drugs (see p. 400–1). Resistance also occurs in other protozoal infections, although it is happily uncommon in some of them, including giardiasis and trichomoniasis. The danger is that very few safe and effective alternatives exist in these infections.

The latest drug to be licensed as an antiprotozoal agent is nitazoxanide, a nitrothiazole derivative of niclosamide (see p. 323). It was developed by Romark Laboratories in Florida, a company founded in 1993 by the French scientist Jean-François Rossignol and his business partner Marc Ayers. Rossignol first synthesized nitazoxanide while working at the University of Lille in France in the mid-1970s. It exhibits anthelminthic activity and was marketed in France and Switzerland for the treatment of tapeworms in dogs and cats. The first exploratory tests in human therapy were similarly on children and adults with *Taenia saginata* and *Hymenolepis nana* infections (186). However, nitazoxanide turned out to be another of those remarkable agents in which useful activity extends well beyond that for which it was originally designed. The spectrum of activity extends not only to intestinal helminths and, possibly, the liver fluke *Fasciola hepatica*, but also to various protozoa and bacteria that share the feature of anaerobic metabolism (187). It is now on sale in some countries for the treatment of giardiasis (and cryptosporidiosis, an occasional pathogen of the immunosuppressed), but its eventual place remains to be properly defined.

Helminth infections

Thanks to the importance of worm infections in animals, prospects for human helminth infection have also been transformed. Astonishingly, most human worm infections can be now treated with just three relatively safe drugs: albendazole, ivermectin, and praziquantel. Resistance is presently not a major problem. Fortunately, drug resistance does not arise as easily in helminths as in bacteria, protozoa, fungi, or viruses, partly because many helminths do not multiply in the human host. None the less, examples of infection with several types of worm that are refractory to standard therapy are well documented (188). For the present most concern exists among animal parasites, but examples also exist for human worm infections and the implications for human infections of the development of resistance in animal parasites are clear.

The challenge for the twenty-first century is to make antiparasitic drugs available to the millions who bear the burden of the most serious parasitic illnesses. They are the people in greatest need of these drugs. Yet they are the ones who are generally deprived of ready access to medical care and are least able to afford treatment for their ailments.

References

1. Maegraith BG (1972). History of the Liverpool School of Tropical Medicine. *Med Hist* **16**, 354–68; Power HJ (1999). *Tropical medicine in the twentieth century. A history of the Liverpool School of Tropical Medicine 1898–1990*. Kegan Paul International, London.

2. Manson-Bahr P (1956). *History of the School of Tropical Medicine in London (1899–1949)*. HK Lewis, London.

3. James RR (1994). *Henry Wellcome*. Hodder and Stoughton, London.

4. Beer JJ (1958). Coal tar dye manufacture and the origins of the modern industrial research laboratory. *Isis* **49**, 123–31.

5. Dünschede H-B (1971). *Tropenmedizinische Forschung bei Bayer* p. 18–22. Michael Triltsch Verlag, Düsseldorf.

6. Duggan AJ (1977). Bruce and the African trypanosomes. *Am J Trop Med Hyg* **26**, 1080–3.

7. Emmerich E, Hallenberger O (1919). Sind Trypanosomiasis und Syphilis vewandte Krankheiten? *Archiv für Schiffs- und Tropen-Hygiene* **23**, 1–17.

8. Yorke W (1921). The treatment of a case of Rhodesian sleeping sickness by the preparation known as 'Bayer 205'. *Ann Trop Med Parasitol* **15**, 479–82.

9. Dünschede H-B (1971). *Tropenmedizinische Forschung bei Bayer*, pp. 15–54. Michael Triltsch Verlag, Düsseldorf.

10. Huxley J (31 December 1923). Probing the secrets of life. *Daily Herald* 1923. Cited by Dünschede H-B (1971). *Tropenmedizinische Forschung bei Bayer*, p. 51. Michael Triltsch Verlag, Düsseldorf.

11. Lesch JE (2007). *The first miracle drugs. How the sulfa drugs transformed medicine*, pp. 72–81. Oxford University Press, New York.

12. Breinl A, Todd JL (1907). Atoxyl in the treatment of trypanosomiasis. *Lancet* **1**, 132–4.

13. Cook AR (1907–1908). On sleeping sickness as met with in Uganda, especially with regard to its treatment. *Trans Soc Trop Med Hyg* **1**, pp. 25–43.

14. Barrowcliffe M, Pyman FL, Remfry FGP (1908). Aromatic arsonic acids. *J Chem Soc, Trans* **93**, 1893–1901.

15. Ollivier G, Legros D (2001). Trypanosomiase humaine africaine: histoire de la thérapeutique et de ses échecs. *Trop Med Int Health* **6**, 855–63.

16. The War Office (1941). *Memoranda on medical diseases in tropical and sub-tropical areas*, p. 217. His Majesty's Stationery Office, London.

17. Prescott JF, Baggot JD, Walker RD (2000). *Antimicrobial therapy in veterinary medicine*, 3rd edn., p. 360. Iowa State University Press, Ames.

18. Bendiner E (1992). Louise Pearce: a 'magic bullet' for African sleeping sickness. *Hospital Practice (office edition)* **27**, 207–12, 214–5, 218 and 221.

19. Jacobs WA (1923–1924). The chemotherapy of protozoan and bacterial infections. *The Harvey Lectures* **19**, 67–95.

20. Jacobs WA, Heidelberger M (1919). Chemotherapy of trypanosome and spirochete infections: chemical series. I. *N*-phenylglycine amide-*p*-arsonic acid. *J Exp Med* **30**, 411–5; Brown WH, Pearce L (1919). Chemotherapy of trypanosome and spirochete infections: biological series. I–IV. *J Exp Med* **30**, 417–96.

21. Pearce L (1921). Studies on the treatment of human trypanosomiasis with tryparsamide (the sodium salt of *N*-phenylglycineamide-*p*-arsonic acid. *J Exp Med* **34** (Suppl.), 1–104.

22. Chesterman CC (1923). Tryparsamide in sleeping sickness. A study of forty cases, with special reference to the cerebrospinal fluid. *Trans R Soc Trop Med Hyg* **16**, 394–408.

23. Chesterman CC (1924). Tryparsamide in sleeping sickness II. *Trans R Soc Trop Med Hyg* **18**, 131–7.

24. Power HJ (1999). *Tropical medicine in the twentieth century. A history of the Liverpool School of Tropical Medicine 1898–1990*, pp. 79–103. Kegan Paul International, London.

25. Yorke W, Murgatroyd F, Glyn-Hughes F, Lester HMO, Ross AOF (1936). A new arsenical for the treatment of syphilis and trypanosomiasis. *BMJ* **1**, 1042–8.

26. Chesterman C (1979). Dr Ernest AH Friedman. A tribute on his eightieth birthday. *Trans R Soc Trop Med Hyg* **73**, 597–8.

27. Friedheim EAH. (1959). Some approaches to the development of chemotherapeutic compounds. *Ann Trop Med Parasitol* **53**, 1–9.

28. Friedheim EAH (1949). Mel B in the treatment of human trypanosomiasis. *Am J Trop Med Hyg* **29**, 173–80.

29. Apted FIC (1953). The treatment of advanced cases of Rhodesian sleeping sickness by Mel B and arsobal. *Trans R Soc Trop Med Hyg* **47**, 387–98.

30. Dale H (1943). A prospect of therapeutics. *BMJ* **2**, 411–6.

31. Grischow JD (August 2004). Tsetse and trypanosomiasis in the Gold Coast 1924–1954. Working Papers on Ghana: historical and contemporary studies Nr 5. Available at: http://www.helsinki.fi/~hweiss/wopag/wopag5new.pdf

32. Saunders GFT (1941). Preliminary report on the treatment of sleeping sickness by 4:4′-diamidino diphenoxy pentane. *Ann Trop Med Parasitol* **35**, 169–74.

33. Bacchi CJ, Ciaccio EI, Koren LE (1969). Effects of some antitumor agents on growth and glycolytic enzymes of the flagellate *Crithidia*. *J Bacteriol* **98**, 23–8.

34. Bacchi CJ, Lipschik GY, Nathan HC (1977). Polyamines in trypanosomatids. *J Bacteriol* **131**, 657–61.

35. Bacchi CJ, Nathan HC, Hutner SH, McCann PP, Sjoerdsma A (1980). Polyamine metabolism: a potential therapeutic target in trypanosomes. *Science* **210**, 332–4.

36. Sjoerdsma AG (10 December 2000). Medical miracle frustrated. A wonder drug for sleeping sickness is not available to patients in Africa. *Baltimore Sun*. Available from the paper's archives at: http://www.baltimoresun.com/

37. Van Nieuwenhove S, Schechter PJ, Declercq J, Boné G, Burke J, Sjoerdsma A (1985). Treatment of gambiense sleeping sickness in the Sudan with oral DFMO (DL-alpha-difluoromethylornithine), an inhibitor of ornithine decarboxylase; first field trial. *Trans R Soc Trop Med Hyg* **79**, 692–8.

38. Snow RW (2000). The burden of malaria: understanding the balance between immunity, public health and control. *J Med Microbiol* **49**, 1053–5.

39. Greenwood D (1995). Conflicts of interest: the genesis of antimalarial agents in peace and war. *J Antimicrob Chemother* **36**, 857–72.

40. Bruce-Chwatt LJ, de Zulueta J (1980). *The rise and fall of malaria in Europe*, pp. 89–105. Oxford University Press, Oxford.

41. Low GC, Gregg AL (1925). "Smalarina" in malaria. *Lancet* **1**, 1339–441.

42. Schönhöfer F (1965). 40 Jahre Plasmochin. *Arzneimittelforschung* **15**, 1256–8.

43. Dünschede H-B (1971). *Tropenmedizinische Forschung bei Bayer*, p. 63. Michael Triltsch Verlag, Düsseldorf.

44. Kopanaris P (1911). Die Wirkung von Chinin, Salvarsan und Atoxyl auf die Proteosoma (*Plasmodium praecox*) Infektion des Kanarienvogels. *Archiv für Schiffs- und Tropen-Hygiene* **15**, 586–96.

45. Bishop A (1942). Chemotherapy and avian malaria. *Parasitology* **34**, 1–54.

46. Whitrow M (1990). Wagner-Jauregg and fever therapy. *Med Hist* **34**, 294–310.

47. Bruce-Chwatt LJ (1973). Malaria Reference Laboratory. *BMJ* **2**, 181.

48. Anonymous (1931). A drug which prevents malaria. *Lancet* **1**, 1248–9.

49. Editorial (1975). A final curtain. *BMJ* **2**, 578; Cox F (2003). Marjorie Ethel Maryon 1914–2002 *Bull Trop Med Int Health* **10**, 5.

50. Martindale WH (ed.) (1932). *The extra pharmacopoeia of Martindale and Westcott*, 20th edn., p. 744. HK Lewis, London.

51. Mühlens P (1926). Die Behandlung der natürlichen menschlichen Malariainfektionen mit Plasmochin. *Archiv für Schiffs- und Tropenhygiene* **30** (Beiheft 3), 25–35.

52. Cordes W (1926). Experiences with plasmochin in malaria. *Annual Report of the United Fruit Company Medical Department*, pp. 72–3.

53. Sinton JA, Bird W (1928). Studies in malaria with special reference to treatment. Part IX. Plasmoquine in the treatment of malaria. *Indian J Med Res* **16**, 159–77.

54. Report (1933). The therapeutics of malaria. Third general report of the Malaria Commission. *Q Bull Health Organ League Nations* **2**, 181–228.

55. Shortt HE, Garnham PCC (1948). The pre-erythrocytic development of *Plasmodium cynomolgi* and *Plasmodium vivax*. *Trans R Soc Trop Med Hyg* **41**, 785–95.

56. Napier LE, Das Gupta BM (1932). Atebrin: a synthetic drug for the treatment of malaria. *Indian Med Gazette* **67**, 181–6.

57. Green R (1932). A report of fifty cases of malaria treated with atebrin. *Lancet* **1**, 826–9.

58. Briercliffe R (1935). The Ceylon malaria epidemic 1934–35. Report of the Director of Medical and Sanitary Services. Ceylon Government Press, Columbo; Fernando PB, Sandarasegaram AP (1935). A clinical study of 647 patients treated for malaria during the Ceylon epidemic of 1934–1935. *Ceylon Journal of Science Section D. Med Sci* (Part 4) **3**, 195–233.

59. Menk W, Mohr W (1950). Sontochin (Nivaquine) in seiner therapeutischen Wirkung bei Malaria. *Zeitschrift für Tropenmedizin und Parasitologie* **2**, 351–61.

60. Loshak D (1994). *From ICI to Zeneca*. Zeneca Pharmaceuticals, Wilmslow.

61. Anonymous (1957). *Pharmaceutical research in I.C.I. 1936–1957*, pp. 2–3. Imperial Chemical Industries Ltd.

62. Fairley NH (1945). Chemotherapeutic suppression and prophylaxis in malaria: experimental investigation undertaken by medical research teams in Australia. *Trans R Soc Trop Med Hyg* **38**, 311–65.

63. Fenner F, Sweeney AW (1998). Malaria in New Guinea during the Second World War: the Land Headquarters Medical Research Unit. *Parassitologia* **40**, 65–8.

64. Sweeney AW (1996). The possibility of an "X" factor. The first documented drug resistance of human malaria. *Int J Parasitol* **26**, 1035–61.

65. Beadle C, Hoffman SL (1993). History of malaria in the United States Naval forces at war: World War I through the Vietnam conflict. *Clin Infect Dis* **16**, 320–9.

66. Bruce-Chwatt LJ (1981). Introduction. In: Bruce-Chwatt LJ, ed. *Chemotherapy of malaria*, 2nd edn., pp. 9–19. World Health Organization, Geneva.

67. Liebenau J (1987). The British success with penicillin. *Soc Stud Sci* **17**, 69–86.

68. Curd FHS, Davey DG, Rose FL (1945). Studies on synthetic antimalarial drugs. X. Some biguanide derivatives as new types of antimalarial substances with both therapeutic and causal prophylactic activity. *Ann Trop Med Parasitol* **39**, 208–16.

69. Hawking F (1947). Activation of Paludrine in vitro. *Nature* **159**, 409.

70. Carrington HC. Crowther AF, Davey DG, Levi AA, Rose FL (1951). A metabolite of 'Paludrine' with high antimalarial activity. *Nature* **168**, 1080.

71. Curd FHC, Davey DG (1950). Antrycide, a new trypanocidal drug. *Br J Pharmacol Chemother* **5**, 25–32.

72. Wiselogle FY (1946). *A survey of antimalarial drugs 1941–1945*, Vols. 1 and 2. JW Edwards, Ann Arbor, Michigan.

73. Sweeney AW (2000). Wartime research on malaria chemotherapy. *Parassitologia* **42**, 33–45.

74. Most H, London IM, Kane CA, Lavietes PH, Schroeder EF, Hayman JM (1946). Chloroquine for treatment of acute attacks of vivax malaria. *JAMA* **131**, 963–7. Reprinted in: *JAMA* 1964; **251**, 2415–9.

75. Coatney GR (1963). Pitfalls in a discovery: the chronicle of chloroquine. *Am J Trop Med Hyg* **12**, 121–9.

76. Elderfield RC, Gensler WJ, Head JD, *et al.* (1946). Alkylaminoalkyl derivatives of 8-aminoquinolines. *J Am Chem Soc* **68**, 1524–9.

77. Alving AS, Arnold J, Robinson DH (1952). Mass therapy of subclinical vivax malaria with primaquine. *JAMA* **149**, 1558–62.

78. Alving AS, Craige B, Pullman TN, Whorton CM, Jones R, Eichelberger L (1948). Procedures used at Stateville Penitentiary for the testing of potential antimalarial agents. *J Clin Invest* **27** (3, Part 2), 2–5.

79. Hornblum AM (1997). They were cheap and available: prisoners as research subjects in twentieth century America. *BMJ* **315**, 1437–41.

80. Falco EA, Hitchings GH, Russell PB, VanderWerff H (1949). Antimalarials as antagonists of purines and pteroylglutamic acid. *Nature* **164**, 107–8; Hitchings GH (1988). Selective inhibitors of dihydrofolate reductase. Nobel Lecture. Available at: http://nobelprize.org/medicine/laureates/1988/hitchings-lecture.pdf

81. Falco EA, Goodwin LG, Hitchings GH, Rollo IM, Russell PB (1951). 2:4-diaminopyrimidines—a new series of antimalarials. *Br J Pharmacol* **6**, 185–200.

82. Goodwin LG (1952). Daraprim (B.W. 50–63)—a new antimalarial. Trials in human volunteers. *BMJ* **1**, 732–4.

83. Archibald HM (1951). Preliminary field trials on a new schizonticide. *BMJ* **2**, 821–3.

84. McGregor IA, Smith DA (1952). Daraprim in treatment of malaria. A study of its effects in falciparum and quartan infections in West Africa. *BMJ* **1**, 730–2.

85. Rollo IM (1955). The mode of action of sulphonamides, proguanil and pyrimethamine on *Plasmodium gallinaceum*. *Br J Pharmacol* **10**, 208–14.

86. Hurly MGD (1959). Potentiation of pyrimethamine by sulphadiazine in human malaria. *Trans R Soc Trop Med Hyg* **53**, 412–3.

87. Eyles DE, Coleman N (1952). Tests of 2,4 diaminopyrimidine on toxoplasmosis. *Public Health Rep* **67**, 249–52.

88. Beadle C, Hoffman SL (1993). History of malaria in the United States Naval forces at war: World War I through the Vietnam conflict. *Clin Infect Dis* **16** 320–9.

89. Trenholme GM, Williams RL, Desjardins RE, *et al.* (1975). Mefloquine (WR 142,490) in the treatment of human malaria. *Science* **190**, 792–4.

90. Cosgriff TM, Boudreau EF, Pamplin CL, Doberstyn EB, Desjardins RE, Canfield CJ (1982). Evaluation of the antimalarial activity of the phenanthrenemethanol halofantrine (WR 171,669). *Am J Trop Med Hyg* **31**, 1075–9.

91. Magerlein BJ, Kagan F (1969). Lincomycin. VIII. 4'-Alkyl-1'-demethyl-4'-depropylclindamycins, potent antibacterial and antimalarial agents. *J Med Chem* **12**, 780–4.

92. Schmidt LH, Harrison J, Ellison R, Worcester P (1970). The activities of chlorinated lincomycin derivatives against infections with *Plasmodium cynomolgi* in *Macaca mulatta*. *Am J Trop Med Hyg* **19**, 1–11.

93. Klayman DL (1975). Qinghaosu (artemisinin): an antimalarial drug from China. *Science* **228**, 1049–55.

94. Hien TT, White NJ (1993). Qinghaosu. *Lancet* **341**, 603–8.

95. Pereira J (1854). *The elements of materia medica and therapeutics*, 4th edn., Vol. 1, pp. 741–2. Longman, Brown, Green and Longmans, London; Adams S (2004). *Dudley, Sir Robert (1574–1649)*. Oxford Dictionary of National Biography, Oxford University Press, http://www.oxforddnb.com/view/article/8161

96. McCallum RI (1999). *Antimony in medical history*. Pentland Press, Edinburgh.

97. Watson T (1857). *Lectures on the principles and practice of physic*, 4th edn., Vol. 2, pp. 98–9. John W Parker and Son, London.

98. Vianna G (1912). Untitled (meeting presentation). *Archivos Brasileiros de Medicina* **2**, 426–8.

99. Di Cristina G, Caronia G (1915). Sulla therapia della leishmaniosa interna. *Bulletin de la Société de Pathologie Exotique et de ses Filiales* **23**, 81–2.

100. Di Cristina G, Caronia G (1915). The treatment of internal leishmaniasis. *J Trop Med Hyg* **18**, 118–9.

101. Rogers L (1915). Tartar emetic in kala-azar. *BMJ* **2**, 197.

102. Dünschede H-B (1971). *Tropenmedizinische Forschung bei Bayer*, p. 93. Michael Triltsch Verlag, Düsseldorf.

103. Smyly HJ, Young CW, Brown C (1926). Experimental kala azar in a hamster, *Cricetulus griseus* M. Edw. *Am J Hyg* **6**, 254–75.

104. Mayer M (1929). Tierversuche mit *Leishmania tropica* (orientbeule). *Dermatologische Wochenschrift* **8**, 286–8.

105. Adler S (1948). Origin of the golden hamster *Cricetus auratus* as a laboratory animal. *Nature* **162**, 256–7.

106. Goodwin LG (1995). Pentostam® (sodium stibogluconate): a 50-year personal reminiscence. *Trans R Soc Trop Med Hyg* **89**, 339–41.

107. Furtado TA (1959–1960). Clinical results in the treatment of American leishmaniasis with oral and intravenous amphotericin. *Antibiot Ann* **7**, 631–7.

108. Peters W (1985). Antiprotozoal agents. In: Greenwood D, O'Grady F, eds. *The scientific basis of antimicrobial chemotherapy*, pp. 99–132. Cambridge University Press, Cambridge.

109. Neal RA (1968). The effect of antibiotics of the neomycin group on experimental leishmaniaisis. *Ann Trop Med Parasitol* **62**, 54–63.

110. El-On J, Jacobs JP, Witztum E, Greenblatt CL (1984). Development of topical treatment for cutaneous leishmaniasis caused by *Leishmania major* in experimental animals. *Antimicrob Agents Chemother* **26**, 745–51.

111. Bryceson ADM, Murphy A, Moody AH (1994). Treatment of 'Old World' leishmaniasis with aminosidine ointment: results of an open study in London. *Trans R Soc Trop Med Hyg* **88**, 226–8.

112. http://www.dndi.org/; http://www.oneworldhealth.org/

113. Croft SL, Neal RA, Pendergast W, Chan JH (1987). The activity of alkyl phosphorylcholines and related derivatives against *Leishmania donovani*. *Biochem Pharmacol* **36**, 2633–6.

114. Sundar S, Rosenkaimer F, Makharia MK, *et al.* (1998). Trial of oral miltefosine for visceral leishmaniasis. *Lancet* **352**, 1821–3.

115. Main PT, Bristow NW, Oxley P, *et al.* (1960). Entamide. *Ann Biochem Exp Med* **20** (Suppl.), 441–8.

116. McVay LV, Lairs RL, Sprunt DH (1949). Preliminary report of successful treatment of amebiasis with aureomycin. *Science* **109**, 590–1.

117. McCowen MC, Callender ME, Lawlis JF (1951). Fumagillin (H-3), a new antibiotic with amebicidal properties. *Science* **113**, 202–3.

118. Diesenhouse MC, Wilson LA, Corrent GF, Visvesvara GS, Grossniklaus HE, Bryan RT (1993). Treatment of microsporidial keratoconjunctivitis with topical fumagillin. *Am J Ophthalmol* **115**, 293–8; Conteas CN, Berlin OGW, Ash LR, Pruthi JS (2000). Therapy for human intestinal microsporidiosis. *Am J Trop Med Hyg* **63**, 121–7.

119. Editorial (1978). The nitroimidazole family of drugs. *Br J Venereal Dis* **54**, 69–71.

120. Cosar C, Julou L (1959). Activité de l'(hydroxy-2-éthyl)-1-méthyl-2-nitro-5-imidazole (8823 R.P.) vis-à-vis des infections expérimentales à *Trichomonas vaginalis. Annales de l'Institut Pasteur* **96**, 238–41.

121. Durel P, Roiron V, Siboulet A, Borel LJ (1960). Systematic treatment of human trichomoniasis with a derivative of nitro-imidazole, 8823 R.P. *Br J Venereal Dis* **36**, 21–6.

122. Schneider J (1961). Traitement de la giardiase (lambliase) par le métronidazole. *Bulletin de la Société de Pathologie Exotique et ses Filiales* **54**, 83–95.

123. Powell SJ, MacLeod I, Wilmot AJ, Elsdon-Dew R (1966). Metronidazole in amoebic dysentery and amoebic liver abscess. *Lancet* **2**, 1329–31.

124. Shinn DLS (1962). Metronidazole in acute ulcerative gingivitis. *Lancet* **1**, 1191.

125. Farthing MJG (1996). Giardiasis. In: Cox FEG, ed. *Illustrated history of tropical diseases*, pp. 248–55. Wellcome Trust, London.

126. Findlay GM (1947). The toxicity of mepacrine in man. *Trop Dis Bull* **44**, 763–79.

127. Brumpt L (1937). Traitement expérimental de la lambliase. *Comptes Rendu des Séances de la Société de Biologie et des ses Filiales* **124**, 1040–2.

128. Galli-Valério B (1937)La lambliase et son traitement par l'atébrine. *Schweizerische Medizinische Wochenschrift* **67**, 1181–2.

129. Page F (1951). Treatment of lupus erythematosus with mepacrine. *Lancet* **2**, 755–8.

130. Zipper J, Kessel E (2003). Quinacrine sterilization: a retrospective. *Int J Gynecol Obstet* **83** (Suppl. 2), S7–11.

131. Korth C, May BCH, Cohen FE, Prusiner SB (2001). Acridine and phenothiazine derivatives as pharmacotherapeutics for prion diseases. *Proc Natl Acad Sci U S A* **98**, 9836–41.

132. Miles MA (1996). New World trypanosomiasis. In: Cox FEG, ed. *Illustrated history of tropical diseases*, pp. 192–205. The Wellcome Trust, London.

133. Lewinsohn R (1981). Carlos Chagas and the discovery of Chagas's disease (American trypanosomiasis). *J R Soc Med* **74**, 451–5; Lewinsohn R (1982). Chagas's disease. *J R Soc Med* **75**, 470.

134. Fornaciari G, Castagna M, Viacava P, Tognetti A, Bevilacqua G, Segura EL (1992). Chagas' disease in Peruvian Inca mummy. *Lancet* **339**, 128–9; Guhl F, Jaramillo C, Yockteng R, Vallejo GA, Cárdenas-Arroyo F (1997). *Trypanosoma cruzi* DNA in human mummies. *Lancet* **349**, 1370.

135. Collier HOJ (1954). *Chemotherapy of infections*, pp. 197–8. Chapman and Hall, London.

136. Gönnert R (1972). Nifurtimox: causal treatment of Chagas' disease. *Arzneimittelforschung* **22**, 1563.

137. Grunberg E, Beskid G, Cleeland R, *et al.* (1968). Antiprotozoan and antibacterial activity of 2-nitroimidazoles. In: Hobby GL, ed. *Antimicrobial agents and chemotherapy–1967*, pp. 513–9. American Society for Microbiology, Ann Arbor, Michigan.

138. Manson-Bahr PH (1966). *Manson's tropical diseases*, 16th edn., p. 961. Baillière, Tindall and Cassell, London.

139. Govier WM (1984). A helminthic tale. *Perspect Biol Med* **28**, 104–6.

140. Campbell WC (1986). Historical introduction. In: Campbell WC, Rew RS, eds. *Chemotherapy of parasitic diseases*, pp. 3–21. Plenum Press, New York.

141. Goodwin LG (1980). New drugs for old diseases. *Trans R Soc Trop Med Hyg* **74**, 1–7.

142. Fayard C (1949). Ascaridiose et piperazine. Thèse, Paris. Abstract, *La Semaine des Hôpitaux, Paris* **35**, 1778; cited in: Editorial (1960). Piperazine as an anthelminthic. *Lancet* **1**, 1177.

143. Swatrtzwelder JC, Frye WW, Muhleisen JP, *et al.* (1957). Dithiazanine, an effective broad-spectrum anthelmintic; results of therapy of trichuriasis, strongyloidiasis, enterobiasis, ascariasis, and hookworm infection. *J Am Med Assoc* **165**, 2063–7.

144. Gill GV, Bell DR (1979). *Strongyloides stercoralis* infection in former Far East prisoners of war. *BMJ* **2**, 572–4.

145. Perroncito E (1880). Helminthological observations upon the endemic disease developed among the labourers in the tunnel of Mount St. Gothard. *J Queckett Microscop Club* **6**, 141–8.

146. Ashford, BK, Gutierrez Igaravidez P (1911). *Uncinariasis (hookworm disease) in Porto Rico. A medical and economic problem*. Government Printing Office, Washington.

147. Goodwin LG, Beveridge E, Gorvin JH (1998). *Wellcome legacies*, pp. 38 and 82–4. The Wellcome Trust, London.

148. Neghme RA (1939). The effect of acridine (mepacrine) on tapeworms. *Revista Chilena de Historia Natural Pura y Aplicada* **43**, 97–9. Cited in: Grove DI (1990). A history of human helminthology. CAB International, Wallingford. Available at: http://www.users.on.net/~david.grove/BOOK.PDF

149. Culbertson JT (1940). The elimination of the tapeworm *Hymenolepis fraterna* from mice by the administration of atabrine. *J Pharmacol Exp Ther* **70**, 309–14.

150. Hoekenga MT (1951). Treatment of *T. saginata* and *H. nana* infections with Atebrine. *Am J Trop Med* **31**, 420–2.

151. Gönnert R, Schraufstätter E (1960). Experimentelle Untersuchungen mit N-(2'-chlor-4'-nitro-phenyl)-5-chlorsalicylamid, einem neuen Bandwurmmittel. 1. Mitteilung: chemotherapeutische Versuche. *Arzneimittelforschung* **10**, 881–4.

152. Austin WC, Courtney W, Danilewicz JC, *et al.* (1966). Pyrantel tartrate, a new anthelmintic effective against infections of domestic animals. *Nature* **212**,1273–4.

153. Bell WJ, Gould GC (1971). Preliminary report on pyrantel pamoate in the treatment of human hookworm infection. *East Afr Med J* **48**, 143–51.

154. Campbell WC (2005). Serendipity and new drugs for infectious disease. *Inst Lab Anim Res J* **46**, 352–6.

155. Lionel ND, Mirando EH, Nanayakkara JC, Soysa PE (1969). Levamisole in the treatment of ascariasis in children. *BMJ* **4**, 340–1.

156. Woolley DW (1944). Some biological effects produced by benzimidazole and their reversal by purines. *J Biol Chem* **152**, 225–32.

157. Brown HD, Matzuk AR, Ilves IR, *et al.* (1961). Antiparasitic drugs. IV. 2-(4'-Thiazolyl) benzimidazole, a new anthelmintic. *J Am Chem Soc* **83**, 1764–5.

158. Venkatesen P (1998). Albendazole. *J Antimicrob Chemother* **41**, 145–7.

159. Zhong, HL, Cao WJ, Rossignol JF, *et al.* (1986). Albendazole in nematode, cestode, trematode and protozoan (Giardia) infections. *Chin Med J* (English language version) **99**, 912–5.

160. Manson P (1903). *Tropical diseases. A manual of the diseases of warm climates*, 3rd edn., p. 615. Cassell, London.

161. Fairley NH (1951). Schistosomiasis and some of its problems. *Trans R Soc Trop Med Hyg* **45**, 279–306.

162. Christopherson JB (1918). The successful use of antimony in bilharziosis. *Lancet* **2**, 325–7.

163. Lasbrey FO, Coleman RB (1921). Notes on one thousand cases of bilharziasis treated by antimony tartrate. *Lancet* **1**, 299–301.

164. McDonagh JER (1915). *The biology and treatment of venereal diseases: and the biology of inflammation and its relationship to malignant disease*, p. 349. Harrison, London.

165. Farley J (1991). *Bilharzia. A history of imperial tropical medicine*, pp. 97–115 and 188–200. Cambridge University Press, Cambridge.

166. Khalil M, Betache MH (1930). Treatment of bilharziasis with a new compound "fouadin". *Lancet* **1**, 234–5.

167. Farley J (1991). *Bilharzia. A history of imperial tropical medicine*, pp. 286–7. Cambridge University Press, Cambridge.

168. Kikuth W, Gönnert R, Mauss H (1946). Miracil, ein neues Chemotherapeuticum gegen die Darmbilharziose. *Naturwissenschaften* **33**, 253.

169. Goodwin LG, Beveridge E, Gorvin JH (1998). *Wellcome's legacies*, p. 37. The Wellcome Trust, London.

170. Schmidt P, Wilhelm M (1966). A new group of antischistosomal compounds. *Angewandte Chem* (International Edition) **5**, 857–62.

171. Foster R (1973). The preclinical development of oxamniquine. *Revista do Instituto de Medicina Tropical de São Paulo* **15** (Suppl. 1), 1–9.

172. Groll E (1984). Praziquantel. *Adv Pharmacol Chemother* **20**, 219–38.

173. Seubert J, Pohlke R, Loebich F (1977). Synthesis and properties of praziquantel, a novel broad spectrum anthelmintic with excellent activity against schistosomes and cestodes. *Experientia* **33**, 1036–7.

174. Reynolds LA, Tansey EM (2001). *British contributions to medical research and education in Africa after the Second World War*, pp. 18 and 76. The Wellcome Trust, London. Available at: http://www.ucl.ac.uk/histmed/PDFS/Publications/Witness/wit10.pdf

175. Van hoof L, Henrard C, Peel E, Wanson M (1947). Sur la chimiothérapie de l'onchocercose. *Annales de la Société Belge de Médecine Tropicale* **27**, 173–7.

176. Sarkies JWR (1952). Antrypol in the treatment of onchocerciasis. *Trans R Soc Trop Med Hyg* **46**, 435–6.

177. Hewitt RI, Kushner S, Stewart HW, White E, Wallace WS, SubbaRow Y (1947). Experimental chemotherapy of filariasis III. Effect of 1-diethylcarbamyl-4-methylpiperazine hydrochloride against naturally acquired filarial infections in cotton rats and dogs. *J Lab Clin Med* **32**, 1314–29.

178. Ōmura S (1986). Philosophy of new drug discovery. *Microbiol Rev* **50**, 259–79.

179. Frost L, Reich MR, Fujisaki T (2002). A partnership for ivermectin: social worlds and boundary objects. In: Reich MR, ed. *Public-private partnerships for public health*, pp. 87–114. Harvard University Press. Available at: http://www.hsph.harvard.edu/hcpds/partnerbook/chap5.PDF

180. Aziz MA, Diallo S, Diop IM, Lariviere M, Porta M (1982). Efficacy and tolerance of ivermectin in human onchocerciasis. *Lancet* **2**, 171–3.

181. Collins K (2004). Profitable pills. A history of the Merck Mectizan® donation programme and its implications for international health. *Perspect Med Biol* **47**, 100–9.

182. Anonymous (29 June 2006). Brian Duke (Obituary) *The Times*.

183. Cao WC, Van der Ploeg CP, Plaisier AP, van der Sluijs IJ, Habbema JD (1997). Ivermectin for the chemotherapy of bancroftian filariasis: a meta-analysis of the effect of single treatment. *Trop Med Int Health* **2**, 393–403.

184. Hoerauf A, Nissen-Pahle K, Schmetx C, *et al.* (1999). Tetracycline therapy targets intracellular bacteria in the filarial nematode *Litomosoides sigmodontis* and results in filarial infertility. *J Clin Invest* **103**, 11–18.

185. Hoerauf A, Volkmann L, Hamelmann C, *et al.* (2000). Endosymbiotic bacteria in worms as targets for a novel chemotherapy in filariasis. *Lancet* **355**, 1242–3.

186. Rossignol JF, Maisonneuve H (1984). Nitazoxanide in the treatment of *Taenia saginata* and *Hymenolepis nana* infections. *Am J Trop Med Hyg* **33**, 511–2.

187. Dubreuil L, Houcke I, Mouton Y, Rossignol JF (1996). In vitro evaluation of activities of nitazoxanide and tizoxanide against anaerobes and aerobic organisms. *Antimicrob Agents Chemother* **40**, 2266–70.

188. Coles GC (1999). Anthelmintic resistance and the control of worms. *J Med Microbiol* **48**, 323–5.

Chapter 8

The poor relations: fungi and viruses

It is a melancholy truth that even great men have their poor relations ... they visit their richer cousins and get into debt when they can, and live but shabbily when they can't.

Charles Dickens, *Bleak House*, Chapter 28

While protozoa and helminths benefited from historical precedent, the exigencies of war and colonial rule, and the importance of parasites in animal husbandry, fungi, and viruses remained in limbo. In the cases of fungi, this was partly because little notice was paid to them. The only fungal infections that attracted much attention before the mid-twentieth century were ringworm (infection of the skin, hair, or nails by a group of fungi collectively called dermatophytes) and thrush (infection of the mucosa with yeasts, normally *Candida albicans*). Neither is life threatening, though ringworm can on occasions be quite severe. Serious fungal infections including mycetoma—a mutilating condition that often affects the foot and may be caused not only by fungi, but also by certain mould-like bacteria—were encountered in the tropics, but were overshadowed by the importance of such widespread diseases like malaria, sleeping sickness, bilharzia, and kala-azar. In United States, several systemic fungal infections including blastomycosis, histoplasmosis, and the tongue-twistingly named coccidioidomycosis, all of which are caused by dimorphic fungi (see p. 13–14) had been described by 1920 (1), but were rarely seen outside the endemic areas. Cryptococcal meningitis, which is caused by the yeast, *Cryptococcus neoformans*, is almost invariably fatal if untreated, but is mercifully rare.* Serious systemic infections with fungi in general hospital practice were uncommon (and, when they occurred, were frequently unrecognized) before the advent of powerful immunosuppressive drugs that undermine the body's ability to withstand infection with opportunist micro-organisms including fungi.

So far as viruses were concerned, little was known about them until the development of electron microscopy and tissue culture techniques (see p. 9–13). Viral diseases that could

---

* Although meningitis caused by yeasts was described over 100 years ago, it was only in the mid-twentieth century that the nomenclature of the causative organism was sorted out. The disease was earlier described as 'European blastomycosis' or 'torula meningitis' (*see* Mitchell TG, Perfect JR (1995). Cryptococcosis in the era of AIDS—100 years after the discovery of *Cryptococcus neoformans*. *Clin Microbiol Rev* **8**, 515–48.)

have serious, even catastrophic, implications, polio, measles, chickenpox, mumps, and rubella among them, were common enough, but the aetiology was obscure. Smallpox was largely under control where Jennerian vaccination was practised. Theories abounded in the early twentieth century about the role in infectious diseases of ultramicroscopic particles able to pass through fine bacterial filters, but they were highly contentious. Filterable viruses were, for example, advanced to explain the disastrous pandemic of influenza in 1918–20, but techniques were lacking to prove the point. The limitations of contemporary virology are highlighted by the findings of a Medical Research Council investigation into the cause of the epidemic. The study, carried out by the Scottish bacteriologist James McIntosh, newly appointed to the Chair of Pathology in the Middlesex Hospital's Bland–Sutton Institute, included a consideration of claims of a viral aetiology. Data assembled by McIntosh strongly implicated a small Gram-negative bacillus described in 1892 by the military bacteriologist Richard Pfeiffer, which had been given the misleading name *Bacillus* (later *Haemophilus*) *influenzae*. McIntosh concluded that 'no evidence was obtained in support of the view that influenza is due to a filter-passing virus (2).'

The low profile of the branches of microbiology dealing with fungi and viruses did not help to encourage the notion that these micro-organisms were worthy of more serious consideration. Among medical microbiologists, the traditional stereotype of mycology was that of a minority pursuit populated by amusing oddballs with a penchant for botanizing. Though fungi came in a fascinating variety of colourful forms, they were slow to grow and the specialty was considered tedious and taxonomically driven, with little impact on everyday management of infectious diseases. In any case, nothing much was available in the way of treatment except for the topical therapy of superficial fungal infections. Virology was similarly viewed as a highly specialized activity with little practical impact. It was often caricatured as an exercise in retrospective futility, since the techniques were slow—colleagues teasingly claimed that they merely confirmed what the patient had recovered or died from—and the therapeutic cupboard was depressingly bare.

This situation started to change in the last decades of the twentieth century as serious fungal diseases were seen with greater frequency, especially among immunocompromised patients, and virology became an important discipline in its own right. Ironically, antibacterial antibiotics contributed to the increased prevalence of fungal infections—in particular vaginal thrush—by eliminating beneficial bacteria that helped to keep these micro-organisms at bay. As fungi and viruses started to move centre stage, more rapid molecular techniques began to come on stream to provide more timely diagnosis and important advances were made in the development of antifungal and antiviral agents.

Antifungal agents

Early remedies: borax, benzoic acid, x-rays, and dyes

Before the twentieth century ringworm was treated with the usual plethora of herbal and chemical nostrums, a few of which, including heavy metal salts and sulphur compounds—sulphur baths was one popular suggestion—may have conferred some benefit. Thrush was recognized as a disease that chiefly affected the mouths of young infants and was often treated with applications of borax, a naturally occurring salt of boric acid containing, as the name suggests, the element boron. The popular Victorian lecturer Thomas Watson taught his students that 'for the local affection of the tongue and mouth, the *mel boracis* [a preparation of borax, glycerine, and honey] is a capital application. It may be painted on the aphthous parts with a camel's-hair pencil (3).' He did not explain how this was to be achieved with a screaming infant.

Watson recognized that thrush (aphthae) also occurred in debilitated adults, but it was some time before it was realized that the yeasts found in oral thrush were also responsible for a common form of vaginal discharge in women. Since (male) doctors frequently dismissed vaginal discharges as trivial complaints of women of a 'nervous temperament' they were more often than not treated with sedatives. Those that took the condition more seriously prescribed vaginal douches often with potassium permanganate (Condy's fluid)* a purple stain with antiseptic properties that no doubt had lasting consequences for the woman's under linen.

From the early twentieth century ringworm of the skin (tinea corporis) and the groin (tinea cruris) was effectively treated with benzoic acid preparations, most notably with Whitfield's ointment, a preparation that also contains salicylic acid. Benzoic acid is widely used in the preservation of food, a property that was already recognized in the nineteenth century. Although its antimicrobial activity was discovered empirically, a biochemically rational basis for the antifungal action of benzoic acid was later elucidated by an Anglo–Spanish team led by no less a person than the Nobel laureate Hans Krebs, discoverer of the Krebs citric acid cycle in cellular metabolism (4).† The eponymous inventor of Whitfield's ointment was Arthur Whitfield, Professor of Dermatology at King's College Hospital, London, and a leading authority on the treatment of skin diseases. The ointment was first described in the first edition of his book *A Handbook of Skin Diseases and their Treatment*, published in 1907. It (or a similar lotion, containing alcohol and acetone to aid penetration of the horny layers of skin on the feet, also developed by Whitfield) became the most popular treatment for fungal diseases until it was replaced by less messy alternatives in the second half of the century. As late as 1955, the dermatologist David Williams was able to write in an appreciation of Whitfield:

'...after some 50 years it is very doubtful whether in practice there is any fungicidal preparation better than Whitfield's ointment (5)'

When ringworm occurred on the scalp (tinea capitis), the consensus among nineteenth and early twentieth century dermatologists was that it was necessary to remove all the infected hair. This entailed plucking it out by the roots. Most of the affected individuals were young children and one blanches at what they were made to undergo by way of

* Condy's fluid was developed and patented around 1857 by Henry Bollmann Condy of Condy Brothers, a firm of vinegar manufacturers in Battersea that later branched out into essential oils and pharmaceutical products.
† This paper, published in early 1983, was one of Hans Krebs' last: he died in November 1981.

treatment. It is said that in the clinic of the celebrated Viennese dermatologist Ferdinand von Hebra, diseased children were encouraged to tear out each other's hair. On learning of this practice, Hebra's contemporary Friedrich Küchenmeister, a pioneering helminthologist (and theological scholar) from Dresden, commented (one hopes sardonically) that it 'is, no doubt, very recommendable and saves time to the physician (6).' Küchenmeister was himself no stranger to controversy. During the 1850s, he demonstrated a crucial feature of the life cycle of tapeworms by feeding measly pork to criminals condemned to death and then dissecting the developing worms from their intestines after they had been executed (7).

Manual removal of the hair was bad enough, but because the process is extremely tedious preparations intended to loosen the hair were frequently preferred. One such treatment, rightly denounced by some as barbaric, was application to the entire scalp of powerful irritants such as pitch plaster (made from resins such as turpentine) or croton oil (obtained from the seeds of *Croton tiglium*, a small tree found in India and the Far East), procedures liable to leave extensive inflammation and ulceration. Towards the end of the nineteenth century, X-rays were found to cause the hair to fall out and the French dermatologist, Raymond Sabouraud,* one of the founders of medical mycology and a specialist in diseases of the scalp, pioneered the development of the technique in the treatment of tinea capitis (8). By the 1920s, X-rays were in common use for scalp ringworm and elaborate equipment was devised to reduce the danger of excessive irradiation, which was known to carry the risk of permanent baldness if not more serious consequences: several early advocates of the treatment, including Henri Noiré, a colleague of Sabouraud in Paris, died from exposure to X-rays.

As a painful, but effective alternative to X-rays, Arthur Whitfield was still recommending several days' application of preparations of croton oil in the 1920s; he advocated delivering the drug into persistently infected follicles with the eye end of a sterilized fine sewing needle (9). Another alternative to X-rays, which also remained in use until the Second World War, was oral thallium acetate, a substance more commonly employed as rat poison. Sabouraud had noted around the turn of the twentieth century that thallium salts cause hair to fall out and the chemical became popular among dermatologists. The depilatory effect is temporary if the dosage is carefully controlled, but the dangers of its use were well known and it seems astonishing that young children with ringworm were commonly exposed to the poison.

Treatment of fungal infections of the finger or toenails presented even greater problems since getting antifungal chemicals to penetrate adequately into the horny structure of nails was a fruitless exercise. The solution most commonly adopted was to remove the whole nail under anaesthetic and dress the exposed area with a fungistatic ointment—often salicylic acid and chrysarobin, a substance extracted from the bark of a South American tree *Andira araroba* and known in early pharmacopoeias as araroba or Goa powder; it featured in many early dermatological preparations.

....

* Sabouraud, famous for devising the standard culture medium for fungi, was also a talented painter and sculptor who exhibited regularly in Paris. See Institut Pasteur archives: Raimond Sabouraud (1864–1938): http://www.pasteur.fr/infosci/archives/sab0.html.

Colourful dyes, such as gentian (crystal) violet or malachite green were also widely used in the treatment of cutaneous and mucus membrane infections; indeed, they are still sometimes suggested as cheap remedies for that purpose. The much-travelled Italian physician, Aldo Castellani, devised one popular preparation—known as Castellani's paint—while he was Professor of Tropical Medicine in Ceylon (now Sri Lanka) from 1903 to 1915, a period he himself described as 'the happiest years of my life' (10). The coloured component of the paint was the red dye basic fuchsin, which was omitted from some subsequent formulations without obvious detriment to its effectiveness—unsurprisingly, since the other constituents of the concoction, ethyl alcohol, boric acid, phenol, acetone, and resorcinol, are enough to deter the hardiest of fungi.

Simple topical remedies like Whitfield's ointment and Castellani's paint satisfactorily filled the bill for many of the common fungal diseases encountered by dermatologists and general practitioners in the first half of the twentieth century. In the 1940s they were supplemented by preparations containing fatty acids with some antifungal activity, such as propionic acid. The antifungal action of fatty acids had been recognized since the turn of the century and investigated in an agricultural context. Interest was revived in 1945 by the microbiologist, Orville Wyss and his colleagues in the research department of Wallace and Tiernan Products in Belleville, New Jersey, a company founded in 1913 to manufacture water chlorination plants. Wyss's group investigated a large range of fatty acids and found activity against a variety of fungi, including some responsible for ringworm (11). One of these compounds, the mono-unsaturated fatty acid, undecylenic (undecenoic) acid, became very popular for the topical treatment of athlete's foot and similar conditions. Although they are of limited efficacy they remain available in proprietary antifungal products.

Aside from these preparations there was nothing effective on offer for patients with mycoses until two remarkable American women—looking in contemporary photographs every inch the stereotype of well-groomed elderly American matrons familiar from Hollywood movies of the time—discovered the first antifungal antibiotic in 1950. The women were Elizabeth Lee Hazen and Rachel Fuller Brown; the antibiotic was nystatin, named after the New York Department of Health, where the discovery was made. It was the first of a series of antifungal antibiotics known from of a feature of their complex structure as polyenes.

Polyenes

Nystatin

Elizabeth Hazen was born, in 1885 or 1888,* to a farming family living in Mississippi just east of the river. Her parents both died while she was still an infant and she was brought up with the family of her uncle and aunt, Robert and Laura Hazen who lived a few miles away.

---

* Many sources, including the United States Social Security Death Index (available on the Family Search website) gave Hazen's date of birth as 1888 and she herself gave this date in her application for the post at the New York Department of Health in 1931. However, Hazen's biographer Richard Baldwin (reference 12, p. 36 and 42–3) claims that the correct date is 1885.

After a rudimentary education in local schools she was given private tuition in Memphis, 60 miles to the north and in 1905 was enrolled in the Mississippi Industrial Institute and College at Columbus (now the Mississippi University for Women) where free tuition was available for Mississippi girls. There she developed an interest in science and after a spell in teaching, moved to Columbia University, New York to pursue postgraduate studies, including a course at the College of Physicians and Surgeons that introduced her to medical bacteriology. After a stint during and after the war working as a laboratory technician, Elizabeth returned to Columbia and eventually completed her PhD in 1927. In 1931 she was recruited by Augustus Wadsworth, Director of the Division of Laboratories and Research of the New York State Department of Health, and put in charge of the branch laboratory in New York City. The headquarters of the Division was over 150 miles away up the Hudson valley in Albany, the state capital. It had been established in 1914 and modelled loosely on the German 'hygiene institutes' with the twin functions of offering diagnostic bacteriology services (including the production of therapeutic vaccines in much the same way as Almroth Wright's Inoculation Department at St Mary's in London) and fostering microbiological research (12).

In 1944, the year before his retirement, Wadsworth became concerned about the neglect of mycological facilities within the Division and Hazen spent part of her time at the nearby Columbia University and the associated Presbyterian Hospital laboratories familiarizing herself with the subject. She started to build up a collection of fungi and to supervise services for the diagnosis of fungal disease and the identification of moulds within her laboratory. Stimulated by the publicity surrounding penicillin and streptomycin as well as the excitement over bacitracin at Columbia of which she would have been very aware, Hazen also began to test fungal isolates and streptomycetes for antifungal activity. As test organisms she chose the yeasts *Candida albicans*, the cause of thrush, and *Cryptococcus neoformans*, which is responsible for a rare, but usually fatal form of meningitis. In 1946, Albert Schatz, the co-discoverer of streptomycin (see p. 153–4), was briefly recruited to this project and assisted in the screening of soil micro-organisms for antibiotic activity.* Gilbert Dalldorf[†] who replaced Wadsworth as director on his retirement in 1945 encouraged the enterprise and during 1948 offered the services of Rachel Brown an organic chemist in his Albany headquarters to help with the extraction and purification of promising antibiotic substances.

Rachel Brown's route to the New York State Department of Health laboratories was scarcely less circuitous than that of Elizabeth Hazen. She was born in Springfield, a city in West Massachusetts on the Connecticut River. The family moved to Missouri when Rachel was six, but her mother took her back to Springfield in 1912 after her husband

---

* Schatz was employed to assist with virological studies, but also collaborated with Hazen on her antibiotic work.

[†] Gilbert Dalldorf is best remembered as a virologist who, in collaboration with Grace Sickles, discovered a new group of viruses in the faeces of children suffering from polio. The viruses were first described in 1948 and were given the name 'Coxsackie' after the small town on the Hudson River from where the first specimens had been obtained.

had abandoned the family. On leaving school the generosity of a family friend, Henrietta Dexter, allowed her to enrol at Mount Holyoke, a women's College in South Hadley, Massachusetts, founded in 1837 by the early campaigner for female education, Mary Lyon, as the *Mount Holyoke Female Seminary*. At Mount Holyoke, Rachel concentrated on her preferred subject, history, but had additionally to select an obligatory basic science course and chose chemistry. Enthused by her experience of chemical analysis she went on to Chicago to gain a Master's degree in organic chemistry, with bacteriology as a subsidiary subject. After a brief flirtation with teaching, and a spell at Harvard, Rachel returned to Chicago in 1924 to pursue research for a PhD, which was completed in 1926, but not formally awarded until 1933 owing to an administrative delay in arranging the oral examination. Having finished the PhD work, Rachel Brown applied to Augustus Wadsworth's department in Albany on the suggestion of an old friend from Holyoke and was taken on to the staff late in 1926 (12).

In pursuing the antibiotic research, Hazen and Brown established a routine in which Elizabeth Hazen's group in New York performed the preliminary screening tests; cultures exhibiting antibiotic activity were sent to Rachel Brown in Albany for extraction of the active component; and crude extracts were returned to Hazen for further tests in animals. By the time Albert Schatz left the New York State Department of Health laboratories in 1947 to move on to the Sloane Kettering Cancer Center, nothing substantial had been achieved, as the sole paper he published with Elizabeth Hazen reveals (13). Microbial products displaying antifungal activity had certainly been found, but all proved highly toxic to mice. The breakthrough came soon after Hazen and Brown joined forces in 1948, with a micro-organism bearing the laboratory number 48240.

In common with antibiotic investigators everywhere, Elizabeth Hazen had enlisted the help of colleagues and friends in the collection of soil samples that could be investigated for organisms exhibiting antibiotic activity. It was, however, a sample that she had dug up with her own hands that yielded culture 48240. She had collected it in a field while visiting the farm of a friend, Walter B. Nourse, in Warrenton, Virginia, south-west of Washington DC. When the organism turned out to be a new species of *Streptomyces*, it was named *Streptomyces noursei* in her friend's honour.

Rachel Brown succeeded in extracting two substances with antibiotic activity from culture 48240. One was a highly soluble substance secreted into the culture broth and was probably responsible for most of the activity Elizabeth Hazen had detected in her screening test. The component was called 'fraction N' since it had little activity against *Candida albicans*, but inhibited *Cryptococcus neoformans*. Perhaps seeking to explain the unexpectedly selective activity of this compound, Brown went on to isolate a second, insoluble substance from the matted growth of the streptomycete. This extract inhibited the growth of both organisms and was called 'fraction AN'. Fraction N proved to be identical to cycloheximide (Actidione) an antibiotic that had already been described in 1947 by scientists in the antibiotic research laboratories of the Upjohn Company in Kalamazoo, Michigan, including the mycologist Alma Whiffen (on marriage in 1952, Alma Barksdale) (14). Cycloheximide, which was discovered as a secondary product of a streptomycin-producing strain of *Streptomyces griseus*, is far too toxic for human use but has selective activity against various types of fungi and has found application in such diverse niches as the treatment of golf course greens and in the prevention of unwanted contaminants of culture media for the laboratory isolation of pathogenic fungi.

The name proposed for the insoluble fraction AN produced by *Streptomyces noursei* was fungicidin, but when it was discovered that this was already in use for another substance it was changed to nystatin. The first laboratory results were unveiled at a regional meeting of the National Academy of Sciences in Schenectady, north-west of Albany, in October 1950, with a paper in *Proceedings of the Society of Experimental Biology and Medicine* following in early 1951 (15). Press coverage of the Albany conference aroused the interest of the drug companies in the new antifungal agent, though no clinical trials had at that time being done. Dalldorf was soon seeking ways of developing and exploiting the discovery, which were plainly beyond the resources of his laboratory.

The solution came through an agreement with Research Corporation, a non-profit organization founded in 1912 by the scientist and philanthropist Frederick Cottrell, which handled patenting and licensing issues for academic institutions and similar bodies, with monies accruing from licensing arrangements going to grants for scholarly research. The agreement reached between Dalldorf and Research Corporation involved handing over-all rights to the invention in exchange for a 50 percent share in any subsequent royalties, which were to paid to a special fund—the Brown–Hazen Fund—set-up to disburse money for scientific research. The deal was signed on 21 February 1951 and within a week an exclusive 5-year licence agreement had been reached with Squibb. A patent application was rushed through (under United States law it had to be presented within 1 year of public disclosure, which had taken place at the Schenectady meeting) and Squibb set about producing enough material at its New Brunswick plant for preliminary clinical trials to start in 1952. In August 1954, the Squibb preparation received approval from the Food and Drug Administration (FDA) and within a month tablets were on the market as Mycostatin.

Nystatin is very toxic when administered by injection, but it is very poorly absorbed when given orally and this was the original route of administration. Creams, ointments, powders, and vaginal pessaries soon followed. At the time of the appearance of nystatin, concern was mounting about *Candida* infections, including serious intestinal overgrowth, in patients receiving broad-spectrum antibiotics, notably tetracyclines. Consequently tablets of nystatin were commonly prescribed together with tetracyclines to forestall this complication and Squibb were soon promoting a product, Mysteclin, which contained a mixture of nystatin and tetracycline. This and similar products, were later discontinued because of disquiet about the use of fixed-dose combinations of antibiotics and lack of evidence that they were necessary or effective. Topical treatment of skin, mouth, and vaginal candidiasis became the predominant role for nystatin and remains so today.

Amphotericin B

Squibb had already been working on potential antifungal antibiotics when they took over the development of nystatin in 1951. Whether or not the antibiotic later known as amphotericin B was already under study at this time is unclear, but if so, it was temporarily put on the back burner as Hazen and Brown's discovery took precedence.

Amphotericins A and B were unveiled at the third annual symposium on antibiotics held in Washington DC in early November 1955. The producer organism, later identified as a new species of streptomycete, *Streptomyces nodosus*, was isolated by Joseph Pagano, Richard Donovick, and their colleagues from the soil obtained from Temblador, near the Orinoco River delta in Venezuela (16). Both antibiotics are highly insoluble in water, but they were readily separated by their differential solubility in various solvents and most of the antifungal activity was found to reside in amphotericin B. Preliminary laboratory studies of amphotericin B outside the company were carried out by the dermatologist Thomas Sternberg and his colleagues at the University of California Medical Center, Los Angeles. The first tentative clinical studies were reported at the 1956 antibiotics symposium (17). Oral treatment proved ineffective as the drug is poorly absorbed from the gut; a particulate suspension fared little better, but the Squibb scientists persisted and in 1956 produced a formulation consisting of a colloidal suspension in the bile salt sodium desoxycholate. Trials of this preparation showed it to be very effective against yeasts, dimorphic fungi, and filamentous fungi, such as *Aspergillus fumigatus*, but at the expense of considerable toxicity. Indeed the propensity of the drug to cause serious toxicity, including irreversible damage to the kidneys, earned it the nickname 'amphoterrible' (18). In the absence of anything safer, amphotericin B became an important part of the therapeutic armamentarium against serious systemic fungal diseases, albeit one that needed to be used with great care.

During the 1980s techniques were developed to entrap amphotericin and other drugs within artificial phospholipid vesicles—liposomes. The biophysicist Alec Bangham first described liposomes in England in1965; indeed, in the early days they were often colloquially described as 'bangasomes'. The idea of using them as drug delivery systems by wrapping toxic drugs within the lipid structure was popularized in the United Kingdom by Gregory Gregoriadis at the Medical Research Council's Clinical Research Centre in Harrow and later at the School of Pharmacy in London. The first speculative experiments with liposome-entrapped amphotericin B were carried out by John Graybill and his colleagues at the University of Texas Health Science Center at San Antonio around 1982 (19), but it was not until the mid-1990s that they came into regular therapeutic use, by which time there were several competing (and expensive) formulations available (20). Use of lipid formulations of amphotericin B reduces the toxicity without affecting the antifungal activity. Despite the availability of less toxic alternatives (see below) they have helped to sustain the popularity of amphotericin B, which remains the most reliable agent for the treatment of severe systemic fungal infections.

Other polyenes

By the time amphotericin B was launched several other polyenes had appeared on the scene. In 1952 Syogo Hosoya and his colleagues at the University of Tokyo described trichomycin (later known as hachimycin) (21). The producer organism, *Streptomyces hachijoensis*, had been isolated from soil on Hachijo-jima a volcanic island, about 180 miles south of Tokyo. It has activity against *Trichomonas vaginalis* as well as yeasts and is still marketed in Japan for the non-specific treatment of vaginal discharge.

Two other polyenes were described at about the same time: Richard Hickey of the Commercial Solvents Corporation, Terre Haute, Indiana, isolated a substance called ascosin from a culture contaminant, *Streptomyces canescens*; and Hubert Lechevalier working with Selman Waksman at Rutgers described candicidin, an antibiotic with fungicidal properties from *Streptomyces griseus*. There was a brief flurry of interest in these compounds, but both were soon discarded.

Numerous polyene antibiotics were subsequently described, but few attracted much attention. Of those that did, pimaricin (also called natamycin) was among the most prominent. It was isolated in 1955 by A. P. Struyk and his colleagues at the Dutch firm of Gist in Delft.* The producer organism was *Streptomyces natalensis* found in soil from Pietermaritzburg in Natal (now KwaZulu-Natal) (22). The same antibiotic, under the name tennecetin, was isolated a few years later from *Streptomyces chattanoogensis* found in soil in Tennessee. Like trichomycin, it was claimed to have activity against *Trichomonas vaginalis*, but its chief use has been in veterinary medicine and in food production to control microbial growth on the surface of cheeses and meat products. The only surviving use in human medicine is as eye drops for keratomycosis, a disease more common in horses than human beings.

Further progress against yeasts

Flucytosine

This detection of the activity of the pyrimidine analogue, flucytosine (5-fluorocytosine), against yeasts—it has no useful activity against filamentous fungi—was an episode in which Lady Luck and commercial doggedness had an equal share. In the late 1950s and early 1960s, Robert Duschinsky at Hoffmann-La Roche in Nutley, New Jersey and Charles Heidelberger of the University of Wisconsin were collaborating on the investigation of nucleic acid analogues as possible anticancer compounds. The first of these, fluorouracil, synthesized by Heidelberger in 1956 was marketed by Roche in 1962. Another candidate, synthesized in 1957 and subsequently rejected as being devoid of cytostatic activity, was 5-fluorocytosine. In the course of routine screening of such compounds in 1962, activity against yeasts was discovered (23). The results were not encouraging, since activity in laboratory cultures was very poor, but the Roche team decided go ahead anyway with a trial of the substance in an experimental model of candidiasis in mice. These results were also far from convincing: treatment with 5-fluorocytosine failed to clear up subcutaneous *Candida* infection and had no effect on *Histoplasma capsulatum* or *Blastomyces dermatitidis*; bloodstream infection with *Cryptococcus neoformans* responded, but the organism was still recoverable from heart and brain cultures (24). Such unpromising findings would normally have sufficed to consign the substance to the dustbin of history, but the prize of a relatively safe, orally administered compound that might be useful in cryptococcal meningitis evidently persuaded the Roche scientists to persevere. Had

---

* Struyk had earlier been involved in the clandestine production of penicillin in the Netherlands during Second World War (see p. 108).

they known that 5-fluorocytosine acts by being metabolized to the cytotoxic agent fluorouracil they might reasonably have thought again about its potential as a candidate for antimicrobial therapy.

It eventually emerged that 5-fluorocytosine itself has little antifungal activity. As Richard Giege and Jacques-Henry Weil of the University of Strasbourg found in 1969, yeasts that possess the enzyme cytosine deaminase convert it to 5-fluorouracil, which is then incorporated into the ribonucleic acid (RNA) of the yeast, interfering with its function. Yeasts lacking this enzyme are resistant (25). However, the mechanism of action of 5-fluorocytosine in yeasts was not at first properly understood in Nutley, New Jersey. By good fortune it turns out that mammalian cells are deficient in cytosine deaminase while yeasts have adopted the enzyme as a useful, though not indispensable tool in nucleic acid formation.

Clinicians were understandably reluctant to use flucytosine (as it came to be known) as antifungal therapy. It was not until March 1967 that John Utz of the Medical College of Virginia ventured to test the new drug in patients suffering from cryptococcosis. The results were encouraging: of 15 patients treated, three with pulmonary disease improved; one with multiple subcutaneous lesions died, but was microbiologically cured; and nine of 11 patients with cryptococcal meningitis responded well, although four subsequently relapsed (26). The findings of this trial spurred others to use the drug in serious *Candida* infections and in cryptococcal meningitis. The value of the drug in human infections was confirmed, but frequent side effects were noted. A considerable boost to flucytosine came in 1971, when Gerald Medoff and his colleagues at Washington University School of Medicine, St Louis, Missouri showed that the drug interacts synergically with amphotericin B (27), opening the way for these two toxic compounds to be used in lower doses. Combined use also increases the likelihood of effective therapy for these difficult clinical infections and lowers the known risk of resistance to flucytosine emerging during treatment.

Tackling the dermatophytes

The polyenes and flucytosine represented a significant advance in the treatment of yeast and systemic fungal infections, but they have little useful activity against the dermatophytes causing the various forms of ringworm. Significant progress in this area came with the availability of griseofulvin, an antibiotic that came in tablet form and was active against all the major causes of hair, skin, and nail ringworm. It was later joined by terbinafine, a synthetic chemical that also displays potent activity against these troublesome fungi.

Griseofulvin

Griseofulvin was first identified in 1938 by a team led by Harold Raistrick at the London School of Hygiene and Tropical Medicine (28). It emerged during an extensive study of the biochemistry of fungi as a metabolic product of *Penicillium griseofulvum*. Raistrick, despite his eminence, seems to have had a genius for appearing on the periphery of antibiotic discovery (see p. 93) for he seems to have had no inkling that griseofulvin might have any therapeutic purpose.

Just after the Second World War a study was under-way at ICI's Butterwick Research Laboratories* in Welwyn, Hertfordshire to examine why the growth of conifers on Wareham Heath in Dorset was unexpectedly poor. Percy Brian, a physicist turned plant physiologist and mycologist, led the investigation (29). The roots of trees, like most other plants are colonized by fungi that exist in a symbiotic relationship—known as a mycorrhiza—whereby the fungus scavenges trace elements from the surrounding soil to the benefit of the plant in return for ready-made sugar molecules. Brian's team started to look for micro-organisms in the soil of Wareham Heath that might be interfering with development of the mycorrhiza. During this investigation a *Penicillium* fungus was isolated which produced a substance affecting growth of the hyphae of *Botrytis allii*, a plant pathogen that was being used as test organism. The fungus was *Penicillium janczewskii* and Brian called the substance that it produced 'curling factor', a graphic, but not very instructive term (30). In 1947 two of Brian's colleagues at the Butterwick Laboratories, John Grove and John McGowan, showed that 'curling factor' was identical to Raistrick's griseofulvin (31). Brain then went on to show that griseofulvin was widely active in protecting plants from certain fungal infections (32) and both ICI and Glaxo began to take an interest in it as a possible systemic fungicide for agricultural use.

Percy Brian wrote several other papers in the immediate post-war period about products of moulds that exhibited biological activity against other fungi, but he and the drug companies with which he collaborated seem to have had more interest in possible agricultural applications of his work, rather than any medical use. In the event, hopes that griseofulvin might be exploited in the control of diseases of plants were frustrated by the cost and a failure to demonstrate that it was better than established antifungal agents (33). It was left to the Scottish mycologist James Clark Gentles in Glasgow—where Brian was later (in 1963) appointed Regius Professor of Botany before moving on to Cambridge in 1968—to take the first steps towards bringing griseofulvin to medical attention. Gentles had succeeded in establishing experimental infections in guinea pigs with dermatophyte fungi that caused human infections. In August 1958, a decade after Brian's initial discovery, he showed that oral griseofulvin provided by Glaxo was able to free the animals of the fungal infection (34). Ironically, almost identical studies were by then independently underway in ICI's Alderley Park laboratories, and soon after Gentles published his work the biologist A. R. Martin of ICI described similar findings (35).

By chance, at the time of the appearance of Gentles' paper in *Nature*, a dermatologist at the University of Miami School of Medicine, Harvey Blank had under his care a rare case of disseminated infection with the dermatophyte *Trichophyton rubrum* which appeared likely to be fatal. He managed to obtain some griseofulvin, and used it to achieve a dramatic cure (36). Meanwhile in King's College Hospital, London, David Williams was

---

* In 1954, ICI changed the name to the Akers Research Laboratory after the death of their former Director of Research, Wallace Alan Akers, who had masterminded the development after the Second World War. The facility was closed in 1961.

using Gentles' new drug to treat more mundane dermatophyte infections and the derma-tologist Gustav Riehl* in Vienna was conducting similar trials. After a brief scare about possible mutagenic effects, both Glaxo and ICI soon had griseofulvin on the market. The drug was launched at two international symposia: the first at the University of Miami in October 1959; the other 6 months later in London, organized by the St John's Hospital Dermatological Society (37).

A unique feature of griseofulvin, as Gentles discovered in collaboration with Karl Fantes at Glaxo, was that the drug was actually deposited in the keratin of the skin and hair, which represented the site of infection (38).† More importantly, adequate quantities of the drug are incorporated into growing nail, so that if treatment is sufficiently pro-longed, a new, uninfected nail should eventually replace the infected tissue. Treatment of slow-growing toenails often took 12 months or more, and treatment failures or relapses were common, but it was the first time that chemotherapeutic cures of nail dermato-phyte infections had been achieved.

Terbinafine

Like griseofulvin, terbinafine has the valuable property of being incorporated into growing nail, where it exerts a potent antifungal action. It belongs to a group of com-pounds described chemically as allylamines. They first came to notice in 1974 during a project being carried out in the Sandoz-Wander laboratories in Berne into potential drugs with central nervous system activity. One of the compounds unexpectedly gener-ated during a routine synthesis turned out to have an unusual structure (39). In keeping with the company policy to screen all such novel molecules for possible antimicrobial activity it was passed on to the Sandoz Research Institute in Vienna, where a team led by the dynamic Jürgen Drews found it to have good activity against certain pathogenic fungi, including various dermatophytes (40). In 1981 one of the institute's chemists, Neil Ryder, discovered that the compound, given the generic name naftifine, preferen-tially inhibited an early step in the biosynthesis of ergosterol; this is the major sterol in fungal, but not mammalian cell membranes, where cholesterol predominates. Naftifine thus had the necessary selective toxicity for a systemically administered human drug, but it was insufficiently active when given orally to infected guinea pigs and it was eventually decided to market it in 1985 for the topical treatment of superficial fungal infections.

Although naftifine was far from being a significant breakthrough in the treatment of fungal infections, it provided the lead compound for further developments pursued at the Sandoz Research Institute by Anton Stütz and his colleagues. By 1979 a particular alteration in the molecular configuration had been found to dramatically improve anti-fungal activity and in January 1980 the compound developed as terbinafine had been

---

* Son of a famous dermatologist and syphilologist, Gustav Riehl senior.

† Coincidentally the paper appears on the same page of the issue of *Nature* in which Ralph Batchelor and his colleagues reported 6-aminopenicillanic acid (see p. 123).

synthesized (41). In standard protection tests in guinea pigs, the activity of terbinafine exceeded that of naftifine by a factor of 100 and that of griseofulvin by a factor of 10. After the usual extensive pharmacological and toxicological testing, clinical trials were initiated and the first preliminary results presented at the 14th International Congress of Chemotherapy held in Kyoto, Japan in 1985 (42). More extensive studies followed and terbinafine was found to be well tolerated, more reliable than griseofulvin in dermatophyte infections—some toenail infections that were refractory to griseofulvin treatment cleared up in 3–6 months—and to have a broader usefulness in certain other types of fungal infection. By the end of the decade the commercial possibilities of terbinafine had become clear. In 1991 it was launched in the United Kingdom and received FDA approval the following year in the United States.

Broad-spectrum breakthrough

The notion that azole derivatives might have useful antifungal activity dates back to the work of Wayne Woolley at the Rockefeller Institute in the 1940s (see p. 325). In 1958, Chemie Grünenthal, a family owned firm founded in 1946 in Germany,* marketed an antifungal imidazole called chlormidazole for cutaneous application, but it made little impression. It was not until 1969, with the description of clotrimazole (Fig. 8.1) by a group led by Manfred Plempel in the Bayer laboratories in Wuppertal (43), and miconazole, developed by Paul Janssen's team in Belgium (44), that the potential of these chemicals as chemotherapeutic agents distinguished by an unusual broad spectrum of antifungal activity began to be appreciated.

Both clotrimazole and miconazole were on the market by 1973 and soon became popular, chiefly for the treatment of oral and vaginal thrush. A similar compound, econazole quickly followed from the Janssen stable. Like the allylamines, these drugs act to disrupt

Clotrimazole   Fluconazole

Fig. 8.1 Structures of the two main types of azole antifungal drugs: clotrimazole (an imidazole) and fluconazole (a triazole).

---

* The company established itself by manufacturing penicillin under licence, but suffered a major setback at the end of the 1950s when thalidomide, a drug that they had developed and marketed as a sedative turned out to cause severe birth defects.

ergosterol synthesis in fungi and they appeared relatively safe in toxicological studies, but poor absorption when administered by mouth prevented their use in systemic fungal infections. An injectable formulation of miconazole was marketed, but clinical results were disappointing and it was later withdrawn. Numerous imidazoles appeared during the next 15 years: Robert Fromtling of the Merck Institute in New Jersey in a comprehensive review written in 1988, was able to survey 21 different antifungal azoles of which 13 were already on the market (45). Most of these drugs were copycat compounds aimed at the market for the topical treatment of vaginal thrush or cutaneous ringworm; one, tioconazole, first described from Pfizer in the United Kingdom in 1979 (46) and marketed there in 1989, was formulated in a keratin-penetrating vehicle and sanguinely claimed to cure nail infections.

The big prize for the drug companies was an antifungal imidazole that was well absorbed and effective when given orally. It was once again Paul Janssen's group in Beerse, Belgium that came up with goods with the synthesis of the chemically complex piperazine derivative, ketoconazole, in 1976. Independent laboratory studies and clinical trials were quickly put in train and preliminary details of the new compound were revealed in 1979 (47). An international symposium devoted to the new drug, organized in Medellin, Columbia in late November 1979, signalled the start of a big publicity drive. It paid off. The drug was enthusiastically received (48) and in 1981 it was approved for use in the United States.

Ketoconazole ruled the roost for a decade as the most active antifungal agent for the oral treatment of many fungal infections. Despite occasional reports of liver damage and other side effects it was clearly less toxic than amphotericin B, though it was considerably less effective against some life-threatening fungal infections including those caused by filamentous fungi like *Aspergillus fumigatus*.

In 1982, Ken Richardson, a Nottingham University graduate who had pursued postdoctoral research with the Nobel laureate Bob Woodward at Harvard, but had by then moved on to Pfizer Central Research in Sandwich, Kent, took out a patent on a new azole derivative, fluconazole. Details of the discovery were disclosed after investigation of the drug's potential 3 years later (49). Fluconazole differs from earlier compounds of this type by having an additional nitrogen atom in the azole ring, making it a triazole, rather than an imidazole derivative; in fact, fluconazole has two triazole rings so that it is properly described as a bis-triazole (Fig. 8.1). Compared with ketoconazole it is more reliably absorbed when administered by mouth and more slowly eliminated in the urine. More importantly, serious side effects are less common and, unlike ketoconazole, the drug is able to cross the blood-brain barrier in sufficient concentration to treat cryptococcal meningitis.

Not surprisingly, fluconazole emerged as the preferred azole drug for many serious systemic fungal infections after it was introduced in the late 1980s and the popularity of ketoconazole was eclipsed. Janssen's team, however, already had another drug in development, which was to maintain their competitive challenge. The new substance was itraconazole, also a triazole compound, synthesized in 1980 and first described by

Jan Heeres, Leo Backx, and Jan Van Cutsem in 1984 (50). It immediately caused a stir of medical interest since it was the first antifungal agent to show convincing activity against infections with filamentous fungi, which, although uncommon, were being seen with greater frequency among debilitated patients. By 1989 itraconazole was on the market in some European countries and the drug received approval for restricted indications in the United States in 1992. Opinions differ about the relative merits of fluconazole and itraconazole, but the former is certainly superior in the treatment of central nervous system infections, while itraconazole is more effective against filamentous fungi.

Not to be outdone, Pfizer responded by further modification of the fluconazole molecule to produce a new derivative, voriconazole, which includes *Aspergillus fumigatus* and some other moulds in its spectrum. It was first described at the 1995 Interscience Conference on Antimicrobial Agents and Chemotherapy (ICAAC) in San Francisco by Chris Hitchcock, Peter Troke, and their colleagues, and received approval for clinical use in the European Union and in the United States in 2002.

The best of the rest

The paucity of resources with which to treat fungal diseases during the glory days of antibacterial antibiotics brought forth a rash of compounds that might not otherwise have received serious consideration. In the United States, antiprotozoal diamidines (see p. 282–3), such as propamidine, stilbamidine, and the somewhat less toxic 2-hydroxystilbamidine were briefly used for indigenous life-threatening infections with dimorphic fungi, such as blastomycosis before amphotericin B came along to offer equally toxic, but a more reliable therapy. There was also a short flirtation with an antibiotic, saramycetin, a peptide antibiotic produced by *Streptomyces saraceticus* discovered in the laboratories of Hoffmann-La Roche in Nutley, New Jersey by Emanuel Grunberg and Edith Titsworth and first described in 1961 (51). Apart from these short-lived compounds a rash of topical agents appeared and there was a doggedly persistent interest in a group of antibiotics with antifungal activity, the echinocandins, which was to pay-off with a compound introduced into human medicine several decades later.

Topical antifungal agents

In addition to polyenes and the allylamine, naftifine (see above), various synthetic chemicals that display antifungal activity appeared between 1960 and 1990. They include: tolnaftate—discovered by Teruhisa Noguchi and his colleagues at the Nippon Soda Company in Japan around 1962 and brought to market by the Schering Corporation in America (52); the iodinated trichlorphenol, haloprogin—another Japanese discovery from Meiji Seika Kaisha Ltd in Yokohama in the early 1960s (53), taken up in the United States by Mead Johnson in Evansville, Indiana (54); the synthetic pyridine derivative, ciclopirox olamine, developed by Hoechst in Germany in the mid-1970s; the morpholine derivative, amorolfine from Hofmann-La Roche in Basel in the early 1980s; and the benzylamine butenafine, synthesized by Tetsuya Maeda and his colleagues at the Kaken Pharmaceutical Company, Tokyo in 1987. These compounds are far too toxic to be used systemically.

Their place in therapy is similar to that of the topical antibacterial antiseptics and, like them, they have played only a peripheral role in the therapeutic revolution of the twentieth century.

Echinocandins

Interest in the echinocandins as potential antifungal agents dates back at least as far as 1974 when chemists from the Ciba-Geigy research laboratories in Basel together with colleagues at the Technische Hochschule (Technical University) in Zürich, described an antibiotic produced by a fungus identified as *Aspergillus nidulans* var. echinulatus isolated from the leaves of beech trees (55). The antibiotic, echinocandin B, one of a group of closely related antibiotics produced by the fungus, displayed good activity against yeasts, including *Candida albicans*. In 1976, Camilla Keller-Juslén and her colleagues at Sandoz in Basel described a new antibiotic from *Aspergillus rugulosus* that turned out to be identical to Ciba-Geigy's echinocandin B. The antibiotic was soon realized to be too toxic for human use, but interest nevertheless continued in natural or semisynthetic derivatives that might provide useful leads. Eli Lilly in the United States was one of the firms that took an interest in this group of compounds and in the early 1980s, scientists at Lilly thought they had come up with a chemically modified derivative of echinocandin B that combined high activity with low toxicity in animal experiments (56). The substance, which was given the generic name cilofungin, briefly reached clinical trial, but the intravenous preparation contained polyethylene glycol, which not surprisingly caused unacceptable toxicity and trials were abandoned.

In 1985 a sample of pond water from River Lozoya valley in Central Spain was examined in the laboratories of the Centro de Investigación Básica de España, the research centre run by Merck, Sharp, and Dohme in Madrid where the antibacterial antibiotic fosfomycin had earlier been discovered (see p. 246–7). A fungus originally identified as *Zalerion arboricola*, but since reclassified as *Glarea lozoyensis* was recovered from which scientists at Merck in Rahway, New Jersey isolated an antibiotic closely related to the echinocandins. Various congeners obtained from mutant strains of the original producer organism were examined for antimicrobial activity and one designated L-671,239 showed excellent activity against *Candida* species and was selected for further development (57). At the time that this work was undertaken, the AIDS epidemic was reaching its height in the United States and an organism called *Pneumocystis carinii* was causing many deaths from pneumonia among those affected. The new antibiotic was tested against the organism (no easy task: *Pneumocystis carinii* cannot be grown in artificial culture and a rat model was used) and found to be active (58). Sensing a market opening, the company declared the compound to be a pneumocandin, rather than an echinocandin in order to stress its dual activity.

Pneumocystis carinii (now called *Pneumocystis jirovecii*) has a chequered history. It was first mistakenly described as a trypanosome by Carlos Chagas in Brazil in 1909, the same year in which he also described the trypanosome that causes what became known as Chagas' disease (see p. 317). The following year Antonio Carini, an Italian working at the

Pasteur Institute in São Paolo in Brazil found the same parasites in lung tissue of rats and sent samples to the Pasteur Institute in Paris. There Pierre Delanoë and his wife Eugénie recognized that the organism was a new species and proposed the name *Pneumocystis carinii* in recognition of Carini's role. Its taxonomic place remained unknown for many years, though it was commonly thought to be some kind of protozoon. Its classification remains controversial, though it is now generally accepted on the basis of genetic evidence to be a fungus. *Pneumocystis carinii* came to prominence at the end of the Second World War, when it was incriminated in pneumonia in malnourished children in Europe. Persistent reports from the United States in the early 1980s of pneumonia caused by the organism in homosexual men was one of the main factors that alerted public health authorities to the existence of what became known as the acquired immune deficiency syndrome (AIDS).

Established *Pneumocystis carinii* pneumonia is difficult to treat. Surprisingly, the antibacterial combination, co-trimoxazole (see p. 255) is effective, but serious side effects are commonly caused by the high doses required. Alternative treatments are also poorly tolerated and prevention rather than cure became the preferred strategy. With the availability of effective retroviral drugs, *Pneumocystis carinii* pneumonia has become much less common, at least in rich countries of the world, but in the early stages of the development of the pneumocandins, it played a crucial part in the decision to progress these compounds. In the event, L-671,239 did not make the grade, but a related derivative synthesized by the Merck chemists, given the generic name caspofungin, received restricted regulatory approval in the United States in January 2001. Ironically, this representative of the pneumocandin family—a name chosen to reflect activity against *Pneumocystis* and *Candida*—received its licence for the treatment of neither infection, but for the so-called 'salvage' therapy of invasive aspergillosis in patients unresponsive or intolerant of other drugs.

A related echinocandin derivative, micafungin, developed by the Japanese firm, Fujisawa, was licensed for use in deep-seated fungal infections in Japan in December 2002 and received FDA approval in the United States the following year. Others are under development. These compounds, though welcome, are unlikely to prove to be a major breakthrough in the treatment of systemic fungal diseases. Despite the progress that has been made during the past 50 years, therapeutic resources for infections with pathogenic fungi still lag far behind those available for bacterial diseases.

Antiviral agents

Views on the prospects for effective antiviral therapy in the antibiotics heyday of the 1950s and 1960s mirrored the gloomy prognostications that were made about antibacterial agents shortly before sulphonamides and penicillin proved them to be wide of the mark (see p. 64). Viruses, it was said, are far too intimately bound up with the metabolism of cells for selective action against them to be possible. Moreover, massive viral reproduction takes place before symptoms become evident so that timely therapeutic intervention would be difficult to achieve. Immunization was the way forward, since viruses are antigenically simple and a powerful long-lasting antibody response was evident in many viral infections.

While subsequent events have, to some extent, confounded these predictions—selectively active antiviral agents have emerged and vaccines against some viruses have proved difficult to devise—the fundamental premises of the argument remain valid. Viruses do subvert the cellular machinery and there are relatively few points in the viral life cycle, from attachment to and penetration in the cell to the production and release of new viral particles, that are open to selective attack. A problem does exist with delivering antiviral agents in a therapeutically timely manner. Prevention remains more reliable than cure and in this immunization has often been spectacularly successful, as parents who are spared the fear of regular outbreaks of poliomyelitis—and, of course, the even grimmer epidemics of the deadly bacterial disease, diphtheria—can testify.

The ease with which vaccines can be developed diminishes with the complexity of the target organism. The least problematic vaccines have been devised against viruses, such as smallpox, polio, measles, mumps, rubella, and yellow fever, or bacterial toxins, such as those of diphtheria and tetanus. Successful vaccines against bacteria—meningococcal, haemophilus, and pertussis vaccines are good examples—have also been produced, but have presented bigger challenges. There are, as yet, no adequate vaccines against protozoal diseases, at least for human use. Vaccines against fungi or helminths such as schistosomes present the greatest challenge of all. Vaccines have played such an important part in the control of viral diseases that it would be a dereliction to omit a brief account of their history.

Antiviral vaccines

Smallpox

A form of vaccination against smallpox—paradoxically one of the most complex viruses—has been practised for centuries in China in the form of variolation: use of material from pustules of mild cases of smallpox to inoculate unaffected individuals. News of the method had travelled along the Silk Route and by the eighteenth century it was established as far west as Turkey. Reports of the practice soon filtered through to the Royal Society in London, but it was Lady Mary Wortley Montagu (née Pierrepont) who championed use of the method in Britain after observing it at close hand in Constantinople (Istanbul). Born in London within living memory of the great plague of 1665, but raised in the family seat, Thoresby Hall,* in Nottinghamshire, Mary contracted smallpox at the age of 26, ruining her widely admired beauty. She had earlier eloped with Edward Wortley Montagu, and set off with him in 1716 (the year after she contracted smallpox) on a year-long diplomatic mission to Turkey. There she observed the practice of variolation and arranged for her 4-year-old son to be inoculated. He developed mild symptoms and about 100 spots, but quickly recovered (59).

---

* The original Thoresby Hall was destroyed by fire in 1745. The present mansion was built in 1865–75 to replace a smaller house constructed in 1767–71.

On her return to England, Lady Mary Wortley Montagu campaigned vigorously for the introduction of variolation, incurring much vilification as 'an unnatural mother' for submitting her own children to the practice. No doubt, history would have agreed if things had gone wrong, but fortunately they did not. However, variolation was to have only a short vogue. The real breakthrough came later in the century when it was discovered that inoculation with matter from lesions caused by the less virulent cowpox could offer a much safer form of protection. It was Edward Jenner, the country doctor from Berkeley, Gloucestershire who famously established the validity of the technique by formal experimentation. On 14 May 1796 Jenner took material from a cowpox pustule on the hand of Sarah Nelmes, daughter of a local farmer, and introduced the matter into the arm of a young boy, James Phipps. A few weeks later, on 1 July, the boy was inoculated with material from a smallpox lesion and, as Jenner had predicted, it produced no effect (60). In fact, Jenner's work had been anticipated by a Dorset farmer, Benjamin Jesty. Aware that milkmaids who had contracted cowpox rarely developed smallpox, Jesty inoculated his wife and two children with material from an infected cow's udder during a smallpox epidemic in 1774. Both Jenner and Jesty received as many brickbats as bouquets for their actions, but it was Jenner, the doctor with London connections, who had conducted a scientific (albeit ethically dubious) enquiry who rightly received most of the credit from those who recognized the value of the procedure (61).

The public reception of Jennerian vaccination is reminiscent of present-day debate over genetically modified food: a highly vociferous campaign, fuelled by the propagation of misleading fears, drowning out convincing evidence of the advantages. Fortunately, in the nineteenth century, the verdict of the public health authorities in Britain prevailed against bitter opposition. An Act of Parliament made vaccination mandatory in 1853, but the ruling was not strictly enforced. Jennerian vaccination was introduced in the United States largely through the pioneering work of Benjamin Waterhouse and James Smith and by the mid-nineteenth century, the procedure had been made compulsory in many countries. The incidence of the infection plummeted in countries where vigorous vaccination programmes were introduced. By the twentieth century the threat of smallpox had largely been removed from many countries, but it was not until the World Health Assembly adopted a Soviet proposal, put forward in 1959, to pursue a policy of global eradication that the first faltering steps began to be taken towards controlling sporadic epidemics among the poorer populations of the world. It took another 12 years for the eradication programme to begin in earnest. Despite many problems and setbacks, the last naturally acquired case of smallpox, Ali Maow Maalin of Somalia, was diagnosed in 1977;* the World Health Organization declared that the goal of global eradication had been achieved on 26 October 1979 (62).

----

* The last death from smallpox occurred in 1978, when Janet Parker, a medical photographer in the Department of Anatomy at Birmingham University acquired the disease while working in a darkroom situated on the floor above a research laboratory where the virologist Henry Bedson was working on the virus. He subsequently suffered severe depression and committed suicide.

The vaccine used for this outstanding accomplishment was not Jenner's cowpox, but vaccinia virus, the origins of which are obscure (63).

From Pasteur to the Second World War

The recognition of the value, first of variolation and then Jennerian vaccination, against smallpox was the result of astute observation and empirical trial at a time when the nature of the disease was totally incomprehensible. Success with other vaccines had to await the birth of medical microbiology in the second half of the nineteenth century and Louis Pasteur's ground-breaking experiments with anthrax in cattle and human rabies. Pasteur's approach was to produce live vaccines from microbes that had been attenuated—much reduced in virulence—by repeated subculture in the laboratory. Naturally, he was unable to grow a rabies germ in artificial culture, but he correctly inferred that the disease must be due to some form of infective micro-organism. His rabies vaccine was a crude extract prepared by his assistant Émile Roux from the desiccated spinal cords of rabbits that had been serially inoculated with the virus. Just how effective it could have been has been hotly disputed, but Pasteur achieved some apparently miraculous cures, starting with the celebrated case of 9-year-old Joseph Meister in July 1885, which brought him instant popular adulation.

The principle of inoculation to cure microbial disease received a major boost from Emil von Behring and Shibasaburo Kitasato's work with anti-diphtheria and anti-tetanus sera in the 1890s, creating hopes that many other life-threatening diseases could be controlled by similar means. Though whole industries grew up around the production of both protective and therapeutic vaccines—including Almroth Wright's Inoculation Department at St Mary's Hospital (see p. 60)—evidence for benefit from most of them was sparse. Some, like Koch's tuberculin (see p. 145) turned out to be disastrous, for most of the rest chemotherapy effectively put paid to their popularity. A few prophylactic vaccines for bacterial diseases, such as those against cholera, typhoid fever and, most successfully, Bacille Calmette Guérin for tuberculosis (see p. 142–4) remained in use, but were at best only partially protective; more effective bacterial vaccines did not emerge until scientific understanding of the immune response to bacterial antigens had become more refined.

For viruses, vaccination remained the most attractive option. The examples of smallpox and rabies did not, however, provide useful precedents, since understanding of the nature of viruses lagged far behind the advances made in bacteriology. The first success did not come until the 1930s when Max Theiler, a South African working at the International Health Division of the Rockefeller Foundation in the United States, devised a vaccine against yellow fever. Theiler and his colleagues settled a long-standing dispute about the cause of yellow fever, showing it to be a filterable virus. Together with Hugh Smith, Theiler went on to show that the virus could be grown in the brains of white mice (much more expensive monkeys had formerly been used) and subsequently by the newly described technique of tissue culture. By 1937 they had produced a vaccine from an attenuated virus grown in tissue culture, which they called strain 17D, initially intended for the protection of laboratory workers. After initial trials in monkeys, Theiler, Smith, and several other volunteers were given the vaccine to test the immune response (64). In field trials conducted in Brazil the vaccine proved generally safe, though a few incidents of reversion to virulence occurred and it transpired that preparations quickly lost their potency on storage. In 1942, when the vaccine was used to protect 2.5 million United States troops, vaccine stabilized by suspension in human serum was used. It proved to be a dreadful mistake: more than 20,000 of the troops went down with infectious hepatitis, caused by a then unknown virus (65).

Protection for children

For those of us who can remember parental fears of life-threatening summer epidemics and the heart-rending sight of young children imprisoned in cumbersome 'iron lungs', one of the greatest achievements of the twentieth century was the virtual elimination of infantile paralysis—poliomyelitis. The prototype iron lung had been developed by Philip Drinker and Louis Shaw at Harvard in 1927 and improved upon by a medical device manufacturer closely associated with Harvard, John Emerson in 1931.[*] Iron lungs were still in use in the late 1950s. They kept many victims alive during the acute paralytic phase of the disease, but affected children were often left with permanent disabilities. It was a vaccine devised at the University of Pittsburgh Medical School by Jonas Salk, son of Russian–Jewish immigrants, that was to turn the tide with the help of money provided by the 'March of Dimes' campaign.[†] President Franklin Delano Roosevelt, who had himself been struck down with polio as an adult in 1921, had established the fund to support research into polio in 1938.

Although the viral nature of polio had been suspected since the early twentieth century and was formally proven through the work of the Polish-born émigré, Albert Sabin and his associates at the Rockefeller Institute in 1936, work on a vaccine was hampered by the lack of a suitable means of propagating the virus. It was only after John Enders and his colleagues succeeded in growing the virus in tissue culture in 1949 (see p. 11)—an achievement that had been given crucial momentum by the availability of antibiotics to prevent bacterial contamination—that prospects for production of a vaccine became a reality. Both Salk and Sabin (by then at the University of Cincinnati) were in the race, as were Herald Cox and his colleague, the multi-talented Polish-born Hilary Koprowski at Lederle, but it was the more impulsive Salk who won, with a formalin-inactivated vaccine announced in 1953 (66). Extensive field trials—among the largest ever conducted—masterminded by the medical virologist at the University of Michigan, Thomas Francis, were carried out in the United States, Canada, and Finland and their success announced by Francis at a legendary news conference in April 1955. Media coverage of the results of the vaccine trial made Salk a public hero. Even an early tragedy when 214 vaccine recipients or their contacts developed polio caused by live virus contaminating a commercially-produced batch of the vaccine failed to dent his popular reputation. Salk milked the adulation and

---

[*] Emerson's improved respirator triggered an unedifying battle over patent rights.

[†] Originally the 'National Foundation for Infantile Paralysis', the 'March of Dimes' was coined by the comedian Eddie Cantor in a radio appeal for funds. The title played on 'The March of Time', a popular newsreel feature in this period.

his attitude antagonized his fellow doctors and scientists. Others who had been involved received scant credit. None deserved recognition more than Tom Francis, who had prior experience of vaccine work at the Rockefeller Institute in the 1920s and had introduced Jonas Salk to the techniques of vaccine production, but Salk was in no mood to acknowledge anyone who might deflect attention from his achievement.

Meanwhile, Albert Sabin and Herald Cox at Lederle were pursuing a live attenuated vaccine that could be administered by mouth. Hilary Koprowski moved in 1957 to the Wistar Institute, a medical research unit in Philadelphia, and also continued work there on an attenuated vaccine. By 1954, Sabin had succeeded in isolating avirulent variants of each of the three antigenic types of virus responsible for polio (67). Injecting an inactivated poliovirus was one thing, giving children a live vaccine with the possibility of reversion to virulence was quite another. Salk's vaccine had effectively stopped polio in its tracks in the United States and there was no appetite for a trial of Sabin's substitute. Moreover mass vaccination with Salk's vaccine had generated a population already rendered immune, making the validation of Sabin's alternative version difficult. An oral vaccine for mass polio prevention campaigns in other countries was, however, an attractive proposition. In 1957, the World Health Organization decided to support a trial of Sabin's vaccine in Russia, Holland, Mexico, Chile, Sweden, and Japan. In the meantime, Cox and Koprowski also had oral vaccines ready for clinical testing. Cox's trial was carried out in Latin America, while Koprowski initiated trials in the Congo, giving rise to a later theory, now discredited by most authorities, that the AIDS pandemic originated in a vaccine prepared in monkey kidney cells contaminated with simian immunodeficiency virus and used in Africa. The WHO-sponsored trial was the most extensive and gave impressive results. By 1961 Sabin's vaccine had become the standard for polio vaccination in many countries, though inactivated virus vaccines manufactured in government laboratories continued in use in the Netherlands and Scandinavia (68).

Although Sabin's vaccine has been largely responsible for the near eradication of poliomyelitis throughout the world, Salk has had the last laugh. The disease has become so rare that the risk of administration of Sabin's live attenuated vaccine now outweighs the benefits of protection and the Salk vaccine is again officially recommended for childhood vaccination programmes. The two scientists remained bitter enemies until the end and this may have contributed to the astonishing fact that neither received the Nobel Prize for their achievements.

Vaccines for other viral diseases of childhood—measles, mumps, rubella, and chickenpox—were soon being considered. Measles, which can be severe, even fatal, was the first priority. Once again it was John Enders and his colleagues in Boston who came up with the goods in 1960 with an attenuated strain of the measles virus grown in tissue culture (69). The vaccine was licensed in the United States in 1963 and by 1968 the incidence of measles had fallen from a yearly average of about 500,000 cases a year to around 25,000 cases with a concomitant decline in deaths and serious complications. By the end of the century less than 100 cases a year were being reported, most of them from abroad or linked to imported cases (70). Similar falls in incidence occurred in other developed countries after introduction of the vaccine.

Vaccines against mumps and german measles (rubella) followed despite vigorous debate when they first appeared about the necessity, or even wisdom, of protecting young children against these diseases: both are trivial diseases in early childhood and it was argued that it is best to let the viruses circulate freely. In the case of rubella, which can cause birth defects during pregnancy, it was reasoned that vaccination should be reserved for young women shown to be non-immune as they approached child-bearing age. A combined vaccine providing protection against measles, mumps, and rubella (MMR) is now offered routinely in infancy alongside vaccines against polio and bacterial diseases including diphtheria, pertussis, tetanus, and certain types of meningitis. Despite periodic scares about side effects of some vaccines, the policy has contributed to a marked decline in these diseases wherever it has been instituted. The need for continued vigilance was highlighted in the United Kingdom in 1995, when a possible link was proposed between the MMR vaccine and the development of autism and inflammatory bowel disease. Although the claim was extensively investigated and convincingly shown to be unjustified, public confidence in the vaccine was dented triggering concern about the return of diseases that had been successfully controlled.

Vaccines galore

The stunning success of vaccines in controlling viral and bacterial diseases of childhood underlines their unique role in the control of infectious diseases. However, viruses have proved much more amenable to the vaccine approach than bacteria. Numerous vaccines have been produced over the years for the protection of animals or people, especially those at special risk, and many of these are for viral diseases. The path is not always smooth, as experience with attempts to develop a vaccine against human immunodeficiency virus (HIV) show. Vaccines against influenza have to be revised regularly to keep up with the changing antigenic make-up of the circulating virus.

The intensive work needed to develop and test vaccines has been prosecuted in many laboratories, both academic and commercial and it would be invidious to select out for mention individual names from the legions of those who have been responsible for the many advances that have been made. However, an exception can certainly be made for one man, the American microbiologist, Maurice Hilleman, who during a long and productive career did more than most to provide safe and effective vaccines for the world. Hilleman's first job after graduation during the Second World War was with Squibb, where he helped to develop a vaccine against Japanese B encephalitis for the Far East war effort. He moved to the Walter Reed Army Institute of Research from 1948–57, working on respiratory viruses, and spent the rest of his career with Merck in New Jersey. In all, Hilleman was intimately involved with the development of around 40 animal and human vaccines. It was his work at Merck that was instrumental in perfecting John Enders' measles vaccine and he was also involved with, among others, mumps (he isolated the most widely used vaccine strain from his daughter's throat during an episode of mumps and gave it her name, Jeryl Lynn, in her honour), rubella, chickenpox, hepatitis A and, perhaps most famously, hepatitis B, first licensed in the United States in 1981. Hilleman additionally initiated crucial work on influenza vaccines and was among the first to investigate the antigenic changes that make the virus such an elusive enemy (71).

Antiviral drugs

Set against the achievements of antiviral vaccines, the search for drugs for the treatment of viral disease has met with modest success. Hopes of finding naturally occurring antiviral substances to match the success of antibiotics have been singularly unsuccessful. It has not been for want of trying, although in the post-Second World War antibiotic gold rush, antiviral agents were not pursued with the same enthusiasm as antibacterial and antifungal compounds. A few early reports of natural products with antiviral activity appeared in the literature at regular intervals, but none of them came to anything. One such substance was isolated by the celebrated American virologist Richard Shope, discoverer in 1931 of swine influenza and in 1933 of the Shope papilloma virus. The antiviral compound was produced by 'a penicillium isolated from the isinglass cover of a photograph of my wife, Helen, on Guam, near the end of the war in 1945'. It was named Helenine 'out of recognition of the good taste shown by the mold producing the substance in locating on the picture of my wife (72).' Helenine aroused considerable interest for a while, but was eventually abandoned. It was later shown to act by inducing a natural antiviral defence protein of the body, interferon, a compound which itself led to premature talk of an antiviral penicillin after its discovery in 1957.

Interferon

Interferon was the outcome of research into a mysterious phenomenon known as 'viral interference' discovered in the 1930s. The essence of the observation was that animals infected with one virus were often found to be refractory for a period of hours or days to infection with an unrelated virus. While investigating the phenomenon at the Medical Research Council laboratories at Mill Hill, North London in 1957, Glasgow-born Alick Isaacs and a Swiss visitor to the laboratory, Jean Lindenmann infected the chorio-allantoic membrane of chicken eggs with influenza virus. They found that material harvested from the membranes and freed of virus could prevent infection of a second batch of eggs with fresh virus. A substance had been produced during the first infection that seemed to have the ability to inhibit viral replication. They named the substance 'the interferon' (73).

It was soon shown that the activity of interferon was non-specific, acting against various unrelated viruses. Expectations were high that a breakthrough had been made that had profound implications for the treatment of viral disease. Disclosure of the discovery precluded patenting in the United Kingdom and many other countries, but patent applications were filed in the United States, Canada, and Germany, where the rules were more relaxed. In 1958 the Medical Research Council entered into an unprecedented partnership with ICI, Glaxo, and Wellcome to investigate and develop the new wonder drug (74). It was soon clear that there were major difficulties. The distinguished virologist David Tyrrell, Director of the Common Cold Research Unit in Salisbury, showed that interferon was species-specific; that is, it was most active in the animal species from which it had been harvested and had poor activity in other unrelated species. Moreover, yields of interferon by the methods then available were very poor and it was difficult to purify. Nonetheless, sufficient active material had been obtained by 1962 for a small clinical trial in volunteers. The trial looked at the effect of prior injection with interferon from Rhesus monkey kidney cells on the success of smallpox vaccination with vaccinia virus. A definite effect was observed in that vaccination took in all but one of 38 volunteers receiving a dummy injection compared to only 14 of those given interferon (75). Interferon enthusiasts were elated by the results, none more so than Alick Isaacs, but the drug firms were insufficiently impressed to commit further resources to the project.* In 1967 Alick Isaacs died after a stroke that had left him suffering from manic depression (76) and bitter at the failure of the drug companies to understand the importance of his discovery. But in truth only one miraculous cure had been reported, in 1960: a character in a strip cartoon of the popular fictional hero, Flash Gordon (74).

Interferon survived through intensive research that continued worldwide. The major stumbling block of inadequate supplies of purified interferon was overcome during the 1970s through a number of important contributions. One of the first advances was made by Kari Cantell at the Central Public Health Laboratory in Helsinki, Finland, who showed that sendai virus—an important pathogen of rodents, but not of man—could induce relatively abundant amounts of human interferon in leucocytes harvested from transfusion blood. Many early trials of interferon in the treatment of cancer used interferon provided by Cantell's group, but the technique was clearly limited by the availability of discarded transfusion blood. Between 1974 and 1979 a team at the National Institutes of Health in Bethesda, Maryland led by the protein chemist and Nobel laureate, Christian Anfinsen, born in Monessen, Pennsylvania of Norwegian parents, succeeded in purifying and establishing the structure of human interferon. The discovery allowed the production of purified interferon in much larger quantities that had hitherto been possible and led to renewed interest in the substance (77). Anfinsen's group used virus-infected Namalwa cells† a technique originally devised by Norman Finter and his colleagues at the Wellcome Laboratories in Beckenham. By the early 1980s industrial scale manufacture of interferon was made possible by using techniques of genetic engineering to induce the bacterium *Escherichia coli* to produce the pure substance. Meanwhile, further research showed that 'interferon' was actually a family of substances that play an important part in the economy of the body not only as a response to viral infection, but also as modulators of the immune system.

....

* John Beale and Karl Fantes of Glaxo and Norman Finter of ICI later joined Wellcome and continued the interferon work there with much enthusiasm, but little support. The work culminated in 1977 in the production of a commercial produce, Wellferon (Finter N. The Wellferon story: part 2. Wellferon moves into the lead. *Wellcome World* November/December 1993, pp. 13–7.

† Namalwa cells are human tumour cells adapted to continuous growth in the laboratory. The original cell line was established by the Hungarian-born pathologist and tumour biologist George Klein at the Karolinska Institute in Stockholm. It was developed from a piece of tissue obtained in 1967 for diagnostic purposes from a 3-year-old Ugandan girl called Namalwa suffering from Burkitt's lymphoma.

As early as 1969, the Yale educated scientist, Ion Gresser and his colleagues at the Institut de Recherches Scientifique sur le Cancer at Villejuif, South of Paris, had found evidence that interferon might have activity against certain tumours (78). Virtually abandoned as an antiviral agent, new hope was fostered that interferon might still have a future as the long-awaited cure for cancer. These claims, too, proved premature, but new therapeutic uses were uncovered as the structure and functions of the various types of interferon were elucidated. Though interferon is far from being the wonder drug of the early dreams, the types classified as interferon-α and interferon-β have established themselves as useful niche products for a variety of viral and non-viral conditions ranging from several types of cancers to multiple sclerosis and viral hepatitis. Ironically, the effectiveness in viral hepatitis probably owes more to the immunomodulatory effects of interferon than any antiviral properties.

Faltering steps

A few other stirrings of hope among the general antiviral gloom are discernable in the 1950s. By the end of the following decade, by which time United States was embroiled in a war in Vietnam and much of the world's youth was preoccupied with anti-war protest, the fantasies of flower power and the extravagances of Beatlemania, the first tentative steps had been taken towards effective therapy for virus diseases. Progress was painfully slow, but it was in this period that the foundations were laid for many of the successful developments that were to come later in the century. Among the compounds to emerge was methisazone, a compound that, ironically, is primarily active against smallpox—a virus that had been successfully eliminated from rich countries and was already earmarked for eradication elsewhere. Another was idoxuridine, the first of what was to become a diverse family of antiviral agents aimed at disrupting the synthesis of viral nucleic acid.

Methisazone. The seeds of the discovery of methisazone (methylisatin thiosemicarbazone) were sown in 1949 at the Squibb Institute for Medical Research in New Brunswick, where Dorothy Hamre and Richard Donovick were following up Gerhard Domagk's work on thiosemicarbazones as antituberculosis agents (see p. 170–2). In 1949 Hamre married another Squibb employee, the Middlesbrough-born, Cambridge-educated statistician, Kenneth Brownlee and in 1950 they developed together a model for testing antiviral agents against vaccinia virus in embryonated hen's eggs (79). Experimental antituberculosis compounds provided by the company chemists, Jack Bernstein and W. A. Lott, were tested in the new model and various derivatives of benzaldehyde thiosemicarbazone showed promising activity, although, disappointingly, subsequent tests in mice showed them to be active only near the maximum tolerated dose (80).

Squibb seems to have taken no further interest in the antiviral activity of thiosemicarbazones, but George Hitchings in the Burroughs Wellcome Laboratories in Tuckahoe, New York took up the finding. Together with Randall L. Thompson he synthesized and tested various derivatives and demonstrated high anti-vaccinia activity in a mouse protection test with a compound called isatin thiosemicarbazone. No one at this stage seems to have thought it worthwhile to test thiosemicarbazones against the related smallpox virus, but this oversight was corrected by John Bauer at the Wellcome Laboratories of Tropical Medicine in London. In collaboration with Peter Sadler of the Courtauld Institute of Biochemistry at the Middlesex Hospital Medical School, isatin thiosemicarbazone derivatives were synthesized and tested against the so-called 'Schofield' strain of the smallpox virus—derived from a case of alastrim, the milder form of the disease—obtained from the smallpox expert Keith Dumbell. In 1960 Bauer and Sadler reported in *The Lancet* that ethylisatin thiosemicarbazone displayed good activity against the smallpox virus in mice (81).

Ethylisatin thiosemicarbazone was too insoluble for injection, but the methyl derivative—later called methisazone—was found to be suitable. In 1963, a clinical trial was setup in Madras (now Chennai) with the help of the Scottish virologist, Alan Downie, Professor of Virology in Liverpool. The Breslau-born paediatrician, Henry Kempe, at the University of Colorado (perhaps better known for his work on child abuse) had established a laboratory in Madras with which Downie collaborated and it was here that Bauer and Kempe's colleague, Leone St Vincent, organized the trial that demonstrated the ability of the new compound to protect contacts of smallpox from acquiring the disease (82). Subsequent trials in India and Brazil, confirmed the protective effect of methisazone, but unfortunately the drug was unable to alter the course of the disease once it had been contracted. In any case, by the time that adequate evidence of safety and efficacy had been assembled, smallpox was on the way out and the chief reason for retention of the drug was for the treatment of the rare, but serious side effect of vaccination, generalized vaccinia. When mass vaccination was abandoned in most countries in the 1970s, so too was methisazone.

Targeting nucleic acid. In 1959, William Prusoff working at Yale University, New Haven Connecticut, synthesized a compound called 5-iodo-2″-deoxyuridine (later abbreviated to idoxuridine), an analogue of the nucleic acid constituent, thymidine (83). The substance is an example of a nucleoside analogue; nucleosides being purine or pyrimidine bases linked to a sugar, which in mammalian nucleic acid is ribose (RNA), or deoxyribose (deoxyribonucleic acid; DNA). Prusoff was looking for compounds with potential anticancer activity and this one attracted attention because it interfered with the development of Ehrlich ascites carcinoma cells—a widely used model in cancer research—by being incorporated in cellular DNA. He had been engaged in work with compounds of this type since joining Yale in 1953 as part of a programme exploring possible anticancer compounds.

Surprisingly, idoxuridine turned out also to possess antiviral activity. In 1961, working in a laboratory housed in a condemned building of the Massachusetts Eye and Ear Infirmary in downtown Boston, the ophthalmologist Herbert Kaufman decided to use idoxuridine to test a theory that a drug which prevented the synthesis of functional viral DNA might be used to treat eye infections caused by herpes viruses. A sample of idoxuridine was obtained commercially from Nutritional Biochemicals Corporation and incorporated into eye drops that could be used for animal experiments. Forty years on,

Kaufman described the experiment in his lecture on the occasion of receiving the 2001 Weisenfeld Award* of the Association for Research in Vision and Ophthalmology. Rabbits were infected with the virus and, working in shifts, Kaufman and his assistants, Emily Varnell and Anthony Nesburn, administered idoxuridine eye drops round the clock: hourly during the day and two-hourly during the night (84). It worked (85).

It was a useful advance, but scarcely a major breakthrough. Yet it had a much wider significance in awakening interest in nucleic acid mimics as antiviral agents. Kaufman himself, together with Charles Heidelberger in Wisconsin, went on in 1964 to show that another thymidine analogue, trifluridine (trifluorothymidine), was an improvement on idoxuridine (86). In the same year, Michel Privat de Garilhe and Jean de Rudder from the Centre de Recherches des Laboratoires Diamant in La Plaine-St Denis, North of Paris, described the inhibitory activity against the viruses of herpes and vaccinia of vidarabine (adenine arabinoside or 9-β-arabinofuranosyladenine; otherwise known simply as ara-A) (87). Vidarabine represents another variation on the nucleoside analogue theme in which the purine base, adenine is linked, not to ribose as in mammalian nucleic acid, but to the molecularly identical, but sterically different sugar, arabinose. The idea had arisen through research in the 1950s by Werner Bergmann and Robert Feeney at Yale, which had first revealed these unusual nucleosides in marine sponges from the Caribbean (88). Interest in arabinosides was at first focused on their use as potential anticancer agents and one of these compounds, cytosine arabinoside (cytarabine; ara-C), synthesized in 1959 by Charles Dekker, and his co-workers in the biochemistry department of the University of California, Berkeley, was developed and marketed as a cytotoxic drug. Vidarabine had also been synthesized around this time with the same purpose in view (89). Cytarabine was briefly proposed as an antiviral agent, but was soon abandoned for that purpose because of its toxicity.

By coincidence, scientists at the Southern Research Institute in Birmingham, Alabama were already working on vidarabine at the time of the appearance of Privat de Garilhe and de Rudder's first paper. Activity against herpes simplex virus had been independently discovered in a concentrate of a streptomycete fermentation culture and the active component was later identified as vidarabine (90). Realization that it was the same compound that the French workers had described seems to have caused consternation in Alabama. Several papers were rapidly prepared for presentation at the October 1968 ICAAC in New York and Frank Schabel, director of chemotherapy research at the Southern Research Institute, rushed a summary of his colleagues' data into print in the Swiss journal *Chemotherapy* earlier in the same year (91). The haste was no doubt prompted by Parke, Davis in Detroit, who had supported the Southern Research Institute work and subsequently developed the compound commercially.

Vidarabine was the first antiviral compound to be sufficiently non-toxic to allow systemic administration. It was Charles Alford, Richard Whitley, and their colleagues at the University of Alabama at Birmingham, who in the early 1970s pioneered the use of this

---

* Named for Mildred Weisenfeld, founder in 1946 of Fight for Sight (now part of Prevent Blindness America).

compound in severe herpes simplex infections in immunocompromised patients and disseminated infections in newborn infants that would otherwise have almost certainly been fatal (92).

Amantadine. In 1964 scientists from DuPont's Stine Laboratory—the company's agricultural and veterinary research facility in Newark, Delaware—announced the discovery of a new agent with antiviral activity, 1-adamantanamine, or amantadine (93). Amantadine is derived from adamantane, an unusual molecule based on a cage-like nucleus composed entirely of carbon atoms, reminiscent of the crystal lattice of natural diamonds.* Adamantane was first isolated in Czechoslovakia in 1933 from a distillate of petroleum. When its chemistry was explored it became the source of numerous derivatives, including polymers, lubricants, and explosives. It was no doubt for these purposes that amantadine was first synthesized and sent to the Stine Laboratory for routine biological screening with no expectation of success.

Subsequent testing of the antiviral activity of amantadine showed that useful activity was virtually restricted to just one of the viruses responsible for influenza epidemics, influenza A. With memories of the Asian influenza pandemic of 1957 still vivid, and the virus still circulating, commercial prospects for a new treatment against this plague were considered to be good. Unfortunately, the compound was already in the public domain and could not be patented, but a patent for the medical application were successfully pursued and the drug was given FDA approval for use in the treatment of the Asian flu. In 1968, a new wave of influenza caused by the so-called Hong Kong variant made its appearance and amantadine was also use to combat the new pandemic strain. Activity of amantadine against measles and rubella viruses was also recognized, but came to nothing.

Amantadine—and, not long afterwards, a very similar compound, rimantadine, which emerged from research in the former Soviet Union—was a useful addition to the therapeutic armoury. However, because it is active only against influenza A strains, has to be given before or soon after infection, and is prone to encourage the emergence of variant viruses that are resistant to its action, it has found limited application. There have been claims that the drug is useful in Parkinson's disease and multiples sclerosis, but the effects at best are modest. Other adamantine derivatives continue to be investigated for antiviral activity, but have not generated much interest so far.

Ribavirin. In 1973, a group led by Robert Sidwell at the Nucleic Acid Research Institute of ICN Pharmaceuticals† in Irvine, California, described a new nucleic acid analogue with antiviral activity (94). The compound, ribavirin, was synthesized in 1970 by Roland K. Robins and Joseph Witkowski. Small scientific enterprises are always looking for the one product that will kick-start their fortunes. And so it was with ICN and ribavirin. Extravagant claims were made for its broad-spectrum activity against viruses that use

---

* The word adamant is derived from a Greek term applied to diamonds and other very hard stones.

† Founded in 1960 as International Chemical and Nuclear Corporation; since 2003, known as Valeant Pharmaceuticals International.

DNA as the basis of their genetic information as well as those that rely on RNA. Much interest was shown in its potential anti-influenza activity and there were unrealistic hopes that it might provide a silver bullet for many virus diseases from smallpox to the common cold. Animal experiments encouraged further development and clinical trials were started in 1975. The results were uniformly disappointing, but against all the odds the drug survived.

In 1983, the husband and wife team of Caroline and William Hall together with colleagues at the University of Rochester showed, after a pilot study in young adult volunteers, that aerosolized ribavirin instilled into the airways was useful in infants suffering from bronchiolitis caused by respiratory syncytial virus (95). The drug received FDA approval in the United States for the treatment of respiratory syncytial virus infection in young children in 1986. The following year it was licensed in the United Kingdom under the generic name, tribavirin because of potential confusion with an unrelated asthma product, Rybarvin, which has since been withdrawn (96). In the course of time ribavirin found other uses: it is the only drug to have shown much promise in the treatment of haemorrhagic fevers like Lassa fever, and it has proved to be useful in combination with interferon in hepatitis C infection.

Inosiplex. A similar story to that of ribavirin attends another putative antiviral drug, inosiplex (inosine pranobex; Isoprinosine). Found to have broad-spectrum antiviral activity by Eric Brown and Paul Gordon at the University of Chicago Medical School around 1970 (97), it was developed by Newport Pharmaceutical International, Newport Beach, California (later Newport Pharmaceuticals Inc.), the company that had financed the research in Chicago. Unfortunately, the drug failed to live up to its promise in preliminary clinical trials. Any activity it may have seems to be exerted through a stimulatory effect on the immune system, but few physicians are persuaded that it has much benefit. It is sometimes used in combination with interferon in a condition known as subacute sclerosing panencephalitis, a late complication of measles, which it is hoped will virtually disappear as the disease is controlled by vaccination.

A new age dawns

With the start of the AIDS pandemic in the 1980s Cinderella was at last invited to the ball: the big pharmaceutical companies scented an important and lucrative new market and drug development strategies worldwide were revised to focus research on the emerging threat. But even before that there was renewed optimism among virologists when a new compound surfaced that turned out to have the elusive selective toxicity that had formerly been considered unattainable. The compound was aciclovir.

Aciclovir and its relatives. Aciclovir emerged from the same sort of research that produced idoxuridine and flucytosine: the hunt for anticancer agents that might target the DNA of cancer cells without doing too much harm to the patient. Many research groups were pursuing this line of investigation, among them the formidable team of George Hitchings and Gertrude Elion at Burroughs Wellcome in the United States. Elion was first alerted to possible antiviral applications of her purine work when she was working on diaminopurine in the late 1940s. In 1968, when talk of the antiviral activity of vidara-bine was in the air, she asked her colleague Jane Rideout to synthesize the corresponding diaminopurine arabinoside. It was sent to John Bauer in the Wellcome Laboratories in Beckenham, Kent, who found it to be active and relatively non-toxic in animals infected with herpes simplex or vaccinia virus. However, the properties of the compound were not sufficiently attractive to warrant commercial development (98).

In 1970 Burroughs Wellcome moved their research base in the United States from New York to the Research Triangle Park in North Carolina and Howard Schaeffer was appointed head of organic chemistry with the task of synthesizing analogues of the nucleoside adenosine. Although the work was directed chiefly at potential antitumour compounds, newly synthesized substances were also routinely screened for antiviral activity. One adenosine derivative in which the ribose component had been modified by opening the ring structure of the sugar surprisingly showed activity against herpes simplex virus that was slightly superior to that of vidarabine. Alerted to the potential of acyclic derivatives, Schaeffer and his co-worker Lilia Beauchamp went on to synthesize similar nucleosides (99). One, an acyclic version of deoxyguanosine, first synthesized in 1974, was tested by John Bauer and Peter Collins at the Wellcome Laboratories in Beckenham and found not only to display high activity against herpes simplex virus, but also to have remarkably low toxicity in animal tests (100). The new compound was given the generic name acyclovir later changed to aciclovir by a bureaucratic whim of the World Health Organization's Expert Advisory Panel on the International Pharmacopoeia and Pharmaceutical Preparations, which recommends International Non-proprietary Names.* Aciclovir is often called acycloguanosine, a name coined by John Bauer, but it is actually a derivative of a deoxygenated version of guanosine (Fig. 8.2) and should properly be given the more cumbersome appellation, acyclodeoxyguanosine.

Since nucleoside analogues achieve their effect by incorporation into genetic material the marked lack of toxicity of aciclovir was at first a puzzle. Trudy Elion's team in the

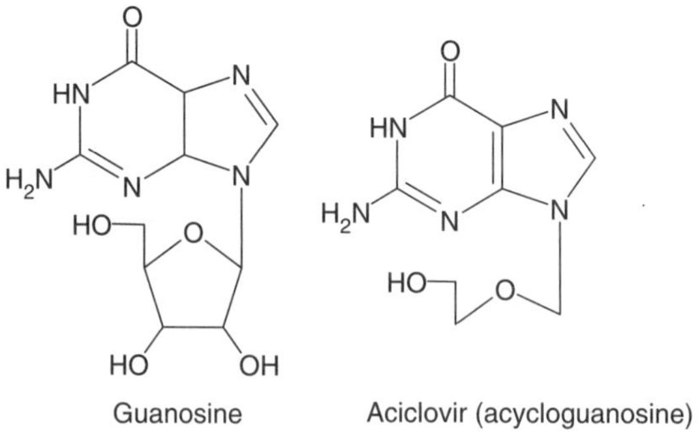

Fig. 8.2 The structures of guanosine and aciclovir.

Guanosine   Aciclovir (acycloguanosine)

----

* The WHO has pronounced that to facilitate translation and pronunciation 'i' should be used instead of 'y' (but mycin suffixes are still allowed), 't' should replace 'th' and 'f' should replace 'ph'. This leads to some unfamiliar names like meticillin (for methicillin) and cefalotin (for cephalothin), which have not found universal acceptance. (See http://www.who.int/druginformation/vol16num2_2002/annexproplist87.pdf).

United States quickly found the reason behind this novel feature by elucidating the basis for the selective action. Before nucleosides can be incorporated into nucleic acids, they must first be converted into triphosphates. Addition of the three phosphate groups takes place sequentially and it turns out that the first phosphorylation of acyclovir is carried out very much more efficiently by an enzyme produced by certain viruses—notably herpes simplex virus—than by the corresponding cellular enzyme (101). The upshot of this is that aciclovir is activated to the form that halts DNA synthesis only in cells already infected by the virus.

Once the extraordinary properties of aciclovir had been uncovered, clinical studies rapidly followed. The drug proved to be more effective than vidarabine or idoxuridine in herpetic eye infections and—much more importantly from a commercial perspective—it could be successfully and safely used in common 'cold sores' on the lips and elsewhere, provided it was applied in the early stages of the recurrent eruptions. Successful use in genital herpes, shingles (a localized reactivation of latent chickenpox), and herpes encephalitis sealed the reputation of aciclovir as the first really safe and effective antiviral drug.

The main disadvantages of aciclovir were its restricted spectrum—it was active only against the few viruses that could perform the necessary phosphorylation step—and poor absorption when given by mouth. Attempts to improve on these shortcomings led to further developments in this class of drugs. First on the scene rejoiced in the name bromovinyldeoxyuridine, usually abbreviated to BVDU. It was synthesized around 1978 by a PhD student, Philip Barr, in the chemistry department of Birmingham University under the guidance of two outstanding nucleic acid researchers, Stanley Jones and Richard Walker. Although BVDU differs from aciclovir in that it is not an acyclic nucleoside derivative, it is also activated by a viral enzyme. It is more active than aciclovir against the chickenpox virus and, although it is not widely available, it has been used topically and orally in shingles.

In 1982 the continued search for acyclic guanosine analogues yielded a compound called dihydroxypropoxymethylguanine, mercifully soon renamed ganciclovir. It was synthesized in the research laboratories of Syntex (now part of the Roche group), a company in Palo Alto, California closely associated with Stanford University. A group including John Martin, Julian Verheyden, Donald Smee, and Thomas Matthews developed the compound (102). Wellcome scientists independently synthesized the molecule around the same time, but Syntex claimed priority and was granted the patent.

Ganciclovir is characterized by useful activity against cytomegalovirus (CMV), another virus of the herpes group that sometimes causes serious infections in immunocompromised patients, including a sight-threatening retinitis. In a similar manner to the activation of aciclovir by herpes simplex virus, CMV produces an enzyme which efficiently phosphorylates ganciclovir. Unfortunately the version of the enzyme normally present in mammalian cells also phosphorylates the compound, which is therefore more toxic than aciclovir. None the less ganciclovir was licensed in the United Kingdom in 1988 and received FDA approval in the United States the following year. It is a useful addition to the antiviral armoury, often saving the sight, and sometimes the life, of immunocompromised individuals with severe CMV infection.

Research workers at Beecham's Biosciences Research Centre in Epsom, Surrey were also on the hunt for aciclovir-like compounds. In the mid-1980s they turned their attention to a compound that was already described in the literature, which their chemists, Michael Harnden and Richard Jarvest were able to obtain in a pure state. They called the derivative penciclovir; it closely resembled aciclovir in activity, but turned out to be even less well absorbed when given by mouth (103). Harnden and his colleagues came up with the solution to the oral bioavailability problem in 1986 by synthesizing an ester of penciclovir—given the name famciclovir—which acted as a prodrug (see p. 125), efficiently releasing penciclovir into the circulation across the intestinal mucosa (104). In truth it was not a great advance on aciclovir, but the convenience of oral administration was a useful selling point. Famciclovir was marketed in the United States and the United Kingdom in 1994; a topical formulation of penciclovir itself followed in 1996. Not surprisingly, the Wellcome researchers in Beckenham had been thinking along similar lines and by 1993 had perfected an oral prodrug of aciclovir, the valyl ester, which they called valaciclovir (105). The compound received approval on both sides of the Atlantic in 1995.

Antiretroviral agents. Recognition of AIDS in the United States in the early 1980s, and the discovery in 1983 of HIV as the causative agent by Luc Montagnier of the Institut Pasteur in Paris,* triggered an intensive search for effective vaccines and chemotherapeutic compounds. A vaccine has proved elusive, but there has been more success in the search for useful drugs to control progression of the disease.

At the time of the discovery of HIV there were only six antiviral agents licensed for clinical use and only one, aciclovir that could be claimed to be of unequivocal benefit in the conditions for which it was prescribed. Less than 20 years later, the number of antiviral compounds had risen to more than 25, around two-thirds of them intended for the treatment of patients with HIV infection. Although none of them is curative or free from side effects, they have had a major impact on the disease. Present concerns about treatment of HIV infection focus more on the dangers of the emergence of resistant strains and on ways in which effective treatment can be made available to the millions of sufferers in the poor countries of the world.

HIV is a retrovirus. That is, its genetic information is contained in single-stranded RNA, which must be converted into DNA by a viral enzyme, reverse transcriptase, to allow the virus to replicate itself. Since host cells have no need of a reverse transcriptase, this process offers a potential target for selective chemotherapy. The first antiretroviral drugs were therefore sought among nucleoside analogues similar to those that had been used in herpes virus infections and in cancer.

The first compound to hit the market in 1987 was azidothymidine, also known as zidovudine or AZT. Jerome Horwitz of the Detroit Institute of Cancer Research had originally synthesized the molecule as a possible anticancer agent in 1964, but it had been

---

* Robert Gallo of the National Institute of Health's National Cancer Institute in Bethesda, Maryland also claimed in 1984 to have discovered the causative virus sparking an unedifying dispute over priority. Montagnier and Gallo settled their differences and agreed to share the credit in 1987.

rejected as ineffective and toxic. The drug came under renewed scrutiny with the emergence of AIDS and was among the compounds tested in a programme of research initiated in 1983 at the Burroughs Wellcome Laboratories in North Carolina by a group led by David Barry. By November 1984, activity against retroviruses had been established in the laboratory. Testing and licensing of the compound proceeded under great pressure from American AIDS sufferers and the drug was eventually approved and released into the market in 1987 after a randomized trial that later came under criticism for breaches of the protocol.

Meanwhile, Wellcome successfully applied for a patent for zidovudine in the United States as a treatment for AIDS. This was granted in 1988, but scientists at the National Cancer Institute and Duke University, where much of the development work had been undertaken under contract from Wellcome, contested the decision in a letter to the *New York Times* in 1989 claiming that their role as co-inventors had been ignored (106). Two generic drug companies with plans to undercut Wellcome, Barr Laboratories, Pomona, New York and Novopharm Inc., Schaumburg, Illinois, subsequently brought a case to court, claiming that the patent was invalid because it had failed to acknowledge the contribution of the National Cancer Institute's scientists. Fortunately for Wellcome, a United States District Court ruled in the company's favour in July 1993 and the judgement was later upheld in the United States Supreme Court on appeal (107).

AZT was a commercial success for Wellcome (later Glaxo Wellcome and then GlaxoSmithKline), but its widespread use revealed serious problems of toxicity and fears of the emergence of resistant variants of the virus. Further doubts emerged in 1993 and 1994 when results of an Anglo–French trial suggested that use of the drug to prevent progression to AIDS in HIV-positive individuals conferred no benefit (108).

For several years Wellcome's AZT had the field to itself, but a flood of nucleoside analogues that acted as reverse transcriptase inhibitors started to emerge from other companies during the 1990s and continued into the new millennium (Table 8.1). In 1987, Samuel Broder, Hiroaki Mitsuya (both of whom had been signatories to the letter of complaint against Wellcome over the zidovudine patent), and colleagues at the National Cancer Institute demonstrated the activity of dideoxyinosine (didanosine or DDI) in laboratory studies (109). By August 1988 clinical assessment was underway led by Robert Yarchoan from Broder's group (110) and further extensive trials were conducted with the help of Bristol-Myers Squibb in New York. The results were fast-tracked by the FDA and the Health Protection Branch of Canada's Department of National Health and Welfare and approval was granted simultaneously on both countries in October 1991. Marketing in the United Kingdom followed in 1994. Other nucleoside analogues quickly emerged aided in the United States by the FDA's accelerated drug review policy. Later several structurally diverse chemical entities were uncovered that also inhibited HIV reverse transcriptase. To distinguish them from nucleoside mimics they became known generically by the cumbersome designation 'non-nucleoside reverse transcriptase inhibitors'.

Meanwhile other avenues were being explored to attack the virus. One fruitful approach was to target a specific viral enzyme responsible for a late event in the replication cycle. Several essential HIV proteins are initially manufactured as a single polypeptide,

Table 8.1 Antiretroviral agents and date of approval for use in the United States

Nucleoside reverse transcriptase inhibitors	Date	Non-nucleoside reverse transcriptase inhibitors	Date	Protease inhibitors	Date	Fusion inhibitors	Date
Zidovudine (AZT) (Burroughs Wellcome)	1987	Nevirapine (Boehringer Ingelheim)	1996	Saquinavir (Hoffmann-La Roche)	1995	Enfuvirtide (Duke University)	2003
Didanosine (ddI) (National Cancer Institute)	1991	Delavirdine (Pharmacia and Upjohn)	1997	Ritonavir (Abbott)	1996		
Zalcitabine (ddC) (Hoffmann-La Roche)	1992	Efavirenz (DuPont Pharmaceuticals)	1998	Indinavir (Merck)	1996		
Stavudine (d4T) (Bristol Myers Squibb)	1994			Nelfinavir (Agouron Pharmaceuticals)	1997		
Lamivudine (3TC) (Biochem Pharma)	1995			Amprenavir (Vertex Pharmaceuticals)	1999		
Abacavir (Glaxo Wellcome)	1998			Lopinavir (Abbott)	2000		
Tenofovir[a] (Gilead Sciences)	2001			Atazanavir (Bristol-Myers Squibb)	2003		
Emtricitabine (Gilead Sciences)	2003			Tipranavir (Boehringer Ingelhem)	2005		

[a] Strictly, a nucleotide rather than a nucleoside analogue.

Abbreviations in brackets are often used to describe these compounds. They are derived from the chemical structures: didanosine is 2′,3′-dideoxyinosine; lamivudine is 2′-deoxy-3′-thiacytidine; stavudine is 2′,3′-didehydro-3′deoxythymidine; zalcitabine is 2′,3′-dideoxycytidine; zidovudine is 3′-azido-2′,3′-dideoxythymidine.

Names in brackets indicate where the compound was first developed as an antiretroviral agent.

which must be split into its components by a viral protease before further development can continue (111). Such processes were already well described in other viruses. In 1987 the Belgium-born molecular geneticist Christine Debouck and her colleagues at SmithKline French (later GlaxoSmithKline) in King of Prussia, Pennsylvania identified an HIV protease and suggested that it might offer a suitable target for a selectively active drug (112). Saquinavir, the first of these protease inhibitors to survive clinical trial to reach the market place, received approval from the FDA in the United States in December 1995. It was synthesized by a team at Hoffmann-La Roche's British laboratories at Welwyn Garden City led by Joseph Martin and Noel Roberts. Other firms climbed on the bandwagon and several HIV protease inhibitors with very complex and diverse structures were added to the antiretroviral arsenal during the next decade (Table 8.1).

In the early 1990s, Dani Bolognesi, Thomas Matthews, and their colleagues at Duke University Medical Center, Durham, North Carolina devised a different approach to the therapy of HIV. They synthesized a peptide mimicking a region of the outer envelope of HIV that was involved in viral infection of cells and subsequent cell-to-cell fusion mediated by the virus. The peptide, subsequently called enfuvirtide, efficiently prevented these processes in laboratory studies (113). In 1993, Bolognesi and Matthews set-up a company, Trimeris, in Durham to exploit the discovery. The results of preliminary clinical trails encouraged a collaborative agreement between Trimeris and Hoffmann-La Roche in 1999 to develop and market the drug. It received accelerated approval from the FDA in 2003 and full approval the following year, shortly before Matthews died prematurely of a brain tumour.

The availability of many different antiretroviral agents offered new ways of approaching therapy of infection with HIV. In particular, the possibility of resistant variants of the virus emerging could be minimized by the tried and tested method of combination therapy aimed at different targets in the viral replication cycle. Various combinations were investigated and found to be successful, ushering in the confident, but somewhat euphemistic concept of highly active antiretroviral therapy (HAART) for this incurable disease. Attention soon focused on simplifying the complicated treatment protocols necessary for the control of HIV, in mitigating the numerous side effects of the drugs used and in tailoring regimens to individual sufferers.

Influenza revisited

The viruses that cause influenza are, by viral standards, relatively complex, but such is the importance of the disease, which is responsible for global pandemics that periodically cause great loss of life, that it has always been an attractive area of research for virologists. Indeed, more is known about the structure and function of influenza viruses than almost any other microbe. Among prominent structures of the influenza virus particle are two proteins seen as surface spikes in electron micrographs: a haemagglutinin—so-called because it causes the agglutination of certain red blood cells in laboratory tests—and neuraminidase, an enzyme that acts on a complex sugar present on the surface of mammalian cells. Both proteins are essential for the establishment and spread of the virus in the respiratory tract and offer suitable targets for an anti-influenza compound. Neuraminidase inhibitors had been sought as early as 1966 (114), but it was not until the 1990s that two safe and effective compounds emerged: zanamivir and oseltamivir. The developments were hailed as a triumph of technological advances that allowed rational drug design.

Influenza virus haemagglutinin and neuraminidase are antigenically variable structures. Indeed, it is variations in these molecules that make pandemics possible and challenges the timely provision of effective vaccines.* In the early 1980s, Peter Colman and

* There are 15 different haemagglutinin (H) antigens and nine types of neuraminidase (N). Influenza virus strains are classified according to the type of H and N antigens that they possess. Thus the 'Asian flu' epidemic of 1957 was recognized as caused by a strain designated H_2N_2 and the Hong Kong bird flu of 1997 as H_5N_1. Annual vaccines are prepared on the basis of evidence of circulation of particular antigenic types.

Joseph Varghese of the Commonwealth Scientific and Industrial Research Organization's Biomolecular Research Institute in Parkville, Victoria, Australia started to investigate influenza virus neuraminidases in collaboration with Graeme Laver of the John Curtin School of Medicine at the Australian National University. Colman already had extensive experience of X-ray crystallography and by 1983 this powerful technique had enabled the group to build up a three-dimensional picture of the viral neuraminidase. The scientists were surprised to discover that although neuraminidases of various influenza strains differed in their structure as expected, certain regions buried within the molecule were invariable in all the strains that they examined. It was soon realized that a corollary to this finding was that a molecule blocking access to this site might be able to inhibit the growth of all epidemic types of influenza virus (115).

In collaboration with Mark von Itzstein and Wen-Yang Wu of the Victorian School of Pharmacy in Monash University substances were sought that might block the invariable region of influenza virus neuraminidase. Computer modelling was used to select molecules with the appropriate three-dimensional structure to lock into the target region of the molecule. The programme started in 1986; by 1988 compounds had been developed that worked in ferrets (the favoured animal model of human influenza) and by early 1990 the substance now known as zanamivir had been synthesized and tested. The discovery was described in *Nature* in 1993; the paper bore the names of 18 authors, underlining the teamwork that had gone into bringing the investigation to a successful conclusion (116).

Development of zanamivir as a marketable drug required the involvement of a commercial organization. As early as 1986, a young Melbourne entrepreneur, Mark Crosling, had spotted the potential of the anti-influenza drug research. He formed a company, Biota Holdings, in Melbourne and acquired rights to substances discovered in the course of the investigations at Monash. In 1990, when compounds with commercial potential had started to emerge, Biota reached an agreement with Glaxo to carry out clinical trials and provide financial support for the research. Volunteer studies and formal clinical trials in naturally acquired influenza began in 1994. By 1999 sufficient data had been accumulated to convince the regulatory authorities in the European Union and Australasia to license the drug for use, but to the dismay of Biota and Glaxo, the FDA in the United States delayed approval because of a dispute over the statistical significance of clinical trials results.

Progress achieved in Australia naturally attracted attention in other countries. Investigation of neuraminidase inhibitors was enthusiastically pursued in a number of laboratories, but it was a research group at Gilead Sciences in California led by Choung U Kim that came up with a compound that was set to rival zanamivir in its efficacy and ease of application. Preliminary information on the drug, later given the generic name oseltamivir, was unveiled at the annual ICAAC held in New Orleans in September 1996. The active compound, originally known by its laboratory code GS 4071, is, like zanamivir, poorly absorbed when given orally. To overcome this problem the ethyl ester was synthesized creating a well-absorbed prodrug that released the active compound into the bloodstream (117). The same principle is used for certain antibacterial antibiotics (see p. 125) and some other antiviral compounds (see p. 378). As with zanamivir, the marketing of oseltamivir was entrusted to a big name player, in this case, Roche. The delay in licensing zanamivir in the States, combined with the benefit of the FDA's fast-track policy enabled Roche to catch up with its competitor. Oseltamivir was approved for use in the United States in 1999 and was licensed in Europe the following year.

Oral absorption provided oseltamivir with a potential advantage over its rival, which is administered by inhalation of a dry powder—a benefit that has been fully exploited in the marketplace. Consequently early sales of zanamivir fell below expectation much to the chagrin of the directors of Biota, who promptly sued GlaxoSmithKline for failure to adequately support the drug during development and after its launch.*

Zanamivir and oseltamivir are safe and effective compounds that offer new hope for the prevention and treatment of influenza (118). Unlike amantadine and rimantadine they are active against influenza B strains as well as influenza A and resistance does not seem to emerge as readily. Nevertheless, doubts remain about the best way to use these valuable compounds. It is still too early to assess with confidence the incidence of adverse reactions; the impact of the drugs on person-to-person spread; and the potential for the emergence of resistance variants. Should the drugs be used for prevention, or reserved for treatment? If for prevention, which groups should receive prophylaxis? If for treatment, can the diagnosis be confidently made sufficiently early for therapy to make a difference? 'Flu-like' illness is common in the community, but few cases are due to influenza viruses except in epidemic years. These and other questions are not easy to address.

Antiviral miscellany

The upsurge of research interest in new antiviral compounds that followed the appearance of HIV naturally concentrated on antiretroviral compounds, but a rash of other substances of greater or lesser importance appeared in their train. Some are 'failed' antiretroviral agents that found another niche; others were aimed at opportunistic infections to which immunocompromised individuals, such as those with AIDS, are prone. A few have emerged as new approaches to old diseases.

Investigations of some compounds were underway before the appearance of AIDS, but subsequent development was heavily influenced by the opportunistic infections that AIDS victims often suffer. As early as 1973, scientists at Abbott Laboratories in North Chicago announced that a random tissue culture screening programme had unearthed a simple phosphonic acid derivative, phosphonoacetic acid that was effective in experimental animals infected with herpes simplex virus (119). The compound was not new, having been described in 1924 in a wide-ranging article on phosphorus derivatives by the Swedish chemist, Paul Nylén (120). Perhaps because of this and because further investigation uncovered toxicity problems, the drug was not progressed.

In February 1978 a group from Michigan State University and the United States Agriculture Department Poultry Research Laboratory in Michigan reported the activity

* Mark Crosling, Biota's founder, had already sold many of his shares without the knowledge or consent of his bank and had pocketed the money. He received a 2-year prison sentence in 2001 for his pains.

of a related compound—also previously described by Nylén—phosphonoformate, later called foscarnet (121). The lead author of the report, John Reno, was investigating phosphonic acid derivatives as part of a PhD project.* An independent report of the same compound from a team at the Swedish pharmaceutical firm, Astra, in collaboration with scientists from Nylén's former University, Uppsala in Sweden, followed a few months later (122).† Astra eventually brought the drug to market in 1990 for the treatment of CMV retinitis in AIDS patients despite its manifest toxicity.

The physician and molecular biologist, Paul Zamecnik, pioneered an alternative approach to the treatment of viral, and possibly other diseases, at Harvard Medical School in Massachusetts. The idea was appealingly simple. Viruses, like all cells, produce short-lived single-stranded messenger RNA (mRNA) carrying the blueprint for the manufacture of proteins. Some viruses use single-stranded RNA to store the basic genetic information. Zamecnik reasoned that if short strands of nucleic acids complementary to regions of the mRNA could be constructed, they would bind to these single-stranded molecules and prevent them from carrying out their function. Such artificial nucleic acids were termed 'antisense' oligonucleotides. Together with his colleague Mary Louise Stephenson, Zamecnik set about testing the antisense theory and in 1978 described their first positive results. Techniques for establishing the sequence of specific mRNAs and for the construction of synthetic nucleic acid strands were by then already available and the sequence of Rous sarcoma virus had recently been described. An antisense molecule 13 nucleotides long and complementary to a sequence found at either end of Rous sarcoma virus RNA was synthesized. To their delight, it inhibited virus multiplication in chick embryo cells in tissue culture (123).

Translating a brilliant idea into a marketable therapeutic compound proved more difficult. For several years nothing of value emerged from attempts to exploit the antisense concept. In 1990, Zamecnik helped to set up a biotechnology company, Hybridon in Cambridge, Massachusetts, but it was a rival concern, ISIS Pharmaceuticals, established the previous year in Carlsbad California, that succeeded in developing a viable antisense product, fomivirsen. Like foscarnet, fomivirsen was found to be effective in CMV retinitis and FDA approval for the drug was obtained in 1998. Worldwide marketing rights were licensed to Novartis.

Two of the antivirals to emerge in the AIDS era, adefovir and cidofovir, are like their sister compound, tenofovir (see above), nucleotides. They are all based on a molecule, dihydroxypropyladenine (DHPA), originally synthesized and investigated in 1978 as a prospective broad-spectrum antiviral agent by Antonín Holý of the Institute of Organic Chemistry and Biochemistry in Prague in collaboration with the ebullient and indefatigable Belgian virologist, Erik de Clercq of the Rega Institute for Medical Research of the Katholieke Universiteit, Leuven (Louvain) (124).

----

* The degree was awarded in 1980 (see State University of Michigan library records).

† The paper by Reno et al. (121) appeared after the report from Sweden had been submitted for publication confirming that the discoveries were indeed made independently.

All three compounds were developed by Gilead Sciences in the United States with the intention of launching them on the lucrative antiretroviral market. In the event, only tenofovir made it into the anti-HIV armoury. Fortunately adefovir and cidofovir were known to display activity against other viruses and the firm was able to fall back onto alternative uses to try to recoup their investment. Adefovir was denied FDA approval as an antiretroviral drug in 1999 on the grounds of toxicity, but won a subsequent application for use in patients with chronic hepatitis B infection in 2002. Cidofovir was similarly approved for CMV retinitis, a potentially blinding infection in patients with AIDS, in 1996.

The success of the anti-HIV nucleoside analogue lamivudine (see above) as a safe and effective treatment for chronic infection with quite a different virus, hepatitis B, prompted Richard Colonno and his colleagues at Bristol-Myers Squibb in Wallingford, Connecticut to pursue a similar line of research (125). The substance they came up with, entecavir, was eventually launched for the treatment of chronic hepatitis B in 2005.

A couple of topical antiviral compounds also appeared towards the end of the millennium, imiquimod (imidazoquinolinamine), and docosanol (behenyl alcohol). Imiquimod is a product of 3M Health Care Group, one of the diverse companies that evolved in due course from the Minnesota Mining and Manufacturing Company.* The parent company was founded in 1902 by a group of local men in Two Harbors, a small town on the edge of Lake Superior, to mine, manufacture, and sell abrasives for grinding wheels. Imiquimod was originally developed in the mid-1980s by scientists at Riker Laboratories, which had been acquired by 3M in 1970. It was optimistically intended as a topical agent able to modify the immunological response to herpes simplex infections, but was later shown to have useful activity on genital warts, a common and difficult to treat sexually transmitted infection. The FDA granted a licence for imiquimod cream to be used for this indication in 1997. The drug subsequently also received approval for the topical treatment of certain types of skin cancer.

Docosanol was developed by David Katz and his colleagues at Lidak Pharmaceuticals a small company established in 1988 in La Jolla California (the name was later changed to Avanir Pharmaceuticals).† It is a long chain alcohol with activity against herpes simplex virus. Alcohols of various chain lengths had been shown to exert antiviral activity in the late 1970s, but were too toxic for therapeutic use. Katz and his co-workers revisited the activity by synthesizing alcohols of longer chain length than had previously been investigated and were able to report in 1991 that docosanol, with a chain length of 22 carbons, displayed good activity (126). There were reasons to suppose that the longer chain might lack the toxic effects of the earlier alcohols and these were borne out in clinical trials. The FDA granted approval in 2000 for a cream formulation to be used without prescription in the treatment of cold sores.

---

* One 3M's most celebrated products is the sticky transparent cellophane tape, Scotch tape, invented in 1930 by Richard G. Drew, a laboratory worker with the firm. It was a development of a masking tape that he had earlier prepared, in 1925, for painters.

† Katz was Chief Executive Officer of the Lidak until 1998, when he left and was promptly sued by the company for abuse of power during his tenure. The case was settled out of court.

Whither antiviral chemotherapy?

Despite the advances that have been made in recent years, the scope of antiviral chemotherapy is still severely circumscribed. There is nothing resembling a truly broad-spectrum antiviral agent—ribavirin is the nearest example—and most antivirals carry with them considerable problems of toxicity. On the other hand the relative simplicity of viruses makes complete understanding of their structure and the identification of vulnerable points in their replication cycle simpler than is the case with other infective agents. This fact is underlined by the greater success that has been achieved in designing antiviral molecules than has been possible with other categories of antimicrobial compounds. But there is more to a successful antimicrobial drug than elegant targeting of essential microbial functions: the resultant compound must be free from unwanted side effects, easily manufactured and stable in pharmaceutical formulations. Success will be short lived if the compound is widely used and resistant microbial variants are easily selected. In addition, the agent must be able to act in a timely manner to control symptoms once they have developed. It is this last feature that makes therapy of viral diseases especially problematical, since the crisis point of the disease is often reached around the time that clear symptoms manifest themselves. In virus diseases above all, prevention is better than cure and vaccines still provide the best defence.

References

1. Espinal-Ingrofff A (1996). History of medical mycology in the United States. *Clin Microbiol Rev* **9**, 235–72.
2. McIntosh J (1922). *Studies in the aetiology of epidemic influenza*. Medical Research Council Special Report Series No. 63. His Majesty's Stationery Office, London.
3. Watson T (1857). *Lectures on the principles and practice of physic; delivered at King's College, London*, 4th edn., Vol. 1, pp. 819–20. John W Parker and Son, London.
4. Krebs HA, Wiggins D, Stubbs M, Sols A, Bedoya F (1983). Studies on the mechanism of the antifungal action of benzoate. *Biochem J* **214**, 657–63.
5. Williams DI (1955). The Whitfield tradition of therapy. *BMJ* **2**, 453–5.
6. Cited in: Ainsworth GC (1986). *Introduction to the history of medical and veterinary mycology*, p. 91. Cambridge University Press, Cambridge.
7. Cox FEG (2002). History of human parasitology. *Clin Microbiol Rev* **15**, 595–612.
8. Ainsworth GC (1986). *Introduction to the history of medical and veterinary mycology*, pp. 88–103. Cambridge University Press, Cambridge.
9. Whitfield A (1927). The treatment of ringworm. In: *Modern technique in treatment*, Vol. 1, pp. 93–102. Lancet, London.
10. Castellani A (1960). *Microbes, men and monarchs. A doctor's life in many lands*, pp. 54–78. Victor Gollancz, London.
11. Wyss O, Ludwig BJ, Joiner RR (1945). The fungistatic and fungicidal action of fatty acids and related compounds. *Arch Biochem* **7**, 415–25.
12. Baldwin RS (1981). *The fungus fighters. Two women scientists and their discovery*. Cornell University Press, Ithaca and London.
13. Schatz A, Hazen EL (1948). The distribution of soil microorganisms antagonistic to fungi pathogenic to man. *Mycologia* **40**, 461–77.

14. Leach BE, Ford JH, Whiffen AJ (1947). Actidione, an antibiotic from *Streptomyces griseus. J Am Chem Soc* **69**, 474.

15. Hazen EL, Brown R (1951). Fungicidin, an antibiotic produced by a soil actinomycete. *Proc Soc Exp Biol Med* **76**, 93–7.

16. Gold W, Stout HA, Pagano JF, Donovick R (1956). Amphotericins A and B, antifungal antibiotics produced by a streptomycete. I. In vitro studies. In: Welch H, Marti-Ibañez F, eds. *Antibiotics annual 1955–1956*, pp. 579–86. Medical Encyclopedia Inc., New York.

17. Sternberg TH, Wright ET, Oura M (1956). A new antifungal antibiotic, amphotericin B. In: Welch H, Marti-Ibañez F, eds. *Antibiotics annual 1955–1956*, pp. 566–73. Medical Encyclopedia Inc., New York.

18. Bennett JE (1992). Developing drugs for the deep mycoses: a short history. In: Bennett JE, Hay RJ, Peterson PK, eds. *New strategies in fungal disease*, pp. 3–12. Churchill Livingstone, Edinburgh.

19. Graybill JR, Craven PC, Taylor RL, Williams DM, Magee WE (1982). Treatment of murine crypto-coccosis with liposome-associated amphotericin B. *J Infect Dis* **145**, 748–52.

20. Graybill JR (1996). Lipid formulations of amphotericin B: does the emperor need new clothes? *Ann Intern Med* **124**, 921–3.

21. Hosoya S, Komatsu N, Soeda M, Sonoda Y (1952). Trichomycin, a new antibiotic produced by *Streptomyces hachijoensis* with trichomonicidal and antifungal activity. *Jpn J Exp Med* **22**, 505–9.

22. Struyk AP, Hoette I, Drost G, Waisvisz JM, van Eek T, Hoogerheide JC (1958). Pimaricin, a new anti-fungal antibiotic. In: Welch H, Marti-Ibañez F, eds. *Antibiotics annual 1957–1958*, pp. 878–85. Medical Encylopedia, Inc., New York.

23. Malbica J, Sello L, Tabenkin B, *et al.* (1962). Some biological properties of 5-fluorocytosine (FC) and its derivatives. *Federation Proceedings* **21** (Abstract), 384.

24. Grunberg, E, Titworth E, Bennett M (1964). Chemotherapeutic activity of 5-fluorocytosine. In: Sylvester JC, ed. *Antimicrobial agents and Chemotherapy-1963*, pp. 566–8. American Society for Microbiology, Ann Arbor, Michigan.

25. Giege R, Weil JH (1970). Étude des tRNA de levure ayant incorporé du fluorouracile provenant de la désamination in vivo de la 5-fluorocytosine. *Bulletin de la Société de Chimie Biologique* **52**, 135–44.

26. Utz JP, Tynes BS, Shadomy HJ, Duma RJ, Kannan MM, Mason KN (1969). 5-Fluorocytosine in human cryptococcosis. In: Hobby GL, ed. *Antimicrobial agents and chemotherapy–1968*, pp. 344–6. American Society for Microbiology, Bethesda, Maryland.

27. Medoff G, Comfort M, Kobayashi GS (1971). Synergistic action of amphotericin B and 5-fluorocy-tosine against yeast-like organisms. *Proc Soc Exp Biol Med* **138**, 571–4.

28. Oxford AE, Raistrick H, Simonart P (1939). Studies in the biochemistry of micro-organisms. LX. Griseofulvin. $C_{17}H_{17}O_6Cl$, a metabolic product of *Penicillium griseo-fulvum* Dierckx. *Biochem J* **33**, 240–8.

29. Garrett SD (1981). Percy Wragg Brian 5 September 1910–1917 August 1979. *Biographical memoirs Fellows R Soc* **27**, 102–30.

30. Anonymous (1967). Griseofulvin. *BMJ* **4**, 608–9.

31. Grove JF, McGowan JC (1947). Identity of griseofulvin and 'curling factor'. *Nature* **160**, 574–5.

32. Brain PW (1949). Studies on the biological activity of griseofulvin. *Ann Bot* **13**, 59–77.

33. Anonymous (1960). Symposium on griseofulvin. *BMJ* **1**, 1804–5.

34. Gentles JC (1958). Experimental ringworm in guinea pigs: oral treatment with griseofulvin. *Nature* **182**, 476–7.

35. Martin AR (1959). The systemic and local treatment of experimental dermatophytosis with griseo-fulvin. *J Invest Dermatol* **32**, 525–8.

36. Editorial (1960). Griseofulvin. *Lancet* **1**, 1175–6.

37. Campbell AH (1964). Chemotherapy of dermatophytes. In: Schnitzer RJ, Hawking F, eds *Experimental chemotherapy*, Vol. III, pp. 461–80. Academic Press, New York.

38. Gentles JC, Barnes MJ, Fantes KH (1959). Presence of griseofulvin in hair of guinea pigs after oral administration. *Nature* **183**, 256–7.

39. Stütz A (1990). Allylamine derivatives—inhibitors of squalene epoxidase. In: Borowski E, Shugar D, eds. *Molecular aspects of chemotherapy*, pp. 205–13. Proceedings of the 2nd international symposium on molecular aspects of chemotherapy, Gdansk, Poland, July 5–8 1988. Pergamon Press, New York.

40. Georgopoulos A, Petranyi G, Mieth H, Drews J (1981). *In vitro* activity of naftifine, a new antifungal agent. *Antimicrob Agents Chemother* **19**, 386–9.

41. Stütz A (1999). A Viennese success story. In: *Novartis Forschunsinstitut Austria*. Available at: http://www.novartis.com/downloads/homepage/NFI_english.pdf.

42. Stephen A, Ganzinger U, Czok R (1985). SF 86-327: results of phase II studies with a new antifungal agent for oral and topical application. In: Ishigami J, ed. *Proceedings of the 14th International Congress of Chemotherapy, Kyoto, Japan*, pp. 1946–7. University of Tokyo Press, Tokyo.

43. Plempel M, Bartmann K, Büchel KH, Regel E (1970). Bay b 5097, a new orally applicable antifungal substance with broad-spectrum activity. In: Hobby GL, ed. *Antimicrobial agents and chemotherapy–1969*, pp. 271–4 American Society for Microbiology, Bethesda Maryland.

44. Godefroi EF, Heeres J, Van Cutsem J, Janssen PAJ (1969). The preparation and antimycotic properties of derivatives of 1-phenethylimidazole. *J Med Chem* **12**,784–91.

45. Fromtling RA (1988). Overview of medically important antifungal azole derivatives. *Clin Microbiol Rev* **1**, 187–217.

46. Jevons S, Gymer GE, Brammer KW, Cox DA, Lemming MRG (1979). Antifungal activity of tioconazole (UK-20,349), a new imidazole derivative. *Antimicrob Agents Chemother* **15**, 597–602.

47. Thienpoint D, Van Cutsem J, Van Gerven F, Heeres J, Janssen PAJ (1979). Ketoconazole—a new broad spectrum orally active antimycotic. *Experientia* **35**, 606–7.

48. Graybill JR, Drutz DJ (1980). Ketoconazole: a major innovation for treatment of fungal disease. *Ann Intern Med* **93**, 921–3.

49. Richardson K, Brammer KW, Marriott MS, Troke PF (1985). Activity of UK-49,858, a bis-triazole derivative, against experimental infections with *Candida albicans* and *Trichophyton mentagrophytes*. *Antimicrob Agents Chemother* **27**, 832–5.

50. Heeres J, Backx LJ, Van Cutsem J (1984). Antimycotic azoles. 7. Synthesis and antifungal properties of a series of novel triazol-3-ones. *J Med Chem* **27**, 894–900.

51. Grunberg E, Berger J, Titsworth E (1961). Chemotherapeutic studies on a new antifungal agent, X-5079C, effective against systemic mycoses. *Am Rev Respir Dis* **84**, 504–6.

52. Weinstein MJ, Oden EM, Moss E (1965). Antifungal properties of tolnaftate in vitro and in vivo. In: Sylvester JC, ed. *Antimicrobial Agents and Chemotherapy—1964*, pp. 595–601 American Society for Microbiology, Ann Arbor, Michigan.

53. Seki S, Nomiya B, Koeda T, Umemura K, Oda M, Ogawa H (1964). Laboratory evaluation of M-1028 (2,4,5- trichlorophenyl-γ-iodopropargyl ether), a new antimicrobial agent. In: Sylvester JC, ed. *Antimicrobial agents and chemotherapy-1963*, pp. 569–72. American Society for Microbiology, Ann Arbor, Michigan.

54. Harrison EF, Zwadyk P, Bequette RJ, Hamlow EE, Tavormina PA, Zygmunt WA (1970). Haloprogin: a topical antifungal agent. *Appl Microbiol* **19**, 746–50.

55. Benz F, Knüsel F, Nüesch J, *et al.* (1974). Echinocandin B, ein neuartiges polypeptid-antibioticum aus *Aspergillus nidulans* var. *echinulatus*. *Helvetica Chimica Acta* **57**, 2459–77.

56. Gordee RS, Zeckner DJ, Ellis LF, Thakkar AL, Howard LC (1984). In vitro and in vivo anti-candida activity and toxicology of LY121019. *J Antibiot* **37**, 1054–65.

57. Schwartz RE, Giacobbe RA, Bland JA, Monaghan RL (1989). L-671,239, a new antifungal agent. I. Fermentation and isolation. *J Antibiot* **42**, 163–7.

58. Schmatz DM, Romancheck MA, Pittarelli LA, *et al.* (1990). Treatment of *Pneumocystis carinii* pneumonia with 1,3-β-glucan synthesis inhibitors. *Proc Natl Acad Sci USA* **87**, 5950–4.

59. Grundy I (1999). *Lady Mary Wortley Montagu. Comet of the Enlightenment.* Oxford University Press, Oxford.

60. Jenner E (1978). An inquiry into the causes and effects of the variolae vaccinae, a disease discovered in some western counties of England, particularly Gloucestershire, and known by the name of The Cow Pox. Sampson Low, London. Abridged version reproduced in: Brock T, ed. *Milestones in microbiology*, pp. 121–5. American Society for Microbiology, Washington, 1961.

61. Fisher RB (1991). *Edward Jenner 1749–1823.* André Deutsch, London.

62. Behbehani AM (1983). The smallpox story: life and death of an old disease. *Microbiol Rev* **47**, 455–509.

63. Baxby, D (1977). The origins of vaccinia virus. *J Infect Dis* **156**, 453–5.

64. Theiler M, Smith HH (1937). The use of yellow fever virus modified by in vitro cultivation for human immunization. *J Exp Med* **65**, 787–800.

65. Mortimer PP (2002). The control of yellow fever: a centennial account. *Microbiol Today* **29**, 24–5.

66. Salk JE (1953). Studies in human subjects on active immunization against poliomyelitis. I. A preliminary report of experiments in progress. *JAMA* **151**, 1081–98.

67. Sabin AB, Hennessen WA, Winsser J (1954). Studies on variants of poliomyelitis virus: I. Experimental segregation and properties of avirulent variants of three immunologic types. *J Exp Med* **99**, 551–76.

68. Blume S, Geesink I (2000). A brief history of polio vaccines. *Science* **288**, 1593–4.

69. Enders JF, Katz SL, Milovanovic MV, Holloway A (1960). Studies on an attenuated measles-virus vaccine. I. Development and preparations of the vaccine: technics for assay of effects of vaccination. *N Engl J Med* **263**, 153–9 (first of a comprehensive series of eight papers on the subject published concurrently in *N Engl J Med* **263**, 153–84).

70. Centers for Disease Control and Prevention (2002). *MMWR* **51**, 120–3.

71. Obituary (19 April 2005). Maurice Hilleman. *The Times*, p. 53.

72. Shope RE (1953). An antiviral substance from Penicillium funiculosum. I. Effect upon infection in mice with swine influenza virus and Columbia SK encephalomyelitis virus. *J Exp Med* **97**, 601–25.

73. Isaacs A, Lindenmann J (1957). Virus interference. I. The interferon. *Proc R Soc London. Series B. Biological Sciences* **147**, 258–67.

74. Finter N (September/ October 1993). The Wellferon story: Part 1. From 'virus interference' to Namalwa. *Wellcome World*, pp. 7–11.

75. Report (1962). Effect of interferon on vaccination in volunteers : a report to the Medical Research Council from the Scientific Committee on Interferon. *Lancet* **1**, 873–5.

76. Dixon B (1997). Interferon reexamined. *Am Soc Microbiol News* **63**, 242–3.

77. Bridgen PJ, Anfinsen CB, Corley L, Bose S, Zoon KC, Rüegg UT (1977). Human lymphoblastoid interferon. Large scale production and partial purification. *J Biol Chem* **252**, 6585–7; Zoon KC, Smith ME, Bridgen PJ, Zur Nedden D, Miller DM, Anfinsen C (1980). Human lymphoblastoid interferon: purification, amino acid composition, and amino-terminal sequence. *Ann NY Acad Sci* **350**, 390–8.

78. Gresser I, Bourali C, Lévy JP, Fontaine-Brouty-Boyé D, Thomas MT (1969). Increased survival in mice inoculated with tumor cells and treated with interferon preparations. *Proc Natl Acad Sci USA* **63**, 51–7.

79. Brownlee KA, Hamre D (1951). Studies on chemotherapy of vaccinia virus. I. An experimental design for testing antiviral agents. *J Bacteriol* **61**, 127–34.

80. Hamre D, Brownlee KA, Donovick R (1951). Studies on the chemotherapy of vaccinia virus. II. The activity of some thiosemicarbazones. *J Immunol* **67**, 305–12.

81. Bauer DJ, Sadler PW (1960). New antiviral chemotherapeutic agent active against smallpox infection. *Lancet* **1**, 1110–1.

82. Bauer DJ, St Vincent L, Kempe CH, Downie AW (1963). Prophylactic treatment of smallpox contacts with N-methylisatin β-thiosemicarbazone (compound 33T57, Marboran). *Lancet* **2**, 494–6.

83. Prusoff WH (1959). Synthesis and biological activity of idoxuridine, an analogue of thymidine. *Biochimica et Biophysica Acta* **32**, 295–6.

84. Kaufman HE (2002). Can we prevent recurrences of herpes infections without antiviral drugs? The Weisenfeld Lecture. *Investigative Ophthalmology and Visual Science* **43**, 1325–9. Available at: http://www.iovs.org/cgi/content/full/43/5/1325.

85. Kaufman HE (1962). Clinical cure of herpes simplex keratitis by 5-iodo-2′-deoxyuridine. *Proc Soc Exp Biol Med* **109**, 251–2.

86. Kaufman HE, Heidelberger C (1964). Therapeutic antiviral action of 5-trifluoromethyl-2′-deoxyuridine. *Science* **145**, 585–6.

87. Privat de Garilhe M, de Rudder J (1964). Effet de deux nucléosides de l'arabinose sur la multiplication des virus de l'herpès et de la vaccine en culture cellulaire. *Comptes rendus hebdomadaires des séances de l'Académie des sciences* **259**, 2725–8; de Rudder J, Privat de Garilhe M (1966). Inhibitory effect of some nucleosides on the growth of various human viruses in tissue culture. In: Hobby GL, ed. *Antimicrobial agents and chemotherapy—1965*, pp. 578–84. American Society for Microbiology, Ann arbour, Michigan.

88. Bergmann R, Feeney RJ (1950). The isolation of a new thymine pentoside from sponges. *J Am Chem Soc* **72**, 2809–10.

89. Lee WW, Benitez A, Goodman L, Baker BR (1960). Potential anticancer agents XL. Synthesis of 9-β-anomer of 9-(D-arabinosyfuranosyl)-adenine. *J Am Chem Soc* **82**, 2648–9.

90. Shannon WM (1975). Adenine arabinoside: antiviral activity in vitro. In: Pavan-Langston D, Buchanan RA, Alford CA, eds. *Adenine arabinoside: an antiviral agent*, pp. 1–43. Raven Press, New York.

91. Schabel FM (1968). The antiviral activity of 9-β-arabinofuranosyladenine (ARA-A) *Chemotherapy* **13**, 321–38.

92. Ch'ien LT, Cannon NJ, Charamella LJ, *et al.* (1973). Effect of adenine arabinoside on severe herpesvirus hominis infections in man. *J Infect Dis* **128**, 658–63; reprinted: 2004 **190**, 1362–7.

93. Davies WL, Grunert RR, Haff RF, *et al.* (1964). Antiviral activity of 1-adamantamine (amantadine) *Science* **144**, 862–3.

94. Sidwell RW, Huffman J, Khare GP, Allen LB, Witkowski JT, Robins RK (1972). Broad-spectrum antiviral activity of Virazole: 1-β-D-ribofuranosyl-1,2,4-triazole-3-carboxamide. *Science* **177**, 705–6.

95. Hall CB, McBride JT, Walsh EE, *et al.* (1983). Aerosolized ribavirin treatment of infants with respiratory syncytial viral infection. A randomized double-blind study. *N Engl J Med* **308**, 1443–7.

96. Thompson F (2001). Where do generic and brand names come from? *Pharmaceutical J* **267**, 223–4.

97. Brown ER, Gordon P (1970). Inosine-alkylamino alcohol complexes: antiviral actions. *Federation Proceedings* **29**, 684; Gordon P, Brown ER, Ronsen B (1971). NPT-10381: novel basis for antiviral action. *Federation Proceedings* **30**, 242.

98. Elion GB (1988). The purine path to chemotherapy. Nobel Lecture. Available at: http://nobelprize.org/medicine/laureates/1988/elion-lecture.pdf.

99. Elion GB (1993). Acyclovir: discovery, mechanism of action, and selectivity. *J Med Virol* **41** (Suppl. 1), 2–6.

100. Schaeffer HJ, Beauchamp L, de Miranda P, Elion GB, Bauer DJ, Collins P (1978). 9-(2-hydroxyethoxymethyl) guanine activity against viruses of the herpes group. *Nature* **272**, 583–5.

101. Elion GB, Furman PA, Fyfe JA, de Mirando P, Beauchamp L, Schaeffer HJ (1977). Selectivity of action of an antiherpetic agent, 9- (2-hydroxyethoxymethyl)guanine. *Proc Natl Acad Sci USA* **74**, 5716–20.

102. Smee DF, Martin JC, Verheyden JPH, Matthews TR (1983). Anti-herpesvirus activity of the acyclic nucleoside 9-(1,3-dihydroxy-2-propoxymethyl)guanine. *Antimicrob Agents Chemother* **23**, 676–82.

103. Boyd MR, Bacon TH, Sutton D, Cole M (1987). Antiherpesvirus activity of 9-(4-hydroxy-3-hydroxy-methylbut-1-yl)guanine (BRL 39123) in cell culture. *Antimicrob Agents Chemother* **31**, 1238–42; Boyd MR, Bacon TH, Sutton D (1988). Antiherpesvirus activity of 9-(4-hydroxy-3-hydroxymethylbut-1-yl) guanine (BRL 39123) in animals. *Antimicrob Agents Chemother* **32**, 358–63.

104. Vere Hodge, RA, Sutton D, Boyd MR, Harnden MR, Jarvest RL (1989). Selection of an oral prodrug (BRL 42810; famciclovir) for the antiherpesvirus agent BRL 39123 [9-(4-hydroxy-3-hydroxy-methylbut-l-yl)guanine; penciclovir]. *Antimicrob Agents Chemother* **33**, 1765–73.

105. Purifoy DJ, Beauchamp LM, de Miranda P, *et al.* (1993). Review of research leading to new anti-herpesvirus agents in clinical development: valaciclovir hydrochloride (256U, the L-valyl ester of acyclovir) and 882C, a specific agent for varicella zoster virus. *J Med Virol* (Suppl. 1), 139–45.

106. Mitsuya H, Weinhold K, Yarchoan R, Bolognesi D, Broder S (28 September 1989). Credit Government Scientists With Developing Anti-AIDS Drug (1989). *New York Times.*

107. Cochrane JMT (2000). Zidovudine's patent history. *Lancet* **356**, 1611–2.

108. Aboulker J-P, Swart AM (1993). Preliminary analysis of the Concorde trial. *Lancet* **341**, 889–90; Concorde Coordinating Committee (1994). Concorde: MRC/ANRS randomised double-blind controlled trial of immediate and deferred zidovudine in symptom-free HIV infection. *Lancet* **343**, 871–81.

109. Ahluwalia G, Cooney DA, Mitsuya H, *et al.* (1987). Initial studies on the cellular pharmacology of 2′,3′-dideoxyinosine, an inhibitor of HIV infectivity. *Biochem Pharmacol* **36**, 3797–800.

110. Yarchoan R, Mitsuya H, Thomas RV, *et al.* (1989). In vivo activity against HIV and favorable toxicity profile of 2′,3′-dideoxyinosine. *Science* **245**, 412–5.

111. Debouck C (1992). The HIV-1 protease as a therapeutic target for AIDS. *AIDS Res Hum Retroviruses* **8**, 153–64.

112. Debouck C, Gorniak JG, Strickler JE, Meek TD, Metcalf BW, Rosenberg M (1987). Human immunodeficiency virus protease expressed in *Escherichia coli* exhibits autoprocessing and specific maturation of the gag precursor. *Proc Natl Acad Sci USA* **84**, 8903–6.

113. Wild C, Oas T, McDanal C, Bolognesi D, Matthews T (1992). A synthetic peptide inhibitor of human immunodeficiency virus replication: correlation between solution structure and viral inhibition. *Proc Natl Acad Sci USA* **89**, 10537–41.

114. Edmond JD, Johnston RG, Kidd D, Rylance HJ, Sommerville RG (1966). The inhibition of neuraminidase and antiviral action. *Br J Pharmacol Chemother* **27**, 415–26.

115. Colman PM (1994). Influenza virus neuraminidase: structure, antibodies, and inhibitors. *Protein Sci* **3**, 1687–96.

116. von Itzstein M, Wu WY, Kok GB, *et al.* (1993). Rational design of potent sialidase-based inhibitors of influenza virus replication. *Nature* **363**, 418–23.

117. Lew W, Chen X, Kim CU (2000). Discovery and development of GS 4104 (oseltamivir): an orally active influenza neuraminidase inhibitor. *Curr Med Chem* **7**, 663–72.

118. Gubareva LV, Kaiser L, Hayden FG (2000). Influenza virus neuraminidase inhibitors. *Lancet* **355**, 827–35.

119. Shipkowitz NL, Bower RR, Appel RN, *et al.* (1973). Suppression of herpes simplex virus infection by phosphonoacetic acid. *Appl Microbiol* **26**, 264–7.

120. Nylén P (1924). Beitrag zur Kenntnis der organischen Phosphorverbindungen. *Chemische Berichte* **57B**, 1023–38.

121. Reno JM, Lee LF, Boezi JA (1978). Inhibition of herpesvirus replication and herpesvirus-induced deoxyribonucleic acid polymerase by phosphonoformate. *Antimicrob Agents Chemother* **13**, 188–92.

122. Helgstrand E, Eriksson B, Johansson NG, *et al.* (1978). Trisodium phosphonoformate, a new antiviral compound. *Science* **201**, 819–21.

123. Zamecnik PC, Stephenson ML (1978). Inhibition of Rous sarcoma virus replication and cell transformation by a specific oligodeoxynucleotide. *Proc Natl Acad Sci U S A* **75**, 280–4.

124. De Clercq E, Descamps J, De Somer P, Holý A (1978). (S)-9-(2,3-Dihydroxypropyl)adenine: an aliphatic nucleoside analog with broad-spectrum antiviral activity. *Science* **200**, 563–5.

125. Innaimo SF, Seifer M, Bisacchi GS, Standring DN, Zahler R, Colonno RJ (1997). Identification of BMS-200475 as a potent and selective inhibitor of hepatitis B virus. *Antimicrob Agents Chemother* **41**, 1444–8.

126. Katz DH, Marcelletti JF, Khalil MH, Pope LE, Katz LR (1991). Antiviral activity of 1-docosanol, an inhibitor of lipid-enveloped viruses including herpes simplex. *Proc Natl Acad Sci U S A* **88**, 10825–9.

Chapter 9

The spectre at the feast

Our inquiry has been an alarming experience. Misuse and overuse of anti biotics are now threatening to undo all their early promises and success in curing disease. But the greatest threat is complacency, from Ministers, the medical professions, the veterinary service, the farming community, and the public at large. Our report is a blueprint for action. It must start now, if we are not to return to the bad old days of incurable diseases before antibiotics were available.

> Lord Soulsby, Chairman, *House of Lords Select Committee*
> *on Resistance to Antibiotics*, 1998 (1).

In 1969, the United States Surgeon General, William H. Stewart, famously told the US Congress that it was 'time to close the books on infectious diseases.' Stewart had, in 1965, been the surprise nomination for the Surgeon General's office (2). He resigned in 1969 shortly after making his controversial statement, though there seems to be no suggestion that the two events were connected. Stewart's intention had been to contrast the stunning success of antibiotics, vaccines, and public health measures in the fight against infectious diseases, with the unsolved problems of heart disease and cancer. Still, he must have lived to regret the statement about infection, for it has been repeated ad nauseam by those wishing to stress misplaced optimism as a contributory factor to the problem of antimicrobial drug resistance.

Today, Cassandras are peddling the contrary prophecy of disaster. The talk is of 'superbugs' (they are no such thing; they are just ordinary bugs trying, like the rest of us, to survive in a hostile environment) and of the 'post-antimicrobial era' (3). What is lacking, as usual, is balance and perspective. The doom-mongers, while paying lip service to the extraordinary advances in the treatment of infectious disease during the twentieth century, seem to have no grasp of history. Doctors before 1935 stood virtually helpless at the bedsides of patients with serious infections like pneumonia, septicaemia, meningitis, and tuberculosis—many of them children or young adults—whose only hope of survival lay in their immune systems' ability to win a bitterly fought internal battle. Barring some cataclysmic upheaval in the world, or the possible emergence of a highly infectious and rapidly lethal virus, such times are extremely unlikely to return whatever the ingenuity of microbes. Our ability to prevent and treat infection, especially bacterial infection, has simply moved too far ahead of the threat.

This is not to preach complacency. There are plenty of problems and far too little political will to face them in many countries. But nothing is gained by exaggerating the present situation or by predicting a doomsday scenario that denies reality. There is much to be done to minimize the impact of antimicrobial drug resistance, but common sense must replace hysteria if the problems are to be solved.

The problem of resistance

In a wonderful essay that won *The Lancet's* first Wakely Prize in 1996, Imre Loeffler, a Hungarian surgeon working in Kenya, summed up the problems that lead to antimicrobial drug resistance:

> Surgeons, who regard the most trivial wound infection as a slight on their skill, are in the forefront of prophylactic use, and use such treatment even if the consequences of an infection would be negligible; physicians give long courses on suspicion of possible infection. In the meantime the public demands antibiotics, injections, ointments, powders and capsules, and since doctors are not paid for advice but for procedures and because writing a prescription is the fastest way to part with a patient, the unholiest of alliances is at work: consumer demand based on misinformation, mercantile interest, and the insecurity and cynicism of the middlemen. In the developing world it is not necessary to go to a doctor and get a prescription for an antibiotic. Time and money can be saved. One can go to the market and buy collections of antibiotics sealed in little envelopes and labelled "strong medicine". Chemotherapy is not limited to human use. There is hardly a domestic animal that has not been treated with an antibiotic, and chicken and goldfish are given daily prophylaxis with their food. Small animal clinics (the paediatric units of suburbia) are the leaders of the trend (4).

Loeffler's colourful language may oversimplify the problem, but he succeeds in neatly encapsulating the main elements that have led to the present difficulties: overuse of antimicrobial drugs in human medicine and in animals; unrestricted availability and unprincipled promotion of these drugs in many countries of the world; and uninformed public demand for prescriptions for trivial infections.

The criticisms are not new. As the medical historian, James Whorton, pointed out in a survey of antibiotic misuse in America, the famous Canadian physician William Osler* had raised many of the same fears about the overprescription and promotion of drugs long before antibiotics were discovered (5). In the 1950s, Maxwell Finland, the diminutive giant of antibiotic studies at the Harvard Medical School, fulminated against doctors who regarded antimicrobial drugs as 'omnibiotics' (6), and started to collect the data that were to provide chapter and verse for the dangers of overprescribing (7). In Britain in 1952, an editorial in the *British Medical Journal†* observed:

....

* Although William Osler, one of the most influential physicians of his day, was born in Canada and qualified in medicine there, he was recruited as one of the first medical appointments at the new Johns Hopkins Hospital in Baltimore in 1888. In 1905 he moved to England to become Regius Professor of Medicine at Oxford.

† Lawrence Paul Garrod, Professor of Bacteriology at St. Bartholomew's Hospital, London, wrote the editorial. See: Waterworth PM (ed.) L. P. Garrod on antibiotics. A selection of his *British Medical Journal* editorials. *Journal of Antimicrobial Chemotherapy* 1985; 15 (Supplement B).

All the newer antibiotics are slowly wasting assets...but if they were restricted to their proper fields we could enjoy them for many years longer. Let anyone tempted to use one of them for, say, a common cold reflect that this type of use may abolish its effect in a patient with septicaemia at some time in the future (8).

Although overprescribing of antimicrobial agents for trivial complaints—especially use of antibacterial drugs for conditions likely to be caused by viruses—is always to be condemned, it is in hospitals and nursing homes rather than the community at large where the major problems arise, at least in countries in which drug availability is well-regulated and antibiotics can be obtained only on a doctor's prescription. In the wider community, so long as there are tight controls on the availability of antibiotics, and they are prescribed and used correctly, resistance is unlikely to become widespread and general. Few individuals (relative to the size of the population) are likely to be receiving therapy with a particular antimicrobial drug at any one time and if resistance arises the overwhelming dilution effect of sensitive organisms within the collective bacterial flora ensures that, in the absence of further selective pressure, resistant organisms will not be advantaged. Good environmental hygiene also hinders the spread within the community of resistant variants that survive.

Sadly, these conditions are not met everywhere, particularly in the poorer countries of the world. Consequently, multiresistant strains of the age-old bacterial enemies, such as *Mycobacterium tuberculosis*, salmonellae that cause typhoid fever, shigellae responsible for severe bacillary dysentery, and venereal pathogens like *Neisseria gonorrhoeae*, have become common in many parts of the world. It is here that the burden of antimicrobial drug resistance is most severely felt. Nor is the problem restricted to bacteria: indeed multidrug resistant malaria remains one of the most serious threats in countries in which the disease is endemic.

For industrially developed nations it is hospitals with their populations of seriously ill patients—especially in high-dependency units—that provide the breeding ground for resistance. The combination of highly vulnerable patients, some with grossly depleted immune systems, liberal use of broad-spectrum antimicrobial agents, lack of isolation facilities, and, sometimes, failure of staff to observe cross-infection control procedures, provides the ideal milieu for the development and dissemination of multiresistant micro-organisms. Most of these multiresistant bacteria are so-called 'opportunists', organisms of generally low virulence that are able to strike when the defences are down. They include species such as *Klebsiella aerogenes*, *Pseudomonas aeruginosa*, *Acinetobacter baumannii*, *Clostridium difficile* (an organism that flourishes as a consequence of antibacterial therapy), and *Streptococcus faecalis*, which pose little threat to healthy individuals and may indeed be harmlessly carried as part of the normal bacterial flora. But the most notorious of the opportunists is a true primary pathogen, *Staphylococcus aureus*. Despite the fact that all the aforementioned bacterial species can cause serious and intractable problems in units affected by them, most publicity has been given to methicillin-resistant *Staphylococcus aureus* (MRSA) an organism that has become the evil demon of all debate about antimicrobial drug resistance in the developed world.

Areas of special concern

Staphylococcus aureus and MRSA

Staphylococcus aureus is unquestionably an organism that should be taken seriously. Although it is often carried harmlessly on the skin and in the nose, the species can produce a formidable battery of virulence factors that enable it to establish and spread through human tissues. It is a lethal pathogen and was much feared before the appearance of antibiotics. In fact, fatality rates from MRSA need to be interpreted with some caution since sensitive strains of *Staphylococcus aureus* can also kill despite appropriate therapy and death is not necessarily attributable to the lack of suitable antibacterial drugs.

Nearly all antimicrobial agents that have appeared on the market over the years, exhibit useful activity against *Staphylococcus aureus* (Table 9.1), but strains of this versatile bacterium have the capacity to develop resistance to each of them. Until 1997, when a strain with reduced susceptibility was reported from Japan (9), the only antibiotic to which *Staphylococcus aureus* seemed unable to develop resistance was vancomycin. This has given rise to the belief that vancomycin (or the related glycopeptide antibiotic, teicoplanin) is the sole drug with which MRSA can normally be treated. In fact, strains resistant to all available antistaphylococcal agents except vancomycin are, if they occur at all, extremely uncommon, although it is true that glycopeptides are often the drugs of first choice for multiresistant strains.

The particular significance of resistance to methicillin is that it also applies to all other β-lactam agents—i.e. all penicillins, cephalosporins, and carbapenems—rendering impotent many of the agents that physicians would prefer to use. If the strain is also resistant to aminoglycosides, tetracyclines, and macrolides, as they often are, first-line therapeutic options are further constrained. Add on to this, traits that enhance the ability of the strain to disseminate, and enable it to colonize more easily those (patients or staff) to whom it spreads, and the scene is set for a serious problem of hospital-acquired infection. In such cases prevention of colonization is crucial to the containment of the outbreak.

Table 9.1 Activity of antibacterial agents against *Staphylococcus aureus*

Antibacterial agents with intrinsic activity			Agents lacking useful activity
Aminoglycosides	Fosfomycin	Oxazolidinones	Monobactams
Carbapenems	Fusidic acid	Penicillins[a]	Nalidixic acid[b]
Cephalosporins	Glycopeptides	Rifamycins	Nitrofurans
Chloramphenicol	Lincosamides	Streptogramins	Nitroimidazoles
Daptomycin	Macrolides	Sulphonamides	Spectinomycin
Diaminopyrimidines	Mupirocin	Tetracyclines	
Fluoroquinolones	Novobiocin		

[a] Except mecillinam and temocillin.

[b] Including other early quinolones such as oxolinic acid and cinoxacin.

The epithet 'methicillin-resistant *Staphylococcus aureus*' originates from the fact that methicillin, the first of the antistaphylococcal penicillins that were developed when resistance to benzylpenicillin became common (see p. 123–4), is (or was) commonly used to test the generic resistance of such strains to all β-lactam antibiotics in the laboratory. Methicillin has long been superseded in therapy and is no longer available, so that these strains would be better designated 'multiresistant *Staphylococcus aureus*', which would leave the acronym intact and would indicate that the strains are also resistant to other types of drug.

Mary Barber at the Royal Postgraduate Medical School, Hammersmith Hospital, West London, showed in 1961 that resistance to methicillin could be induced in staphylococci by exposing them to low concentrations of the antibiotic in laboratory experiments (10). The first clinical isolate was reported in the same year by Patricia Jevons of the Staphylococcus Reference Laboratory at the Central Public Health Laboratory, Colindale (now part of the Health Protection Agency). She had examined over 5000 strains of *Staphylococcus aureus* that had been submitted to the laboratory for phage typing (a technique used to establish the relatedness of strains) during October and November 1960, a year after methicillin was first marketed (11). Three strains were found to be methicillin-resistant, all from the same hospital in Guildford, Surrey: a patient with a nephrectomy wound; a nurse from the same ward with an infected skin lesion; and a patient with eczema, who regularly attended the hospital and was thought to be the source. A follow-up study two years later of over 22,000 staphylococcus strains, carried out with the help of Tom Parker, then freshly appointed to the post of director of a newly established Cross-Infection Reference Laboratory at Colindale, yielded 102 methicillin-resistant isolates (12). Since resistance in this very widespread pathogen seemed relatively uncommon, was unrelated to the enzymic activity that was responsible for resistance to other penicillins, and was difficult to induce under laboratory conditions, it was thought unlikely that it would pose a major threat. The optimism was supported by an unusual feature of methicillin resistance: the bacteria expressed their resistance fully only under laboratory conditions far removed from those that exist in infection, viz. when tested in the presence of a high concentration of salt or at a low, non-physiological temperature.

For a while, the initial optimism appeared justified. A trickle of methicillin-resistant strains was reported in the United Kingdom over the next few years, but the overall prevalence remained very low. However, more disturbing news soon began to emerge. Somewhat higher frequencies of resistance to methicillin and instances of multidrug resistance were reported from hospitals in France, Denmark, and Switzerland (13). Eriksen in Denmark described in 1964 a methicillin-resistant strain of *Staphylococcus aureus* that appeared during treatment with the drug (14); by 1967, he was reporting to the 5th International Congress of Chemotherapy in Vienna that 10 per cent of isolates from Danish cases of staphylococcal septicaemia were resistant. In 1968, Max Finland and his colleagues at the Boston City Hospital in the United States described 22 strains of *Staphylococcus aureus* that were not only resistant to methicillin, but in most cases also exhibited resistance to erythromycin, tetracyclines, and chloramphenicol (15).

Vigorous infection control measures successfully limited the spread of MRSA in European and American hospitals during the 1970s. Small outbreaks occurred in some units from time to time, but the problem did not become persistent or widespread. Renewed concerns began to be expressed in the early1980s, when a worrying increase in the incidence of MRSA was reported from several countries, including the United States, Ireland, and England. In Australia an epidemic of multiresistant *Staphylococcus aureus* strains was noted in hospitals in the state of Victoria leading to the startling suggestion that such infections were in danger of becoming untreatable (16). The Australian experience attracted considerable media attention in the country and there were frantic efforts to control and monitor the developing situation (17). There were repercussions around the world, where closer scrutiny of the situation revealed an escalating problem and little consensus on how it should be dealt with.

An intriguing aspect of MRSA is the varying prevalence in different countries. Since 1998 surveillance of MRSA in Europe has been coordinated in the Netherlands as part of the European Antimicrobial Resistance Surveillance System (EARSS), which is sponsored by the European Commission and the Dutch Rijksinstituut voor Volksgezondheid en Milieu (National Institute for Public Health and the Environment). A survey of over 50,000 *Staphylococcus aureus* isolates from blood cultures (and hence presumptively causing a life-threatening septicaemia) collected from around 500 hospitals in 27 countries between 1999 and 2002 showed that overall 20 per cent were categorized as MRSA. However, the national prevalence rates varied from less than 1 per cent in Scandinavia and the Netherlands to over 40 per cent in Greece, Ireland, Italy, and the United Kingdom. Most surprisingly, the prevalence rates for the Netherlands and neighbouring Belgium and Germany were 0.6 per cent, 23.6 per cent, and 13.8 per cent,* respectively (18). Microbes have no respect for boundaries, and free movement occurs across the borders between these countries, so national policies of prevention and containment clearly seem to have some impact on infection rates.

So far the major problem with MRSA has been largely confined to hospitals, but carriage of MRSA in the nose or on the skin and episodes of associated infection are increasing in nursing homes and even within the population at large, at least in countries with high hospital prevalence rates (19).

Pneumococci

For three decades after benzylpenicillin was introduced into general use, it remained uniformly active against strains of pneumococci and was always the drug of first choice in the absence of penicillin allergy. It therefore came as a considerable shock when in 1977, penicillin-resistant strains were found in children being treated in Soweto's Barangwanath Hospital near Johannesburg in South Africa. Similar strains were found in Durban around the same time and a number of children died despite what would normally have been

---

* The criterion by which an isolate is judged resistant to methicillin in Germany is slightly lower than that used in most other European countries, so the figure for Germany may be a little inflated.

regarded as curative treatment. There had been earlier reports of penicillin-resistant pneumococci—in an aboriginal child at the Ernabella hospital in South Australia in 1967; and in 15 New Guineans from Anguganak, New Guinea in 1969 (20)—but the level of resistance in some of the South African strains was of a higher level and, even more alarmingly, a few of the strains were resistant not only to penicillin, but also to chloramphenicol and some other drugs (21). At first it was hoped that these were isolated occurrences, but further reports soon emerged in Europe, America, and elsewhere and by the 1990s penicillin-resistant pneumococci began to be taken seriously everywhere.

As with MRSA, there is considerable geographical variation in the prevalence of penicillin-resistant pneumococci, but the problem is rather different. In pneumococci, the most frequent form of resistance is manifested by a relatively small decline in susceptibility, so that the high doses of penicillin that are ordinarily used are still sufficient to treat the infection, except in the relatively uncommon, but devastating pneumococcal meningitis, where penetration of drug into the meninges may be inadequate. Moreover, multidrug resistance is less of a problem with pneumococci than with MRSA so more therapeutic options exist, provided the susceptibility profile is known.

Mycobacterium tuberculosis

Multidrug resistance in *Mycobacterium tuberculosis* is something of a misnomer, since any strain resistant to more than one drug may be categorized as multiresistant. However, the term usually refers to strains resistant to rifampicin and isoniazid, the two most useful agents in standard antituberculosis regimens. Given that alternative treatment regimens are much less satisfactory the 'multiresistant' epithet is probably justified. Latterly, strains have emerged that are resistant not only to rifampicin and isoniazid, but also to many second line drugs. These strains are thus truly multiresistant and to distinguish them they have been labelled extensively drug resistant, or XDR-TB (22).

In the United Kingdom and other countries of Western Europe, multidrug resistant tuberculosis has not gained a major foothold, but elsewhere in the world, including Africa, south-east Asia and countries of the former Soviet Union, prevalence rates are much higher. It is tuberculosis brought into the country from these areas of high prevalence that poses the chief threat to developed nations. In a survey carried out in Britain in the final years of the twentieth century around 1 per cent of isolates of *Mycobacterium tuberculosis* were found to be resistant to rifampicin and isoniazid (23). They were almost exclusively found in urban areas, most notably, and unsurprisingly, among immigrant communities in London. Similar figures have been reported from the United States (24). Resistance to isoniazid alone is somewhat more common and, since variants resistant to rifampicin can flourish if they are not suppressed by the other agents used concomitantly (see p. 184), it is important that the susceptibility of the infecting strain is established without undue delay. For this reason routine susceptibility testing of all isolates of *Mycobacterium tuberculosis* is recommended, and rapid detection methods for this slow-growing organism are increasingly used.

With such a system in place and with good surveillance, contact tracing, and supervised treatment schemes in operation, it is hoped that the spread of multidrug resistant tuberculosis will be successfully contained. Such an outcome seems likely in the rich nations of the world, but it would be optimistic to suppose that rapid progress is likely to be made in poorer countries, where around 2 million people die of tuberculosis each year whether the infecting organism is resistant or not.

Malaria parasites

Although a succession of antimalarial drugs arrived on the scene during the course of the twentieth century (see Chapter 7), it was perhaps inevitable that resistance should emerge to each of them in its turn and spread inexorably. Strangely, quinine, which has been used extensively for over 350 years—often in ways in which it might be supposed that the development of resistance would have been unwittingly encouraged—is an exception to this rule. Resistance to quinine in malaria parasites is not unknown, but it is uncommon and has not disseminated in the way that other types of resistance have done. The most likely reason is that quinine has never been heavily used among indigenous populations in hyperendemic areas, so that the parasites have not been subjected to the intense selective pressure that drives resistance, but there may also be something intrinsic to the drug that hinders the ready development of resistance (25).

Resistance to mepacrine, the earliest synthetic antimalarial drug to be of practical value in prophylaxis and treatment, was first detected in the late stages of the Second World War among Australian troops operating in the highly malarious area between Aitape and Wewak on the northern coast of New Guinea. Despite strict enforcement of orders to ensure daily administration of mepacrine (Atebrin) to prevent malaria, cases of malaria continued to occur among the Australian soldiers even when the daily dosage was increased. That this was due to mepacrine resistance rather than avoidance of prophylaxis, was subsequently demonstrated by experiments among soldier volunteers, carried out by Neil Hamilton Fairley's team at the Australian army's Medical Research Unit at Cairns in Northern Queensland (26).

Resistance to mepacrine did not develop into a long-term worry, since it was largely abandoned as an antimalarial agent after the end of the war, when better drugs, including the antifolate compounds, proguanil and pyrimethamine, and, most importantly, the 4-aminoquinoline compounds, chloroquine and amodiaquine, became available. Resistance to the antifolates was soon encountered, but this did not come as a great surprise, because laboratory experiments by Ann Bishop and Betty Birkett at the Molteno Institute in Cambridge (27), and by Emmanuel Lourie's group at the Liverpool School of Tropical Medicine (28), had revealed as early as 1947 that resistance to proguanil emerged readily in chicken malaria. However, when resistance to chloroquine was detected in south-east Asia and in South America in the late 1950s and early 1960s it was a serious blow.

There is a strong suspicion that chloroquine resistance was hastened by a misguided scheme instigated in Brazil in the 1950s by Mário Pinotti, director of the Brazilian Endemic Diseases Programme, to prevent malaria by adding subtherapeutic doses of chloroquine to table salt (29). Encouraged by the reduction in the incidence of malaria that Pinotti's method seemed to achieve, a medicated salt programme was introduced by workers at the Pasteur Institute in Phnom Penh in a highly malarious area in Kampuchea

(Cambodia) on the border with Thailand, between 1960 and 1962. At first pyrimethamine was used in the French scheme, but chloroquine was substituted in 1961 when pyrimethamine resistance emerged (30). A similar strategy for the mass distribution of medicated pyrimethamine was started in Irian Jaya (Papuan Indonesia) in 1959. As in the Kampuchean programme, chloroquine was substituted after the rapid development of pyrimethamine resistance and the policy is thought to have given rise to the extensive multidrug resistance that is now found in the region.

Once established, resistance to chloroquine rapidly spread to the heartland of malaria in tropical Africa and has become a major problem wherever falciparum malaria occurs. Unfortunately, it is much more common in the highly lethal *Plasmodium falciparum* than in other malaria species, though it has also been found in the less dangerous *Plasmodium vivax*. Inevitably, resistance has emerged to a greater or lesser degree to other synthetic antimalarial agents as they have appeared, but so far it has not been detected in derivatives of artemisinin (31), which like quinine, is a natural compound.

Sharing the blame

Who is at fault for the rise in antimicrobial drug resistance? Doctors and veterinarians who over-prescribe, patients who unreasonably insist on antibiotic treatment for themselves and their children, an unscrupulous pharmaceutical industry, a self-interested agricultural lobby, and somnolent government health departments have all been held responsible for the present state of affairs.

Clearly, each of these groups must take some share of the blame. Prescribers have undoubtedly been profligate in their use of antibiotics; patients demand treatment and are often indignant if they feel that the curative pills are being withheld. Following the lead of William Osler, James Whorton has correctly maintained that:

> ...it is with the doctor that the buck has to stop. Patients can demand unnecessary medication, and manufacturers can aggressively advertise their product, but the doctor writes the prescription (5).

While this is undoubtedly true in countries in which prescription by a doctor is the norm, unfortunately this does not apply in much of the world where drugs—many of them counterfeit—are openly available without prescription. Moreover, in marketing their products in the Third World, pharmaceutical companies have been rightly castigated for practices that sometimes overstep accepted ethical bounds (32). In these countries it is up to governments to put in place the necessary legislation to control the availability of drugs, to stamp out unethical manufacturing and promotional practices, and to ensure that the rules are properly enforced.

Understanding the problem

Concerns about the ability of micro-organisms to develop resistance to potent antimicrobial drugs have been voiced since the early days of chemotherapy. Paul Ehrlich himself investigated the phenomenon of resistance in his early researches into the effects of dyes and arsenicals on trypanosomes, and, moreover, postulated combination therapy aimed at disabling different targets within the parasite, as a means of avoiding resistance (33).

Once antibiotics became available, microbiologists and infectious disease physicians were quick to observe the potential of microbes to circumvent or negate the antibiotic attack. Edward Abraham and Ernst Chain recognized as early as 1940 that some bacteria could produce an enzyme that inactivated penicillin. In Fleming's Nobel lecture in December 1945, he drew attention to the danger of misuse (in his view, underdosing with this virtually non-toxic drug) leading to untreatable infection:

> But I would like to sound one note of warning. Penicillin is to all intents and purposes non-poisonous so there is no need to worry about giving an overdose and poisoning the patient. There may be a danger, though, in underdosage. It is not difficult to make microbes resistant to penicillin in the laboratory by exposing them to concentrations not sufficient to kill them, and the same thing has occasionally happened in the body.
>
> The time may come when penicillin can be bought by anyone in the shops. Then there is the danger that the ignorant man may easily underdose himself and by exposing his microbes to non-lethal quantities of the drug make them resistant. Here is a hypothetical illustration. Mr. X has a sore throat. He buys some penicillin and gives himself, not enough to kill the streptococci but enough to educate them to resist penicillin. He then infects his wife. Mrs. X gets pneumonia and is treated with penicillin. As the streptococci are now resistant to penicillin the treatment fails. Mrs. X dies. Who is primarily responsible for Mrs. X's death? Why Mr. X whose negligent use of penicillin changed the nature of the microbe (34).

Evidence that fears about resistance were fully justified, quickly emerged. In 1947, Mary Barber, then Lecturer in Clinical Bacteriology* at the Royal Postgraduate Medical School in West London, reported that the incidence of resistance to penicillin (caused by the enzyme that Abraham and Chain had described) in staphylococci isolated at the school's Hammersmith Hospital had nearly tripled from around 12-14 per cent in 1946, to 38 per cent in 1947 (35); by the following year more than half of all staphylococci isolated were resistant (36). Similar reports were quickly forthcoming from other centres round the world. Furthermore it soon became plain that resistance to other antibiotics was also on the cards.

The trouble was, the spectacular cures achieved by sulphonamides, penicillin, streptomycin, tetracyclines, and chloramphenicol, had led to these antimicrobial agents being used with great abandon, often unnecessarily and sometimes illogically (37). Such indiscriminate use took little account of the needless risks of side effects to which patients were exposed or the selective pressures that fostered bacterial resistance. Changing prescribing habits in the face of antibiotic euphoria and public expectation was never going to be easy.

Fortunately, wiser counsels were on hand to warn against complacency. Voices were raised against the use of blunderbuss therapy with broad-spectrum agents and antibiotic combinations rather than targeted treatment that sought to preserve the normal bacterial ecology as much as possible. Prominent infectious disease experts such as Louis Weinstein

---

* Later Reader and eventually, from 1964 until her untimely death in a traffic accident the following year, Professor.

and Maxwell Finland in Boston, and Harry Dowling in Chicago were among the early critics who warned of the dangers of rash and irrational prescribing (38). Ernest Jawetz, the distinguished Viennese Professor of Microbiology at the University of California, San Francisco, who did much to put the use of antimicrobial drug combinations on a rational footing, laconically summarized the prevailing attitude as late as 1967:

> Apparently there is a feeling among doctors that, if one antimicrobial drug is good, two should be better, and three should cure virtually everybody of virtually everything (39).

There was even talk in the United States of a 'crusade' for the rational use of antibiotics, though it was fuelled as much by concerns about adverse reactions as by the fear that over-use would render the drugs impotent (40). In 1957, the CIBA Foundation, at the suggestion of Sir Charles Harington, director of the National Institute for Medical Research in Britain, dedicated one of its celebrated symposia to the subject of antibiotic resistance (41). The initiative was timely, since the problem of hospital-acquired infection with staphylococci resistant to the new 'miracle drugs' was by then giving grave cause for concern.

Antibiotics and agriculture

It was not only resistance in staphylococci that was ringing alarm bells. By the mid-1950s resistance was becoming widespread to one of the most useful and widely used group of broad-spectrum antibiotics: the tetracyclines. A contributory factor in the dissemination of tetracycline-resistant organisms was strongly suspected to be the rapidly increasing use of tetracyclines in animal feeds as growth promoters (see p. 229).

The effect of tetracycline in enhancing the growth of farm animals was first discovered accidentally by the combative biochemist, molecular biologist, and nutritionist, Thomas Jukes. Jukes was born in Hastings, England, but emigrated to Canada at the age of 18, eventually obtaining a PhD in biochemistry from the University of Toronto in 1933. After a spell at the University of California, he worked for Lederle from 1942 until 1949, when he moved back to the University of California, Berkeley. In 1948 Jukes was looking for an inexpensive source of 'animal protein factor' a mysterious, but essential ingredient in the animal diet, later identified by scientists at Merck as vitamin B_{12}. The source of Merck's vitamin proved to be *Streptomyces griseus*, and Jukes persuaded his boss Wilbur 'Weed'* Malcolm to provide him with a sterilized sample of a *Streptomyces aureofaciens* fermentation, which he thought might also provide the elusive dietary factor. The sample was given experimentally to chickens, and as part of the procedure they were weighed at intervals. Laboratory records showed that Jukes himself weighed the chickens on Christmas Day 1948, carrying on the festive tradition observed by Gerhard Domagk (see p. 68). The Aureomycin fermentation product exhibited the expected vitamin activity, but remarkably, the chicks also grew more rapidly than those given liver extract as an alternative source of the dietary factor (42).

---

* See footnote p. 224.

Further experimentation was clearly called for and Jukes obtained more of the by-products of Aureomycin production containing the so-called 'animal protein factor' and sent them for testing to colleagues and friends elsewhere, including Tony Cunha, who had just been appointed head of the Department of Animal Science at the University of Florida, Gainesville. Cunha succeeded in tripling the growth rate of pigs by feeding them material provided by Jukes. By early 1950, Jukes had established that it was the antibiotic Aureomycin that was responsible for animals' weight gain. At first, the growth supplement was marketed as 'animal protein factor' neatly circumventing problems of registration as an antibiotic in the United States. By the time it was announced in 1950 that Aureomycin was the agent responsible, addition of the substance to feed lots was well established and the Food and Drug Administration were persuaded to accept the usage as a fait accompli.

During the next few years use of tetracyclines—and soon other antibiotics—in animal husbandry was taken up with great enthusiasm all over the world, considerably inflating drug company profits, even though patents were disregarded in many countries. Anxiety began to be expressed about the impact of such use on the pool of resistant bacteria in the environment, with possible consequences for the treatment of human infections. A joint committee of the Agricultural and Medical Research Councils in the United Kingdom was set up in 1960 with the brief 'to examine the possible consequences of the feeding of antibiotics to farm animals and to consider whether this use constitutes any danger to human or animal health.' The committee, under the chairmanship of Lord Netherthorpe submitted its report in 1962, coming to the conclusion that there was no persuasive reason to halt the use of permitted feed additives, including tetracyclines.

Continued disquiet and a review of the evidence led to the issue being revisited in 1968. To the forefront of those speaking out was the irascible but brilliant bacteriologist E.S. ('Andy') Anderson, director of the Enteric Reference Laboratory at the Central Public Health Laboratory, Colindale, and pioneer of the use of genetic methods in epidemiological studies of bacterial drug resistance. In 1965 he published a landmark paper with his colleague Malcolm Lewis in which they presented evidence linking the development of antibiotic resistance in animals to an outbreak of human salmonellosis that had led to six deaths (43). Partly as a result of Anderson's pressure a new committee chaired by Professor Michael Swann was convened to examine the evidence. The Swann report, published in 1969 (44), reversed the Netherthorpe judgement by concluding that the administration of antibiotics, including tetracyclines, to farm livestock, particularly at subtherapeutic levels, posed hazards to human and animal health. It was recommended that only antibiotics with little or no therapeutic value in man or animals should be used for growth promotion and that antibiotics should be used for the treatment of infection in animals only when prescribed by a registered veterinary surgeon. Antibiotics that the Swann committee regarded as unsuitable for use for growth promotion included the tetracyclines, penicillin, tylosin (a macrolide antibiotic related to erythromycin), and sulphonamides. In contrast, surveys in the United States, by the National Academy of Sciences found no reason to curb the use of antibiotics in food animals. An attempt by the Food and Drug Administration to limit animal use was blocked by political opposition.

The Swann report was widely praised, but had limited impact, even in Britain, partly because farmers exploited the grey area between the use of antibiotics for growth promotion, prophylaxis, or treatment, and partly because of dubious practices such as the diversion of antibiotics intended for sick animals to general animal feedstuff. Black market trading undoubtedly also added to the problem.

Pressure for effective legislation continued none the less. In 1999, the European Union belatedly banned use of most antimicrobial agents for growth promotion in animals, with a view to phasing out all use by the year 2006. There were howls of protest from the pharmaceutical industry, but they lost a court case brought against the ruling. In countries of Scandinavia, which have been to the forefront in restricting use of antibiotics as growth promoters, no major adverse effects on animal health and productivity have been observed, probably because of improved methods of animal husbandry in the past 50 years. However, therapeutic use of antibiotics has increased and arguments continue to rage as to whether banning use in animals translates into significant clinical benefits in human medicine (45).

Unravelling the genetics of resistance

At first, the focus of research into the ways in which antibiotic resistance developed and spread, concentrated on standard laboratory studies based on classic genetic principles. By 1950, bacterial geneticists like Vernon Bryson and Milislav Demerec at the Carnegie Institution, Cold Spring Harbor, were trying to unravel why resistance to some antibiotics seemed to emerge through a series of small cumulative steps, while in other cases—streptomycin being the prime example—a single mutation seemed able to cause very high levels of resistance (46). Others, unconvinced that mutation alone could account for the experimental findings, were seeking to explain some forms of resistance by adaptive changes occurring within the bacterial cell. Curiously, the most prominent proponents of these theories were not microbiologists: they included the physical chemist and Nobel laureate, Sir Cyril Hinshelwood working with his colleague Alistair Dean in Oxford (47) and the nutritionist John Yudkin (48). The genetic camp undoubtedly won the debate, and the phenomenon of adaptive (phenotypic) resistance has since been neglected, though examples of it certainly occur.

Microbial genetics at this time was going through its own golden age in which immense strides were being made. Pioneers of the subject, such as Joshua Lederberg (who was awarded a Nobel Prize for his work in 1958) in the United States and the Irishman, William Hayes working at the Postgraduate Medical School at Hammersmith Hospital in London, had elucidated the mechanism by which genetic characteristics can be transferred between bacterial cells in a quasi-sexual process called conjugation involving donor ('male') and recipient ('female') cells. This had an immediate impact on the understanding of acquired antibiotic resistance, and paved the way for a discovery made in Japan in1959 that sent shivers of apprehension through the antibiotic world: that bacteria could simultaneously acquire resistance to several unrelated antibiotics in a single genetic event.

Bacillary dysentery caused by particularly virulent species of *Shigella* had long been a problem in Japan; the advent of sulphonamides, chloramphenicol, and tetracyclines had revolutionized the treatment, but by the mid-1950s resistance was undermining this success. Close monitoring of the epidemiology of the resistance revealed the puzzling observation that fully sensitive and multiresistant variants of the same strain of *Shigella* could sometimes be isolated from a single patient. Even more disturbingly, treatment with chloramphenicol of patients harbouring fully sensitive *Shigella* strains sometimes led to the appearance of isolates of *Shigella*—and of *Escherichia coli* cohabiting in the gut—that were resistant not only to chloramphenicol itself, but also to unrelated antibiotics. These observations led K. Ochiai in Nagoya and, independently, Tomoichiro Akiba and his colleagues in Tokyo to postulate, and subsequently show in laboratory tests, that resistance to several antibiotics could be transferred en bloc between bacteria of the same or different species. The results were published in 1959, but they originally appeared in Japanese and although the findings were mentioned in papers in English by Tsutomu Watanabe and Toshio Fukasawa of Keio University, Tokyo in 1961 (49), they came to general attention only through a lengthy exposition of the original experiments in a review by Tsutomu Watanabe published in *Bacteriological Reviews* in 1963 (50).

It turned out that the genes encoding these resistance determinants were carried on circular pieces of DNA that existed in the cell independently of the bacterial chromosome. Such elements were originally given the name 'episomes', but became universally known as 'plasmids', a term coined by Joshua Lederberg of the University of Wisconsin in 1952 (51). What the Japanese scientists had uncovered was that transfer by conjugation of plasmids carrying sets of genes responsible for resistance to several unrelated antibiotics was allowing sensitive recipient organisms to acquire multiresistance at one fell swoop. This was alarming enough, but in the mid-1970s it emerged that another important factor had to be taken into account. It was revealed that genes—and sometimes packets of genes—could be transposed between plasmids and the bacterial chromosome (or vice versa) allowing them to turn up in unexpected places. These elements were officially called 'transposons' but soon acquired the descriptive epithet 'jumping genes'.

The distinguished American geneticist Barbara McClintock first discovered transposable genetic elements in 1948 during her studies on maize at the Cold Spring Harbor laboratories. The finding was highly controversial and when the results were eventually presented at the institute's annual symposium in 1951 they were received with indifference. It was only when European research revealed similar elements in bacteria and viruses that the significance of her major contribution came to be generally recognized (52). Belatedly, McClintock was awarded the Nobel Prize in physiology or medicine at the age of 81 in 1983.

The finding that genes determining antimicrobial drug resistance could assemble themselves in groups on transmissible plasmids and, moreover, could hop from plasmid to plasmid or between plasmid and chromosome (53), set the cat among the pigeons. Coming at a time when new mechanisms of resistance were regularly being reported and the versatility of Gram-negative bacilli in producing enzymes capable of inactivating penicillins and cephalosporins* was fast being recognized, alarm bells were ringing loud and clear. Suddenly, the ingenuity of microbes, to which microbiologists were fond of paying lip service, seemed to have been grossly underestimated and people began to wonder if the astonishing progress that had been made in antibacterial therapy was as secure as had been assumed.

Tackling the problem

Wake-up calls

In January 1981 a group of scientists at the International Plasmid Conference on Molecular Biology, Pathogenicity, and Ecology of Bacterial Plasmids, held in Santo Domingo, Dominican Republic, issued a statement raising public health concerns over the spread of antibiotic resistance genes (54). The prime mover behind the statement was the ebullient and irrepressible Professor of Medicine and Molecular Biology at Tufts University, Boston, Stuart Levy. Levy, a tireless communicator of fears about antibiotic resistance, went on to found the *Alliance for the Prudent Use of Antibiotics* in 1981 with the laudable aim of raising public awareness of the problems and promoting proper use of antimicrobial drugs.

Microbiologists, in particular microbial geneticists and those engaged in monitoring antimicrobial drug resistance, were now in no doubt of the dangers, but the message was slow to get through to prescribers and legislators throughout the world. Antimicrobial agents continued to be used profligately; pharmaceutical houses continued to promote antimicrobial agents for inappropriate indications and in ineffective combinations; and nothing was done to restrict the availability of antibiotics in the many countries where they were freely available.

The World Health Organization (WHO) was sufficiently aware of the dangers to set up a working group to address the problem of antibiotic resistance (55). Stimulated by the working group's report, another indefatigable fighter for rational antimicrobial therapy, Calvin Kunin, the genial Professor of Internal Medicine at Ohio State University, issued a call to arms in 1983 in an editorial in *Annals of Internal Medicine*, the influential journal of the American College of Physicians (56). Less populist in his approach than Levy, Kunin has had an equally profound influence on his fellow prescribers through his incisive writings and trenchant analysis of the problems, perhaps best typified by his 1993 article, also in *Annals* (57).

Other initiatives followed, culminating in a meeting in Freiburg in September 1988, sponsored by the WHO's Regional Office for Europe. A select group of delegates (including

---

* Staphylococci produce only a few, closely related kinds of these enzymes—β-lactamases—but Gram-negative bacilli like *Escherichia coli* and *Klebsiella* species can produce several different families of enzyme with vastly different properties. Dozens of variants of most common type, the so-called TEM enzyme (the designation derives from the first letters of the name of a patient in Athens from whom an isolate of *Escherichia coli* with this type of resistance was first isolated), have been described.

Kunin and Levy) from around the world met to address the burgeoning problems arising from the use and abuse of antimicrobial agents, with particular emphasis on the Third World, where antibiotic availability and use were virtually unregulated. The lack of adequate surveillance data and guidelines for antibiotic use were highlighted and recommendations for the appropriate choice of antibacterial therapy of specific bacterial infections were tentatively formulated (58).

But in the climate of the 1980s few were listening. Resistance had been acknowledged as a threat since the earliest days of sulphonamides, penicillin, and streptomycin—indeed, since Ehrlich—but the pharmaceutical industry had always responded with new and ever more powerful agents. Throughout the 1980s antibacterial agents continued to proliferate, with agents designed to overcome prevalent forms of resistance appearing regularly from the pharmaceutical company conveyor belt. There seemed little incentive for prescribers—always vigorous defenders of their professional independence to judge what is best for their patients—to change their ways. Arguments about the non-medical uses of antimicrobial agents had similarly fallen on deaf ears and the possibility of stimulating the political will to control drugs more effectively in countries with lax regulations seemed as remote as ever. It was only when the pharmaceutical industry switched its priorities from bacteria to the more lucrative field of antiviral agents as they reacted to the acquired immune deficiency syndrome (AIDS) pandemic in the 1990s that notice began to be taken of the potential gravity of the situation. The figures for new antimicrobial drugs marketed in 3-year periods since 1990 tell their own story (Table 9.2). In 2005 the number of new antibacterial drugs marketed in the United Kingdom reached zero: the antibacterial bonanza was over.

In August 1992 the widely-read American journal *Science* published a series of articles on antibiotic resistance, led by a provocative paper by Mitchell Cohen of the Centers for Disease Control in Atlanta, Georgia, on the epidemiology of drug resistance (3). These articles reinvigorated the debate among doctors and scientists and had a profound influence on the general perception of the problem of antimicrobial drug resistance. The

Table 9.2 Antimicrobial agents newly marketed in the United Kingdom in three-year periods 1990–2004

Period	Antibacterial agents	Antiviral agents[a]	Antifungal agents	Antiparasitic agents
1990–1992	10	1	2	2
1993–1995	7	4	1	1
1996–1998	3	9	1	1
1999–2001	2	8	0	1
2002–2004	3	5	2	0

Source: Data from Greenwood D, Finch RG, Davey PD, Wilcox MH. *Antimicrobial Chemotherapy*, 5th edn. Oxford University Press, 2007.

[a] Predominantly anti-HIV agents.

media, which had hitherto taken only a desultory interest in tales of antibiotic use and misuse, scented a story of professional complacency and official incompetence. Television and radio programmes, and newspaper articles began to proliferate, spreading the usual mixture of sense and nonsense, and the topic emerged for the first time into public consciousness. By the end of the decade, resistance was high on the agenda at infectious disease conferences and symposia, antibiotic resistance monitoring programmes had been set up in various countries, expert committees were being convened and many other initiatives were being explored.

Action stations

Highlighting the problem of antimicrobial drug resistance was one thing; doing something about it was another. Predictably the initial response was the time-honoured one: 'when in doubt, set up a committee of inquiry' and this was done in a big way in many countries throughout the 1990s.

In the United Kingdom, that much-underestimated assemblage of assorted expertise, the House of Lords, carried out one of the most comprehensive inquiries into the problem of antimicrobial drug resistance during 1997 and 1998. Following on from an earlier survey by the Parliamentary Office of Science and Technology in 1994 (59) the Lords' Select Committee on Science and Technology set up a sub committee under the Chairmanship of Lord Soulsby of Swaffham Prior, Emeritus Professor of Animal Pathology at the University of Cambridge and a distinguished veterinarian, to look into the problem of antibiotic resistance in depth. Professors Harold Lambert and Richard Wise were appointed as specialist advisers to the inquiry, written submissions from all interest groups were invited, expert witnesses were summoned for questioning by the committee and visits were arranged to various relevant institutions, including several in the United States. The report, issued in March 1978 (60) together with the evidence on which it was based (61), generated a great deal of media interest and public debate. Following the publication of the government's response outlining its strategy for implementing the recommendations (62), renewed efforts were made in the United Kingdom to promote sensible prescribing, educate the public on the dangers of overprescribing of antibiotics and to encourage control of infection measures in hospitals. In June 2000, the Department of Health issued its action plan to tackle antimicrobial drug resistance (63).

Similar attempts to devise strategies to curb the spread of drug resistant microbes have been made in many other countries of the developed world. In the United States both the American Society for Microbiology (in 1994) (64) and the Food and Drug Administration (in 2000) (65) organized expert task forces to examine the problem of antibiotic resistance and Congress's Office of Technology Assessment considered the matter shortly before the office was dissolved in 1995 (66). In the European Union a conference was convened in Copenhagen in September 1998 to formulate recommendations for dealing with what it termed 'the microbial threat' (67). A follow-up conference to review progress took place in Visby, Sweden in June 2001, and further meetings were held in Brussels in November 2001 and in Rome in November 2003.

Most of these efforts have made a serious attempt to grapple with the problem and devise constructive proposals. Various welcome initiatives have been set in train to improve surveillance of antibiotic resistance and to promote rational prescribing. In addition, legislation to curtail antibiotic use in agriculture, particularly for growth promotion in food animals, has been enacted in the European Union (see p. 405); the United States is slowly moving in the same direction.

But a striking feature of all the reports that have emanated from Europe and North America has been their insular focus on problems arising from the use of antibiotics in the developed world. Clearly, it has been the development of multiresistant bacteria in vulnerable patients in high-dependency units of hospitals that has generated the most intense unease, notwithstanding the fact that most of these organisms—MRSA is, perhaps, an exception—are opportunist pathogens of low intrinsic virulence that pose little hazard to the community at large. The urgent problems of resistance in the Third World have received much less attention. Furthermore, non-bacterial infections hardly get a mention in most reports, although fungi, protozoa, and viruses—for which therapeutic resources are already much scarcer than for bacterial infection (see Chapters 7 and 8)— also affect seriously ill and immunocompromised individuals, and one of the most pressing problems of drug resistance in the world is in falciparum malaria.

It has been left to the WHO to tackle these issues. In September 2001 the WHO launched its Global Strategy for Containment of Antibiotic Resistance with an ambitious programme designed to involve consumers, prescribers, veterinarians, national governments, the pharmaceutical industry, professional societies, and international agencies (68). Crucial to the strategy, but most difficult to implement, are proposals urging all national governments to introduce legislation and policies governing the development, licensing, distribution, and sale of antimicrobial agents. It is a tall order, but until such legislation is in place and enforced, problems of antimicrobial drug resistance in countries where the majority of the world's population live, will stand little chance of a lasting solution.

Envoi

Ronald Hare, who was an eyewitness to much of Fleming's work with penicillin at St Mary's Hospital, describes in the opening chapter of his book, *The birth of penicillin and the disarming of microbes*, the life of his father, a general practitioner in a mining village in north-east England at the turn of the twentieth century. There was infection aplenty, but little that could be done, except smallpox vaccination, the newfangled antitoxin treatment for diphtheria and the removal of patients with contagious diseases to a local fever hospital or, if they were among the lucky few, a tuberculosis sanatorium. He dispensed only four medicines: a cough mixture consisting of bromide of ammonia and belladonna flavoured with camphor for respiratory diseases of all kinds; sodium bicarbonate and extract of rhubarb for intestinal diseases; peppermint water, Epsom salt, and magnesium carbonate for less serious intestinal problems; and teething powders containing mercury and chalk for infants and young children (69). No doubt other nostrums were being prescribed in Harley Street, but few had any consistent effect in infectious disease. Hare's father could have had no conception of the remarkable changes that were to occur during his son's lifetime. By the time Ronald Hare died in 1986, riches beyond belief were available for the treatment of virtually every type of infection and the days of medical impotence were a distant memory.

It is well to remember the days before the antimicrobial revolution at a time when there is so much talk of a return to the pre-antibiotic era. Although microbes continue to surprise us by their ingenuity in surviving the antibiotic onslaught, the chances that microbial disease will once more become regularly untreatable is exceedingly remote. That said, resistance is a real and urgent threat that must be addressed if reliable therapy with first-line agents is to remain the norm. When patients cannot be treated with a reasonable expectation of success without recourse to time-consuming laboratory tests to establish the susceptibility status of the offending pathogen, much unnecessary death and suffering will necessarily ensue, especially in areas where there is no ready access to laboratory facilities.

It is not the nuisance of drug resistance in the high-tech hospitals of the developed world that should be the prime concern: in principle that can be managed by good control of infection practices, careful prescribing, and effective policies of antibiotic use. It is the problem of resistance to drugs used in the treatment of the classic infectious diseases such as typhoid fever, tuberculosis, malaria, and bacillary dysentery that should be commanding our urgent attention. These diseases, and others, still affect millions of the most disadvantaged people in the world. The most pressing challenge is to make the twentieth century miracle of antibiotics as available to these people as it is for the affluent minority.

References

1. House of Lords Select Committee on Science and Technology (23 April 1998). Resistance to antibiotics and other antimicrobial agents. Press release.

2. United States Department of Health & Human Services, William H Stewart (1965–1969). http://www.surgeongeneral.gov/library/history/biostewart.htm

3. Cohen ML (1992). Epidemiology of drug resistance: implications for a post-antimicrobial era. *Science* **257**, 1050–5.

4. Loeffler IJP (1996). Microbes, chemotherapy, evolution, and folly. *Lancet* **348**, 1703–4.

5. Whorton JC (1980). "Antibiotic abandon": the resurgence of therapeutic rationalism. In: *The history of antibiotics—a symposium*, pp. 125–36. American Institute of the History of Pharmacy, Madison, Wisconsin.

6. Finland M (1954). Clinical uses of the presently available antibiotics. In: Welch H, Marti-Ibañez F, eds. *Antibiotics annual 1953–1954*, pp. 10–26. Medical Encyclopedia Inc., New York.

7. Finland M, Jones WF, Barnes MW (1959). Occurrence of serious bacterial infections since introduction of antibacterial agents. *JAMA* **170**, 2188–97.

8. Editorial (1952). Abuse of antibiotics. *BMJ* **2**, 1301–2.

9. Hiramatsu K, Hanaki H, Ino T, Yabuta K, Oguri T, Tenover FC (1997). Methicillin-resistant *Staphylococcus aureus* clinical strain with reduced vancomycin susceptibility. *J Antimicrob Chemother* **40**, 135–6.

10. Barber M (1961). Methicillin resistance in staphylococci. *J Clin Pathol* **14**, 385–93.

11. Jevons MP (1961). "Celbenin"-resistant staphylococci. *BMJ* **1**, 124–5.

12. Jevons MP, Coe AW, Parker MT (1963). Methicillin resistance in staphylococci. *Lancet* **1**, 904–7.

13. Benner EJ, Kayser FH (1968). Growing clinical significance of methicillin-resistant *Staphylococcus aureus*. *Lancet* **2**, 741–4.

14. Eriksen KR (1964). Methicillin-resistance in *Staphylococcus aureus* apparently developed during treatment with methicillin. *Acta Pathol Microbiol Scand* **61**, 154–5.

15. Barrett FF, McGehee RF, Finland M (1968). Methicillin-resistant *Staphylococcus aureus* at the Boston City Hospital. *N Engl J Med* **279**, 441–8.

16. Pavillard R, Harvey K, Douglas D, *et al.* (1982). Epidemic of hospital-acquired infection due to methicillin-resistant *Staphylococcus aureus* in major Victorian hospitals. *Med J Aust* **1**, 451–4.

17. Turnidge J, Lawson P, Munro R, Benn R (1989). A national survey of antimicrobial resistance in *Staphylococcus aureus* in Australian teaching hospitals. *Med J Aust* **150**, 65–72; Turnidge JD, Nimmo GR, Francis G (1996). Evolution of resistance in *Staphylococcus aureus* in Australian teaching hospitals. *Med J Aust* **164**, 68–71.

18. Tiemersma EW, Bronzwaer SLAM, Lyytikäinan O, *et al.* (2004). Methicillin-resistant *Staphylococcus aureas* in Europe 1999–2002. *Emerg Infect Dis* **10**, 1627–34.

19. Grundmann H, Aires-de-Sousa M, Boyce J, Tiemersma E (2006). Emergence and resurgence of meticillin-resistant *Staphylococcus aureus* as a public-health threat. *Lancet* **368**, 874–85.

20. Hansman D, Glasgow HN, Sturt J, Devitt L, Douglas RM (1971). Pneumococci insensitive to penicillin. *Nature* **230**, 407–8.

21. Jacobs MR, Koornhof HJ, Robins-Browne RM, *et al.* (1977). Emergence of multiply resistant pneumococci. *N Engl J Med* **299**, 735–40.

22. World Health Organization (2007). XDR-TB. Extensively drug-resistant tuberculosis. Available at: http://www.who.int/tb/xdr/en/; Centers for Disease Control and Prevention (2006). Emergence of *Mycobacterium tuberculosis* with extensive resistance to second-line drugs—worldwide 2000–2004. *Morb Mortal Wkly Rep* **55**, 301–5.

23. Djuretic T, Herbert J, Drobniewski F, *et al.* (2002). Antibiotic-resistant tuberculosis in the United Kingdom: 1993-1999. *Thorax* **57**, 477–82.

24. Anonymous (2004). Trends in tuberculosis—United States 1998–2003. *Morb Mortal Wkly Rep* **53**, 209–14. Available at: http://www.cdc.gov/mmwr/preview/mmwrhtml/mm5310a2.htm

25. Meshnick SR (1997). Why does quinine still work after 350 years of use? *Parasitol Today* **13**, 89–90.

26. Sweeney AW (1996). The possibility of an "x" factor. The first documented drug resistance of human malaria. *Int J Parasitol* **26**, 1035–61.

27. Bishop A, Birkett B (1947). Acquired resistance to paludrine in *Plasmodium gallinaceum*. Acquired resistance and persistence after passage through the mosquito. *Nature* **159**, 884–5.

28. Williamson J, Bertram DS, Lourie EM (1947). Effects of Paludrine and other antimalarials. *Nature* **159**, 885–6.

29. Pinotti M (1954). Um novo método de profilaxia da malaria associação de uma droga antimalárica ao sal de cozinea. *Revista Brasileira de Malariologia e Doenças Tropicalis* **6**, 5–12.

30. Verdrager J (1986). Epidemiology of the emergence and spread of drug-resistant falciparum malaria in south-east Asia and Australasia. *J Trop Med Hyg* **89**, 277–89.

31. White NJ (2004). Antimalarial drug resistance. *J Clin Invest* **113**, 1084–92.

32. Melrose D (1982). *Bitter pills. Medicines and the Third World poor*. Oxfam, Oxford; Chetley A (1990). *A healthy business? World health and the pharmaceutical industry*. Zed Books, London; Chetley A (1995). *Problem drugs*. Health Action International, Amsterdam.

33. Ehrlich P (1913). Chemotherapeutics: scientific principles, methods and results. *Lancet* **2**, 445–51.

34. Fleming A (11 December 1945). Nobel lecture. Available at: http://nobelprize.org/medicine/laureates/1945/fleming-lecture.html

35. Barber M (1947). Staphylococcal infection due to penicillin-resistant strains. *BMJ* **2**, 863–5.

36. Barber M, Rozwadowska-Dowzenko M (1948). Infection by penicillin-resistant staphylococci. *Lancet* **2**, 641–4.

37. Whorton JC (1980). "Antibiotic abandon": the resurgence of therapeutic rationalism. In: Parascandola J, ed. *The history of antibiotics—a symposium*, pp. 125–36. American Institute for the History of Pharmacy, Madison, Wisconsin.

38. Weinstein L (1964). Superinfection: a complication of antimicrobial therapy and prophylaxis. *Am J Surg* **107**, 704–9; Finland M (1954). Clinical use of the presently available antibiotics. In: Welch H, Marti-Ibañez F, eds. *Antibiotics annual 1953–1954*, pp. 10–26. Medical Encyclopedia Inc., New York; Dowling HF (1954). The effect of the emergence of resistant strains on the future of antibiotic therapy. In: Welch H, Marti-Ibañez F, eds. *Antibiotics annual 1953–1954*, pp. 27–34. Medical Encyclopedia Inc., New York.

39. Jawetz E (1968). Combined antibiotic action: some definitions and correlations between laboratory and clinical results. In: Hobby GL, ed. *Antimicrobial agents and chemotherapy—1967*, pp. 203–9. American Society for Microbiology, Ann Arbor, Michigan.

40. Hussar AE (1955). A proposed crusade for the rational use of antibiotics. In: Welch H, Marti-Ibañez F, eds. *Antibiotics annual 1954–1955*, pp. 379–3. Medical Encyclopedia Inc., New York.

41. Wolstenholme GEW, O'Connor CM (eds.) (1957). *Drug resistance in micro-organisms. Mechanisms of development*. J & A Churchill Ltd., London.

42. Jukes JH (1985). Some historical notes on chlortetracycline. *Rev Infect Dis* **7**, 702–7.

43. Anderson ES, Lewis MJ (1965). Drug resistance and its transfer in *Salmonella typhimurium*. *Nature* **206**, 579–83.

44. Report (1969). *Joint committee on the use of antibiotics in animal husbandry and veterinary medicine* (Swann MM, Chairman). Her Majesty's Stationery Office, London.

45. Singer RS, Finch R, Wegener HC, Bywater R, Walters J, Lipsitch M (2002). Antibiotic resistance—the interplay between antibiotic use in animals and human beings. *Lancet Infect Dis* **3**, 47–51.

46. Bryson V, Demerec M (1950). Patterns of resistance to antimicrobial agents. *Ann N Y Acad Sci* **53**, 283–9.

47. Dean ACR, Hinshelwood C (1957). Aspects of the problem of drug resistance in bacteria. In: Wolstenholme GEW, O'Connor CM, eds. *Drug resistance in micro-organisms. Mechanisms of development*, pp. 4–29. J & A Churchill Ltd., London.

48. Yudkin J (1953). Origin of acquired drug resistance in bacteria. *Nature* **171**, 541–5.

49. Watanabe T, Fukasawa T (1961). Episome-mediated transfer of drug resistance in Enterobacteriaceae. I. Transfer of resistance factors by conjugation. *J Bacteriol* **81**, 669–78.

50. Watanabe T (1963). Infective heredity of multiple drug resistance. *Bacteriol Rev* **27**, 87–115.

51. Lederberg J (1952). Cell genetics and hereditary symbiosis. *Physiol Rev* **32**, 403–30.

52. United States National Library of Medicine. Profiles in medicine. *The Barbara McClintock papers*. Available at: http://profiles.nlm.nih.gov/LL/

53. Cohen SN (1976). Transposable genetic elements and plasmid evolution. *Nature* **263**, 731–8.

54. Anonymous (1981). Saving antibiotics from themselves. *Nature* **292**, 661.

55. World health Organization Scientific Working Group on Antibacterial resistance (1983). Control of antibiotic-resistant bacteria: memorandum from a WHO meeting. *Bull World Health Organ* **61**, 423–33.

56. Kunin CM (1983). Antibiotic resistance—a world healthy problem we cannot ignore. *Ann Intern Med* **99**, 859–60.

57. Kunin CM (1993). Resistance to antimicrobial drugs—a worldwide calamity *Ann Intern Med* **118**, 557–61.

58. CM, Johansen KS, Worming AM, Daschner FD (1990). Report of a symposium on use and abuse of antibiotics worldwide. *Rev Infect Dis* **12**, 12–19.

59. Border P (1994). *Diseases fighting back—the growing resistance to TB and other bacterial diseases to treatment*. Parliamentary Office of Science and Technology, London.

60. House of Lords Select Committee on Science and Technology (1998). *Resistance to antibiotics and other antimicrobial agents. Report.* The Stationery Office, London. Available at: http://www.parliament.the-stationery-office.co.uk/pa/ld199798/ldselect/ldsctech/081vii/st0701.htm

61. House of Lords Select Committee on Science and Technology (1998). *Resistance to antibiotics and other antimicrobial agents.* Evidence. The Stationery Office, London.

62. Government response to the House of Lords Select Committee on Science and Technology report: Resistance to antibiotics and other antimicrobial agents. (1998). The Stationery Office, London.

63. Department of Health (2000). UK antimicrobial resistance strategy and action plan.

64. American Society for Microbiology (1994). Report of the ASM task force on antibiotic resistance. ASM, Washington.

65. United States Food and Drug Administration (December 2000). FDA task force on antimicrobial resistance. Key recommendations and report. Available at: http://www.fda.gov/oc/antimicrobial/taskforce2000.html

66. U.S. Congress, Office of Technology Assessment (1995). Impacts of antibiotic resistant bacteria (OTA-H-629). Washington, DC. Available at: http://www.wws.princeton.edu/~ota/disk1/1995/9503_n.html

67. Rosdahl VT, Pedersen KB (eds.) (1998). The Copenhagen recommendations. Report from the invitational EU conference on the microbial threat. Copenhagen Denmark, 9–10 September 1998. Ministry of Health, Ministry of Food, Agriculture and Fisheries, Denmark. Available at: http://www.im.dk/publikationer/micro98/index.htm

68. World Health Organization Fact Sheet No. 194 (Revised January 2002). Antibiotic resistance. Available at: http://www.who.int/mediacentre/factsheets/fs194/en/

69. Hare R (1970). *The birth of penicillin and the disarming of microbes*, pp. 15–28. George Allen and Unwin, London.

Drug register

Neomycin B 180
Neosalvarsan (neoarsphenamine) 59, 61, 62
Neostam (*see* stibamine glucoside)
Neostibosan 308
Neoteben 175
Netilmicin 232
Nevirapine 380
Niclosamide 322, 323
Nicotinamide 172, 174, 197
Nifuratel 252
Nifurtimox 252, 318
Nifurtoinol 252
Nilodin (*see* lucanthone)
Niridazole 329–30
Nisin 213
Nitazoxanide 326, 336
Nitrofurantoin 251, 252, 258
Nitrofurazone 250–1, 317
Nocardicin A 134
Norfloxacin 258–9
Novobiocin (cathomycin, streptonivicin)
    240, 241, 396
Nystatin 158, 349–52

Oil of chenopodium 30, 318, 322
Olamufloxacin 260
Oleandomycin 238
Omnacillin 109
Omnadin 109
Opium 43
Optochin (ethyl hydocupreine) 63
Orbifloxacin 260
Oritavancin 241
Orsanin 280
Oseltamivir 381, 382–3
Osteogrycin 244
Oxacillin 124
Oxamniquine 329–30
Oxantel 324
Oxaphenarsine (mapharsan) 62
Oxolinic acid 258
Oxytetracycline 225–7, 229

Paludrine (*see* proguanil)
Pamaquine 286–90, 292, 294–5, 300
Panipenem–betamipron 133
para–Aminobenzylpenicillin 122
para–Aminophenylarsonate (Soamin) 277, 280
para–Aminosalicylic acid 49, 144, 164–70, 249
Paromomycin (aminosidine, catenulin) 234–5,
    309–10, 312, 323
Patulin 113
Pazufloxacin 260
Pefloxacin 259
Penciclovir 378
Penicillin F (pentenylpenicillin) 106n
Penicillin G (benzylpenicillin) 106n,
    119, 121, 123, 124
Penicillin K (n–heptylpenicillin) 106n
Penicillin N (cephalosporin N, adicillin,
    synnematin B) 117
Penicillin V (phenoxymethylpenicillin) 119–21, 123

Penicillin X
    (*p*–hydroxybenzylpenicillin) 106n
Pennotin 110
Pentamidine 283, 285, 309, 332
Pentaquine 300
Pentostam (*see* sodium antimony gluconate)
Phenacetin 49
Phenbenicillin 123
Phenethicillin 123
Phenol 50
Phenoxymethylpenicillin (penicillin V) 120–1
Phosphonoacetic acid 383
Phosphonoformate (*see* foscarnet)
Phosphonomycin (*see* fosfomycin)
Picromycin 236
Pimaricin (natamycin) 354
Pipemidic acid 258–9
Piperacillin 126, 132
Piperaquine 305
Piperazine 319–20
Pirlimycin 242
Piromidic acid 258
Pivampicillin 125
Pivmecillinam 126
Plasmoquine (plasmochin; *see* pamaquine)
Polymyxin A 217, 218
Polymyxin B 213, 217, 218
Polymyxin C 217, 218
Polymyxin D 217, 218
Polymyxin E *see* Colistin
Polymyxin M 217
Polypeptin 213
Potassium antimony tartrate (tartar emetic) 272,
    277, 280, 327–8
    filarial worms 332
    leishmaniasis 305–7
Potassium arsenite 55
Potassium dichromate 51
Potassium iodide 6
Potassium permanganate 347
Praziquantel 323, 326, 330–1, 337
Primaquine 300–1
Pristinamycin 244–5
Proactinomycin 236
Probenecid 121
Procaine penicillin 121
Proflavine 63
Proguanil (Paludrine; chlorguanide) 253,
    297, 301, 400
Promin (Promamide) 147, 155, 164, 169, 195–6
Promizole (thiazosulphone) 147, 156, 164, 196
Prontosil 66–74, 78–9, 92, 109, 147, 150, 170, 247
Prontylin 75
Propamidine 283, 360
Propicillin 123
Propionic acid 349
Propoquine (*see* amopyroquine)
Protionamide 174, 198, 201
Prulifloxacin 260
Pseudomonic acid (*see* mupirocin)
Pulvis Warwicensis 306
Pyocyanase 29

Subject Index